Nutrition and Traumatic Brain Injury

Improving Acute and Subacute Health Outcomes in Military Personnel

This book is due for return on or before the last date shown below.

19/11/2014.

Committee on Nutrition, Trauma, and the Brain

Food and Nutrition Board

Institute of Medicine

INSTITUTE OF MEDICINE
OF THE NATIONAL ACADEMIES

THE NATIONAL ACADEMIES PRESS
Washington, D.C.

www.nap.edu

THE NATIONAL ACADEMIES PRESS 500 Fifth Street, N.W. Washington, DC 20001

NOTICE: The project that is the subject of this report was approved by the Governing Board of the National Research Council, whose members are drawn from the councils of the National Academy of Sciences, the National Academy of Engineering, and the Institute of Medicine. The members of the committee responsible for the report were chosen for their special competences and with regard for appropriate balance.

This study was supported by Contract No. W911QY-10-C-0010 between the National Academy of Sciences and the Department of Defense. Any opinions, findings, conclusions, or recommendations expressed in this publication are those of the author(s) and do not necessarily reflect the view of the organizations or agencies that provided support for this project.

International Standard Book Number-13: 978-0-309-21008-9
International Standard Book Number-10: 0-309-21008-9

Additional copies of this report are available from the National Academies Press, 500 Fifth Street, N.W., Lockbox 285, Washington, DC 20055; (800) 624-6242 or (202) 334-3313 (in the Washington metropolitan area); Internet, http://www.nap.edu.

For more information about the Institute of Medicine, visit the IOM home page at: **www.iom.edu**.

Cover credit: "Pavement" created by Matthew A. Ping (www.visionaryveteran.blogspot.com) for Vet Art Project.

The serpent has been a symbol of long life, healing, and knowledge among almost all cultures and religions since the beginning of recorded history. The serpent adopted as a logotype by the Institute of Medicine is a relief carving from ancient Greece, now held by the Staatliche Museen in Berlin.

Suggested citation: IOM (Institute of Medicine). 2011. *Nutrition and Traumatic Brain Injury: Improving Acute and Subacute Health Outcomes in Military Personnel*. Washington, DC: The National Academies Press.

"Knowing is not enough; we must apply.
Willing is not enough; we must do."
—Goethe

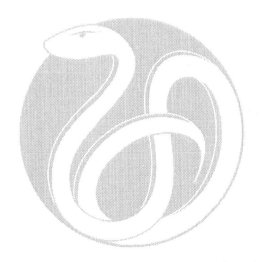

INSTITUTE OF MEDICINE
OF THE NATIONAL ACADEMIES

Advising the Nation. Improving Health.

THE NATIONAL ACADEMIES
Advisers to the Nation on Science, Engineering, and Medicine

The **National Academy of Sciences** is a private, nonprofit, self-perpetuating society of distinguished scholars engaged in scientific and engineering research, dedicated to the furtherance of science and technology and to their use for the general welfare. Upon the authority of the charter granted to it by the Congress in 1863, the Academy has a mandate that requires it to advise the federal government on scientific and technical matters. Dr. Ralph J. Cicerone is president of the National Academy of Sciences.

The **National Academy of Engineering** was established in 1964, under the charter of the National Academy of Sciences, as a parallel organization of outstanding engineers. It is autonomous in its administration and in the selection of its members, sharing with the National Academy of Sciences the responsibility for advising the federal government. The National Academy of Engineering also sponsors engineering programs aimed at meeting national needs, encourages education and research, and recognizes the superior achievements of engineers. Dr. Charles M. Vest is president of the National Academy of Engineering.

The **Institute of Medicine** was established in 1970 by the National Academy of Sciences to secure the services of eminent members of appropriate professions in the examination of policy matters pertaining to the health of the public. The Institute acts under the responsibility given to the National Academy of Sciences by its congressional charter to be an adviser to the federal government and, upon its own initiative, to identify issues of medical care, research, and education. Dr. Harvey V. Fineberg is president of the Institute of Medicine.

The **National Research Council** was organized by the National Academy of Sciences in 1916 to associate the broad community of science and technology with the Academy's purposes of furthering knowledge and advising the federal government. Functioning in accordance with general policies determined by the Academy, the Council has become the principal operating agency of both the National Academy of Sciences and the National Academy of Engineering in providing services to the government, the public, and the scientific and engineering communities. The Council is administered jointly by both Academies and the Institute of Medicine. Dr. Ralph J. Cicerone and Dr. Charles M. Vest are chair and vice chair, respectively, of the National Research Council.

www.national-academies.org

COMMITTEE ON NUTRITION, TRAUMA, AND THE BRAIN

JOHN W. ERDMAN (*Chair*), Professor Emeritus, Department of Food Science and Human Nutrition, University of Illinois at Urbana-Champaign

ELDON WAYNE ASKEW, Professor and Director, Division of Nutrition, University of Utah, Salt Lake City

BRUCE R. BISTRIAN, Professor, Harvard Medical School, Boston, Massachusetts

JOSEPH G. CANNON, Professor, College of Allied Health Sciences, Georgia Health Sciences University, Augusta

XIANG GAO, Research Scientist and Assistant Professor, Departments of Nutrition and Medicine, Harvard School of Public Health, Boston and Harvard Medical School, Boston, Massachusetts

MICHAEL S. JAFFEE, Past National Director, Defense and Veterans Brain Injury Center, Wilford Hall Medical Center, San Antonio Uniformed Services Health Education Consortium, Texas

ROBIN B. KANAREK, Professor, Department of Psychology, Tufts University, Medford, Massachusetts

CATHY W. LEVENSON, Associate Professor, Department of Biomedical Sciences and Program in Neuroscience, Florida State University College of Medicine, Tallahassee

ESTHER F. MYERS, Chief Science Officer, Research & Strategic Business Development, American Dietetic Association, Chicago, Illinois

LINDA J. NOBLE, Professor, Departments of Neurological Surgery and Physical Therapy and Rehabilitation Science, University of California, San Francisco

ROSS D. ZAFONTE, Professor and Chair, Department of Physical Medicine & Rehabilitation, Harvard Medical School, Boston, Massachusetts

Study Staff

MARIA ORIA, Study Director
LAURA PILLSBURY, Associate Program Officer
GUI LIU, Senior Program Assistant
LEANN BARDEN, Intern
ANTON BANDY, Financial Officer
GERALDINE KENNEDO, Administrative Assistant, Food and Nutrition Board
LINDA D. MEYERS, Director, Food and Nutrition Board

Consultant

HILARY RAY, Copyeditor

Reviewers

This report has been reviewed in draft form by individuals chosen for their diverse perspectives and technical expertise, in accordance with procedures approved by the National Research Council's Report Review Committee. The purpose of this independent review is to provide candid and critical comments that will assist the institution in making its published report as sound as possible and to ensure that the report meets institutional standards for objectivity, evidence, and responsiveness to the study charge. The review comments and draft manuscript remain confidential to protect the integrity of the deliberative process. We wish to thank the following individuals for their review of this report:

Luke R. Bucci, Vice President of Research, Schiff Nutrition International, Salt Lake City, Utah

David X. Cifu, Chair and Professor, Department of Physical Medicine & Rehabilitation Medical Director, Rehabilitation and Research Center, Virginia Commonwealth University, Richmond

William C. Franke, Associate Director, Center for Advanced Food Technology, Rutgers, The State University of New Jersey, New Brunswick

Robert I. Grossman, Professor and Dean, Department of Radiology, New York University School of Medicine, New York

Ainsley Malone, Nutrition Support Dietitian, Pharmacy Department, Mt. Carmel West Hospital, New Albany, Ohio

Ronald G. Riechers II, Neurologist, Louis Stokes Cleveland Veterans Affairs Medical Center, Ohio

Hilaire Thompson, Assistant Professor, Biobehavioral Nursing and Health Systems, University of Washington, Seattle

Katherine L. Tucker, Professor and Chair, Department of Health Sciences, Northeastern University, Boston, Massachusetts

Jacob W. VanLandingham, Assistant Professor, Biomedical Sciences, Florida State University School of Medicine, Tallahassee

Steven H. Zeisel, Professor, Departments of Nutrition and Pediatrics, University of North Carolina at Chapel Hill

Although the reviewers listed above have provided many constructive comments and suggestions, they were neither asked to endorse the conclusions or recommendations nor did they see the final draft of the report before its release. The review of this report was overseen by **Johanna Dwyer,** Director, Frances Stern Nutrition Center at Tufts University, and **Floyd E. Bloom,** chairman emeritus, Department of Neuropharmacology at Scripps Research Institute. Appointed by the National Research Council and Institute of Medicine, they were responsible for making certain that an independent examination of this report was carried out in accordance with institutional procedures and that all review comments were carefully considered. Responsibility for the final content of this report rests entirely with the authoring committee and the institution.

Contents

Part III: Recommendations

Appendixes

Preface

This Institute of Medicine report was the result of a request by the Department of Defense's (DoD's) Military Nutrition Division of the U.S. Army Research Institute of Environmental Medicine (USARIEM) to the Institute of Medicine (IOM) to review the potential role of nutrition in improving the outcomes of traumatic brain injury (TBI) at the acute stage. As background, the committee was to include an overview of types of TBI that are most commonly associated with combat operations. The committee also was asked to identify research needed in promising areas.

Active military service members experience a high percentage of traumatic brain injury ranging from severe to mild cases. The biological mechanisms of TBI are still not fully understood, and it involves a cascade of events resulting in a diversity of adverse effects in many realms of an individual's health. In fact, brain injury has been the topic of several National Academies studies in the past decade, many of them revealing the paucity of answers in regard to treating or preventing the injury. To date, there is no single standardized or effective approach for managing TBI and targeting a single aspect of the injury cascade following TBI has largely been unsuccessful. Because of the evidence that nutrition can modulate brain function in the healthy and injured population, nutrient approaches have been proposed as a way to provide resilience prior to TBI and as an adjuvant to other treatments after injury. The U.S. military forces are currently deployed in areas that present new challenges, such as the use of new types of warfare that increases the risk of experiencing blast injuries. In addition, since 2001, the number of troops deployed and the frequency and length of deployments augment the demands on our troops. The numbers of military personnel being affected by TBI in its various types (concussion/mild, mild, moderate, severe, penetrating, or blast) have frequently reached the news. As awareness of this public health problem increases, the military has devoted more resources in technology, research, diagnosis, and treatment to manage this disease.

A committee of 11 experts was formed with extensive knowledge across both military and civilian populations in the areas of neurology; nutritional sciences, clinical nutrition and dietetics; physiology; physical medicine and rehabilitation; psychiatry and behavior;

biochemical and molecular neuroscience; epidemiology/methodology; and the pathobiology of traumatic brain injury. In addition to its reviews of literature and discussions in closed meetings, the committee had the opportunity to have rich discussion with other experts in clinical care and research during two public workshops. On behalf of the committee, I sincerely thank the participants and speakers who contributed to the two workshops held to inform this study (see Appendix A) and to address topics critical to the completion of the committee's work. Their presentations served as essential references and resources for the committee.

The majority of the committee recommendations direct DoD to conduct research. It is the opinion of the committee that nutrition is a promising component of managing TBI, but many answers are still needed before any nutrition intervention can be utilized.

I would like to express my appreciation to Andrew Young, Chief of the Military Nutrition Division for his help in clarifying the task of the committee and being available to answer questions. I also would like to gratefully acknowledge the effort and skill that committee members brought to this report. Their backgrounds and experience made it possible to integrate nutritional science and neuroscience and to think forward about improving the outcomes of TBI. Finally, I thank the project staff of the National Academies: Maria Oria, study director, Laura Pillsbury, associate program officer, and Gui Liu, senior program assistant for their tireless dedication to the production of this report.

TBI also is a major health concern for the civilian population, and the actual burden of TBI in the United States is underestimated. It is my hope that this report assists not only DoD in its efforts to improve outcomes from TBI but also the public health community as a whole. I envision that this report will encourage different groups to work together toward answering the many answers still remaining.

John W. Erdman, *Chair*
Committee on Nutrition, Trauma, and the Brain

Summary

The U.S. military has seen significant advances in the prevention and treatment of wartime injuries. Science, medicine, and engineering have progressed to the point that the number of casualties of current wars is at a historic low compared with the wars of the past century. Today's warfighters benefit from multiple protections against penetrating injury. However, more widespread use of weapons like improvised explosive devices (IEDs) is leading to a higher number of nonpenetrating head and neck wounds, particularly traumatic brain injury (TBI). Mild single and recurrent injuries are especially worrisome because they might be silent—and consequently not treated—for months or years, only later becoming symptomatic and jeopardizing optimal health and performance. Although estimates of incidence vary, TBI has emerged as an important concern for the military, which in 1992 established the Department of Defense (DoD)/Department of Veterans Affairs (VA) Defense and Veterans Brain Injury Center to serve the military through clinical care, research initiatives, and educational programs.

Any injury to the brain, the main center for receiving and processing information and response, will likely result in a complex disease or condition. The military defines TBI as a traumatically induced structural injury or physiological disruption of brain function resulting from an external force that is indicated by new onset or worsening of symptoms involving level of consciousness, memory, mental or neurological states, or intracranial lesion (DOD, 2009). TBI has also been categorized as an ongoing process that affects multiple organs and systems and that may cause or accelerate other diseases and disorders that can reduce life expectancy (Masel and DeWitt, 2010). Although the characteristics of the disease will vary with the individual and injury and the sequence of events is not yet completely understood, there are several common pathobiological processes, including intracranial hemorrhage, excitotoxicity, ionic disturbances, decreased cerebral blood flow, edema, oxidative stress, inflammation, and damage and death of brain cells that occur during the acute (i.e., within minutes) and subacute (i.e., within 24 hours) phases. Other effects will manifest much later after the injury, although they will still be a consequence of the initial insult. In this longer-term phase, TBI has been associated with neurological disorders, neurodegenerative disorders (e.g., Alzheimer's disease, Parkinson's disease, and chronic traumatic encephalopathy), neuroendocrine disorders, psychiatric and psychological diseases, nonneurological disorders, and musculoskeletal dysfunction. Managing this multifaceted disease is a challenge. Given TBI's complex pathobiology and acute, subacute, and long-term effects, both the timing and duration of administration of any potential interventions are important to consider.

Nutrition has emerged as a possible approach for the prevention of or therapy for injuries to the brain, including neurodegenerative disorders and ischemia. DoD requested that the Institute of Medicine (IOM) convene an ad hoc committee to review the existing evidence for the potential role of nutrition in providing resilience or treating the acute and subacute effects of neurotrauma, with a focus on TBI.

SCOPE OF THE STUDY AND APPROACH OF THE COMMITTEE

This report reviews nutritional approaches that show promise in providing resilience or treating the acute and subacute effects of TBI. The committee was not asked to evaluate the role of nutritional therapies in the rehabilitation phase or the potential role of nutrition in ameliorating long-term effects of TBI. It is important to note that the chronological boundaries of acute, subacute, and long-term effects are not clear. For example, an event such as angiogenesis, which is typically associated with long-term wound healing, is initiated within the brain during the acute phase. This report therefore includes some studies that also evaluate seemingly long-term outcomes that may be initiated in the acute and subacute phases of the disease. This report does not address other outcomes such as neurodegenerative (e.g., Alzheimer's disease, Parkinson's disease), neuroendocrine, psychiatric, and other nonneurological disorders that appear later in life and may be associated with TBI but for which a causal relationship with the original injury has not been clearly established.

In spring of 2010, the IOM appointed a committee of 11 experts with extensive knowledge in the areas of neurology; nutritional sciences, clinical nutrition, and dietetics; physiology; physical medicine and rehabilitation; psychiatry and behavioral science; biochemical and molecular neuroscience; epidemiology/methodology; and the pathobiology of TBI. Two public workshops featuring presentations by civilian and military subject matter experts in TBI provided important information for the committee. A review of the scientific literature was conducted to examine physiological sequelae and metabolic responses to TBI, with the purpose of identifying mechanistic interventions. Nutrients were reviewed for their efficacy on TBI or on brain injuries with pathologies related to TBI, such as hypoxia, epilepsy, and subarachnoid hemorrhage. The committee also reviewed current practice guidelines for specific nutritional approaches to the clinical treatment of TBI on the battlefield, in garrison, or in hospital intensive care units (ICUs). In general, the nutrients were selected based on their potential role in restoring cellular energetics, reducing oxidative stress and inflammation, and repairing and recovering from the injury. The following nutritional interventions were identified for review: energy needs for severe cases of TBI, acetyl coA, antioxidants, branched-chain amino acids, choline, creatine, ketogenic diets, magnesium, nicotinamide adenine dinucleotide (NAD^+), n-3 fatty acids, polyphenols, probiotics, vitamin D, and zinc. Three of the nutritional interventions (i.e., acetyl-L-carnitine, niacin, and probiotics) initially selected were not included in the report because of insufficient evidence to reach conclusions about effectiveness from animal and human studies, or concerns for harm.

CONCLUSIONS AND RECOMMENDATIONS

This report emphasizes the importance of nutrition not only to augment overall defensive mechanisms against the effects of TBI but also as postinjury treatment to lessen the acute and subacute effects of TBI. The committee found that the majority of clinical guidelines for TBI do not specifically address optimal nutritional support for TBI. Based on the literature searches the committee concluded that conducting a review of the nutrition approaches to improve long-term effects of TBI, which was part of the initial task and later excluded because of financial constraints, would also be important (see also workshop papers by Metzger, Gomez-Pinilla, and Sands in Appendix C).

The recommendations were reached by consensus and are a reflection of the gap in data about the efficacy of most of the nutrition approaches reviewed. For this reason, except for early feeding of severe cases, the committee thought it premature to direct DoD to adopt any of them at this time. For the approaches that are supported by enough preclinical and, in some cases, clinical data, the committee sees the potential benefits for TBI patients and reached consensus about research needed in some promising areas. The report includes recommendations for research on the specific nutrition approaches that are promising and warrant further investigation. The research recommended will serve to confirm published results and to refine the protocols (i.e., optimal route of administration, timing, and dose).

The committee made recommendations for updating the evidence-based guidance for severe TBI with the provision of early feeding (Box S-1) as well as for research on continuing the development of animal models and the identification of biomarkers (Box S-2), on assessing nutritional status and intake of military populations (Box S-3), and on promising areas of nutrition research (Boxes S-4 and S-5). Finally, the committee includes a general recommendation to develop and update evidence-based guidance for TBI in the future, as more evidence about the value of nutritional interventions becomes available (Box S-6). The committee offers here its reflections on the prioritization of research based on its opinion of the likelihood of positive results for lessening the effects of TBI. Research on interventions for which human trials to explore the efficacy of improving the outcomes of TBI already exist or are ongoing have been presented as "most promising research" (Box 17-4). Research on interventions for which animal studies in TBI or human studies in associated conditions have shown improvements in outcomes are presented as "other research" (Box 17-5). DoD is encouraged to conduct the research internally, to support extramural research, or to collaborate with others in order to obtain answers more effectively.

The committee recognizes that conducting clinical research on TBI is extremely complex and that the understanding of the differences in pathophysiology between mild and severe

---

BOX S-1
Standardize the Provision of Energy and Protein to Patients with Severe TBI

RECOMMENDATION 6-1. The committee recommends that evidence-based guidelines include the provision of early (within 24 hours after injury) nutrition (more than 50 percent of total energy expenditure and 1–1.5 g/kg protein) for the first two weeks after injury. This intervention is critical to limit the intensity of the inflammatory response due to TBI, and to improve outcome.

BOX S-2
Continue Improving Animal Models and Identifying Biomarkers

RECOMMENDATION 3-1. The committee recommends that DoD, in cooperation with others, refine the existing animal models to investigate the potential benefits of nutrition throughout the spectrum of TBI injuries, that is, mild/concussion, moderate, severe, and penetrating, as well as repetitive and blast injuries. Development of animal models is particularly urgent for concussion/mild TBI and brain injuries due to blast as well as for repetitive injuries. These models also will aid in understanding the pathobiology of TBI, which is particularly needed for concussion/mild TBI, blast, and repetitive injuries.

RECOMMENDATION 3-2. The committee recommends that DoD, in cooperation with others, continue to develop better clinical biomarkers of TBI (i.e., mild/concussive, moderate, severe, penetrating, repetitive, and blast injuries) for the purposes of diagnosis, treatment, and outcome assessment. In addition, the committee recommends the identification of biomarkers specifically related to proposed mechanisms of action for individual nutritional interventions.

---

injuries is continuously evolving. Randomized clinical trials in a TBI population are difficult to carry out, and long-term prospective studies among high-risk populations are costly. Still, the committee emphasizes the need to follow best practices when designing such studies, and the importance of the following: (1) using appropriate biomarkers and animal models (see recommendations 3-1 and 3-2), (2) considering the full spectrum of TBI, (3) recording adverse effects, (4) recording gender and age differences, (5) carefully monitoring the quality of the compounds being tested, (6) using effective chemical forms and sources, based on their bioavailability, metabolism, and ability to reach the target area, (7) optimizing the route and timing of administration and dosage, and (8) recording synergistic and antagonistic effects with nutrients and dietary supplements or other substances in the diets of military personnel.

Energy and Protein Needs in Patients with Severe TBI

The current clinical practice guidelines for patients with TBI or other critical illnesses recommend early feeding, but the elements of the feeding regimen vary substantially, from

---

BOX S-3
Assessing Nutrition Status

RECOMMENDATION 5-1. DoD should conduct dietary intake assessments in different military settings (e.g., when eating in military dining facilities or when subsisting on a predominantly ration-based diet) both predeployment and during deployment to determine the nutritional status of soldiers as a basis for recommending increases in intake of specific nutrients that may provide resilience to TBI.

RECOMMENDATION 5-2. Routine dietary intake assessments of TBI patients in medical treatment facilities should be undertaken as soon after hospitalization as possible to estimate preinjury nutrition status as well as to provide optimal nutritional intake throughout the various stages of treatment.

RECOMMENDATION 5-3. In individuals with TBI, DoD should estimate pre-injury and post-injury dietary intake or status for those nutrients, dietary supplements, and diets that might show a relationship to TBI outcome. For example, based on the current evidence, the committee recommends collecting those estimates for creatine, n-3 fatty acids, choline, and vitamin D. The data could be used to investigate potential relationships between preinjury nutritional intake or status and recovery progress. Such data also would show possible synergistic effects between nutrients and dietary supplements.

BOX S-4
Most Promising Research Recommendations

RECOMMENDATION 6-2. DoD should conduct human trials to determine appropriate levels of blood glucose following TBI to minimize morbidity and mortality. These should be clinical trials of early feeding using intense insulin therapy to maintain blood glucose concentrations at less than 150–160 mg/dL versus current usual care of acute TBI in ICU settings for the first two weeks.

RECOMMENDATION 6-3. DoD should conduct clinical trials of the benefits of insulin therapy for care of acute TBI in inpatient settings with total parenteral nutrition (TPN) alone (or plus enteral feeding) versus enteral feeding alone. The goals for blood glucose in the TPN group should be lower (e.g., less than 120 mg/dL) than in the enteral group (e.g., less than 150–160 mg/dL). Variables to measure include clinical outcomes and incidence of hypoglycemia.

RECOMMENDATION 6-4. DoD should conduct studies to determine the optimal goals for nutrition (e.g., when to begin meeting total energy expenditure for optimal lean tissue maintenance or repletion) after the first two weeks following severe injury.

RECOMMENDATION 8-1. DoD should continue to monitor the literature on the effects of nutrients, dietary supplements, and diets on TBI, particularly those reviewed in this report but also others that may emerge as potentially effective in the future. For example, although the evidence was not sufficiently compelling to recommend that research be conducted on BCAAs, DoD should monitor the scientific literature for relevant research.

RECOMMENDATION 9-1. DoD should monitor the results of the Citicoline Brain Injury Treatment (COBRIT) trial, a human experimental trial examining the effect of CDP-choline and genomic factors on cognition and functional measures in severe, moderate, and complicated mild TBI. If the results of that trial are positive, DoD should conduct animal studies to define the optimal clinical dose and duration of treatment for choline (CDP-choline) following TBI, as well as to explore choline's potential to promote resilience to TBI when used as a preinjury supplement.

RECOMMENDATION 10-1. Based on the evidence supporting the effects of creatine on brain function and behavior after brain injury in children and adolescents, DoD should initiate studies in adults to assess the value of creatine for treating TBI patients.

RECOMMENDATION 13-1. DoD should conduct animal studies that examine the effectiveness of preinjury and postinjury oral administration of current commercial preparations of purified n-3 fatty acids on TBI outcomes.

RECOMMENDATION 13-2. Based on the evidence that fish oil decreases inflammation within hours of continuous administration, human clinical trials that investigate fish oil or purified n-3 fatty acids as a treatment for TBI are recommended. For acute cases of TBI, it should be noted that there are intravenous fish oil formulations available in Europe, but these are not approved by the FDA. Continuous enteral feeding with a feeding formula containing fish oil should provide equivalent effects for this purpose in the early phase of severe TBI when enteral access becomes available.

RECOMMENDATION 16-1. Based on a report showing efficacy in humans, the committee recommends that animal studies be conducted to determine the best practices for zinc administration after concussion/mild, moderate, and severe TBI, such as determining the therapeutic window for zinc administration, the length of treatment time for greatest efficacy, and the optimal level of zinc to improve outcomes. These trials should also evaluate the safety of zinc, based on concerns about toxicity and overload. Results from these studies should be used to design human clinical trials using zinc as a treatment for TBI.

BOX S-5
Other Research Recommendations

RECOMMENDATION 7-1. Based on the literature from animal and human trials concerning stroke and epilepsy, DoD should consider a clinical trial with TBI patients using an array of antioxidants in combination (e.g., vitamins E and C, selenium, beta-carotene) should be considered by DoD.

RECOMMENDATION 11-1. DoD should conduct animal studies to examine the specific effects of ketogenic diets, other modified diets (e.g., structured lipids, low-glycemic-index carbohydrates, fructose), or precursors of ketone bodies that affect energetics and have potential value against TBI. These animal studies should specifically consider dose, time, and clinical correlates with injury as variables. Results from these studies should be used to design human studies with these various diets to determine if they improve outcome against severe TBI. These studies should include time as a variable to determine whether there is an optimal initiation point and length of use.

RECOMMENDATION 11-2. If these studies show benefits, DoD should further investigate whether the potential beneficial effect of such ketogenic or modified diets or precursors to ketone bodies applies to concussion/mild and moderate TBI. Before conducting these studies, DoD should consider the feasibility (i.e., how to ensure compliance with a modified diet) of using diets that affect the metabolic energy available, such as ketogenic diets, for the treatment of TBI.

RECOMMENDATION 14-1. Based on positive outcomes in small-animal models of TBI with curcumin and resveratrol, DoD should consider conducting human trials. In addition, other flavonoids (e.g., isoflavones, flavanols, epicatechin, theanine) should be evaluated in animal models of TBI.

RECOMMENDATION 15-1. The committee recommends more animal studies be conducted to determine if vitamin D enhances the beneficial actions of progesterone in the treatment of TBI. If this synergistic effect is confirmed in animals, then studies in humans should be conducted to evaluate the extent to which vitamin D supplementation might improve the efficacy of progesterone treatment.

RECOMMENDATION 15-2. Based on animal studies showing a requirement of vitamin D for the efficacy of progesterone therapy, future animal studies are recommended to test the efficacy of using vitamin D supplements to improve resilience to TBI. Should the data from animal studies support use of this steroid hormone, human trials should be implemented to test the efficacy of vitamin D in populations at high risk for TBI.

RECOMMENDATION 16-2. Future work is needed in both humans and animal models to determine the extent to which chronic preinjury zinc supplementation can improve resilience in the event of a TBI.

the route of administration to the specific timing of initiation and the optimal method to estimate energy needs.

Based on recent meta-analyses showing that mortality and morbidity of TBI patients are improved by early feeding, the committee strongly supports the provision of energy and protein to patients with severe TBI early after injury. This important recommendation should

BOX S-6
Future Update of Evidence-Based Guidelines

RECOMMENDATION 2-1. Evidence-based nutrition guidelines specific for severe TBI should be updated. These guidelines should address unique nutritional concerns of severe TBI when different from generic critical illness nutrition guidelines (e.g., meeting energy needs and benefits of specific nutrients, food components, or diets). In addition, current guidelines to manage mild and moderate TBI should include recommendations for nutritional interventions. The guidelines should be developed in a collaborative manner with the various key stakeholders (e.g., American Dietetic Association, Department of Veterans Affairs, DoD).

be implemented immediately and will achieve significant positive outcomes by reducing the inflammatory response, which is likely to be at its height during the first 2 weeks after the injury.

Continue Improving Animal Models and Identifying Biomarkers

Appropriate animal study designs and biomarkers of injury and recovery are important components of a research agenda to support any hypothesis about the benefits of nutrition interventions (Box S-2). Reviews of the literature on animal models reveal limitations, especially for animal models of mild/concussion and blast TBI. Likewise, recent reviews on biomarkers for TBI reveal substantial limitations that decrease their value, such as poor discrimination between levels of injury severity, especially mild TBI; limited sensitivity; poor correlation between serum and brain levels; or systemic increases in the absence of TBI. Developing better clinical biomarkers of all types of TBI for the purposes of diagnosis, treatment, and outcome assessment is warranted. Nutrient mechanisms of action in TBI are still being studied, and it would be premature to identify any marker of nutritional interventions. Multiple biomarkers in conjunction with clinical data may offer better predictability of outcome.

Conducting Nutrition Assessments

Conducting nutrition assessments among active duty military personnel is costly and logistically challenging, particularly in combat zones, but collecting such information is necessary because the equivalent of NHANES data (i.e., health and nutritional data for adults and children in the United States) is lacking for the military population. Data on food consumption and nutrient intakes prior to mobilization would be valuable when making nutrition recommendations as a preventive approach. Knowing the nutrition status of TBI patients pre- and postinjury will also be essential to determine whether specific nutrient supplements would improve their health outcomes. The committee makes general recommendations about evaluating nutrition status in the military (Box S-3).

Research Needs on Nutritional Goals for Severe TBI

Although the importance of early feeding for patients with severe TBI is recognized and recommended in this report, there are still key questions, such as determining the optimal blood glucose concentration for the period immediately after a severe injury. The committee concluded that it is important to develop best feeding practices both for the initial period after TBI when the systemic inflammatory response is likely to be at its height, and also after about two weeks when concern about lean tissue maintenance and repletion assumes greater importance and tolerance to feeding is likely to be improved. Both hyperglycemia and hypoglycemia can occur in the critically ill, with the risk of hypoglycemia being higher in brain tissues that have glucose as their required source of energy. A number of recent studies have shown the negative effects of hypoglycemia on the likelihood of mortality in the critically ill, including TBI patients. The concept of permissive underfeeding has been applied to TBI patients in order to reduce the risk of hyperglycemia and its adverse effects. Increasing protein intake while following a lower energy intake regimen will improve the retention of lean tissue and may favorably affect clinical outcome in these patients. Intensive insulin therapy has been widely used to produce normal blood glucose levels, but its use appears most valid for the reduction of inflammation and improvement in morbidity and mortality in surgical patients. The utility of intensive insulin therapy has not been established in medical patients, and although a few human studies have been conducted with intensive insulin therapy in TBI patients, the goals for the level of nutritional support and glucose homeostasis still need to be established (Box S-4).

Research Needs on Nutrients and Dietary Supplements

The existing evidence varies, but not enough has been accumulated on any of the selected nutritional interventions to recommend their provision to increase resilience or ameliorate the acute effects of TBI. For some of the selected interventions, studies have demonstrated benefits in animal models of TBI or related brain injuries, but there are no clinical trials that confirm similar beneficial effects in humans. In other cases, human trials are under way, and the military should review those studies as the results are made public. Depending on the strength of the evidence for resilience or treatment, the committee makes recommendations for research in animal models or humans to confirm efficacy or determine the optimal dose, route of administration, or timing of administration.

Antioxidants

Oxidative stress is identified early after the initial injury, and compounds that intercept the production of reactive oxygen species could be beneficial for TBI outcomes. However, based on the fact that, even in the case of the most-studied compounds such as vitamins C and E, the use of single antioxidants has not been successful in treating oxidative-related diseases, the committee does not recommend any future research with single antioxidants and TBI. The committee's recommendation for further research is based on the limited success of some combinations of antioxidants in treating stroke and cancer.

Branched-Chain Amino Acids

Branched-chain amino acids (BCAAs) are commonly used by military personnel seeking a good source of protein to build muscle mass and reduce fatigue. Although these performance claims for BCAAs are not well supported, the possibility that BCAAs will help TBI patients cannot be discarded. BCAAs are precursors of neurotransmitters and compete with other neurotransmitters for transport through the blood-brain barrier. However, there is no strong evidence from animal or human studies on its effects in brain injury, and the committee suggests that research on BCAAs and TBI should not be a priority for the military until more compelling evidence is collected by other researchers.

Choline

Choline has been shown to act as an anti-inflammatory and antioxidant in other diseases, and also to decrease calcium-mediated cell death, a feature of TBI. Although substantial research has been conducted on choline and treatment of brain injury (stroke), differences in study design and study limitations have produced varying results; no conclusions about its efficacy can therefore be made at this time. There is one ongoing human trial on the effect of CDP-choline on cognition and functional measures on severe, moderate, and complicated mild TBI being led by a member of the committee. The committee recognizes the importance of this trial in that the findings will reveal more insights about the potential for this nutrient and whether there is a need for more human studies.

Part I

Background

1

Introduction

Recognizing the role of nutrition in maintaining optimal mental and physical condition, the military has long been devoted to ensuring adequate nutrition for its personnel. Service members experience a wide range of environmental and physiological circumstances associated with a variety of situations, including training for or performing combat operations. The current combat operations in Afghanistan (referred to as Operation Enduring Freedom [OEF]) and Iraq (referred to as Operation Iraqi Freedom [OIF]) have also presented new wartime challenges. Since 2001, the OEF and OIF conflicts have been characterized by extended and repeated deployments of a smaller, all-volunteer force, new tactics and weapons (such as improvised explosive devices [IEDs]), and higher rates of injury to the head and neck region than in past conflicts (Owens et al., 2008; Tanielian et al., 2008). Although estimates of incidence and prevalence are elusive, the available data indicate that traumatic brain injury (TBI) is a significant cause of mortality and morbidity in the OEF and OIF conflicts (Elder and Cristian, 2009).

Contributing to nearly one-third of all injury-related deaths in the United States, TBI is also a major health concern for the civilian population, especially because the complications of this injury are not always readily apparent (Faul et al., 2010). The Centers for Disease Control and Prevention (CDC) estimates that 1.7 million people in the United States sustain a TBI each year (Faul et al., 2010). In addition, an estimated 207,830 patients with sports-related TBIs were treated in U.S. emergency departments annually between 2001 and 2005 (Schroeder et al., 2007). Because the CDC surveillance system only draws data from hospitalizations and emergency department visits, the actual burden in the United States is underrepresented in this estimate. In fact, when the data on sports-related brain injuries are extrapolated based on cases involving loss of consciousness, they suggest that on an annual basis, only 5.5–13 percent of patients visit hospital emergency departments. It is therefore estimated that 1.6–3.8 million sports-related TBIs actually occur in the United States annually, including those not treated by a health care provider (Langlois et al., 2006; Schroeder et al., 2007).

The increased attention that the issue of head injuries is receiving from sports leagues and the military is generating greater overall awareness about this significant public health problem. However, TBI's mechanisms and its damaging effects on the brain are still not fully understood. The multifactorial injury process of blast injuries—the most frequent cause of TBI in current combat operations—adds to the complexity of TBI. Similarly, multiple clinical trials on the acute treatment of TBI in civilian populations using pharmacological agents targeted at a single aspect of the injury cascade that follows TBI have been largely unsuccessful. Combat-related brain injury and stress disorders (such as posttraumatic stress disorder [PTSD]) as well as sports-related brain injuries have been the topic of several National Academies studies since 2000, including *Returning Home from Iraq and Afghanistan: Preliminary Assessment of Readjustment Needs of Veterans, Service Members, and Their Families* (IOM, 2010); *Gulf War and Health: Volume 7: Long-Term Consequences of Traumatic Brain Injury* (IOM, 2009); *Opportunities in Neuroscience for Future Army Applications* (NRC, 2009); *Systems Engineering to Improve Traumatic Brain Injury Care in the Military Health System Workshop Summary* (NAE/IOM, 2009); *Treatment of Posttraumatic Stress Disorder: An Assessment of the Evidence* (IOM, 2008); *Evaluating the HRSA Traumatic Brain Injury Program* (IOM, 2006a); *Posttraumatic Stress Disorder: Diagnosis and Assessment* (IOM, 2006b); and *Is Soccer Bad for Children's Heads?: Summary of the IOM Workshop on Neuropsychological Consequences of Head Impact in Youth Soccer* (IOM, 2002).

Despite the paucity of evidence on effective treatments for TBI, new information is advancing the understanding of the relationship between nutrition status and brain func-

---

BOX 1-1
Statement of Task

An expert committee will review the existing evidence that supports the potential role for nutrition in providing resilience (i.e., protecting), mitigating, or treating of primary (i.e., within minutes of insult) and secondary (i.e., within 24 hours of insult) associated effects of neurotrauma, with a focus on traumatic brain injury. As a background, it will include an overview of types of central nervous system–related neurotrauma (primary and secondary effects) that are most commonly associated with combat operations. Research in promising areas will also be identified. Specifically the committee will respond to the following questions:

(1) What specific types of CNS-related neurotrauma (primary and secondary effects) are most commonly associated with combat operations? (Developed as an overview for background)
   (a) Compare injury effects of severe neurotrauma produced by a single causative event versus accumulating effects of multiple concussions associated with lower-level events.
   (b) What clinical standards qualitatively and quantitatively define severity of neurotrauma-associated injury?
(2) What biological mechanisms of combat-associated CNS-related neurotrauma injury (primary and secondary effects) are likely to have nutritional implications, vis-à-vis resilience to injury and/or severity of injury?
   (a) What are the metabolic responses to neurotrauma in cells and tissues?
   (b) How do metabolic responses to neurotrauma influence development of physiological sequelae and functional outcomes associated with injury?
   (c) Do biological mechanisms (metabolic and cellular) and physiological sequelae of combat-associated neurotrauma (items 2.a and 2.b, above) exhibit "dose-dependency" such that concussion elicits the same response, albeit quantitatively less pronounced, compared to a single severe neurotrauma, or do the biological mechanisms in response to neurotrauma initiate in a "threshold" manner?
   (d) Do quantitative and temporal relationships among metabolic responses, physiological sequelae, and functional outcomes to neurotrauma provide any useful clinical biomarkers of the severity, progression, or resolution of injury?

tion, and increasingly indicates that nutritional interventions could possibly help with the prevention, resilience, or treatment of the acute events of TBI. Because the literature on the pathophysiology and treatment of TBI still contains significant information gaps, this study effectively raises more research questions than it provides specific recommendations for preventive interventions or acute treatments to mitigate an injury.

PURPOSE AND SCOPE OF THE STUDY

For these reasons, the Institute of Medicine (IOM) was requested to convene an ad hoc expert committee under the oversight of the Committee on Military Nutrition Research to review the potential role of nutrients and dietary supplements in the prevention and treatment of TBI. As requested in the statement of task presented in Box 1-1, this study reviews only the potential nutritional implications for primary and secondary physiological sequelae of neurotrauma. Although the effects of TBI (primary, secondary, and long-term effects) are conceptually expressed according to the amount of time elapsed after the initial insult, the boundaries of these definitions are actually ambiguous, and extrapolating the timing of effects from animal models to humans is not always feasible. That is, some of the early pathogenic events related to cell death may extend into the more chronically injured brain, while other pathogenic events typically associated with wound healing are also initiated—and perhaps resolved—within the more acutely injured brain. Given these challenges, this

(e) Do the metabolic responses to neurotrauma suggest that resilience and susceptibility to neurotrauma might be positively or negatively modulated by metabolic or nutritional status (and hydration) before injury?

(f) If nutritional status does affect resilience and susceptibility, would a preventive nutritional approach be feasible to mitigate the primary or secondary physiological sequelae and functional outcomes of neurotrauma when it does occur?

(3) Do the metabolic and physiological responses to CNS-related neurotrauma (primary and secondary effects) have nutritional implications for optimal clinical treatment?

(a) What nutrition interventions for concussion and other CNS-related neurotrauma are included in current standards of practice, best practice, or clinical practice guidelines for treatment and recovery?

(b) How do regulation of metabolism and physiology in tissues injured by neurotrauma differ from non-injured tissue? Are the differences, if any, "dose-dependent"? Do those differences have nutritional implications for optimizing treatment?

(c) What specific nutritional approaches (e.g., nutrients, diets and nutritional interventions, including enteric and intravenous nutrition) have been shown to enhance efficacy of clinical treatment for patients experiencing CNS-related neurotrauma?

(4) What research is needed to adequately address the questions listed above?

(a) What research methods and models are appropriate for evaluating putative nutritional interventions for neurotrauma (e.g., animal models, epidemiological and clinical studies)?

(b) Are there other injuries (e.g., high pressure nervous syndrome) or situations (e.g., high altitude exposure) that might have similar underlying biological mechanisms as those for brain injury and recovery that could be useful models when exploring nutrition interventions for CNS-related neurotrauma and health disorders?

(c) Are there other populations (e.g., football, boxing, cyclists) that would be useful models for studying how nutrition modulates resilience, susceptibility, and recovery from neurotrauma? What specific nutrients, botanicals, and other nutritional interventions are the highest priority, i.e., most promising, for the military to study for mitigating and treating combat neurotrauma?

report includes a select number of studies that also evaluate outcomes that are seemingly long term but that might be initiated in the acute phase of the disease. In general, however, long-term health disorders associated with neurotrauma, such as PTSD, neurodegenerative diseases (Alzheimer's disease or parkinsonism), neurocognitive deficits, psychosocial health problems (e.g., major depression, impairment of social functioning and ability to work, suicide), epilepsy, pain, and other alterations in personality or behavior that might be affected by the nutritional status of the individual are not reviewed in this study.

It also should be noted that descriptions of diagnostics tools, such as imaging techniques or neuropsychological tests, are not included in this report because such descriptions are beyond the scope of the task. Although genetic factors may be identified as increasing risk of TBI effects in the acute and subacute phases in the future, this report does not include discussion of this consideration because the committee is unaware of research identifying genetics as a risk factor of TBI, and it would therefore be premature to make conclusions or recommendations concerning this possibility.

TRAUMATIC BRAIN INJURY

CDC defines TBI as being caused by a bump, blow, or jolt to the head or a penetrating head injury that disrupts the normal function of the brain.[1] A penetrating brain injury is the result of an object, such as a bullet, shrapnel, or debris, piercing the skull. A closed head injury is caused by blunt-force trauma that does not break through the skull, as in a fall or hitting a car dashboard. Closed head injuries are commonly categorized by the severity of the symptoms, i.e., as mild, moderate, or severe. The definitions of severity are based on the clinical signs listed in Table 1-1. Mild TBI (mTBI), also referred to as concussion, accounts for over 75 percent of TBIs that occur annually in both civilian and military populations. Concussion and mTBI are often used interchangeably in clinical practice guidelines covering the management of TBI and by military and civilian health-care providers. For the purposes of this report, the two terms frequently appear together to recognize their consistent definitions. Much more is known about the effects of moderate to severe brain injuries, however, than those of mild or concussion injuries.

The cellular- and molecular-level events initiated by injury can be roughly characterized according to their sequence during and following injury (as described in Margulies et al., 2009). The complexity of TBI markedly restricts the precision of such characterization because the emergence and duration of pathogenic events are variable, and can even overlap. Primary effects refer to those effects that arise within minutes. The effects that emerge over the next 24 hours are considered secondary, and are believed to exacerbate the primary neurological damage. In this report, primary and secondary effects are also referred to as acute and subacute effects. Finally, long-term or chronic effects are those that are associated with the injury, but that occur weeks to years later. This characterization, described in greater detail in Chapter 3, served as the basis for the committee's review of the effectiveness of select nutrients in treating the complex cascade of events initiated during the acute and subacute phases of TBI.

TBI in the Military

The definition of TBI currently used by the military, which has been modified to include combat-related mechanisms, appears in Box 1-2. Between 2000 and 2010, 195,547 service

---

[1] Available online: http://www.cdc.gov/traumaticbraininjury/ (accessed December 1, 2010).

TABLE 1-1 Severity Ratings of TBI Based on Clinical Signs

Criteria	Mild	Moderate	Severe
Structural Imaging	Normal	Normal or Abnormal	Normal or Abnormal
Loss of Consciousness (LOC)	0–30 min	> 30 min and < 24 hrs	> 24 hrs
Alteration of Consciousness/Mental State (AOC)	≤ 24 hrs	> 24 hrs	> 24 hrs
Posttraumatic Amnesia (PTA)	≤ 24 hrs	> 24 hrs and < 7 days	> 7 days
Glasgow Coma Scale (GCS) (best available score in first 24 hours)	Score 13–15	Score 9–12	Score 3–8

NOTE: Although commonly used in practice, the official DoD definition for TBI does not include GCS.
SOURCE: DoD, 2010.

members were diagnosed with TBI.[2] This number includes injuries sustained in both combat operations and in garrison. The leading causes of TBI in the military are blasts, fragments, bullets, motor vehicle crashes, and falls (DoD, 2010). Figure 1-1 breaks down the incidence of TBI for 2000 through 2010 by severity, according to the clinical classifications listed in Table 1-1.

The epidemiological data for combat-related TBI, especially blast-induced and mild TBI, are still evolving, with some researchers finding that 10–20 percent of returning veterans have sustained a TBI (Hoge et al., 2008; Tanielian et al., 2008; Terrio et al., 2009), while others estimate that TBI accounts for up to one-third of combat-related injuries in Iraq and Afghanistan (Meyer et al., 2008). About 78 percent of the TBIs occurring in 2009 across all military services were classified as mild,[3] which has generated great concern for the military because of their high incidence, persistent health outcomes, and the often unnoticeable effects at the time of injury. The 2009 IOM report on long-term consequences of TBI identified several outcomes that can persist even after mTBI, including unprovoked seizures, depression, aggression, and postconcussion symptoms. These symptoms include headache; dizziness; fatigue; irritability; subjective concentration difficulty; memory impairment; insomnia; and reduced tolerance to stress, emotional excitement, or alcohol. The report also highlighted the research finding of a dose-response relationship with regard to severity of injury and outcome; that is, the more severe the TBI, the more severe the outcome (IOM, 2009).

Concurrent disorders have been found common among TBI patients, particularly posttraumatic stress disorder and other mental health disorders, substance abuse, and risk of suicide (Tanielian et al., 2008; Warden, 2006). The 2010 IOM report on readjustment needs indicated a greater prevalence of many of these health outcomes than in previous conflicts. Furthermore, in a study of more than 2,000 U.S. Army infantry soldiers three to four months after their return from Iraq, Hoge et al. (2008) found the highest prevalence of PTSD occurred among soldiers who had lost consciousness, suggesting a stronger association between TBI and PTSD than other types of injury and PTSD. This relationship is complicated and still not completely understood because of the overlap of symptoms between PTSD, TBI, and postconcussion syndrome.

The increased use of IEDs in the current conflicts has produced more blast-related injuries than previous combat operations. Approximately two-thirds of medical evacuations are blast-induced injuries, and these can often involve concurrent injuries resulting in cognitive, physical, or psychological impairments (commonly referred to as polytrauma), necessitating

---

[2] Available online: http://www.dvbic.org/TBI-Numbers.aspx (accessed February 25, 2011).
[3] Available online: http://www.dvbic.org/TBI-Numbers.aspx (accessed December 1, 2010).

BOX 1-2
Department of Defense Definition of Traumatic Brain Injury (2007)

A traumatically induced structural injury and/or physiological disruption of brain function as a result of an external force that is indicated by new onset or worsening of at least one of the following clinical signs immediately following the event:

- Any period of loss of or a decreased level of consciousness
- Any loss of memory for events immediately before or after the injury (i.e., PTA)
- Any alteration in mental state at the time of the injury (confusion, disorientation, slowed thinking, etc.)
- Neurological deficits (weakness, loss of balance, change in vision, praxis, paresis/plegia, sensory loss, aphasia, etc.) that may or may not be transient
- Intracranial lesion

External forces may include any of the following events:

- Head being struck by an object
- Head striking an object
- Brain undergoing an acceleration/deceleration movement without direct external trauma to the head
- Foreign body penetrating the brain
- Forces generated from events such as blast or explosion, or other force yet to be defined

multiple health-care services (IOM, 2010; Warden, 2006). Of 433 TBI patients from OEF and OIF being treated at Walter Reed Army Medical Center between 2003 and 2005, 19 percent also required an amputation (Warden, 2006; Warden et al., 2005). TBI outcomes can be affected by some of these associated injuries. Significant blood loss and dehydration can produce hypotension, which has been associated with more adverse outcomes. A single

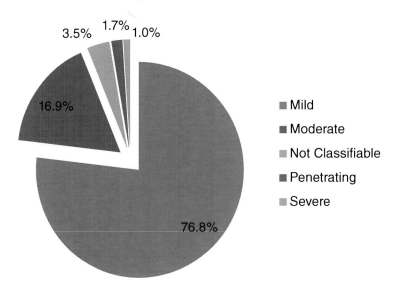

FIGURE 1-1 TBI Categories, 2000–2010Q3.
NOTE: Numbers for the current year are updated on a quarterly basis. 2009–2010Q3 numbers updated as of November 15, 2010.
SOURCE: See http://www.dvbic.org/TBI-Numbers.aspx (accessed December 1, 2010).

hypotensive episode during the prehospital phase of severe TBI has been associated with doubling of mortality and increased morbidity (Fearnside et al., 1993). In polytrauma situations where the other injuries require more immediate medical attention, it can be especially difficult to identify cases of mild or concussion injuries. Similar to the evidence on the detrimental long-term effects of repetitive sports-related concussion injuries and second impact syndrome, exposure to multiple blasts has been linked to increased probability of further injury that can result in long-term physical and psychological impairments (Lew et al., 2006, 2007; Tanielian et al., 2008). The understanding of blast as a contributing mechanism to TBI—and its clinical similarities to and differences from other forms of TBI—continues to evolve. A summary of some recent findings is included in the discussion on pathobiology found in Chapter 3.

The reader is referred to the workshop papers by Col. Michael Jaffee, Dr. Mårten Risling, and Col. Geoffrey Ling in Appendix C for greater detail on the epidemiology of TBI in the military.

Sports-Related Brain Injuries

With nearly half of Americans of all ages participating in non-work-related sports activities annually, there are ample opportunities for sports-related injuries, despite the health benefits of being physically active (Schroeder et al., 2007). Almost 16 percent of all cases of injury in the United States between 2004 and 2005 occurred during sports or exercise (Bergen et al., 2008). Among people under the age of 25, sports injuries are most prevalent, accounting for about 30 percent of all injury episodes (Bergen et al., 2008). The risk for sports-related TBI is likewise particularly high for children and adolescents, who had the highest rates among those treated in hospital emergency departments (Schroeder et al., 2007). Overall, an estimated 1.6–3.8 million sports-related TBIs occur in the United States each year (Langlois et al., 2006).

A review of the literature indicates that the blast-induced brain injuries most commonly seen in the military population have pathological characteristics that differ from other TBIs, despite their similar secondary effects (Cernak and Noble-Haeusslein, 2010). Although more research is needed to differentiate and draw parallels between the various injury mechanisms, much is being shared between the military and sports communities, particularly on the assessment and management of concussions. Because of the parallels between the acute pathological effects of blast-induced brain injuries and other injury mechanisms, the nutrients considered in this report can similarly be considered for sports-related and other civilian brain injuries.

STUDY APPROACH AND ORGANIZATION OF THE REPORT

From patient to patient, brain injuries are remarkably diverse. Apart from differences in the cause and severity of the injury, the insult initiates a complex cascade of mechanistic events, making it impossible for any therapeutic intervention to target a single event. The ability of nutrients to interact with a variety of physiological and metabolic injury responses suggests the advantage of nutritional approaches to the treatment of TBI. The committee believes that nutritional approaches, or interventions, should not been seen as singular therapies but rather as complementary or supportive of other therapies. The committee considers nutritional interventions to range from the clinical support provision of essential nutrients and energy for recovery from major trauma, to individual nutrients or dietary supplements that may uniquely alter the repair process. It is from this perspective that the committee approached its charge.

Initial work for this study began at a June 2008 meeting of the IOM Committee of Military Nutrition Research, with various researchers and neurosurgeons attending. Potential mechanistic targets, such as inflammation or mitochondrial dysfunction, were identified as relevant to the consideration of nutritional interventions for TBI. A preliminary exploration of the published literature was conducted, and several nutrients were selected for further exploration of their effectiveness in alleviating or mitigating various components of the injury process.

In spring of 2010, the IOM appointed a committee of 11 experts with extensive knowledge across both military and civilian populations in the areas of neurology; nutritional sciences, clinical nutrition, and dietetics; physiology; physical medicine and rehabilitation; psychiatry and behavior; biochemical and molecular neuroscience; epidemiology/methodology; and the pathobiology of traumatic brain injury. The committee gathered further information during two public workshops in June and October 2010 that featured presentations by civilian and military subject matter experts on TBI in the military, the pathophysiology of TBI, nutritional considerations in the clinical management of TBI, and various nutritional interventions studied in animal and human models of brain injury or other brain disorders.

The committee conducted a review of the scientific literature to examine physiological sequelae and metabolic responses to TBI. After identifying neuroprotective targets possibly responsive to nutritional interventions, the committee established a search plan to investigate the effect of promising nutrients on outcomes of brain injury, stroke, hypoxia, epilepsy, and subarachnoid hemorrhage. These additional conditions were selected for the literature review because of their pathophysiological similarities to the secondary events associated with TBI. Based on expert consultation, discussions, and their review of the literature, the committee focused on nutritional approaches that have demonstrated some level of efficacy in relevant physiological processes. The details of the committee's approach to identifying the most promising nutrients that may be of benefit for the treatment of or resilience to TBI are described in Chapter 4. As with other ad hoc study reports prepared by The National Academies, the recommendations in the following chapters were reached by consensus.

In their comprehensive examination of the literature, the committee addressed the question of which specific nutritional approaches have been shown to enhance efficacy of treatment for patients experiencing neurotrauma, as well as which nutritional strategies might help with resilience to brain injury. The committee's approach to reviewing the literature for the selected nutritional interventions targeted brain injuries with physiological effects similar to those of TBI (subarachnoid hemorrhage, hypoxia-ischemia, stroke, and epilepsy) because there was not enough evidence solely from TBI models for a thorough evaluation. The review did not include the preventive literature on other areas such as brain health and cognitive function of healthy individuals. The committee also reviewed current practice guidelines for specific nutritional approaches to the clinical treatment of TBI on the battlefield, in garrison, or in hospital intensive care units.

This report has been organized into three major sections based on the breakdown of the committee's charge. Part I provides a background on the acute effects of neurotrauma most commonly associated with combat operations. Chapter 2 reviews the current clinical practice guidelines across all levels of severity of TBI, highlighting those practices that specify nutritional approaches for treatment and recovery. Chapter 3 provides background on the pathophysiological changes that accompany TBI. This review of the physiological mechanisms of TBI serves as the committee's framework for the selection of nutrients, based on functions and mechanisms of action that suggest they might promote resilience and/or be efficacious when provided after TBI. Part II outlines the preliminary selection of nutritional interventions for TBI (Chapter 4), the importance of nutrition in resilience to TBI (Chapter

5), and energy and protein needs during early feeding following TBI (Chapter 6). Chapters 7 through 16 discuss the evidence on the nutrients and dietary supplements reviewed by the committee. Part III presents a summary of the committee's findings and conclusions, and highlights its recommendations on promising areas for future research. Chapter 17 includes a breakdown of research, organized by topic, needed to overcome gaps in information, including assessing nutrition status of military personnel and TBI patients, improving animal models and identifying biomarkers of TBI, and prioritizing research that would address questions of TBI treatment efficacy for the most promising nutrients. Appendixes provide the workshop agenda, relevant nutrition advice in current clinical guidelines, workshop presentations, biographical sketches of committee members and speakers, a glossary of terms, and a list of acronyms and abbreviations.

REFERENCES

Bergen, G., L. H. Chen, M. Warner, and L. A. Fingerhut. 2008. *Injury in the United States: 2007 chartbook.* Hyattsville, MD: National Center for Health Statistics.

Cernak, I., and L. J. Noble-Haeusslein. 2010. Traumatic brain injury: An overview of pathobiology with emphasis on military populations. *Journal of Cerebral Blood Flow and Metabolism* 30(2):255–266.

DoD (Department of Defense). 2010. *Mild traumatic brain injury pocket guide (conus).* Washington, DC.

Faul, M., L. Xu, M. M. Wald, and V. G. Coronado. 2010. *Traumatic brain injury in the United States: Emergency department visits, hospitalizations and deaths 2002–2006.* Atlanta, GA: Centers for Disease Control and Prevention.

Fearnside, M. R., R. J. Cook, P. McDougall, and R. J. McNeil. 1993. The Westmead head-injury project outcome in severe head-injury—A comparative-analysis of prehospital, clinical and CT variables. *British Journal of Neurosurgery* 7(3):267–279.

Hoge, C. W., D. McGurk, J. L. Thomas, A. L. Cox, C. C. Engel, and C. A. Castro. 2008. Mild traumatic brain injury in U.S. soldiers returning from Iraq. *The New England Journal of Medicine* 358(5):453–463.

IOM (Institute of Medicine). 2002. *Is soccer bad for children's heads? Summary of the IOM workshop on neuropsychological consequences of head impact in youth soccer.* Washington, DC: National Academy Press.

IOM. 2006a. *Evaluating the HRSA Traumatic Brain Injury Program.* Washington, DC: The National Academies Press.

IOM. 2006b. *Posttraumatic stress disorder: Diagnosis and assessment.* Washington, DC: The National Academies Press.

IOM. 2008. *Treatment of posttraumatic stress disorder: An assessment of the evidence.* Washington, DC: The National Academies Press.

IOM. 2009. *Gulf War and health: Long-term consequences of traumatic brain injury.* Vol. 7. Washington, DC: The National Academies Press.

IOM. 2010. *Returning home from Iraq and Afghanistan: Preliminary assessment of readjustment needs of veterans, service members, and their families.* Washington, DC: The National Academies Press.

Langlois, J. A., W. Rutland-Brown, and M. M. Wald. 2006. The epidemiology and impact of traumatic brain injury: A brief overview. *Journal of Head Trauma Rehabilitation* 21(5):375–378.

Lew, H. L., J. H. Poole, S. B. Guillory, R. M. Salerno, G. Leskin, and B. Sigford. 2006. Persistent problems after traumatic brain injury: The need for long-term follow-up and coordinated care. *Journal of Rehabilitation Research and Development* 43(2):vii–x.

Lew, H. L., D. Thomander, K. T. L. Chew, and J. Bleiberg. 2007. Review of sports-related concussion: Potential for application in military settings. *Journal of Rehabilitation Research and Development* 44(7):963–973.

Margulies, S., R. Hicks, and Combination Therapies for Traumatic Brain Injury Workshop Leaders. 2009. Combination therapies for traumatic brain injury: Prospective considerations. *Journal of Neurotrauma* 26(6):925–939.

Meyer, K., K. Helmick, S. Doncevic, and R. Park. 2008. Severe and penetrating traumatic brain injury in the context of war. *Journal of Trauma Nursing* 15(4):185–189; quiz 190–181.

NAE/IOM (National Academy of Engineering/Institute of Medicine). 2009. *Systems engineering to improve traumatic brain injury care in the military health system workshop summary.* Washington, DC: The National Academies Press.

NRC (National Research Council). 2009. *Opportunities in neuroscience for future army application.* Washington, DC: The National Academies Press.

Owens, B. D., J. F. Kragh, J. C. Wenke, J. Macaitis, C. E. Wade, and J. B. Holcomb. 2008. Combat wounds in Operation Iraqi Freedom and Operation Enduring Freedom. *Journal of Trauma-Injury Infection and Critical Care* 64(2):295–299.

Schroeder, T., C. Irish, J. L. Annest, T. Haileyesus, K. Sarmiento, and J. Mitchko. 2007. Nonfatal traumatic brain injuries from sports and recreation activities—United States, 2001–2005 *Morbidity and Mortality Weekly Report* 56(29):733–737.

Tanielian, T. L., and L. Jaycox. 2008. *Invisible wounds of war psychological and cognitive injuries, their consequences, and services to assist recovery.* http://site.ebrary.com/lib/natacademies/Doc?id=10246315 (accessed October 26, 2010).

Terrio, H., L. A. Brenner, B. J. Ivins, J. M. Cho, K. Helmick, K. Schwab, K. Scally, R. Bretthauer, and D. Warden. 2009. Traumatic brain injury screening: Preliminary findings in a U.S. Army Brigade Combat Team. *Journal of Head Trauma Rehabilitation* 24(1):14–23.

Warden, D. 2006. Military TBI during the Iraq and Afghanistan wars. *Journal of Head Trauma Rehabilitation* 21(5):398–402.

Warden, D. L., L. M. Ryan, K. M. Helmick, K. Schwab, L. French, W. Lu, W. Lux, G. Ling, and J. Ecklund. 2005. War neurotrauma: The Defense and Veterans Brain Injury Center (DVBIC) experience at Walter Reed Army Medical Center (WRAMC). *Journal of Neurotrauma* 22(10):1163–1258.

2

Nutrition in Clinical Practice Guidelines for Traumatic Brain Injury

Evidence-based guidelines (EBGs) are a common tool used in evidence-based medicine by health-care practitioners. Evidence-based medicine is founded on the following two principles (Guyatt et al., 2000; Sackett et al., 1996): (1) there is a hierarchy of strength of evidence behind recommendations, and (2) the clinician uses judgment when weighing the trade-offs associated with alternative management strategies, including consideration of patient values and preferences as well as societal values.

As will be obvious in Chapters 6–16, much of the available evidence suggesting potential benefits of specific nutritional interventions in traumatic brain injury (TBI) comes from findings in animal models and, in a handful of cases, randomized human trials. The committee has defined a research agenda for the many questions that still remain. This research agenda provides an opportunity for those developing clinical guidelines to be made cognizant of the questions that remain to be elucidated.

This chapter includes a brief summary of the nutrition-related recommendations from selected clinical guidelines for severe trauma patients, including TBI patients, and for patients with mild or moderate TBI.

EVIDENCE-BASED CLINICAL GUIDELINES

Hierarchy of Strength of Evidence

There is a hierarchy of strength of evidence behind recommendations in evidence-based clinical guidelines. The hierarchy of strength of evidence (i.e., which studies are best able to answer the question with certainty) varies, depending on the type of question being asked. Many questions addressed in EBGs are treatment questions best answered by a systematic review of randomized controlled human trials, or by several large, well-designed, randomized controlled human trials designed to answer the specific inquiry with consistent results (Howick et al., 2011). The EBGs are usually based on one or more systematic reviews, and these appear at the top of the hierarchy of evidence for treatment. Other questions are better answered by different types of research designs. For example, systematic reviews of cross-sectional studies would best respond to diagnostic issues. Questions about the likelihood of causing harm would be best answered by either a systematic review of randomized n-of-1 trials for common harms and rare harms, by a systematic review of case-control studies, or by studies revealing dramatic effects. Prognosis questions would be best answered by systematic review of inception cohort studies. There often is no best evidence, but a clinical guideline is still needed by health-care practitioners. Therefore, in addition to attending to the kind of study needed, the reviewer needs to explicitly describe the strength of the evidence supporting a specific guideline. Such description provides the health-care practitioner an indication of the level of certainty of a guideline recommendation (ADA, 2010; Howick et al., 2011). Guidelines with weak supporting evidence need to be updated as new evidence becomes available.

The Bradford-Hill criteria provide a framework for epidemiological research demonstrating causality between environment and disease states (Hill and Bradford, 1965). These criteria can be applied to the development of EBGs because they help determine whether an association between an intervention and an outcome is causal. For the task of this committee, establishing a causal relationship between a nutritional intervention and a TBI outcome would rely on the following: strength of evidence, consistency of evidence, specificity, temporal relationship (temporality), biological gradient (dose-response relationship), plausibility (biological plausibility), coherence with existing knowledge, experimental testing, and analogy (consideration of alternative explanations).

Use of Clinical Judgment

The second principle of evidence-based medicine is that the clinician uses judgment when weighing the trade-offs associated with alternative management strategies, including consideration of patient values and preferences as well as societal values (Guyatt, 2002; Guyatt et al., 2000).

DEVELOPMENT OF EVIDENCE-BASED GUIDELINES

Evidence-based guidelines are developed by professional organizations, health-care organizations, or other nonprofit, disease- or condition-specific organizations (DoD, 2008; Grilli et al., 2000; Knuth et al., 2005; Thomas et al., 1999). There are well-established procedures to systematically review and synthesize the research best suited to answer the clinical questions faced by health-care practitioners. More than 40 clinical guidelines for TBI were identified at the National Guideline Clearinghouse online database.[1] However, many of these guidelines focus on emergency department treatment or evaluating for the presence or absence of TBI in primary care or sports settings, and only a few address nutritional concerns.

In addition to guidelines developed specifically for TBI, generic evidence-based clinical practice guidelines for critical care of adults in intensive care units may also be appropriate in acute TBI. For mild TBI, other EBGs might also be appropriate based on additional conditions, such as obesity.

For this report, EBGs from the following organizations were selected for more comprehensive evaluation because of their relevance to TBI: the American Society of Parenteral and Enteral Nutrition (ASPEN), the Society of Critical Care Medicine (SCCM), the American Dietetic Association (ADA), the Brain Trauma Foundation, the National Neurotrauma Soci-

---

[1] Available online: http://www.guideline.gov/ (accessed October 26, 2010).

ety, the American Association of Neuroscience Nurses (AANN), the Department of Defense (DoD), and the U.S. Department of Veterans Affairs (VA) (ADA, 2006; Bratton et al., 2007; Kattelmann et al., 2006; Knuth et al., 2005; McClave et al., 2009; VA/DoD, 2009). The following section summarizes the nutrition components of these EBGs. For this chapter, the EBGs were divided into two types: those for patients with severe TBI in the acute phase who are in the intensive care unit (ICU) critical-care setting, and those for patients with mild TBI, who are more likely to be outpatients.

EBGS FOR SEVERE TBI IN THE ACUTE STAGES

DoD's *Guidelines for the Field Management of Combat-Related Head Trauma* (Knuth et al., 2005) address assessment of oxygenation and blood pressure, Glasgow Coma Scale, airway, ventilation, fluid treatment, pain management and sedation, triage for transport, and brain-targeted therapy. The only nutrition-related content is the discussion of assessment of nausea as a side effect of pain medication. Nutrition needs are not specifically addressed.

In contrast, other guidelines do recognize the importance of nutrition to accelerate progress in trauma patients. For example, the SCCM/ASPEN *Guidelines for Provision and Assessment of Nutrition Support Therapy in the Adult Critically Ill Patient* include recommendations for timing of initiation of enteral nutrition, use of parenteral nutrition, dosage of enteral feeding, monitoring, intolerance and adequacy of enteral nutrition, selection of appropriate enteral formulation, adjunctive therapies, and maximizing the efficacy of parenteral nutrition, as well as specific recommendations for the following medical conditions: pulmonary failure, renal failure, hepatic failure, acute pancreatitis, and end-of-life treatments (McClave et al., 2009).

The ADA *Critical Illness Evidence-Based Nutrition Practice Guideline* also includes recommendations for assessing nutritional issues in trauma patients. The recommendations address energy expenditure and needs, choosing enteral versus parenteral nutrition, timing of feeding, feeding tube site, use of immune-enhancing formulas, use of blue dye in enteral nutrition to detect aspiration, monitoring criteria and blood glucose control, and special considerations for persons with diabetes (Kattelmann et al., 2006).

The third edition of the *Guidelines for the Management of Severe Traumatic Brain Injury* from the Brain Trauma Foundation includes a recommended time frame for patients to attain adequate energy (within seven days), but concludes there is insufficient evidence to make recommendations on how to determine whether enteral or parenteral nutrition is preferred or whether the use of vitamin, minerals, or other supplements is warranted (Bratton et al., 2007).

Nursing interventions to maintain adequate nutrition are considered in the AANN EGB. The *Nursing Management of Adults with Severe Traumatic Brain Injury* guidelines include four main recommendations for adequate nutrition and glycemic control: timing of feeding, feeding tube site, the effect of certain agents on feeding tolerance, and the administration of intensive insulin therapy (Mcilvoy and Meyer, 2008).

Extracts from these guidelines related to nutrition appear in Appendix B, Table B-1. The following are key recommendations pertinent to TBI patients.

Estimating Energy Needs

The ASPEN and ADA EBGs discuss the need to determine energy requirements at the time of initiation of nutritional therapy. Both indicate that predictive equations should be used with caution and that indirect calorimetry is more accurate in determining resting metabolic rate (ADA, 2006; McClave et al., 2009).

There is no clear consensus, however, on the best method to determine energy needs or how frequently they should be adjusted or remeasured. The ADA EBGs evaluated various formulas for estimating resting metabolic rate in the ICU patient population, and concluded that measurement was preferable to estimation formulas. If estimation is needed, the following formulas for nonobese patients are recommended in the following order, based on their accuracy: the Penn State equation (2003a) is the most accurate, with ~79 percent accuracy,[2] followed by Swinamer (55 percent accuracy) and Ireton-Jones, 1992 (52 percent accuracy). An estimation of resting metabolic rate was considered accurate if it was within 10 percent of the measured rate. These estimation formulas are preferred over the more traditional Harris-Benedict formula (ADA, 2006). The recommendations are summarized in Box 2-1. However, it should be noted that these are recommendations for estimating the resting metabolic rate, and although they present a good starting point for determining total energy needs, they are not specific for TBI patients and do not account for injury factors.

Meeting Energy Needs

Enteral Nutrition

The ASPEN and ADA EBGs recommend enteral feeding be started early, within the first 24–48 hours of admission, and advanced toward optimal nutrition goals over the next 48–72 hours (ADA, 2006; McClave et al., 2009). The European Society for Parenteral and Enteral Nutrition also supports early feeding (< 24 hours if patients are hemodynamically stable and have functioning gastrointestinal tracts); however, they note there are no data to document improvement in relevant outcome parameters associated with early enteral feeding (Kreymann et al., 2006). Continuous intragastric feeding and initiating adequate nutrition within 72 hours of injury are recommended by the AANN to improve feeding tolerance and outcomes, respectively (Mcilvoy and Meyer, 2008). The Brain Trauma Foundation guidelines emphasize the need for feeding at least by the end of the first week postinjury, and indicate that feeding prior to seven days improves outcomes (Bratton et al., 2007). By the end of the first week of hospitalization, it is recommended that patients receive greater than 50 to 65 percent of their energy needs in order to achieve the clinical benefit of enteral nutrition.

Parenteral Nutrition

ASPEN supports the concept of permissive mild underfeeding (i.e., the restriction of nutrient intake, specifically in critically ill patients, over a short term) with a recommendation to meet at least 80 percent of energy requirements as the ultimate goal for patients receiving parenteral nutrition (see Appendix B, Recommendation G.2). As the patient stabilizes, parenteral nutrition may be increased to meet energy needs. The ASPEN guideline has different goals for parenteral feeding than for enteral feeding. A separate recommendation (see Appendix B, Recommendation C.2) is made for enteral feeding that specifies a goal of providing from 50 to 65 percent of calories within the first week to achieve clinical benefit (McClave et al., 2009).

---

[2] The 2003a Penn State equation has been updated since the ADA guidelines were published in 2006.

BOX 2-1
Critical Illness Recommendations from the ADA Evidence Analysis Library[a]
Regarding Determining Resting Metabolic Rate (RMR)

Indirect calorimetry to determine RMR
Indirect calorimetry is the standard for determination of RMR in critically ill patients, because RMR based on measurement is more accurate than estimation using predictive equations.
Rating: Strong[b]
Imperative[c]

RMR predictive equations for nonobese patients
If predictive equations are needed in nonobese, critically ill patients, consider using one of the following, as they have the best prediction accuracy[d] of equations studied (listed in order of accuracy): Penn State, 2003a[e] (79%), Swinamer (55%), and Ireton-Jones, 1992 (52%). In some individuals, errors between predicted and actual energy needs will result in under- or over-feeding.
Rating: Fair[f]
Conditional[g]

Inappropriate RMR predictive equations for this population
The Harris-Benedict (with or without activity and stress factors), the Ireton-Jones, 1997 and the Fick equation should not be considered for use in RMR determination in critically ill patients, as these equations do not have adequate prediction accuracy. In addition, the Mifflin-St. Jeor equation should not be considered for use in critically ill patients, because it was developed for healthy people and has not been well researched in the critically ill population.
Rating: Strong
Imperative

RMR predictive equations for obese patients
If predictive equations are needed for critically ill, mechanically ventilated individuals who are obese, consider using Ireton-Jones, 1992 or Penn State, 1998, as they have the best prediction accuracy of equations studied. In some individuals, errors between predicted and actual energy needs will result in under- or over-feeding.
Rating: Fair
Conditional

---

[a]Available online: http://www.adaevidencelibrary.com/template.cfm?key=1309&cms_preview=1 (accessed November 30, 2010).

[b]A **Strong** recommendation means that the workgroup believes that the benefits of the recommended approach clearly exceed the harms (or that the harms clearly exceed the benefits in the case of a strong negative recommendation), and that the quality of the supporting evidence is excellent/good (grade I or II). In some clearly identified circumstances, strong recommendations may be made based on lesser evidence when high-quality evidence is impossible to obtain and the anticipated benefits strongly outweigh the harms. Practitioners should follow a **Strong** recommendation unless a clear and compelling rationale for an alternative approach is present.

[c]Imperative recommendations "require," or "must," or "should achieve certain goals," but do not contain conditional text that would limit their applicability to specified circumstances.

[d]A formula was considered accurate if it predicted resting metabolic rate within +/– 10% of measured resting metabolic rate.

[e]The 2003a Penn State equation has been updated since these 2006 ADA guidelines.

[f]A **Fair** recommendation means that the workgroup believes that the benefits exceed the harms (or that the harms clearly exceed the benefits in the case of a negative recommendation), but the quality of evidence is not as strong (grade II or III). In some clearly identified circumstances, recommendations may be made based on lesser evidence when high-quality evidence is impossible to obtain and the anticipated benefits outweigh the harms. Practitioners should generally follow a **Fair** recommendation but remain alert to new information and be sensitive to patient preferences.

[g]Conditional statements clearly define a specific situation, while imperative statements are broadly applicable to the target population without restraints on their pertinence.

Serum Glucose Control

ASPEN, ADA, and AANN EBGs discuss serum glucose control. ASPEN recommends moderate glucose control, indicating that 110–150 mg/dL may be most appropriate (McClave et al., 2009). AANN supports the intravenous administration of intensive insulin therapy for elevated serum glucose (greater than 110 mg/dL) to improve glycemic control and possibly even reduce intracranial pressure (Mcilvoy and Meyer, 2008). The ADA recommendation is currently under revision.

Antioxidants and Immune-Enhancing Formulas

ASPEN EBGs recommend that immune-modulating enteral formulations (supplemented with agents such as arginine, glutamine, nucleic acid, omega-3 fatty acids, and antioxidants) be used for appropriate patient populations (including major elective surgery and trauma cases) while urging caution in their use for patients with severe sepsis. ADA indicates that in trauma patients, any benefit of immune-enhancing formulas has not been associated with reduced mortality, reduced length of stay, reduced complications from infections, or fewer days on mechanical ventilation (ADA, 2006). ASPEN recommends that a combination of antioxidant vitamins and trace minerals (specifically including selenium) be provided to all critically ill patients receiving specialized nutrition therapy (McClave et al., 2009). Neither ADA nor ASPEN address the specific needs of TBI patients.

EBGS FOR MODERATE OR MILD TBI AND CONCUSSION

DoD's *Updated Mild Traumatic Brain Injury (mTBI) in Non-Deployed Medical Activities* (2008) addresses the assessment of TBI (and classification into acute [injury to 7 days], subacute [8–90 days], and chronic [> 90 days]), visual complaints, balance and hearing, use of imaging, medication management, and specialty referral and duty restrictions. The guideline recommends a multidisciplinary team with some identified specialties, but does not specify a practitioner with nutrition expertise (e.g., a registered dietitian) as a member of that team.

The VA/DoD *Evidence-Based Clinical Practice Guideline for Management of Concussion/Mild Traumatic Brain Injury* (2009) includes a consensus document with definitions, classification and taxonomy, and guidelines and tools for initial presentation including screening and management of symptoms and follow-up of persistent symptoms for individuals with mild TBI. The guidance acknowledges the two previously developed DoD guidelines for management of mild TBI in theater and in nondeployed circumstances. A summary of the nutrition-related content of this guideline is included in Appendix B, Table B-2. Key recommendations are summarized here.

Nutrition-related assessment factors include nausea and vomiting as well as changes in appetite, taste, or smell. DoD guidance for nondeployed settings also mentions the need to assess weight status and, in cases with a body mass index greater than 30, consider referral to polysomnogram (sleep study) to evaluate for sleep apnea.

Nutritional interventions mentioned in DoD guidance include the use of novel therapy (unspecified nutrition supplements). The VA/DoD guideline addresses limiting caffeine, alcohol, and herbal supplements, specifically some "energy" products that may interact with psychiatric medication and lead to hypertensive crisis. The VA/DoD guideline also mentions that nutritional supplements are being explored for potential treatment applications, and should only be included as part of a research protocol with institutional review board oversight.

Although all of the guidelines acknowledged nausea and vomiting as side effects of medications used in treating TBI, none specifically addressed their impact on weight in the longer term or a need for referral for complete nutritional assessment by a registered dietitian.

CONCLUSIONS AND RECOMMENDATIONS

Medical and nutrition care in the field, military treatment facilities, VA medical facilities, and in the home environment after discharge from medical treatment facilities are increasingly guided by EBGs. The TBI-specific EBGs currently available are extremely limited in their discussion of nutrition assessment, nutrition-specific interventions, and nutrition monitoring and evaluation criteria. The generic critical-illness EBGs that may apply do not specifically identify any unique nutritional concerns of TBI patients. There is general agreement among the existing EBGs on the need to determine energy requirements and to meet those needs in acute TBI early in treatment, the preference of use of enteral nutrition over parenteral nutrition when possible (in U.S. guidelines), and the need to maintain serum glucose control. The consensus is less clear on the use of antioxidants and immune-enhancing formulas, the method or frequency of determining energy requirements, and the percentage of energy needs that should be met in acute TBI treatment.

The body of research to support clinical practice guidelines specific to the nutrition care of TBI patients is extremely limited. To aid those preparing such guidelines, specific questions of interest for future research are included in Appendix C, Table B-3. The questions are based on the recommendations of the committee (Chapters 6–16) and have been tabulated in the Population, Intervention, Comparator, Outcome format. The general topics are:

- Identification of specific nutrients, dietary supplements, and food components that promise benefits in providing resilience or treating TBI and for which nutritional status should be assessed in the military population.
- Determination of optimal feeding regimens (e.g., energy needs and sources, route of administration, novel nutrition therapies) at various points (e.g., less than 24 hours, 24 hours to 7 days, post 7 days, chronic home care) within the nutrition care treatment cycle for varying levels of severity of TBI injury.
- Identification of biomarkers and assessment indicators to reflect level of mitochondrial function and inflammatory responses.

RECOMMENDATION 2-1. Evidence-based nutrition guidelines specific for severe TBI should be updated. These guidelines should address unique nutritional concerns of severe TBI when different from generic critical-illness nutrition guidelines (e.g., meeting energy needs and benefits of specific nutrients, food components, or diets). In addition, current guidelines to manage mild and moderate TBI should include recommendations for nutritional interventions. The guidelines should be developed in a collaborative manner with the various key stakeholders (e.g., ADA, VA, DoD).

REFERENCES

ADA (American Dietetic Association). 2006. *Critical illness evidence-based nutrition practice guideline.* American Dietetic Association. http://www.adaevidencelibrary.com/topic.cfm?cat=2799 (accessed October 26, 2010).

ADA. 2010. *ADA method of creating evidence-based nutrition practice guidelines.* American Dietetic Association. http://www.adaevidencelibrary.com/category.cfm?cid=16&cat=0&library=EBG (accessed October 26, 2010).

Bratton, S. L., R. M. Chestnut, J. Ghajar, F. F. McConnell Hammond, O. A. Harris, R. Hartl, G. T. Manley, A. Nemecek, D. W. Newell, G. Rosenthal, J. Schouten, L. Shutter, S. D. Timmons, J. S. Ullman, W. Videtta, J. E. Wilberger, and D. W. Wright. 2007. Guidelines for the management of severe traumatic brain injury. XII. Nutrition. *Journal of Neurotrauma* 24(Suppl 1):S77–S82.

DoD (Department of Defense). 2008. *Updated mild traumatic brain injury (mTBI) clinical guidance in non-deployed medical activities.* http://www.dvbic.org/images/pdfs/Providers/mTBI_recs_for_ CONUS.aspx (accessed January 19, 2011).

Grilli, R., N. Magrini, A. Penna, G. Mura, and A. Liberati. 2000. Practice guidelines developed by specialty societies: The need for a critical appraisal. *Lancet* 355(9198):103–106.

Guyatt, G. 2002. *Users' guide to the medical literature: Essentials of evidence-based clinical practice.* Chicago, IL: American Medical Association.

Guyatt, G. H., R. B. Haynes, R. Z. Jaeschke, D. J. Cook, L. Green, C. D. Naylor, M. C. Wilson, and W. S. Richardson. 2000. Users' guides to the medical literature: XXV. Evidence-based medicine: Principles for applying the users' guides to patient care. *The Journal of the American Medical Association* 284(10):1290–1296.

Hill, G. B., and A. Bradford. 1965. The environment and disease: Association or causation? Presented at the Proceedings of Royal Society of Medicine.

Howick, J., I. Chalmers, P. Glasziou, T. Greenhalgh, C. Henegham, A. Liberati, I. Moschetti, B. Phillips, H. Thornton, O. Goddard, and M. Hodgkinson. 2011. *The Oxford 2011 table of evidence.* Oxford Centre for Evidence-Based Medicine. http://www.cebm.net/index.aspx?o=5653 (accessed January 19, 2011).

Kattelmann, K. K., M. Hise, M. Russell, P. Charney, M. Stokes, and C. Compher. 2006. Preliminary evidence for a medical nutrition therapy protocol: Enteral feedings for critically ill patients. *Journal of the American Dietetic Association* 106(8):1226–1241.

Knuth, T., P. Letarte, G. Ling, L. Moores, P. Rhee, D. Tauber, and A. Trask. 2005. *Guidelines for the field management of combat-related head trauma.* New York: Brain Trauma Foundation.

Kreymann, K. G., M. M. Berger, N. E. P. Deutz, M. Hiesmayr, P. Jolliet, G. Kazandjiev, G. Nitenberg, G. van den Berghe, J. Wernerman, C. Ebner, W. Hartl, C. Heymann, and C. Spies. 2006. ESPEN guidelines on enteral nutrition: Intensive care. *Clinical Nutrition* 25(2):210–223.

McClave, S. A., R. G. Martindale, V. W. Vanek, M. McCarthy, P. Roberts, B. Taylor, J. B. Ochoa, L. Napolitano, and G. Cresci. 2009. Guidelines for the provision and assessment of nutrition support therapy in the adult critically ill patient: Society of Critical Care Medicine (SCCM) and American Society for Parenteral and Enteral Nutrition (ASPEN). *Journal of Parenteral and Enteral Nutrition* 33(3):277–316.

Mcilvoy, L., and K. Meyer. 2008. *Nursing management of adults with severe traumatic brain injury.* Glenview, IL: American Association of Neuroscience Nurses.

Sackett, D. L., W. M. Rosenberg, J. A. Gray, R. B. Haynes, and W. S. Richardson. 1996. Evidence based medicine: What it is and what it isn't. *British Medical Journal* 312(7023):71–72.

Thomas, L., N. Cullum, E. McColl, N. Rousseau, J. Soutter, and N. Steen. 1999. Guidelines in professions allied to medicine. *Cochrane Database of Systematic Reviews* Issue 1. Art No.:CD000349.

VA/DoD (Department of Veterans Affairs and Department of Defense). 2009. *VA/DoD clinical practice guideline for management of concussion/mild traumatic brain injury.* http://www.healthquality.va.gov/mtbi/concussion_mtbi_full_1_0.pdf (accessed January 19, 2011).

3

Understanding Pathophysiological Changes

Traumatic brain injury (TBI) is characterized by both the primary damage resulting from physical disruption of neural and vascular structures and the early emergence of secondary pathogenic events, which collectively contribute to neurologic deficits (Andriessen et al., 2010; Dash et al., 2010; Marklund et al., 2006). The identification of nutrients, dietary supplements, or specific diets that may provide resilience or treat TBI requires an understanding of the key pathophysiological events that govern both injury and reparative processes. A detailed description of those events for the various types of TBI can be found in the published literature and will not be repeated in this document. The reader is referred to recent reviews addressing the pathophysiology of focal and diffuse TBI including diffuse axonal injury, a common consequence of TBI (Andriessen et al., 2010; Farkas and Povlishock, 2007); moderate, severe, and penetrating TBI (Dash et al., 2010; Maas et al., 2008); blast TBI (Cernak and Noble-Haeusslein, 2010; Desmoulin and Dionne, 2009; Elder and Cristian, 2009; Hicks et al., 2010; Ling et al., 2009; Taber et al., 2006); and mild or concussion TBI, including recurrent injuries (Dash et al., 2010; Elder and Cristian, 2009; Mazzeo et al., 2009; McKee et al., 2009b; Weber, 2007). As background for the report, this chapter includes a brief review of the literature on the pathophysiological changes that accompany TBI. The sequence of events following TBI has been the subject of different classifications. The committee relies on a recent working definition that describes the onset of secondary pathogenic processes after TBI (Margulies et al., 2009). This chapter will refer to primary or acute effects as those effects that begin within the first minutes after injury, secondary or subacute effects as those that arise over the next 24 hours after injury, and long-term or chronic effects as those that are associated with the insult but occur at a later time. The committee recognizes that, as Margulies and colleagues (2009) observe, these definitions are estimates of the emergence of pathogenic events whose duration is likely to be variable and possibly overlapping. Both the cascade of secondary effects and the long-term effects are consequences of the primary insult and are susceptible to interventions to improve resilience or to treat TBI. The chapter also includes a brief review of the animal models and biomarkers used for TBI. Although the information in this chapter is provided as background to this report, the committee acknowledges the importance of developing good animal models and identifying biomarkers of the disease progression and outcomes, and therefore recommendations are made for improving these areas of research.

EXPERIMENTAL MODELS OF TBI

Much of our understanding of the pathobiology of TBI has arisen from animal models that mimic features of human TBI. There are a number of detailed reviews of models of TBI (Artinian et al., 2006; Morales et al., 2005; O'Connor et al., 2005). Some examples of in vivo models are presented in Figure 3-1. The general objective of these models is to replicate certain aspects of human brain injury. It is important to note that there is currently no single model that can accurately reflect the heterogeneity of human TBI, and in each of these models, pathologic and neurologic outcomes vary according to the severity and location of the insult and heterogeneity of the vasculature. Also, there are no good animal models for mild or repetitive TBI.

Here the committee briefly reviews several of the most commonly used animal models of TBI (Morales et al., 2005): the weight-drop model, the controlled cortical impact model, the fluid percussion model, and the impact acceleration model (Figure 3-2). Each of these models produces motor/sensory and cognitive impairments. The weight-drop, midline fluid percussion, and controlled cortical impact models produce focal contusions and, depending on injury severity, may be associated with subarachnoid and intraparenchymal hemorrhages,

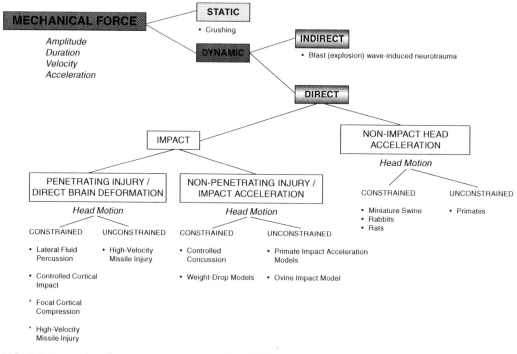

FIGURE 3-1   Classification of in vivo models of TBI.
SOURCE: Cernak, 2005.

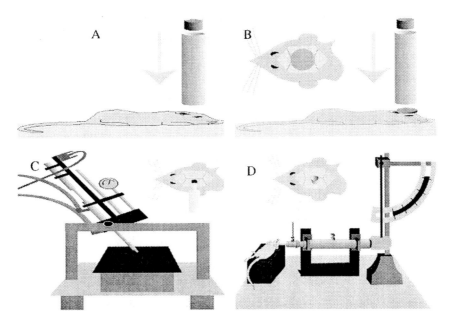

FIGURE 3-2 Rodent models of TBI: (A) weight-drop model, (B) impact acceleration model, (C) controlled cortical impact model, and (D) fluid percussion model.
SOURCE: Morales et al., 2005.

disruption of the blood-brain barrier (BBB), cortical and subcortical cell loss, and diffuse axonal injury. The weight-drop model relies on a free-falling, guided weight that strikes the exposed skull or the dura; the head may be either restrained or unrestrained. The midline fluid percussion injury model entails delivery of a brief pulse of fluid to the intact dura. The skull is exposed and after a craniectomy to expose the dura, an injury is produced by delivery of a fluid bolus, resulting from the release of a pendulum. The controlled cortical impact model utilizes a rigid impactor, controlled by pressurized air, to strike the exposed dura.

The impact acceleration model is characterized by a more diffuse injury that includes hemorrhage (typically intraparenchymal as well as subarachnoid); disruption of the BBB; cortical and subcortical damage; and widespread axonal swelling, damage, or both. This model uses a weight-drop strategy. However, a plate is secured to the skull to distribute the weight and minimize skull fractures. The head is unrestrained and positioned on a cushion with specified properties that allow a defined movement of the head after impact. Finally, it is noteworthy that a modification to the fluid percussion injury, with the insult shifted from midline to a more lateral position, results in both focal and diffuse brain injury.

Models of blast-induced brain injury, developed and characterized in both large and small animals, were reviewed by Cernak and Noble-Haeusslein in 2010. In brief, shock waves are produced by either shock tubes using compressed air or gas, or blast tubes that rely on explosive charges. There is increasing evidence that these models share pathologic and biochemical characteristics seen in the more traditional models of focal and diffuse TBI, including hemorrhage, diffuse axonal injury, cortical and subcortical cell injury, metabolic disturbances/energy failure, inflammation, and oxidative stress. What remains controversial is the extent to which blast-induced brain injuries have unique temporal and spatial profiles of pathogenic events that would distinguish them from other types of TBIs.

MODERATE, SEVERE, AND PENETRATING TBI

As discussed by the National Institutes of Health (NIH) in 2002, while concussion is the most minor and common type of TBI, more severe types of TBI have been described (Chapter 1) as moderate, severe, and penetrating. Moderate, severe, and penetrating TBI will be considered together as one specific type of TBI for the purpose of presenting mechanisms; however, it is important to note that every case will present unique characteristics due to the nature of the insult itself, the location of the injury in the brain, and the individual. Such heterogeneity is a likely determinant of outcome and is considered a major barrier to developing or optimizing therapeutics for the brain-injured patient (Saatman et al., 2008).

This section draws from the 2009 Institute of Medicine (IOM) report *Gulf War and Health: Volume 7: Long-Term Consequences of Traumatic Brain Injury*, which describes the biology of TBI based on animal models and brain-injured patients and from other reviews (Cederberg and Siesjo, 2010; Margulies et al., 2009; Morganti-Kossmann et al., 2007, 2010; Unterberg et al., 2004; Werner and Engelhard, 2007; Ziebell and Morganti-Kossmann, 2010). A schematic hypothesis of the series of events resulting from injury is shown in Figure 3-3. These events will be presented as primary and secondary, depending on the time of appearance. [This background does not present long-term events because they are not included in the statement of task for this study.] Repair and recovery mechanisms that have also been identified as potential targets for interventions are briefly described as well. Finally, the existence of endogenous neuroprotective factors provides another mechanism to influence the health outcomes of TBI, and it is also included here.

Primary or Acute Effects

Primary (i.e., acute) effects are those that occur during the first minutes after the injury (Table 3-1). The primary effects are the result of mechanical damage that includes stretching and/or rupture of cellular membranes, release of intracellular and vascular contents, and alterations of cerebral blood flow and metabolism. Axons may be severely compromised, as evidenced by perturbations in axonal transport, cytoskeletal damage, swelling, and disconnection (Povlishock and Katz, 2005; Smith et al., 2003). Injury to the head often results in damage to the vascular system that can, depending on the extent of the damage, result in serious complications. For example, hemorrhage and intravascular coagulation can develop, potentially leading to hemorrhagic or ischemic stroke. Studies in animals and humans have revealed that focal or global ischemia frequently occurs both early after the injury and in late stages, and suggest that ischemic stroke and TBI share similar mechanisms. Morphological injury, hypotension, inadequate availability of nitric oxide or cholinergic neurotransmitters, and potentiation of prostaglandin-induced vasoconstriction are all mechanisms that result in ischemia.

TBI patients might experience hypoperfusion or hyperfusion; each represents a mismatch between cerebral blood flow and metabolism, and both are pathological conditions with detrimental outcomes. For example, cerebral blood flow that exceeds the metabolic requirement would result in increased cerebral blood volume and intracranial pressure. Intracranial pressure also occurs as a result of swelling of tissues and fluid accumulation. Depending on the injury, metabolic failure also occurs, leading to mitochondrial dysfunction (i.e., reduced respiratory rates and production of adenosine 5′-triphosphate [ATP] and calcium overload) (see also Sullivan in Appendix C). The ischemia pattern and impaired regulation of aerobic metabolism result in greater reliance upon anaerobic metabolism of glucose that in turn results in an accumulation of lactic acid from the accelerated anaerobic

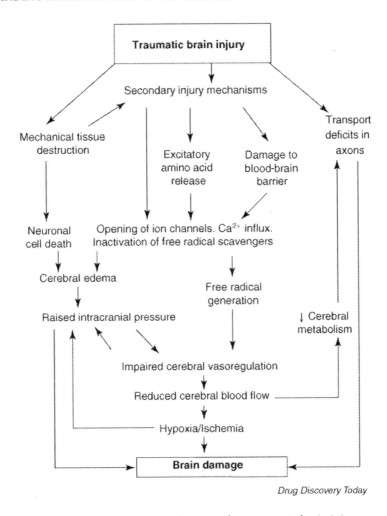

FIGURE 3-3 Cascade of pathophysiological events after traumatic brain injury.
SOURCE: Jain, 2008.

glycolysis. Hypermetabolism and anaerobic glycolysis from glucose occur in an attempt to meet energy needs.

One major event that happens early after insult is the massive ionic influx referred to as traumatic depolarization. Anaerobic glycolysis is inadequate to maintain energy states of the transient transmembrane ionic fluxes and neuroexcitation, and the consequent depletion of ATP results in alterations of ion pumps (i.e., efflux of potassium and influx of sodium and calcium) and the release of neurotransmitters. The release of neurotransmitters, specifically glutamate, into the extracellular compartment results in an overstimulation of glutamate receptors linked to ion channels and creates prolonged membrane depolarization, depletion of ATP stores, and an increase in intracellular calcium derived from both extracellular and intracellular stores, indicating disturbances in mitochondrial function. (For a discussion of the timing of the cascade typically seen in experimental brain injury models and the consequences of the early, high glycolytic rate resulting in ionic pump disturbance, the reader

TABLE 3-1   Initiation of Acute Secondary Events Post-TBI

Within Minutes	Minutes–24 Hours	24–72 Hours
Cell/axon stretching, compaction of neurofilaments, impaired axonal transport, axonal swelling, axonal disconnection	Oxidative damage: increased reactive oxygen and nitrogen species (lipid peroxidation, protein oxidation, peroxynitrite), reduction in endogenous antioxidants (e.g., glutathione)	Nonischemic metabolic failure
Disruption of the blood-brain barrier	Ischemia	
Excessive neuronal activity: glutamate release	Edema: cytotoxic vasogenic	
Widespread changes in neurotransmitters: catecholamines, serotonin, histamine, GABA, acetylcholine	Enzymatic activation: kallikrein-kinins, calpains, caspases, endonucleases, metalloproteinases	
Hemorrhage (heme, iron-mediated, toxicity)	Decreased ATP: changes in brain metabolism (altered glucose utilization and switch to alternative fuels), elevated lactate	
Physiologic disturbances: decreased cerebral blood flow, hypotension, hypoxemia, increased cranial pressure, decreased cerebral perfusion pressure	Cytoskeletal changes in cell somas and axons	
Increased free radical production	Widespread changes in gene expression: cell cycle, metabolism, inflammation, receptors, channels and transporters, signal transduction, cytoskeleton, membrane proteins involved in transcription/translation	
Disruption of calcium homeostasis	Inflammation: Cytokines, chemokines, cell adhesion molecules, influx of leukocytes, activation of resident macrophages	
Mitochondrial disturbances		

SOURCE: Margulies and Hicks, 2009.

is referred to Hovda et al., 1995.) A series of proteases becomes activated by the increase in calcium, resulting in cytoskeletal damage and further BBB breakdown, cell injury, and generation of free radicals. In this sense, a decrease in glutamate transporters in glial cells is also thought to be responsible for the significant increase in glutamate levels early after TBI.

Although there may be direct damage to axons from shear and tensile forces, it is now the prevalent opinion that damage to axons occurs mostly via deformation and changes in permeability that permit the influx of calcium and the opening of calcium channels. This increase in intracellular calcium induces proteolysis by calcium-dependent proteases; calcium may also enter and damage the mitochondria and disrupt ionic homeostasis, leading to more proteolysis and swelling, impaired axonal transport, and disconnection.

After head injury, electroencephalogram recordings show early signs of dysfunction. There is a significant risk of developing recurrent seizures that can start as early as within a week of injury, or as late as years afterward. The hippocampus is particularly vulnerable to TBI, as evidenced in part by immediate mechanically induced damage to interneurons in the dentate granule cell layer of the hippocampus that are remote from the site of insult (Gallyas and Zoltay, 1992; Toth et al., 1997). These morphologic findings correlate with an early selective depolarization of the resting membrane potentiation, attributed to a decrease in the activity of the electrogenic Na$^+$/K$^+$-ATPase, that results in an enhancement of the efficacy of excitatory inputs to these interneurons (Ross and Soltesz, 2000).

Secondary or Subacute Effects

Secondary (i.e., subacute) effects are defined as those experienced up to 24 hours after injury (Table 3-1). There are multiple sources of reactive oxygen and nitrogen species, as mentioned in the process described in the preceding paragraphs. The formation of free radicals is augmented by their own reactivity as lipid, protein, and DNA (deoxyribonucleic acid) oxidation continues. The brain is especially vulnerable to oxidative damage, in part because of its high rate of oxidative activity and relatively low antioxidant capacity. In the setting of TBI, the oxidative cascade overwhelms endogenous antioxidants (e.g., superoxide dismutase and catalase) and low-molecular antioxidants (e.g., glutathione and melatonin, tocopherol, and ascorbic acid), resulting in cell injury and death.

Ischemia may occur at this stage of the injury, leading to further accumulation of lactic acid, depletion of ATP, alteration of membrane function, and release of neurotransmitters. The depolarization of membranes in smooth muscle, release of endothelin and reduced nitric oxide, vasoconstriction, and formation of free radicals may lead to cerebral vasospasm, a condition that determines the outcome of the patient.

The immune response to TBI may promote both pathogenesis and recovery processes; the precise mechanisms underlying the duality of inflammation are not yet clearly defined. The BBB is compromised early after TBI, resulting in the emergence of vasogenic edema and an influx of circulating leukocytes including neutrophils, monocytes, and lymphocytes (Ziebell and Morganti-Kossmann, 2010). These leukocytes release inflammatory mediators such as prostaglandins, free radicals, complement factors, and cytokines, which in turn further support the travel of leukocytes into the brain and mobilize glia to the injury site (Morganti-Kossmann et al., 2007). Cytokines generated in response to TBI likely have multiple roles that may support tissue damage as well as repair mechanisms. For example, interleukin-1, which triggers cell activation by binding to specific membrane receptors, plays a key role in initiating an inflammatory cascade, but interleukin-10, produced by microglia and astrocytes and lymphopoietic cells, appears to play a neuroprotective role by producing anti-inflammatory cytokines. Opposing roles may even be seen in the same cytokine. For example, whether the cytokine tumor necrosis factor, which is released early after injury, will function as a neuroprotectant or neurotoxin seems to be related to concentration and the timing of release. Vasoactive inflammatory molecules promote vascular dilation and trigger vasogenic edema, resulting in decreased oxygen and failure of metabolism. Further damage from inflammation comes directly from the triggering of death receptors leading to apoptotic death, and direct cell death by nitrogen oxide. From a prophylactic point of view, the increased permeability of the BBB during injury presents an opportunity for beneficial nutrients to reach the injury site. Reviews that identify inflammation as a target for interventions conclude that novel treatments should aim at minimizing the secondary injury by modifying the inflammatory response, rather than completely eliminating it.

The cascade of events described (activation of proteases, generation of free radicals, and inflammation) after TBI results in cytoskeletal damage, death of glia and neurons, and white matter degeneration. The two types of cell death that have been most studied are necrosis (due to mechanical or hypoxic tissue damage) and apoptosis (programmed cell death). Necrosis appears within hours to days after injury and is characterized by neurons that initially appear swollen, and over time assume a shrunken eosinophilic phenotype with pyknotic nuclei (Raghupathi, 2004). In contrast to necrosis, cells that die via apoptosis show membrane disintegration, chromatin condensation, and DNA fragmentation. Recent discoveries suggest a less obvious distinction between necrosis and apoptosis, with dying cells showing structural changes that are common to both necrosis and apoptosis (Raghupathi, 2004). Such findings have led to the definition of cell death evolving to reflect a continuum between necrosis and apoptosis. Experimentally, the time course may show a biphasic pattern with peak periods of death occurring at 24 hours and one week after injury (Conti et al., 1998). Activation and deactivation of caspases are important mediators of programmed cell death. It is also believed that the delayed occurrence of cell death may offer opportunity for interventions.

Other important effects of this secondary phase are both vasogenic and cytotoxic brain edema (Unterberg et al., 2004). Vasogenic edema arises from disruption of the BBB and the concurrent ion and plasma protein transfer to the extracellular matrix, and results in accumulation of extracellular water. Cytotoxic edema reflects the intracellular accumulation of water. Cytotoxic edema is partly associated with the early release of glutamate and accumulation of ions and osmotically active solutes, and with failure of the active ion pumps in the neurons and glia. The ion pump system of the membrane cannot compensate for the increase in sodium uptake. This failure of the ion pump to maintain homeostasis and the associated cytotoxic edema is aggravated by mitochondrial structural and functional impairment. Importantly in the setting of TBI, a marked increase in net water content of the brain leads to an increase in tissue volume. With limited ability to expand due to the confines of the intracranial compartment, there is an increase in intracranial pressure and a reduction in perfusion and oxygenation, giving rise to additional ischemic damage.

BIOMARKERS OF INJURY AND OUTCOMES

Excellent reviews on biomarkers for TBI appeared in 2009 and 2010 (Dash et al., 2010; Svetlov et al., 2009). These included consideration of TBI biomarkers, inflammatory biomarkers, small-molecule biomarkers, lipid metabolite biomarkers, and biomarkers for mild and penetrating TBIs, secondary pathologies, predicting outcome, and polytrauma (Dash et al., 2010). Dash et al. (2010) provides a complete listing of these biomarkers, including their diagnostic value. Table 3-2 summarizes those biomarkers of greatest interest in the scientific community (Svetlov et al., 2009): S-100B, neuron-specific enolase, glial fibrillary acidic protein, and myelin basic protein. Cellular localization as well as strengths and limitations for each of these candidate markers are summarized in Table 3-2.

There is also an emerging interest in brain-type fatty acid–binding proteins, phosphorylated neurofilament H and ubiquitin C-terminal hydrolase, and proteolytic breakdown products of cell proteins such as alpha-II spectrin and the microtubule-binding protein tau (Dash et al., 2010). These candidates show general promise in terms of specificity and, in some cases, sensitivity. There is additional ongoing research to address pro- and anti-inflammatory biomarkers and lipid metabolites such as F2-isoprostane and 4-hydroxynonenol (Dash et al., 2010). Although the newest imaging may suggest brain damage after mild traumatic brain injury (mTBI) (Mayer et al., 2010), the committee concluded that there is not enough data yet to demonstrate that the results of imaging can be used as accurate markers of outcome.

Researchers are also interested in blast injury biomarkers in an animal model. Recent studies modeling blast injury show that glial fibrillary acidic protein (GFAP) and neuron-specific enolase (NSE) are increased in blood within the first 48 hours after blast injury. Ubiquitin C-terminal hydrolase-L1 (UCH-L1) shows a similar early increase in blood, and is also detected in cerebrospinal fluid (CSF) throughout 14 days after injury (Svetlov et al.,

TABLE 3-2 Examples of Biomarkers for TBI

Biomarker	Description	Localization	Strengths	Limitations
S-100B	Calcium binding protein. Serum half-life is < 60 minutes.	Astrocytes, Schwann cells, adipocytes, chondrocytes, melanocytes	Readily detected early after injury. Correlated to injury magnitude and outcome.	May be insensitive to mild TBI. Poor correlation between serum and brain levels suggesting that barrier integrity is a determinant of serum levels. Increases after extracranial trauma.
Neuron-specific enolase	Isozyme of enolase. Serum half-life is 24 hours; can be detected within 6 hrs after TBI	Neuronal cytoplasm, platelets, erythrocytes	Serum levels thought to be sensitive indicator of mortality and outcomes.	Possible cross-contamination with blood. May not correlate with injury severity. Limited sensitivity. Systemic increase can occur with trauma in the absence of TBI.
Glial fibrillary acidic protein	Intermediate filament protein	Astrocytes	Specific for brain. Not affected by extra-cranial trauma. Serum levels predictive of mortality, increased intracraneal pressure, and poor Glacow outcome scores.	Not studied in mild or moderate TBI.
Myelin basic protein	Major constituent of myelin	Myelin	Marker of axonal damage—released into serum and CSF after white-matter injury. Specificity in both CSF and serum. May be predictive of outcome.	Limited sensitivity.

2010). Other strategies are being developed to define biomarkers for blast-induced brain injury. Among them is blastomics, an approach involving delineation of a functional interaction map of proteins that are affected by a blast-wave exposure (Svetlov et al., 2009).

While the list of putative biomarkers continues to expand, it is becoming increasingly clear that there may be no single biomarker that can adequately meet the requirements of specificity and sensitivity, and that multiple biomarkers, in conjunction with clinical data, may offer better predictability (Dash et al., 2010). There are new approaches being applied, such as trajectory analysis that takes into account temporal changes in multiple biomarkers (Berger et al., 2010).

ENDOGENOUS NEUROPROTECTIVE TARGETS

The brain produces endogenous substances that protect against insults or neurodegenerative diseases (Leker and Shohami, 2002). Enhancing their activity or increasing their levels is another target for interventions that is already under investigation. Compounds that serve as antioxidants, such as enzymes (e.g., Cu/Zn-superoxide dismutase [SOD], extracellular SOD, Mn-SOD, glutathione peroxidase, catalase) and low-molecular-weight antioxidants (e.g., uric acid and ascorbate), are induced early after ischemia and trauma. Heat shock proteins (i.e., HSP-70, HSP-90, GRP-78, HSP-27) are also induced after ischemia; they mainly prevent protein denaturation. Many growth factors (e.g., bFGF, NGF, BDNF,

TABLE 3-3   Biological Role of Neurotrophins in Axonal Guidance and Nerve Regeneration

Neurotrophins	Action
Nerve Growth Factor (NGF)	Stimulates nerve regeneration Axonal guidance molecule
Neurotrophin-3 (NT-3)	Stimulates neurite outgrowth Stimulates nerve regeneration Axonal guidance molecule Growth cone collapse
Neurotrophin-4/5 (NT-4/5)	Stimulates nerve regeneration
Brain-derived Neurotrophic Factor (BDNF)	Essential condition for nerve regeneration Stimulates nerve generation

SOURCE: Lykissas et al., 2007.

NT-4, TGF-B, GDNF; Table 3-3) and their receptors have been implicated in the repair and recovery phase of injury. However, many questions remain about their control and modulation of repair, and it appears that their effects depend on many determinants, including timing, levels, specific binding to receptors, and interaction with other factors. As mentioned above, inflammatory processes also contribute to resolution of inflammation, and cytokines have been identified that could be targeted as interventions to enhance the reparative processes. One cytokine that has received much attention is erythropoietin, which regulates hematopoiesis as a growth factor and inhibits apoptotic cell death. It is induced in cultured neurons and astrocytes under hypoxic and ischemic conditions, and it has been shown to have neuroprotective properties in various animal models of brain injury. Sex hormones (i.e., estrogen and progesterone) protect the brain from ischemia via both vascular and neuronal mechanisms. In the setting of TBI, progesterone has received more attention. Progesterone functions as a pleiotropic drug; it reduces edema, excitotoxicity, lipid peroxidation, and ischemia, and increases prosurvival growth factors and improves mitochondrial function (Cekic and Stein, 2010). It is currently being investigated in a phase III, multi-center, double-blind, randomized clinical trial for TBI (Cekic and Stein, 2010). Hypoxia-inducible factor 1 is a key regulator in hypoxia and is thought to be an important player in neurological outcomes following ischemic stroke. It regulates the functions of downstream genes that are involved in promoting glucose metabolism, angiogenesis, erythropoiesis, and cell survival. Its effects on neuronal tissue injuries, based on evidence from in vitro and preclinical studies, are still debatable. Understanding the fundamental mode of action and modulation of these potential endogenous neuroprotectants will provide a more complete picture of the pathophysiology of TBI, together with more opportunities for effective therapies, including nutritional therapies.

REPAIR AND RECOVERY MECHANISMS

This section draws from a 2007 review of the topic by Lykissas and colleagues. As a result of the processes described above, repair and recovery mechanisms are initiated concomitantly with the resolution of inflammation and edema. Although much of the information in this section comes from research in the areas of stroke and spinal cord injury, the processes described are also relevant for head injury. Processes that belong to the category of repair and recovery are revascularization of the surviving area (angiogenesis), cell genesis (glio-

and neurogenesis), axonal plasticity, and changes in the neuronal network (synaptogenesis). From a temporal perspective, these mechanisms fall into three consecutive phases: recovery of function and cell repair, axonal growth, and consolidation of new neural networks. Like the events leading to death and damage, repair and recovery processes are amenable to interventions that facilitate them and that might improve functional outcomes beyond what the normal repair mechanisms could achieve. Angiogenesis is prominent after brain injury, and it has a crucial role in supporting wound healing. Among several angiogenesis factors, vascular endothelial growth factor (VEGF) has been the most thoroughly studied. In recent reviews (Greenberg and Jin, 2005; Rosenstein et al., 2010), the authors highlight the neuroprotective role of VEGF and the detrimental effects (e.g., in motor function) of reduced levels of VEGF in animal models. VEGF has been shown to be neuroprotective after experimental TBI models (Thau-Zuchman et al., 2010). Altogether, it appears that VEGF might have two roles in neuroprotection: as a direct neurotrophic agent and as an angiogenic factor stimulating endothelial cells to provide adequate perfusion and neurotrophic factors (Rosenstein et al., 2010).

Neurogenesis, arising within the subventricular zone (SVZ) and the subgranular zone of the dentate gyrus, has led to the speculation that neurons recruited from these regions may contribute to some functional recovery after brain injury. For example, cerebral ischemia and seizures stimulate neurogenesis and the migration of neurons toward the affected zone. TBI induces hippocampal cell proliferation, with many of these cells differentiating into neurons that sometimes extend axonal projections and glia. As in cerebral ischemia, cortical injuries also result in the migration of new cells, generated in the SVZ, to areas of tissue damage. Of particular interest are treatments to enhance neurogenesis to promote cognitive recovery after TBI (Kernie and Parent, 2010).

Neurotrophic factors also may modulate recovery processes. Neutrophins constitute a family of neurotrophic factors (other families include neuropoietic cytokines, including interleukin-6; fibroblast growth factors; transforming growth factors; and insulin-like growth factors) that regulate neuronal survival, growth, and synaptic plasticity and neurotransmission both in the central and peripheral nervous system. They may act in other target organs, in nearby cells, or in the same cell. A discussion of the identification, functions, and interactions of the neurotrophins is beyond the scope of this study, and the reader is referred to existing reviews (Hagg, 2009; Lykissas et al., 2007). Table 3-3 lists examples of neurotrophins with roles in axonal guidance and nerve regeneration. Neurotrophins perform their functions by binding to two different types of receptors, tyrosine kinase receptors and neurotrophic receptor 75. Nerve growth factor (NGF), brain-derived neurotrophic factor (BDNF), and neurotrophin 3 (NT-3) are perhaps the most studied neurotrophic factors in the context of axonal growth. Of these, the role of BDNF has generated interest among nutritionists because it has been suggested that some food components (e.g., docosahexaenoic acid and curcumin) may act as neuroprotectants by affecting the levels of this neurotrophin in the brain (Wu et al., 2004; see also Gomez-Pinilla in Appendix C).

Although in vitro studies of the injured peripheral nerve suggest a role in neuronal regeneration, neurotrophins—BDNF and N/T-4/5 in particular—have the ability to bind both growth-promoting and growth-inhibiting receptors. In vitro experiments also suggest that the timing of the signaling, the level, and the type of neurotrophin are key variables in nerve regeneration. Importantly, in vitro assays may not accurately predict the behavior of these growth factors in the central nervous system, particularly in the complex environment of the injured brain.

MILD TRAUMATIC BRAIN INJURY

The term mild traumatic brain injury (mTBI) is interchangeable with concussion. Mild TBI as defined by the Veterans Affairs/Department of Defense Clinical Practice Guidelines, is classified as structural or physiological disruption of brain function resulting from an external traumatic force. Presentation includes loss of consciousness for < 30 minutes, alteration of mental state for < 24 hours, posttraumatic amnesia for < 1 day, and a Glasgow Coma Score of 13–15 (Maruta et al., 2010). Postconcussion syndrome, which may follow mTBI, is characterized by experiencing numerous cognitive, affective, or somatic symptoms (Table 3-4) for longer than three months, and can lead to chronic disability. Recent data from the military suggest that about five percent of all the mild TBI cases suffer from postconcussion syndrome, which still represents a high number of cases (Ling, 2010).

Mild TBI is difficult to model because the insults, whether produced by fluid percussion, cortical impact, or focal brain contusions, often generate focal damage, diffuse axonal damage, cell loss, and varying degrees of hemorrhage. Nevertheless, there has been a growing effort to refine these models to better approximate the mTBI seen in a clinical setting. Several examples, listed in Table 3-5, demonstrate that although only relatively modest changes are seen in the histopathology, brain-injured animals show cognitive deficits. Of interest, despite negative findings by magnetic resonance imaging (MRI), patterns of neuronal cell loss are apparent by subsequent histological analysis (Henninger et al., 2005). Finally, it is noteworthy that following mTBI, the cortex presents with very early alterations in mitochondrial bioenergetics (Gilmer et al., 2009). Early initiation of strategies to support mitochondrial function may therefore limit the subsequent progression of secondary pathogenesis.

A common feature of TBI is diffuse axonal injury (DAI) (Maruta et al., 2010), which is characterized by a focal alteration of the axolemma, leading to an impairment in axonal transport and the appearance of a local swelling that then detaches from its distal segment (Povlishock and Katz, 2005). The latter culminates in disconnection from its downstream segment. DAI may be an accompanying feature of mTBI (Maruta et al, 2010). Because structural features of DAI are difficult to detect by traditional computed tomography (CT) or magnetic resonance imaging (MRI) scans (Maruta et al, 2010), mTBI is not easily diagnosed in the acute stage, and in fact may go unnoticed until the emergence of postconcussion symptoms (Maruta et al, 2010). Nevertheless, recent advances in neuroimaging using high resolution MRI and diffusion tensor imaging have made it possible to identify axonal damage in the brain after an mTBI (Barkhoudarian et al., 2011). Such advances offer the opportunity to better understand the vulnerability of the brain to a mild insult, and to determine the extent to which indices of damage correlate with measures of functional outcomes.

TABLE 3-4 Symptoms of Postconcussion Syndrome

Cognitive	Somatic	Affective
Memory difficulties	Headache	Irritability
Decreased concentration	Dizziness	Depression
Decreased processing speed	Nausea	Anxiety
	Fatigue	
	Sleep disturbances	
	Blurred vision	
	Tinnitus	
	Hypersensitivity to light/noise	

SOURCE: Maruta et al., 2010.

TABLE 3-5   Animal Models of Mild TBI

Model	Pathologic Findings	Behavioral Findings	Molecular/Biochemical Findings	Reference
Cortical impact (rat)	Neuronal vulnerability in the hippocampus	Deficits in performance on Morris water maze	Involvement of sulfonylurea receptor 1 in hippocampal cell injury	Patel et al., 2010
Fluid percussion injury (rat)		Deficits in performance on Morris water maze	Protein oxidation (elevated protein carbonyls and reduced levels of SOD and Sir2) Reduced levels of BDNF, synapsin I, CREB, CaMKII	Wu et al., 2010
Cortical contusion (rat)			Alterations in mitochondrial respiration	Gilmer et al., 2009
Weight-drop (rat)	Serial MRI: no abnormalities in the cerebrum. Histology: loss of neurons in the frontal cortex and hippocampus, but preserved cytoskeletal architecture	Brief loss of consciousness, extended loss of the corneal and righting reflexes; deficits in performance on Morris water maze		Henninger et al., 2005

RECURRENT MILD HEAD INJURIES/CONCUSSIONS

There is a substantial body of literature to support recognition of second impact syndrome, which results when a mild head injury is followed shortly thereafter by a second one. Such a situation has marked clinical ramifications, including possible death. This has been documented most recently in the sphere of competitive contact sports, where determining the resting time needed before an injured athlete (e.g., a football player) can return to play has been the focus of much debate. Like competitive athletes, military personnel are also subject to recurrent concussions. If these are mild concussions (see definitions in Chapter 1), they may go unrecognized. As part of an effort to manage episodes of recurrent mild TBI, the U.S. military (the Department of Defense [DoD] and Department of Veterans Affairs [VA]) convened an expert committee in 2008 to develop evidence-based guidelines for the management of concussion/mild TBI; the product was the first system-wide codified approach to mTBI (Ling, 2010). DoD's *Policy Guidance for Management of Concussion/ Mild Traumatic Brain Injury in the Deployed Setting* was updated in June 2010, and the 2008 Zurich Consensus Statement on Concussion in Sports (McCrory et al., 2009) has been adapted to determine when a soldier can return to duty, based on a functional assessment of the individual. Among military personnel, there is no epidemiological data available on the incidence of recurrent head injury (Ling, 2010).

Second impact syndrome is a rare complication associated mostly with contact sports but also with active duty military service. There is often no loss of consciousness, but suffering a second concussion before complete recovery from the first can cause cerebral edema and death. It has been suggested that the effect of recurrent mild concussions is synergistic instead of additive. Based on a handful of case reports that involved a second injury within days of the primary event, it is hypothesized that second impact syndrome results from a loss of autoregulation of cerebral blood flow and a resultant vascular engorgement. These authors (Mori et al., 2006) have also postulated that acceleration forces, substantial enough to produce a small acute subdural hematoma in many cases, are the cause of second impact syndrome and hyperemic swelling.

Repetitive mild TBIs have been studied in vitro and in vivo using weight-drop and controlled cortical impact injuries to either the rodent skull or to the dural surface (see Table 3-6 for examples). In vitro studies, such as those that produce a stretch-induced model of injury to murine hippocampal cells, demonstrate that repeated insults produce more pronounced damage to both neurons and glia than single insults (Slemmer and Weber, 2005; Slemmer et al., 2002). Although in vivo findings vary depending on the experimental design, there are also some common characteristics. In general, a single mild injury may show either no or only a modest behavioral phenotype in terms of cognitive or motor sensory impairments, whereas repeated injuries produce a more robust adverse behavioral phenotype. An exception to this is one report that mild repetitive injuries may have a conditioning effect on the brain, with a subsequent severe injury producing no or modest effects on motor control loss when compared to severe injury alone (Allen et al., 2000). Histologic evidence of cell injury or loss and BBB dysfunction after repeated mild injuries is variable, and may reflect differences in the experimental design. There is some evidence for a temporal window of

TABLE 3-6 Examples of Experimental Models of Repetitive TBI

Experimental Model	Experimental Design	Species/Strain/Age/Sex	General Findings
Concussion weight-drop (closed head injury) (DeFord et al., 2002)	1 or 4 mild injuries each separated by 24 hours. Various weight-drop distances (40 and 60 cm) and masses (50, 100, and 150 g) were studied.	Mice/B6C3/9 weeks old/male	No overt cell death or evidence of disruption of the barrier in any groups. Some groups (100 and 150 g masses) showed greater spatial learning deficits than other groups.
Concussion weight-drop (closed head injury) (Laurer et al., 2001)	1 or 2 mild injuries separated by 24 hours.	Mice/C57BL6/10 weeks old/male	More pronounced disruption of the BBB and somatodendritic cytoskeletal damage and motor sensory impairment after a second hit. No cognitive dysfunction or overt cell loss between groups.
Weight-drop injury (exposed dural surface) (Allen et al., 2000)	3 groups: mild, repetitive mild (3 mild injuries separated by 3 days), repetitive mild + severe as above followed by a severe injury between 3 and 5 days after last mild injury, and severe TBI.	Rats/Sprague-Dawley/adult/male	Repetitive mild injuries had little or no effect on motor function, whereas severe injuries showed motor dysfunction. Severe injury preceded by mild injuries showed little or no motor deficits. Cell injury and loss were minimal in mild and repetitive mild, whereas severe and repetitive mild + severe produced a similar-sized necrotic cavity.
Controlled cortical impact (closed head injury) (Longhi et al., 2005)	1 or 2 mild injuries separated by 3, 5, or 7 days.	Mice/C57BL6/6–8 weeks old/male	When injuries were separated by 3 days there were significantly more learning impairment, greater axonal injury and somatodendritic cytoskeletal damage, and prolonged cognitive deficits. No differences in water content or neuronal injury (Fluoro-Jade staining).
Controlled cortical impact (closed head injury) (Manville et al., 2007)	1 versus 2 mild injuries, separated by 1 day.	Mice/C57BL6/adult/male	Single injury did not affect ATP, glucose, or lactate, whereas repetitive injury caused severe depression in cerebral metabolism.

vulnerability, with repeated mild injuries in close temporal proximity producing greater damage than injuries separated by longer periods of time (in the case of rodents, a separation of seven days) (Longhi et al., 2005).

Postmortem studies of athletes have suggested that repetitive head injury is associated with chronic traumatic encephalopathy (CTE) (McKee et al., 2009b). CTE presents memory disturbances, behavioral and personality changes, parkinsonism, and speech and gait abnormalities that may arise long after the last concussion blow. De Beaumont and colleagues (2009) have demonstrated neurophysiological changes in Canadian football players decades after their last game. The neuropathology consists of atrophy of the cerebral hemispheres, medial temporal lobe, thalamus, mammillary body, and brainstem, with ventricular dilation and fenestrated cavum septum pellucidum. At the microscopic level, the pathology of CTE is characterized by a tauopathy where neurofibrillary tangles are found throughout the brain in the relative absence of b-amyloid deposits. A 2010 investigation (McKee et al., 2010) indicated the presence of the DNA-binding protein TDP-43 in the frontal and temporal cortices, medial temporal lobe, basal ganglia, diencephalon, and brainstem among athletes with CTE. An association between the presence of TDP-43 in the spinal cord and CTE cases with a progressive motor neuron disease, amyotrophic lateral sclerosis (ALS), is evidence that repetitive head trauma might be linked to impairments in the motor system. TDP-43 was also found in the cerebral cortex of boxers with CTE, and in cases with a variety of neurodegenerative disorders including frontotemporal lobar degeneration as well as Alzheimer's disease and ALS. It has been hypothesized that ALS develops as an interaction between genetic and environmental factors. Several epidemiological investigations document the incidence of ALS in athletes who had been exposed to repetitive head trauma (Chiò et al., 2005; Chen et al, 2007). Notably, the time between the injury-related events and diagnosis of ALS seems to be less than previously thought (Chiò et al., 2005). Among those who had experienced repetitive head injuries within the previous 10 years, the diagnosis of ALS was calculated to be three times higher than in those with no history of head injury (Chen et al., 2007). A few epidemiological investigations with military personnel reveal similar findings. For example, the risk of ALS among veterans of the 1991 Gulf War was about double the risk among civilians during the 10 years after the war (Horner et al., 2003).

There are many mechanisms by which recurrent head concussions may trigger neuronal degeneration (see above in moderate and severe TBI). As with moderate and severe TBI, in the case of mild concussions, there is an opportunity to investigate interventions that will impede the progress of the pathology. There are also, as with moderate and severe TBI, genetic factors contributing to this pathology that have not been identified. Neural degeneration might be associated with a widespread TDP-43 proteinopathy that contributes to the clinical manifestations of recurrent TBI, such as cognitive and memory loss, behavioral changes, and motor dysfunction. Mechanisms for the involvement of TDP-43 in neuronal degeneration have been hypothesized. For example, loss of TDP-43 activity due to sequestration in inclusions could affect its regulatory function during transcription of neurofilaments, leading to aggregates. Alternatively, abnormal phosphorylation of TDP-43 may disrupt important signaling pathways, leading to neuronal dysfunction (Forman et al., 2007).

In order to ameliorate or treat the effects of concussion, there are many research questions to answer, such as the physiological and biochemical pathways that lead to proteinopathies and tauopathies in recurrent head injuries, and the contribution of genetic or other factors (e.g., age) to outcome. As will be apparent below, an understanding of the effects of exposure to repetitive blasts and the proximity of each exposure is even more incomplete. Although human epidemiological studies are being conducted to address the effect of repetitive blasts (e.g., with Marines) and a longitudinal study is being carried out with combat veterans and retired athletes (see Stern et al., Appendix C), there is also a need for animal models that replicate repetitive TBI in humans.

BLAST INJURIES

Relatively few studies have been conducted to elucidate the mechanisms of blast TBI and even fewer have examined the consequences of exposure to repetitive blast episodes. One 2010 study examined whether exposure to repeated explosions or firing is associated with detection of neurochemical markers of brain damage (Blennow et al., 2011). Biomarkers measured in cerebrospinal fluid were tau and neurofilament protein (for neuron damage), GFAP and S-100b (for glial cell injury), and hemoglobin and bilirubin (for hemorrhage). Serum levels of GFAP and S-100b also were measured. All levels were normal, suggesting that repeated exposure to blasts does not result in neurochemical effects. This study presents some potential limitations, however, such as the timing of sampling and the sensitivity and specificity of the biomarkers. Another study with 12 Iraq war veterans diagnosed with mTBI who reported one or more blast injuries showed decreased cerebral metabolic rate for glucose in the cerebellum, vermis, pons, and medial temporal lobe. Clinical examination revealed impairments in verbal and cognitive abilities (Peskind et al., 2011). At the time of this writing, a two-week controlled study was being conducted with Marines who, during their training to be breachers, are exposed to 50 to 70 blasts of weapons-grade explosives. The outcomes will be measured using magnetic resonance imaging (MRI), functional magnetic resonance imaging (fMRI), electroencephalogram, and neurobehavioral and biochemical testing (Ling, 2010). Although repeated blast exposures below a certain threshold result in no cumulative damage, the long-term impacts of multiple blasts above that threshold are not known (Ling, 2010).

There have been ongoing efforts to correlate some of the emerging clinical data from service members and veterans with blast as a mechanism of injury. Severe TBI from blast has been associated with a greater incidence of traumatic vasospasm (Armonda et al., 2006) than severe nonblast TBI. Evaluation of the performance of severity-matched populations with blast and nonblast injuries using neuropsychological testing did not find any significant difference between these two populations (Belanger et al., 2009). Evaluations of vestibular assessment with blast patients have shown a pattern different from that seen in nonblast injuries (Hoffer et al., 2010). There are some data utilizing neuroimaging techniques such as diffusion tensor imaging, which, in patients whose injuries were matched for severity, has shown a more diffuse pattern of brain injury in patients with blast as part of their contributing mechanism than in those without blast (Moore, 2009). To better understand and determine the role of blast as a mechanism of injury, 75 experts from the Department of Defense, the Department of Transportation, the Department of Veterans Affairs, academia, and industry were gathered from five countries in May 2009 to evaluate evidence from past and ongoing blast research at the International State-of-the-Science Meeting on Non-Impact, Blast-Induced Mild Traumatic Brain Injury. Based on the data reviewed, which included published and unpublished data from human and animal research, the participants determined there was evidence that mild trauma to the brain can occur because of blast and that this injury is different from nonblast injury. From the proceedings, this conclusion was based on evidence that demonstrated:

- Statistically significant differences in diffusion tensor imaging-based fractional anisotropy between service members with documented mTBI associated with blast, and service members with impact-only mTBI.

- Statistically significant differences in event-related potentials between blast and non-blast exposures in human studies.
- Preliminary evidence of disturbed phase synchrony following blast exposure.
- Differences in fMRI between breacher instructors and students (statistically significant fMRI results, statistically nonsignificant neurocognitive results).
- Alterations in inflammatory markers in animal studies.
- Physiological, histological, and/or behavioral differences between blast and nonblast exposures in shock tubes models with rodents.
- Low-level axonal, neuronal, and/or glial damage/reactivity in blast studies (including free field and other) in porcine models.

The existence of comorbidities with psychological stress for those who sustained a TBI involving blast as a mechanism has been another challenge in attempting to compare blast TBI with nonblast (impact) TBI. One attempt to better understand and clinically correlate some of the disparate findings described above is comparison of the total number of domains or symptoms produced by those who have had TBI with a comorbidity of posttraumatic stress disorder (PTSD), those with TBI without a PTSD comorbidity, and those with PTSD but with no history of TBI or concussion. For example, it has been demonstrated (Brenner et al., 2010) that patients who had TBI with a PTSD comorbidity reported more symptoms than patients who had TBI without PTSD or patients who had PTSD without a history of TBI or concussion.

Furthermore, there is an acknowledged lack of data about long-term complications from blast injury (IOM 2009) and about how blast also may have similar effects to emerging data on CTE from recurrent injuries from sports concussions (McKee et al., 2009a).

CONCLUSIONS AND RECOMMENDATIONS

In general, TBI is characterized by its heterogeneity, reflecting the nature, severity and location of the insult. Despite this heterogeneity, there are shared mechanisms of secondary pathogenesis that are potentially amenable to therapeutic intervention. This chapter is written as background and serves as the basis for subsequent chapters in which the committee considers nutrients, dietary supplements, or specific diets whose functions and mechanisms of action suggest they might promote resilience, be efficacious when provided after TBI, or both.

Appropriate animal study designs and biomarkers of injury and recovery are considerable components of the exploration of hypotheses about the benefits of nutritional interventions. Therefore, although not related to nutrition specifically, the committee thought it important to urge the advancing of these experimental tools. There are still significant inadequacies in the current TBI animal models and biomarkers of injury, and greater advances will be realized in TBI management when these are improved. The committee made two general recommendations: first, to continue to develop better animal models, and second, to identify biomarkers of injury and improved brain function.

RECOMMENDATION 3-1. The committee recommends that DoD, in cooperation with others, refine existing animal models to investigate the potential benefits of nutrition throughout the spectrum of TBI injuries, that is, concussion/mild, moderate, severe, and penetrating, as well as repetitive and blast injuries. Development of animal models is particularly urgent for concussion/mild TBI and brain injuries because of blast as well as for repetitive injuries. These models will also aid in understanding the pathobiology of TBI, which is particularly needed for concussion/mild TBI, blast, and repetitive injuries.

RECOMMENDATION 3-2. The committee recommends that DoD, in cooperation with others, continue to develop better clinical biomarkers of TBI (i.e., concussion/ mild, moderate, severe, penetrating, repetitive, and blast injuries) for the purposes of diagnosis, treatment, and outcome assessment. In addition, the committee recommends the identification of biomarkers specifically related to proposed mechanisms of action for individual nutritional interventions.

REFERENCES

Allen, G. V., D. Gerami, and M. J. Esser. 2000. Conditioning effects of repetitive mild neurotrauma on motor function in an animal model of focal brain injury. *Neuroscience* 99(1):93–105.

Andriessen, T. M., B. Jacobs, and P. E. Vos. 2010. Clinical characteristics and pathophysiological mechanisms of focal and diffuse traumatic brain injury. *Journal of Cellular and Molecular Medicine* 14(10):2381–2392.

Armonda, R. A., R. S. Bell, A. H. Vo, G. Ling, T. J. DeGraba, B. Crandall, J. Ecklund, and W. W. Campbell. 2006. Wartime traumatic cerebral vasospasm: Recent review of combat casualties. *Neurosurgery* 59(6):1215–1225.

Artinian, V., H. Krayem, and B. DiGiovine. 2006. Effects of early enteral feeding on the outcome of critically ill mechanically ventilated medical patients. *Chest* 129(4):960–967.

Barkhoudarian, G., D. A. Hovda, and C. C. Giza. 2011. The molecular pathophysiology of concussion brain injury. *Clinics in Sports Medicine* 30(1):33–48.

Belanger, H. G., T. Kretzmer, R. Yoash-Gantz, T. Pickett, and L. A. Tupler. 2009. Cognitive sequelae of blast-related versus other mechanisms of brain trauma. *Journal of the International Neuropsychological Society* 15(1):1–8.

Berger, R. P., M. C. Bazaco, A. K. Wagner, P. M. Kochanek, and A. Fabio. 2010. Trajectory analysis of serum biomarker concentrations facilitates outcome prediction after pediatric traumatic and hypoxemic brain injury. *Developmental Neuroscience* 32(5–6):396–405.

Blennow, K., M. Jonsson, N. Andreasen, L. Rosengren, A. Wallin, P. A. Hellstrom, and H. Zetterberg. 2011. No neurochemical evidence of brain injury after blast overpressure by repeated explosions or firing heavy weapons. *Acta Neurologica Scandinavica* 123(4):245–251.

Brenner, L. A., B. J. Ivins, K. Schwab, D. Warden, L. A. Nelson, M. Jaffee, and H. Terrio. 2010. Traumatic brain injury, posttraumatic stress disorder, and postconcussion symptom reporting among troops returning from Iraq. *Journal of Head Trauma Rehabilitation* 25(5):307–312.

Cederberg, D., and P. Siesjo. 2010. What has inflammation to do with traumatic brain injury? *Childs Nervous System* 26(2):221–226.

Cekic, M., and D. G. Stein. 2010. Traumatic brain injury and aging: Is a combination of progesterone and vitamin D hormone a simple solution to a complex problem? *Neurotherapeutics* 7(1):81–90.

Cernak, I. 2005. Animal models of head trauma. *NeuroRx* 2(3):410–422.

Cernak, I., and L. J. Noble-Haeusslein. 2010. Traumatic brain injury: An overview of pathobiology with emphasis on military populations. *Journal of Cerebral Blood Flow and Metabolism* 30(2):255–266.

Chen, H., M. Richard, D. P. Sandler, D. M. Umbach, and F. Kamel. 2007. Head injury and amyotrophic lateral sclerosis. *American Journal of Epidemiology* 166(7):810–816.

Chiò, A., G. Benzi, M. Dossena, R. Mutani, and G. Mora. 2005. Severely increased risk of amyotrophic lateral sclerosis among Italian professional football players. *Brain* 128(3):472–476.

Conti, A. C., R. Raghupathi, J. Q. Trojanowski, and T. K. McIntosh. 1998. Experimental brain injury induces regionally distinct apoptosis during the acute and delayed post-traumatic period. *Journal of Neuroscience* 18(15):5663–5672.

Dash, P. K., J. Zhao, G. Hergenroeder, and A. N. Moore. 2010. Biomarkers for the diagnosis, prognosis, and evaluation of treatment efficacy for traumatic brain injury. *Neurotherapeutics* 7(1):100–114.

De Beaumont, L., H. Theoret, D. Mongeon, J. Messier, S. Leclerc, S. Tremblay, D. Ellemberg, and M. Lassonde. 2009. Brain function decline in healthy retired athletes who sustained their last sports concussion in early adulthood. *Brain* 132(Pt 3):695–708.

DeFord, S. M., M. S. Wilson, A. C. Rice, T. Clausen, L. K. Rice, A. Barabnova, R. Bullock, and R. J. Hamm. 2002. Repeated mild brain injuries result in cognitive impairment in B6C3F1 mice. *Journal of Neurotrauma* 19(4):427–438.

Desmoulin, G. T., and J. P. Dionne. 2009. Blast-induced neurotrauma: Surrogate use, loading mechanisms, and cellular responses. *Journal of Trauma* 67(5):1113–1122.

Elder, G. A., and A. Cristian. 2009. Blast-related mild traumatic brain injury: Mechanisms of injury and impact on clinical care. *The Mount Sinai Journal of Medicine, New York* 76(2):111–118.

Farkas, O., and J. T. Povlishock. 2007. Cellular and subcellular change evoked by diffuse traumatic brain injury: A complex web of change extending far beyond focal damage. *Progress in Brain Research* 161:43–59.

Forman, M. S., J. Q. Trojanowski, and V. M. Y. Lee. 2007. TDP-43: A novel neurodegenerative proteinopathy. *Current Opinion in Neurobiology* 17(5):548–555.

Gallyas, F., and G. Zoltay. 1992. An immediate light microscopic response of neuronal somata, dendrites and axons to non-contusing concussion head injury in the rat. *Acta Neuropathologica* 83(4):386–393.

Gilmer, L. K., K. N. Roberts, K. Joy, P. G. Sullivan, and S. W. Scheff. 2009. Early mitochondrial dysfunction after cortical contusion injury. *Journal of Neurotrauma* 26(8):1271–1280.

Greenberg, D. A., and K. Jin. 2005. From angiogenesis to neuropathology. *Nature* 438(7070):954–959.

Hagg, T. 2009. From neurotransmitters to neurotrophic factors to neurogenesis. *Neuroscientist* 15(1):20–27.

Henninger, N., S. Dutzmann, K. M. Sicard, R. Kollmar, J. Bardutzky, and S. Schwab. 2005. Impaired spatial learning in a novel rat model of mild cerebral concussion injury. *Experimental Neurology* 195(2):447–457.

Hicks, R. R., S. J. Fertig, R. E. Desrocher, W. J. Koroshetz, and J. J. Pancrazio. 2010. Neurological effects of blast injury. *Journal of Trauma-Injury Infection and Critical Care* 68(5):1257–1263.

Hoffer, M. E., C. Balaban, K. Gottshall, B. J. Balough, M. R. Maddox, and J. R. Penta. 2010. Blast exposure: Vestibular consequences and associated characteristics. *Otology & Neurotology* 31(2):232–236.

Horner, R. D., K. G. Kamins, J. R. Feussner, S. C. Grambow, J. Hoff-Lindquist, Y. Harati, H. Mitsumoto, R. Pascuzzi, P. S. Spencer, R. Tim, D. Howard, T. C. Smith, M. A. Ryan, C. J. Coffman, and E. J. Kasarskis. 2003. Occurrence of amyotrophic lateral sclerosis among Gulf War veterans. *Neurology* 61(6):742–749.

Hovda, D. A., S. M. Lee, M. L. Smith, S. Von Stuck, M. Bergsneider, D. Kelly, E. Shalmon, N. Martin, M. Caron, J. Mazziotta, et al. 1995. The neurochemical and metabolic cascade following brain injury: Moving from animal models to man. *Journal of Neurotrauma* 12(5):903–906.

IOM (Institute of Medicine). 2009. *Gulf War and health: Long-term consequences of traumatic brain injury.* Vol. 7. Washington, DC: The National Academies Press.

Jain, K. K. 2008. Neuroprotection in traumatic brain injury. *Drug Discovery Today* 13(23–24):1082–1089.

Kernie, S. G., and J. M. Parent. 2010. Forebrain neurogenesis after focal ischemic and traumatic brain injury. *Neurobiology of Disease* 37(2):267–274.

Laurer, H. L., F. M. Bareyre, V. Lee, J. Q. Trojanowski, L. Longhi, R. Hoover, K. E. Saatman, R. Raghupathi, S. Hoshino, M. S. Grady, and T. K. McIntosh. 2001. Mild head injury increasing the brain's vulnerability to a second concussion impact. *Journal of Neurosurgery* 95(5):859–870.

Leker, R. R., and E. Shohami. 2002. Cerebral ischemia and trauma-different etiologies yet similar mechanisms: Neuroprotective opportunities. *Brain Research. Brain Research Reviews* 39(1):55–73.

Ling, G. 2010. Explosive blast traumatic brain injury. Presented at the IOM Nutrition and Neuroprotection in Military Personnel Workshop, Washington, D.C.

Ling, G. S. F., F. Bandak, R. Armonda, G. Grant, and J. M. Ecklund. 2009. Explosive blast neurotrauma. *Journal of Neurotrauma* 26(6):815–825.

Longhi, L., K. E. Saatman, S. Fujimoto, R. Raghupathi, D. F. Meaney, J. Davis, A. McMillan, V. Conte, H. L. Laurer, S. Stein, N. Stocchetti, and T. K. McIntosh. 2005. Temporal window of vulnerability to repetitive experimental concussion brain injury. *Neurosurgery* 56(2):364–373.

Lykissas, M. G., A. K. Batistatou, K. A. Charalabopoulos, and A. E. Beris. 2007. The role of neurotrophins in axonal growth, guidance, and regeneration. *Current Neurovascular Research* 4(2):143–151.

Maas, A. I., N. Stocchetti, and R. Bullock. 2008. Moderate and severe traumatic brain injury in adults. *Lancet Neurology* 7(8):728–741.

Manville, J., H. L. Laurer, W. I. Steudel, and A. E. M. Mautes. 2007. Changes in cortical and subcortical energy metabolism after repetitive and single controlled cortical impact injury in the mouse. *Journal of Molecular Neuroscience* 31(2):95–100.

Margulies, S., R. Hicks, and B. Combination Therapies Traumatic. 2009. Combination therapies for traumatic brain injury: Prospective considerations. *Journal of Neurotrauma* 26(6):925–939.

Marklund, N., A. Bakshi, D. J. Castelbuono, V. Conte, and T. K. McIntosh. 2006. Evaluation of pharmacological treatment strategies in traumatic brain injury. *Current Pharmaceutical Design* 12(13):1645–1680.

Maruta, J., S. W. Lee, E. F. Jacobs, and J. Ghajar. 2010. A unified science of concussion. *Annals of the New York Academy of Sciences* 1208:58–66.

Mayer, A. R., J. Ling, M. V. Mannell, C. Gasparovic, J. P. Phillips, D. Doezema, R. Reichard, and R. A. Yeo. 2010. A prospective diffusion tensor imaging study in mild traumatic brain injury. *Neurology* 74(8):643–650.

Mazzeo, A. T., A. Beat, A. Singh, and M. R. Bullock. 2009. The role of mitochondrial transition pore, and its modulation, in traumatic brain injury and delayed neurodegeneration after TBI. *Experimental Neurology* 218(2):363–370.

McCrory, P., W. Meeuwisse, K. Johnston, J. Dvorak, M. Aubry, M. Molloy, and R. Cantu. 2009. Consensus statement on concussion in sport—The 3rd International Conference on concussion in sport, held in Zurich, November 2008. *Clinical Journal of Sport Medicine* 19(3):185–200.

McKee, A. C., R. C. Cantu, C. J. Nowinski, E. T. Hedley-Whyte, B. E. Gavett, A. E. Budson, V. E. Santini, H. S. Lee, C. A. Kubilus, and R. A. Stern. 2009a. Chronic traumatic encephalopathy in athletes: Progressive tauopathy after repetitive head injury. *Journal of Neuropathology and Experimental Neurology* 68(7):709–735.

McKee, A. C. M., R. C. M. Cantu, C. J. A. Nowinski, E. T. M. Hedley-Whyte, B. E. P. Gavett, A. E. M. Budson, V. E. M. Santini, H.-S. M. Lee, C. A. Kubilus, and R. A. P. Stern. 2009b. Chronic traumatic encephalopathy in athletes: Progressive tauopathy after repetitive head injury. *Journal of Neuropathology and Experimental Neurology* 68(7):709–735.

McKee, A. C., B. E. Gavett, R. A. Stern, C. J. Nowinski, R. C. Cantu, N. W. Kowall, D. P. Perl, E. T. Hedley-Whyte, B. Price, C. Sullivan, P. Morin, H. S. Lee, C. A. Kubilus, D. H. Daneshvar, M. Wulff, and A. E. Budson. 2010. TDP-43 proteinopathy and motor neuron disease in chronic traumatic encephalopathy. *Journal of Neuropathology and Experimental Neurology* 69(9):918–929.

Moore, D. F. 2009. *Diffusion Tensor Imaging and mTBI6A Case-Control Study of Blast (+) in Returning Service Members Following OIF and OEF*. Seattle, WA: 61st Annual Meeting of the American Academy of Neurology Platform Presentation.

Moore, D. F., et al. 2010. Diffusion Tensor Imaging and mTBI—A Case-Control Study of Blast (+) in Returning Service Members Following OIF and OEF. Under review *Journal of Neurotrauma*. Platform presentation at American Academy of Neurology, 2009.

Morales, D. M., N. Marklund, D. Lebold, H. J. Thompson, A. Pitkanen, W. L. Maxwell, L. Longhi, H. Laurer, M. Maegele, E. Neugebauer, D. I. Graham, N. Stocchetti, and T. K. McIntosh. 2005. Experimental models of traumatic brain injury: Do we really need to build a better mousetrap? *Neuroscience* 136(4):971–989.

Morganti-Kossmann, M. C., L. Satgunaseelan, N. Bye, and T. Kossmann. 2007. Modulation of immune response by head injury. *Injury* 38(12):1392–1400.

Morganti-Kossmann, M. C., E. Yan, and N. Bye. 2010. Animal models of traumatic brain injury: Is there an optimal model to reproduce human brain injury in the laboratory? *Injury* 41(Suppl. 1):S10–S13.

Mori, T., Y. Katayama, and T. Kawamata. 2006. Acute hemispheric swelling associated with thin subdural hematomas: Pathophysiology of repetitive head injury in sports. *Acta Neurochirurgica. Supplement* 96:40–43.

O'Connor, C. A., I. Cernak, and R. Vink. 2005. Both estrogen and progesterone attenuate edema formation following diffuse traumatic brain injury in rats. *Brain Research* 1062(1–2):171–174.

Patel, A. D., V. Gerzanich, Z. H. Geng, and J. M. Simard. 2010. Glibenclamide reduces hippocampal injury and preserves rapid spatial learning in a model of traumatic brain injury. *Journal of Neuropathology and Experimental Neurology* 69(12):1177–1190.

Peskind, E. R., E. C. Petrie, D. J. Cross, K. Pagulayan, K. McCraw, D. Hoff, K. Hart, C. E. Yu, M. A. Raskind, D. G. Cook, and S. Minoshima. 2011. Cerebrocerebellar hypometabolism associated with repetitive blast exposure mild traumatic brain injury in 12 Iraq war veterans with persistent post-concussion symptoms. *Neuroimage* 54(Suppl. 1):S76–S82.

Povlishock, J. T., and D. I. Katz. 2005. Update of neuropathology and neurological recovery after traumatic brain injury. *Journal of Head Trauma Rehabilitation* 20(1):76–94.

Raghupathi, R. 2004. Cell death mechanisms following traumatic brain injury. *Brain Pathology* 14(2):215–222.

Ross, S. T., and I. Soltesz. 2000. Selective depolarization of interneurons in the early posttraumatic dentate gyrus: Involvement of the Na(+)/K(+)-ATPase. *Journal of Neurophysiology* 83(5):2916–2930.

Rosenstein, J. M., J. M. Krum, and C. Ruhrberg. 2010. VEGF in the nervous system. *Organogenesis* 6(2):107–114.

Saatman, K. E., A. C. Duhaime, R. Bullock, A. I. R. Maas, A. Valadka, G. T. Manley, and P. Workshop Sci Team Advisory. 2008. Classification of traumatic brain injury for targeted therapies. *Journal of Neurotrauma* 25(7):719–738.

Slemmer, J. E., E. J. T. Matser, C. I. De Zeeuw, and J. T. Weber. 2002. Repeated mild injury causes cumulative damage to hippocampal cells. *Brain* 125(Pt 12):2699–2709.

Slemmer, J. E., and J. T. Weber. 2005. The extent of damage following repeated injury to cultured hippocampal cells is dependent on the severity of insult and inter-injury interval. *Neurobiology of Disease* 18(3):421–431.

Smith, D. H., D. F. Meaney, and W. H. Shull. 2003. Diffuse axonal injury in head trauma. *Journal of Head Trauma Rehabilitation* 18(4):307–316.

Svetlov, S. I., S. F. Larner, D. R. Kirk, J. Atkinson, R. L. Hayes, and K. K. W. Wang. 2009. Biomarkers of blast-induced neurotrauma: Profiling molecular and cellular mechanisms of blast brain injury. *Journal of Neurotrauma* 26(6):913–921.

Taber, K. H., D. L. Warden, and R. A. Hurley. 2006. Blast-related traumatic brain injury: What is known? *The Journal of Neuropsychiatry and Clinical Neurosciences* 18(2):141–145.

Thau-Zuchman, O., E. Shohami, A. G. Alexandrovich, and R. R. Leker. 2010. Vascular endothelial growth factor increases neurogenesis after traumatic brain injury. *Journal of Cerebral Blood Flow and Metabolism* 30(5):1008–1016.

Toth, Z., G. S. Hollrigel, T. Gorcs, and I. Soltesz. 1997. Instantaneous perturbation of dentate interneuronal networks by a pressure wave-transient delivered to the neocortex. *Journal of Neuroscience* 17(21):8106–8117.

Unterberg, A. W., J. Stover, B. Kress, and K. L. Kiening. 2004. Edema and brain trauma. *Neuroscience* 129(4):1021–1029.

Weber, J. T. 2007. Experimental models of repetitive brain injuries. *Progress in Brain Research* 161:253–261.

Werner, C., and K. Engelhard. 2007. Pathophysiology of traumatic brain injury. *British Journal of Anaesthesia* 99(1):4–9.

Wu, A., Z. Ying, and F. Gomez-Pinilla. 2004. Dietary omega-3 fatty acids normalize BDNF levels, reduce oxidative damage, and counteract learning disability after traumatic brain injury in rats. *Journal of Neurotrauma* 21(10):1457–1467.

Wu, A. G., Z. Ying, and F. Gomez-Pinilla. 2010. Vitamin E protects against oxidative damage and learning disability after mild traumatic brain injury in rats. *Neurorehabilitation and Neural Repair* 24(3):290–298.

Ziebell, J. M., and M. C. Morganti-Kossmann. 2010. Involvement of pro- and anti-inflammatory cytokines and chemokines in the pathophysiology of traumatic brain injury. *Neurotherapeutics* 7(1):22–30.

Part II

Nutrition and TBI

4

Approach for Selecting Nutritional Interventions: Mechanistic Targets

The relationship between nutrition and brain function continues to be investigated, and there is still much to be discovered about brain function, brain disease processes, and interventions to improve or restore brain function following injury. There are likewise numerous challenges in identifying pharmaceutical interventions to improve resilience or treat traumatic brain injury (TBI). Despite years of pharmaceutical research, there is still no effective drug treatment for TBI (see Hall in Appendix C); since the 1970s, not a single phase III human clinical trial has shown a significant benefit (Maas et al., 2010).

In this second part of the report, the committee presents its core recommendations. In particular, this chapter describes the committee's rationale for selecting specific nutritional interventions for review. Briefly, the committee based its selection on the current understanding of the injury process and of mechanisms of action of specific nutritional interventions. When the function and biochemistry associated with a particular nutritional approach appeared promising, a literature search was initiated. Based on the experience with pharmaceuticals mentioned above, the committee understands that nutrition will not be the sole treatment for TBI, but it is a potentially powerful adjunct to promote metabolic support during wound healing, and may even exert neuroprotection in some instances if provided prior to injury.

GENERAL APPROACH FOR SELECTING NUTRITIONAL INTERVENTIONS

The committee's approach to identifying nutritional interventions of potential use in the treatment of TBI consisted of expert discussions, literature reviews on the pathophysiology of TBI, initial identification of promising nutrients, and reviews of their effectiveness.

Expert Discussions

A public workshop was held June 23–24, 2010, in Washington, DC, where invited civilian and military subject-matter experts (e.g., medical experts, nutritionists, and neuroscientists) presented their findings and experiences on various TBI-related topics, with a focus on potential nutrient interactions with the pathogenic sequelae of TBI. The committee also reviewed the existing literature examining the pathology and metabolic alterations of the insult with the goal of identifying nutrients that had the potential to favorably alter metabolism, oxidative stress, and tissue structure and repair, following and sometimes in advance of TBI.

Review of the Literature on Pathophysiology and Identification of Targets for Nutritional Interventions

As a background to elucidate the committee's rationale, a summary of current knowledge about the pathophysiology of TBI was presented in Chapter 3. Briefly, brain injuries differ dramatically from patient to patient depending upon the location, type, intensity, and duration of the initiating concussion force. One common feature of severe brain injury is reduced blood flow and oxygen deficiency. Neuronal membranes become damaged and ion channels malfunction, leaking proteins and neurotransmitters. Apoptotic genes are activated, brain cells begin to swell, and mitochondrial function diminishes as the brain cells enter a "death spiral" (Scudellari, 2010). Production of free radicals increases and calcium ions are released, resulting in tissue damage and cell death (Mattson and Chan, 2003). For the purposes of this report, TBI pathology has been divided into primary, secondary, and long-term injury mechanisms to permit more specific focus on the timing and locus of the nutrient intervention. Box 4-1 shows a summary listing of adverse physiological responses as well as select potential neuroprotective targets (e.g., control of inflammation, angiogenic and neurogenic repair and recovery) discussed during the June public workshop and committee meetings that might respond to nutritional interventions. Box entries with an asterisk indicate especially promising potential targets for nutritional intervention. These potential nutritional targets and the mechanism or metabolic bridge linking them to TBI treatment or prevention have been grouped into three topic areas and will be discussed briefly in this chapter. Table 4-1 matches these potential nutritional targets with nutrients having relevant mechanisms of action; however, the reader should make no conclusions about the clinical efficacy of any of these nutrients based on this table. The information in this table is not meant to imply that there is any evidence from animal models or human trials showing benefits in ameliorating TBI. The table was constructed to illustrate that those nutrients and food components act on multiple and diverse processes that are common to brain injury, and therefore their effects (beneficial and adverse) should be reviewed.

For most nutrients, more than one mechanism is proposed. The scientific community believes that, based on the variations in injuries, responses, and outcomes after TBI, no single nutritional mechanism will serve as the magic bullet for TBI. The evidence on the ability of these putative nutrients to improve resilience or ameliorate the effects of TBI will be discussed in detail in subsequent chapters (Chapters 6–16).

Review of the Literature on Effectiveness of Nutrients

From its discussions, the committee identified an initial list of search criteria and promising pre- and postinjury nutritional interventions that might be useful adjuncts in the overall medical treatment and prevention of TBI. The committee decided on the search criteria and vocabulary included in Box 4-2.

BOX 4-1
Physiologic Responses to TBI and Protective/Reparative Targets

Physiologic responses
Intracranial hemorrhage
Release of glutamate/excitotoxicity
Ionic disturbances: Efflux of potassium, influx of calcium and sodium
Decreased cerebral blood flow
Vasogenic edema
Cytotoxic edema
Disruption of the blood-brain barrier
Intravascular coagulation
Ischemia
*Decreased ATP (altered glucose metabolism [hyper- followed by hypoglycolysis] and switch to alternative fuels, elevated lactate) cerebral acidosis
Nonischemic metabolic failure
*Mitochondrial disturbances/failure
Reactive oxygen and nitrogen species
Seizures
Vasospasm
*Inflammation
*DNA damage
*Cell injury: apoptosis, necrosis, cytoskeletal changes in cell bodies and processes
Activation of enzymes: e.g., calpains, caspases, endonucleases, metalloproteinases
*Altered neurotransmitters: e.g., catecholamines, serotonin, histamine, acetylcholine, GABA, dopamine

Endogenous Neuroprotective Targets
*Antioxidants (e.g., Cu/Zn-SOD, extracellular SOD, Mn-SOD, glutathione peroxidase, catalase)
Heat shock proteins (e.g., HSP-70, HSP-90, GRP-78, HSP-27)
Hypoxia-inducible-1 factor
*Erythropoietin
Antiapoptotic genes (e.g., XIAP, c-IAP2, Bcl-xL)
Antiapoptotic proteins (e.g., Bcl-2, Bcl-XL)
Growth factors (e.g., bFGF, NGF, BDNF, NT-4, TGF-B, GDNF)
*Anti-inflammatories (e.g., IL-10, IL-18)
Sex hormones (e.g., estrogen, progesterone)

Plasticity/Repair/Recovery Targets
*Neurotrophic factors: (e.g., nerve growth factor, glial-derived neurotrophic factors, neurotrophin 4/5)
*Inflammation
Angiogenesis
*Neurogenesis

---

*Promising mechanistic target areas for nutritional intervention.
SOURCES: Bales et al., 2009; Bazan, 2006; Bazan et al., 2005; Bramlett and Dietrich, 2004; Dietrich and Bramlett, 2010; Dubreuil et al., 2006; Faden, 2002; Graham et al., 2000; Kokiko and Hamm, 2007; Longhi et al., 2001; Maas et al., 2010; Mammis et al., 2009; Margulies et al., 2009; Marklund et al., 1997, 2006; Mattson et al., 2002; Moppett, 2007; Morales et al., 2005; Morganti-Kossmann et al., 2007; Povlishock and Katz, 2005; Raghupathi, 2004; Royo et al., 2003; Schouten, 2007; Stein et al., 2008; Stetler et al., 2010; Thompson et al., 2005, 2006; Unterberg et al., 2004; Werner and Engelhard, 2007; Yi and Hazell, 2006.

TABLE 4-1   Plausible Mechanisms of Action by Selected Nutrients and Food Components That Might Affect TBI Outcomes[a]

Nutrient/Mechanistic Target	Edema	Reduced CBF	Hypoxia	Inflammation	Oxidative Stress	Apoptosis	Ionic Disturbances
Antioxidants (vit E, vit C)				X	X		
Branched-chain amino acids							
Choline	X					X	
Creatine							
Curcumin							
Flavonoids				X	X	X	
Ketogenic diet			X		X		
Magnesium		X					X
n-3 FAs				X	X		
Resveratrol		X		X	X		
Vitamin D + Progesterone	X			X	X	X	
Zinc				X	X	X	

[a]The information in this table does not imply there is any evidence from animal models or human trials showing benefits in ameliorating TBI. The table was constructed to demonstrate that those nutrients and food components act on multiple and diverse processes that are common to brain injury, and therefore their effects (beneficial and adverse) should be reviewed. Summaries of reviews and committee's conclusions and recommendations are found in Chapters 6–16.

BOX 4-2
Literature Search Criteria and Vocabulary

Inclusion Criteria
- Health condition: patients or animal models of TBI (including in the developing brain), subarachnoid hemorrhage, intracranial aneurysm, stroke, anoxic or hypoxic ischemia, epilepsy
- Study designs: (1) randomized controlled trials or clinical controlled studies, (2) epidemiological/observational studies, (3) animal studies, (4) reviews and meta-analyses
- No minimum sample size or age limit in human trials
- Language: limited to articles published in English
- Publication date: 1990 and later
- Dietary supplementation or therapeutic use of nutrient

Search Vocabulary
Health Condition:
- Brain injuries: brain concussion, traumatic brain hemorrhage, chronic brain injury, diffuse axonal injury, posttraumatic epilepsy, pneumocephalus
- Subarachnoid hemorrhage or intracranial hemorrhage
- Intracranial aneurysm
- Hypoxia–ischemia, brain
- Stroke
- Epilepsy

Decreased ATP/ Mitochondrial Dysfunction	Excitotoxicity	Revascularization	Neuroplasticity	Neurogenesis	Neurotrophic Factors	Synapses
			X			X
			X	X		
X						
X	X					
X	X					
X	X					
X	X					
			X			
			X	X	X	X

Intervention:
- Acetyl-L-carnitine
- Amino acids, branched-chain: aminoisobutryic acids, isoleucine, leucine, valine
- Antioxidants
- Ascorbic acid (vitamin C)
- Creatine
- Curcumin
- Cytidine Disphosphate Choline
- Diet therapy or nutritional support
- Fatty acids, n-3
- Flavonoids: anthocyanins, benzoflavones, biflavonoids, catechin, chalcones, flavanones, flavones, flavonoligans, flavonols, isoflavones, proanthocyanidins
- Ketogenic diet
- Magnesium
- Stilbenes (resveratrol)
- Vitamin D
- Vitamin E: tocopherol, tocotrienols
- Zinc

NUTRITIONAL MODIFIERS OF TBI: PROMISING TARGETS

The treatment and recovery of TBI typically involves one or more of the following interventions: fueling hypermetabolism, reestablishment of vascularity, supporting brain plasticity, prevention of posttrauma protein tangle development, and controlling glutamate excitotoxicity. For the purposes of this report, the potential nutritional approaches targeting these interventions and the mechanism or metabolic connection linking them to TBI have been grouped into three target areas: (1) restoration of cellular energetics, (2) reduction of oxidative stress and inflammation and repair of cellular damage, and (3) repair and recovery. Each of these approaches is discussed briefly below, with example(s) of potentially useful nutrients that may have implications across several of these target areas. It is important to note that nutrients typically have multiple modes of action, interacting with various aspects of the potential target areas, so they may be considered in more than one target area.

Restoration of Cellular Energetics

Metabolic characteristics of TBI include cerebral acidosis, hypoxia, decreased adenosine triphosphate (ATP) production, and resultant mitochondrial malfunction followed by apoptotic cell death. Apoptosis can be triggered by many different stimuli such as certain cytokines, toxins, oxidative stress, and calcium influx through damaged plasma membrane channels or release from the endoplasmic reticulum. Mitochondrial calcium dynamics are involved in the regulation of cellular energy metabolism and neurotransmitter release (Mattson and Chan, 2003). Although it is a nutrient, calcium acts in this case as a messenger to coordinate cellular reactions that drive apoptosis. Calcium release is normally under tight physiological control, but this normally close regulation is altered by the events following a traumatic brain injury. Calcium released from the endoplasmic reticulum triggers a mass exodus of cytochrome C from mitochondria in the cell, activating caspases and other nuclease enzymes that finalize cell death (Mattson and Chan, 2003). Many of the hypothetical mechanisms of nutrients included in this report may have the effect of preventing apoptosis. Neuronal apoptosis can be induced by activation of glutamate receptors confined to the postsynaptic membrane of a dendrite, permitting a local influx of calcium that triggers cytochrome C release from mitochondria throughout the dendrites and cell body (Boehning et al., 2003). The series of events that triggers the malfunctioning of mitochondria severely disrupts the energetics of the cell. Thus, restoration of mitochondrial function or providing sources of energy other than glucose is a key objective after a TBI event. In addition, nutrients or food components that counteract or prevent ionic disturbances and excitotoxicity have the potential to improve outcomes of TBI. One such nutrient is magnesium, which plays a role in the pathobiology leading to TBI (Sen and Gulati, 2010). The level of magnesium in the brain has been found to affect the influx of calcium and glutamate to the postsynaptic neuron, one potential mechanism by which magnesium exerts its effects.

Several other food components could potentially ameliorate the described effects on mitochondrial malfunction by augmenting energy metabolism. Creatine, a nitrogenous guanidine compound found naturally in vertebrates, accesses the brain via a creatine transporter. Creatine and the creatine kinase/phosphocreatine system serve to buffer energy in tissues with high and fluctuating energy requirements (e.g., muscle and brain). Since the brain requires significant ATP turnover to maintain membrane potentials and its signaling capacity, creatine metabolism and the creatine kinase/phosphocreatine system are important for normal brain functioning; these may be compromised in diseases of the central nervous system. Studies also suggest that creatine's neuroprotective effects are at least partly due to increased cerebral blood flow and reduction in the processes associated with secondary brain damage, such as an increase in free fatty acid and lactate (Sullivan et al., 2000).

Acetyl-L-carnitine (ALC), another food component, has been shown to confer neuroprotection in models of both global and focal ischemia (see review, Zanelli et al., 2005). It is postulated that ALC serves as an alternative source of acetyl coA, and as such promotes aerobic energy metabolism and reduces tissue acidosis. With reduced tissue acidosis, oxidative stress may likewise be ameliorated. Data further suggest that ALC modulates excitotoxicity, apoptosis, and inflammation. The beneficial effects of ALC may reflect the targeting of multiple pathogenic pathways. However, a review of the literature did not deliver enough evidence for the committee to write a chapter and make recommendations. Only a few studies have been done in animal models of ischemia. In addition, improvements in neurological outcomes were only seen when ALC was administered within 30 minutes after the injury, which might not be feasible in the field. The acetate precursor glyceryl triacetate, a food additive and dietary supplement, has also been found to effectively supply acetyl coA as an alternative energy source in an animal model of TBI (Arun et al., 2010), which can contribute to more immediate energy production for mitochondria than glucose.

Essential nutrients might also be promising in the treatment of TBI. Dietary branched-chain amino acids (BCCAs) are important for de novo synthesis of glutamate, which plays an important role in maintaining synaptic neurotransmitter pools. In an experimental model of TBI, BCAAs (i.e., valine, isoleucine, leucine) were found to be reduced (Cole et al., 2010), and dietary delivery resulted in improved cognitive outcomes that correlated with restored net synaptic efficacy. Although these findings are quite encouraging, further studies, as recommended in the next chapter, are needed to determine if this benefit is sustained over time. It is postulated that BCAAs are beneficial as precursors of neurotransmitters as well as providing an alternative energy source. It is unclear to what extent the synthesis neurotransmitters might contribute to the potential effects of BCAAs in TBI, because BCAAs influence the synthesis of both excitatory and inhibitory neurotransmitters.

Other promising interventions include specific diets rather than a single food component or nutrient. The ketogenic diet is a high-fat, low-carbohydrate diet used as a therapy for epilepsy, especially in children (Beniczky et al., 2010). This diet provides an alternative source of fuel to the brain and enhances energy production in the brain when glucose utilization is impaired. Although the mechanisms of protection in epilepsy are not completely understood, it appears that following a ketogenic diet provides resistance to metabolic stress and may thereby provide protection to the injured brain. Animal studies have shown that ketogenic diets improve mitochondrial antioxidant status and protect the DNA (deoxyribonucleic acid) from oxidative damage by increasing glutathione, a major mitochondrial antioxidant, and by reducing both acetyl coA, an indicator of mitochondrial redox status, and lipoic acid, a thiol antioxidant. One drawback of ketogenic diets is that patient compliance is difficult to maintain. Alternative diets could be developed that are more organoleptically acceptable and have similar effects in the brain.

Reduction of Oxidative Stress and Inflammation and Repair of Cellular Damage

Oxidative stress and chronic inflammation are among the root causes of many diseases, such as cardiovascular disease, insulin resistance, autoimmune diseases like rheumatoid arthritis, and Alzheimer's disease. Brain injuries such as ischemic brain injury and TBI have also implicated oxidative stress as a key pathological factor in secondary injury progression. Mitochondria, the main source of cellular ATP production under normal aerobic conditions, are susceptible to reactive oxygen species (ROS), which generate localized oxidative stress.

Injury to the brain also promotes inflammation, which can eventually lead to further tissue damage if not well regulated and resolved promptly. These observations suggest that dietary antioxidant and anti-inflammatory therapy may be useful approaches to promote protective mechanisms in the injured brain (Wu et al., 2006).

One class of nutrients that could be important to improve TBI outcomes is niacin (i.e., vitamin B3, nicotinamide adenine dinucleotide [NAD$^+$]) and its derivatives, since it plays an important role in maintaining and regulating cellular redox states, calcium ion stores, DNA damage and repair, response to cellular stress, and energy metabolism (Xu and Sauve, 2010). Enhanced oxidative stress can induce DNA strand breaks, which in turn are repaired by activation of poly(ADP-ribose) polymerase (PARP). Under certain pathological conditions such as trauma and resulting sepsis, this process of DNA damage and repair can consume large amounts of NAD$^+$, leading to its cellular depletion, which in turn promotes inflammation (Wendel and Heller, 2010). The nuclear protein poly(ADP-ribose) polymerase-1 (PARP-1) functions as a molecular stress sensor and DNA repair mechanism. Overactivation of PARP-1 followed by NAD$^+$ depletion is a major contributor to ischemic brain damage (Love, 1999). PARP-1 is believed to be a key mediator of cell death in excitotoxicity, ischemia, and oxidative stress (Alano et al., 2010). Reactive oxygen species strongly activate the enzymatic activity of PARP-1 (Altmeyer and Hottiger, 2009). Excessive activation of PARP-1 is believed to be a key link between oxidative stress, glutamate excitotoxicity, and cell death (Ying and Xiong, 2010; Yu et al., 2009). NAD$^+$ links PARP-1 to energy metabolism (Altmeyer and Hottiger, 2009), suggesting that NAD$^+$ depletion, such as that observed in TBI, is a causal event in PARP-1 mediated cell death. Preventing the depletion of cytosolic NAD$^+$ that characterizes the massive disruption of energy metabolism following TBI could therefore ameliorate the chain of events that lead to cell death. Despite this role in regulating redox states, a literature search on niacin did not reveal any study to explore its effects in outcomes of TBI. For this reason, niacin was excluded from the list of promising nutritional approaches.

There are numerous other nutrients and food components that have either antioxidant or anti-inflammatory effects and that could potentially be beneficial in TBI pathology. The committee initially selected some because they have been studied extensively in connection with cardiovascular disease and other chronic diseases having inflammation as one of their etiologies. Vitamin E (alpha-tocopherol) is a potent reactive species scavenger that acts as an inhibitor of lipid peroxidation (Marklund et al., 2006). In a 2010 experimental model of TBI, dietary supplementation with alpha-tocopherol has been shown to reduce protein oxidation, increase levels of the antioxidant superoxide dismutase, and improve cognitive outcome (Wu et al., 2010). Identifying compounds such as alpha-tocopherol or alpha-eleostearic acid that mitigate oxidative stress or regulate the release of apoptosis-releasing factors from the mitochondria may yield important therapeutic approaches for the nutritional treatment of neuronal injury (Kondo et al., 2010).

Brain development and function are reliant upon n-3 fatty acids (Bazan, 2007). This group of fatty acids is of particular interest in the setting of TBI because of its potential role as a modulator of inflammation. Two fatty acids, the n-3s docosahexaenoic acid (DHA—C22:6) and eicosapentaenoic acid (EPA—C20:5), support resolution of inflammation (see review, Kidd, 2007). While their mechanisms of action are currently being elucidated, Serhan and colleagues in Appendix J describe a number of studies that led to this conclusion. A hallmark finding of this research is that DHA is metabolized to resolvins and protectins, which are hypothesized to resolve inflammation and protect the brain from further damage. Endogenous neuroprotectin D1, while elevated in a model of brain ischemia, may not be sufficient to thwart the pro-inflammatory response; exogenous administration (intraventricular infusion), however, may reduce inflammation and result in neuroprotection (Bazan, 2007). Taken together, it appears that the mechanistic effects of diets high in n-3 fatty acids, such as DHA or its analogues, warrant further investigation for ameliorating the adverse effects of TBI.

Many phytochemicals, such as flavonoids, may also exert benefits because of their antioxidant or anti-inflammatory actions. Flavonoids consist of two aromatic rings bound together by three carbons that form an oxygenated heterocycle. Flavonoids can be classified into seven subclasses: flavonols (e.g., quercetin), flavones (e.g., apigenin), flavanones (e.g., hesperetin), flavan-3-ols (e.g., epicatechin), anthocyanins (e.g., cyanidin), polymers (e.g., proanthocyanidins), and isoflavones (e.g., genistein). The flavanol epicatechin was shown to be neuroprotective in a stroke model of brain injury (Shah et al., 2010). It is thought that this flavanol supports antioxidant defense mechanisms in the brain by activating the transcription factor Nrf2. This results in an increase in the enzyme heme oxygenase-1, which confers neuroprotection in part by degrading the prooxidant heme to the antioxidants biliverdin and bilirubin (Chang et al., 2005). In the setting of TBI, where heme arises from the breakdown of hemoglobin as well as the release of heme from dying cells, epicatechin may prove to be beneficial (Doré, 2010).

One food component with anti-inflammatory properties is resveratrol (3,4′,5-trihydroxystilbene). Resveratrol belongs to a class of polyphenolic compounds called stilbenes. Some types of plants produce resveratrol and other stilbenes in response to stress and injury, presumably to aid in their recovery process. Resveratrol has been shown to be neuroprotective in animal models of cerebral ischemia. Its exact mechanism of action is not known; there are several hypotheses, one of which is that it acts indirectly by increasing sirtuin-1 (SIRT1) activity during recovery or by sparing cells via 5′ adenosine monophosphate-activated protein kinase's (AMPK's) elevation of NAD+ levels. The NAD-dependent deacetylase, SIRT1, is an enzyme that deacetylates proteins involved in cellular regulation, including reaction to stressors. Recent evidence suggests that SIRT1 inhibitors may be neuroprotective. Based on in vitro studies, resveratrol is also hypothesized to inhibit the activity of several inflammatory enzymes, including cyclooxygenase and lipoxygenase, resulting in a suppressive effect on inflammatory and oxidative stress (Ghanim et al., 2010). Yet another hypothesis states that resveratrol may also inhibit proinflammatory transcription factors, such as NFκB or AP-1. This is supported by a human randomized controlled trial in which resveratrol was shown to exert anti-inflammatory and antioxidative stress effects in normal humans when measured by blood biomarkers (Ghanim et al., 2010). The suppressive effects of this extract on ROS generation and a range of inflammatory mediators suggest that resveratrol may induce its effects through increased expression of anti-inflammatory cytokines and a reduction in proinflammatory molecules, all potentially beneficial implications for TBI.

Curcumin, a phenolic yellow pigment from the rhizome *Curcuma longa* used as a flavoring and coloring agent, especially in curries, is an antioxidant and an anti-inflammatory agent. Curcumin is a potent inhibitor of the proinflammatory cytokine IL-1β and the transcription factor NFκB that are involved in cellular responses to stimuli such as stress, cytokines, and free radicals (Laird et al., 2010).

One compound that deserves attention because of its potential synergism with progesterone therapy is vitamin D. The hormone progesterone and its metabolites are considered pleiotropic drugs that confer neuroprotection by preventing the expression of inflammatory cytokines in the brain while reducing apoptosis, lipid peroxidation, and cerebral edema (Beauchamp et al., 2008) and stimulating growth-promoting factors that may play a significant role in remyelination of damaged neurons. The dosage of progesterone effective for treatment is too high to be feasibly achieved with current commercial dietary supplements. The committee therefore did not consider it as a potential stand-alone nutritional approach to the treatment of TBI; rather, it considered vitamin D$_3$ as an example of a nutrient that may act synergistically with a pharmaceutical product, progesterone. Cekic and Stein (2010) suggest that vitamin D, a potent modulator of cell cycle, immune function, and calcium homeostasis, can work synergistically with progesterone therapy to reduce post-TBI inflammation.

Although microbial proteases have been used as anti-inflammatory agents (e.g., in wounds and hematomas), a review of their effects using the criteria in Box 4-2 did not identify any active research with proteases and TBI or associated conditions; therefore, they were neither considered as promising interventions nor reviewed in this report.

Repair and Recovery

Studies in the late 1990s showed that the brain has the capacity to generate new cells and that these cells can, under defined conditions, become functional. These findings, together with key studies showing the plasticity of the somatosensory circuits, serve as a foundation for understanding mechanisms of adaptability after a brain injury (see review, Kidd, 2009). Repair and recovery mechanisms likely involve revascularization of damaged tissue, neurogenesis, axonal/dendritic plasticity, and changes in neuronal networks. These events may be susceptible to nutritional augmentation approaches. For example, neurotrophins regulate neuronal survival, growth, and synaptic plasticity and neurotransmission, and protect against neuronal injury. One neurotrophin that has received particular attention is brain-derived neurotrophic factor (BDNF), modulated by diet and exercise. Brain-derived neurotrophic factor has been shown to regulate survival, growth, and differentiation of neurons during development, and is associated with learning and memory skills.

The nutrient vitamin E may act to improve neuroplasticity. Utilizing a fluid percussion model in rats, Wu et al. (2010) found that rats receiving dietary supplementation with vitamin E prior to TBI suffered less loss of BDNF and showed better-preserved brain cognition and synaptic plasticity than rats receiving no vitamin E supplementation. Thus, in addition to its antioxidant activity, vitamin E may exert its action via other targets, such as those supporting neuroplasticity.

Dietary curcumin has also been investigated for its potential to counteract the outcome of TBI on synaptic plasticity and cognition, as well as for its antioxidant properties (Wu et al., 2006). Dietary supplementation reduced oxidative damage and normalized levels of BDNF and cyclic AMP-response element-binding protein. It was therefore suggested that oxidative stress may influence synaptic plasticity and cognitive recovery through its actions on BDNF.

Cytidine 5′-diphosphocholine (citicoline or CDP-choline) is an essential intermediate in the biosynthetic pathway of cell membrane phospholipids. It is naturally present in eggs and liver, and also sold as a dietary supplement. It is readily absorbed by the oral route, with no reported serious side effects, and is subsequently widely distributed throughout the body where it is incorporated into membrane and microsomal phospholipids. The two principal components of CDP-choline, cytidine and choline, can cross the blood-brain barrier where they then become incorporated into lipid membranes (Jain, 2008). CDP-choline has been shown to inhibit apoptosis associated with cerebral ischemia and edema and to potentiate neuroplasticity in experimental models. It exerts neuroprotection in hypoxic and ischemic conditions (Secades and Lorenzo, 2006) as well as in rodent models of TBI (Kokiko and Hamm, 2007; Marklund et al., 2006), and is currently in phase III clinical trials for TBI, sponsored by the National Institute of Child Health and Human Development (NICHD) (Jain, 2008; Zafonte et al., 2009).

The antioxidant effects of flavonoids, polyphenolic compounds found in fruits and vegetables as well as wine, tea, and other beverages, are well known. They also exert a multiplicity of neuroprotective actions within the brain, including a potential to protect neurons against injury induced by neurotoxins; an ability to suppress neuroinflammation; and the potential to promote memory, learning, and cognitive function (Spencer, 2009). Flavonoids are believed to interact with critical protein and lipid kinase signaling cascades in the brain that lead to an inhibition of apoptosis and to a promotion of neuronal survival and synaptic plasticity (Spencer, 2009). Based on their actions, it is possible that flavonoids also hold potential to aid in recovery from brain trauma, although this particular aspect of flavonoid therapy has not been the subject of human clinical trials. Spencer (2009) suggests that flavonoids increase peripheral and cerebral blood flow, which in turn support angiogenesis and neurogenesis. Flavonoids likely have other effects on the injured brain, targeting post-transcriptional factors and gene expression, and scavenging neurotoxic and proinflammatory species. Yao and colleagues (2010) also observed that *Epimedium* (a genus of more than 60 species of herbaceous flowering plants in the family Berberidaceae) flavonoids can have a direct stimulatory effect on neuronal stem cell proliferation and differentiation in a rat cell culture model. Altogether, these observations hold promise for the application of flavonoids to neuroprotection.

SUMMARY

The heterogeneity of TBI, together with prolonged secondary pathogenesis and long-lasting adverse neurological sequelae, makes this disease a challenge to manage. In fact, there has never been a single pharmaceutical that has been successful as a therapeutic agent. Interventions targeting features of the acutely injured brain such as hypoxia and excitotoxicity will differ from those that are directed toward the more chronically injured brain that is characterized in part by the emergence of proteinopathies. Alterations in metabolism early after the injury can result in disorders in the areas of motor function, cognition, and neuropsychiatry. Based on the multifaceted nature of the disease, scientists and clinicians recommend a combinatorial approach to its management. Nutritional interventions should not be viewed as stand-alone therapies but rather as support for other therapies, and can range from the clinical support provision of essential nutrients and energy for recovery from major trauma, to individual nutrients or phytochemicals that may uniquely affect the neuronal repair process.

A number of nutrients, dietary supplements, or specific diets act in biological systems in ways that suggests administration to TBI patients before or after injury could improve patient outcomes. For example, restoring energetics, acting as anti-inflammatory or antioxidant agents, or delaying apoptosis could all contribute to faster recovery from TBI. The mechanisms of action of most nutrients are currently not well understood. The committee centered its attention on those compounds shown to act in relevant physiological processes. As an illustration, based upon the clinical success of progesterone and its mechanism of action, it seems logical to focus upon the same clinical goals, that is, to prevent or modulate the expression of inflammatory cytokines (particularly interleukin-6) in the brain while blocking the mechanisms that trigger apoptosis, such as oxidative stress, excess cellular calcium release, and activation of apoptotic genes. The fact that nutrients can affect various pathological responses presents a real advantage in potential interventions. However, when selecting nutritional interventions and conducting reseach, it is essential to consider that the target population is critically ill (see Chapter 17 for other considerations in study designs). Therefore, it is extremely important that adverse events associated with the nutrients be investigated not only in the healthy population, but also in the critically ill. As an example, although probiotics have shown some benefits for TBI, care should be taken when considering administering these to critically ill persons because of potential adverse effects (Besselink et al., 2008).

Based on the expert opinion of the committee and the target areas identified as relevant for nutrition, the following nutritional interventions were identified for review: energy needs for severe cases of TBI, acetyl-CoA, antioxidants, branched-chain amino acids, choline, creatine, ketogenic diets, magnesium, nicotinamide adenine dinucleotide (NAD^+), n-3 fatty acids, polyphenols, probiotics, vitamin D, and zinc. The committee searched the literature using the database Medline and employing the parameters shown in Box 4-2. Three of the nutritional interventions (i.e., acetyl-L-carnitine, niacin, and probiotics) initially selected were not included in the report because of insufficient evidence from animal and human studies to reach conclusions about their effectiveness, or concerns for harm. Based on the existence of promising data from animal or human studies on TBI (or the associated conditions listed in Box 4-2), the committee selected the following ten nutritional interventions to review in greater detail: energy needs (Chapter 6), antioxidants (i.e., vitamins E and C) (Chapter 7), branched-chain amino acids (Chapter 8), choline (Chapter 9), creatine (Chapter 10), ketogenic and modified diets (Chapter 11), magnesium (Chapter 12), omega-3 fatty acids (Chapter 13), polyphenols (i.e., flavonoids, resveratrol, and curcumin) (Chapter 14), vitamin D (Chapter 15), and zinc (Chapter 16).

REFERENCES

Alano, C. C., P. Garnier, W. Ying, Y. Higashi, T. M. Kauppinen, and R. A. Swanson. 2010. NAD+ depletion is necessary and sufficient for poly(ADP-ribose) polymerase-1-mediated neuronal death. *Journal of Neuroscience* 30(8):2967–2978.

Altmeyer, M., and M. O. Hottiger. 2009. Poly(ADP-ribose) polymerase 1 at the crossroad of metabolic stress and inflammation in aging. *Aging* 1(5):458–469.

Arun, P., P. S. Ariyannur, J. R. Moffet, G. Xing, K. Hamilton, N. E. Grunberg, J. A. Ives, and A. M. Namboodiri. 2010. Metabolic actetate therapy for the treatment of traumatic brain injury. *Journal of Neurotrauma* 27(1):293–298.

Bales, J. W., A. K. Wagner, A. E. Kline, and C. E. Dixon. 2009. Persistent cognitive dysfunction after traumatic brain injury: A dopamine hypothesis. *Neuroscience and Biobehavioral Reviews* 33(7):981–1003.

Bazan, N. G. 2006. The onset of brain injury and neurodegeneration triggers the synthesis of docosanoid neuroprotective signaling. *Cellular and Molecular Neurobiology* 26(4–6):901–913.

Bazan, N. G. 2007. Omega-3 fatty acids, pro-inflammatory signaling and neuroprotection. *Current Opinion in Clinical Nutrition and Metabolic Care* 10(2):136–141.

Bazan, N. G., V. L. Marcheselli, and K. Cole-Edwards. 2005. Brain response to injury and neurodegeneration—Endogenous neuroprotective signaling. *Annals of the New York Academy of Sciences* 1053:137–147.

Beauchamp, K., H. Mutlak, W. R. Smith, E. Shohami, and P. F. Stahel. 2008. Pharmacology of traumatic brain injury: Where is the "golden bullet"? *Molecular Medicine* 14(11–12):731–740.

Beniczky, S., M. Jose Miranda, J. Alving, J. Heber Povlsen, and P. Wolf. 2010. Effectiveness of the ketogenic diet in a broad range of seizure types and EEG features for severe childhood epilepsies. *Acta Neurologica Scandinavica* 121(1):58–62.

Besselink, M. G., H. C. van Santvoort, E. Buskens, M. A. Boermeester, H. van Goor, H. M. Timmerman, V. B. Nieuwenhuijs, T. L. Bollen, B. van Ramshorst, B. J. Witteman, C. Rosman, R. J. Ploeg, M. A. Brink, A. F. Schaapherder, C. H. Dejong, P. J. Wahab, C. J. van Laarhoven, E. van der Harst, C. H. van Eijck, M. A. Cuesta, L. M. Akkermans, and H. G. Gooszen. 2008. Probiotic prophylaxis in predicted severe acute pancreatitis: A randomized, double-blind, placebo-controlled trial. *The Lancet* 371(9613):651–659.

Boehning, D., R. L. Patterson, L. Sedaghat, N. O. Glebova, T. Kurosaki, and S. H. Snyder. 2003. Cytochrome c binds to inositol (1,4,5) trisphosphate receptors, amplifying calcium-dependent apoptosis. *Nature Cell Biology* 5(12):1051–1061.

Bramlett, H. M., and W. D. Dietrich. 2004. Pathophysiology of cerebral ischemia and brain trauma: Similarities and differences. *Journal of Cerebral Blood Flow and Metabolism* 24(2):133–150.

Cekic, M., and D. G. Stein. 2010. Traumatic brain injury and aging: Is a combination of progesterone and vitamin D hormone a simple solution to a complex problem? *Neurotherapeutics* 7(1):81–90.

Chang, E. F., C. P. Claus, H. J. Vreman, R. J. Wong, and L. J. Noble-Haeusslein. 2005. Heme regulation in traumatic brain injury: Relevance to the adult and developing brain. *Journal of Cerebral Blood Flow and Metabolism* 25(11):1401–1417.

Cole, J. T., C. M. Mitala, S. Kundu, A. Verma, J. A. Elkind, I. Nissim, and A. S. Cohen. 2010. Dietary branched chain amino acids ameliorate injury-induced cognitive impairment. *Proceedings of the National Academy of Sciences of the United States of America* 107(1):366–371.

Dietrich, W. D., and H. M. Bramlett. 2010. The evidence for hypothermia as a neuroprotectant in traumatic brain injury. *Neurotherapeutics* 7(1):43–50.

Doré, S. 2010. Mechanisms of Nutritional Neuroprotection: Neuroprotective action of the flavanol (–)-epicatechin. Presented at the IOM Nutrition and Neuroprotection in Military Personnel Workshop, Washington, DC.

Dubreuil, C. I., N. Marklund, K. Deschamps, T. K. McIntosh, and L. McKerracher. 2006. Activation of Rho after traumatic brain injury and seizure in rats. *Experimental Neurology* 198(2):361–369.

Faden, A. I. 2002. Neuroprotection and traumatic brain injury: Theoretical option or realistic proposition. *Current Opinion in Neurology* 15(6):707–712.

Ghanim, H., C. L. Sia, S. Abuaysheh, K. Korzeniewski, P. Patnaik, A. Marumganti, A. Chaudhuri, and P. Dandona. 2010. An antiinflammatory and reactive oxygen species suppressive effects of an extract of polygonum cuspidatum containing resveratrol. *The Journal of Clinical Endocrinology and Metabolism* 95(9):E1–E8.

Graham, D. I., T. K. McIntosh, W. L. Maxwell, and J. A. Nicoll. 2000. Recent advances in neurotrauma. *Journal of Neuropathology and Experimental Neurology* 59(8):641–651.

Jain, K. K. 2008. Neuroprotection in traumatic brain injury. *Drug Discovery Today* 13(23–24):1082–1089.

Kidd, P. M. 2007. Omega-3 DHA and EPA for cognition, behavior, and mood: Clinical findings and structural-functional synergies with cell membrane phospholipids. *Alternative Medicine Review* 12(3):207–227.

Kidd, P. M. 2009. Integrated brain restoration after ischemic stroke—medical management, risk factors, nutrients, and other interventions for managing inflammation and enhancing brain plasticity. *Alternative Medicine Review* 14(1):14–35.

Kokiko, O. N., and R. J. Hamm. 2007. A review of pharmacological treatments used in experimental models of traumatic brain injury. *Brain Injury* 21(3):259–274.

Kondo, K., S. Obitsu, S. Ohta, K. Matsunami, H. Otsuka, and R. Teshima. 2010. Poly(ADP-ribose) polymerase (PARP)-1-independent apoptosis-inducing factor (AIF) release and cell death are induced by eleostearic acid and blocked by alpha-tocopherol and MEK inhibition. *Journal of Biological Chemistry* 285(17):13079–13091.

Laird, M. D., S. Sukumari-Ramesh, A. E. Swift, S. E. Meiler, J. R. Vender, and K. M. Dhandapani. 2010. Curcumin attenuates cerebral edema following traumatic brain injury in mice: A possible role for aquaporin-4? *Journal of Neurochemistry* 113(3):637–648.

Longhi, L., K. E. Saatman, R. Raghupathi, H. L. Laurer, P. M. Lenzlinger, P. Riess, E. Neugebauer, J. Q. Trojanowski, V. M. Y. Lee, M. S. Grady, D. I. Graham, and T. K. McIntosh. 2001. A review and rationale for the use of genetically engineered animals in the study of traumatic brain injury. *Journal of Cerebral Blood Flow and Metabolism* 21(11):1241–1258.

Love, S. 1999. Oxidative stress in brain ischemia. *Brain Pathology* 9(1):119–131.

Maas, A. I. R., B. Roozenbeek, and G. T. Manley. 2010. Clinical trials in traumatic brain injury: Past experience and current developments. *Neurotherapeutics* 7(1):115–126.

Mammis, A., T. K. McLntosh, and A. H. Maniker. 2009. Erythropoietin as a neuroprotective agent in traumatic brain injury review. *Surgical Neurology* 71(5):527–531.

Margulies, S., R. Hicks, and B. Combination Therapies Traumatic. 2009. Combination therapies for traumatic brain injury: Prospective considerations. *Journal of Neurotrauma* 26(6):925–939.

Marklund, N., A. Bakshi, D. J. Castelbuono, V. Conte, and T. K. McIntosh. 2006. Evaluation of pharmacological treatment strategies in traumatic brain injury. *Current Pharmaceutical Design* 12(13):1645–1680.

Marklund, N., K. Salci, A. Lewen, and L. Hillered. 1997. Glycerol as a marker for post-traumatic membrane phospholipid degradation in rat brain. *Neuroreport* 8(6):1457–1461.

Mattson, M. P., and S. L. Chan. 2003. Calcium orchestrates apoptosis. *Nature Cell Biology* 5(12):1041–1043.

Mattson, M. P., W. Z. Duan, S. L. Chan, A. W. Cheng, N. Haughey, D. S. Gary, Z. H. Guo, J. W. Lee, and K. Furukawa. 2002. Neuroprotective and neurorestorative signal transduction mechanisms in brain aging: Modification by genes, diet and behavior. *Neurobiology of Aging* 23(5):695–705.

Moppett, I. K. 2007. Traumatic brain injury: Assessment, resuscitation and early management. *British Journal of Anaesthesia* 99(1):18–31.

Morales, D. M., N. Marklund, D. Lebold, H. J. Thompson, A. Pitkanen, W. L. Maxwell, L. Longhi, H. Laurer, M. Maegele, E. Neugebauer, D. I. Graham, N. Stocchetti, and T. K. McIntosh. 2005. Experimental models of traumatic brain injury: Do we really need to build a better mousetrap? *Neuroscience* 136(4):971–989.

Morganti-Kossmann, M. C., L. Satgunaseelan, N. Bye, and T. Kossmann. 2007. Modulation of immune response by head injury. *Injury* 38(12):1392–1400.

Povlishock, J. T., and D. I. Katz. 2005. Update of neuropathology and neurological recovery after traumatic brain injury. *Journal of Head Trauma Rehabilitation* 20(1):76–94.

Raghupathi, R. 2004. Cell death mechanisms following traumatic brain injury. *Brain Pathology* 14(2):215–222.

Royo, N. C., S. Shimizu, J. W. Schouten, J. F. Stover, and T. K. McIntosh. 2003. Pharmacology of traumatic brain injury. *Current Opinion in Pharmacology* 3(1):27–32.

Schouten, J. W. 2007. Neuroprotection in traumatic brain injury: A complex struggle against the biology of nature. *Current Opinion in Critical Care* 13(2):134–142.

Scudellari, M. 2010. Brain, interrupted. *The Scientist* 24(7):37, http://www.the-scientist.com/2010/7/1/37/1/ (accessed July 19, 2010).

Secades, J. J., and J. L. Lorenzo. 2006. Citicoline: Pharmacological and clinical review, 2006 update. *Methods and Findings in Experimental and Clinical Pharmacology* 28:1–56.

Sen, A. P., and A. Gulati. 2010. Use of magnesium in traumatic brain injury. *Neurotherapeutics* 7(1):91–99.

Shah, Z. A., R. C. Li, A. S. Ahmad, T. W. Kensler, M. Yamamoto, S. Biswal, and S. Dore. 2010. The flavanol (−)-epicatechin prevents stroke damage through the Nrf2/HO1 pathway. *Journal of Cerebral Blood Flow Metabolism* 30(12):1951–61.

Spencer, J. P. E. 2009. Flavonoids and brain health: Multiple effects underpinned by common mechanisms. *Genes and Nutrition* 4(4):243–250.

Stein, D. G., D. W. Wright, and A. L. Kellermann. 2008. Does progesterone have neuroprotective properties? *Annals of Emergency Medicine* 51(2):164–172.

Stetler, R. A., Y. Gan, W. Zhang, A. K. Liou, Y. Gao, G. Cao, and J. Chen. 2010. Heat shock proteins: Cellular and molecular mechanisms in the CNS. *Progress in Neurobiology* 92(2):184–211.

Sullivan, P. G., J. D. Geiger, M. P. Mattson, and S. W. Scheff. 2000. Dietary supplement creatine protects against traumatic brain injury. *Annals of Neurology* 48(5):723–729.

Thompson, H. J., J. Lifshitz, N. Marklund, M. S. Grady, D. I. Graham, D. A. Hovda, and T. K. McIntosh. 2005. Lateral fluid percussion brain injury: A 15-year review and evaluation. *Journal of Neurotrauma* 22(1):42–75.

Thompson, H. J., N. Marklund, D. G. LeBold, D. M. Morales, C. A. Keck, M. Vinson, N. C. Royo, R. Grundy, and T. K. McIntosh. 2006. Tissue sparing and functional recovery following experimental traumatic brain injury is provided by treatment with an anti-myelin-associated glycoprotein antibody. *European Journal of Neuroscience* 24(11):3063–3072.

Unterberg, A. W., J. Stover, B. Kress, and K. L. Kiening. 2004. Edema and brain trauma. *Neuroscience* 129(4):1021–1029.

Wendel, M., and A. R. Heller. 2010. Mitochondrial function and dysfunction in sepsis. *Wiener Medizinische Wochenschrift* 160(5–6):118–123.

Werner, C., and K. Engelhard. 2007. Pathophysiology of traumatic brain injury. *British Journal of Anaesthesia* 99(1):4–9.

Wu, A., Z. Ying, and F. Gomez-Pinilla. 2006. Dietary curcumin counteracts the outcome of traumatic brain injury on oxidative stress, synaptic plasticity, and cognition. *Experimental Neurology* 197(2):309–317.

Wu, A. G., Z. Ying, and F. Gomez-Pinilla. 2010. Vitamin E protects against oxidative damage and learning disability after mild traumatic brain injury in rats. *Neurorehabilitation and Neural Repair* 24(3):290–298.

Xu, P., and A. A. Sauve. 2010. Vitamin B3, the nicotinamide adenine dinucleotides and aging. *Mechanisms of Ageing and Development* 131(4):287–298.

Yao, R. Q., L. Zhang, X. L. Li, and L. Li. 2010. Effects of epimedium flavonoids on proliferation and differentiation of neural stem cells in vitro. *Neurological Research* 32(7):736–742.

Yi, J. H., and A. S. Hazell. 2006. Excitotoxic mechanisms and the role of astrocytic glutamate transporters in traumatic brain injury. *Neurochemistry International* 48(5):394–403.

Ying, W., and Z. G. Xiong. 2010. Oxidative stress and NAD(+) in ischemic brain injury: Current advances and future perspectives. *Current Medicinal Chemistry* 17(20):2152–2158.

Yu, S.-W., Y. Wang, D. S. Frydenlund, O. P. Ottersen, V. L. Dawson, and T. M. Dawson. 2009. Outer mitochondrial membrane localization of apoptosis-inducing factor: Mechanistic implications for release. *ASN Neuro* 1(5).

Zafonte, R., W. T. Friedewald, S. M. Lee, B. Levin, R. Diaz-Arrastia, B. Ansel, H. Eisenberg, S. D. Timmons, N. Temkin, T. Novack, J. Ricker, R. Merchant, and J. Jallo. 2009. The citicoline brain injury treatment (COBRIT) trial: Design and methods. *Journal of Neurotrauma* 26(12):2207–2216.

Zanelli, S. A., N. J. Solenski, R. E. Rosenthal, and G. Fiskum. 2005. Mechanisms of ischemic neuroprotection by acetyl-l-carnitine. *Annals of the New York Academy of Sciences* 1053:153–161.

5

Acquiring Resilience to TBI Prior to Injury

The concept that the brain is a flexible organ that can be affected by its environment has only recently begun to be accepted in the scientific community. As a result, the fields of nutrition and central nervous system function have only started to coalesce within the past few decades, attempting to associate nutrition and diet with improvements in behavior, cognition, and alertness. As demonstrated in Chapter 3, information about the pathological processes of traumatic brain injury (TBI) and their timing is also incomplete, especially when considering the diversity in brain injuries. There are still questions and challenges in attempting to identify promising nutrition interventions to increase resilience to TBI. Still, using nutrition as a preventive intervention is a sensible proposition, since it appears that the presence or absence of a nutrient (see Chapters 6–16) within minutes to hours of the injury may have the potential to influence the outcome.

The problem of identifying promising nutritional interventions for TBI was faced from two different angles: resilience and treatment. The committee uses the term resilience to refer to the effect of interventions that occur before the insult. A nutritional intervention may impart resilience in two general ways, by preventing or interrupting pathological processes postinjury, or by enhancing the damage repair process. This chapter provides the committee's thinking about the importance of nutrition in providing resilience. In addition, the chapter summarizes military nutrition standards and what is known about the diets of military personnel.

INTRODUCTION

Over time, both the North American Dietary Reference Intakes (DRIs) and the Military Dietary Reference Intakes (MDRIs) have shifted their focus from preventing deficiencies to promoting optimal health. Among the nutrients that offer promise in providing resilience and are therefore important to consider are both essential (e.g., vitamins E and C) and non-essential food components (e.g., creatine and resveratrol). This section explores the concept that dietary intake prior to experience of a TBI event affects the outcomes. The evidence, based on studies conducted to investigate the resilience imparted by specific nutrients or food components, is presented in Chapters 6–16.

Research clearly indicates that malnourished patients have longer hospitalizations and poorer surgical outcomes than well-nourished patients (Garrouste-Orgeas et al., 2004; O'Brien et al., 2006; Tremblay and Bandi, 2003). However, research also indicates that in a generally adequately nourished population, short-term reduction of protein and energy intake prior to surgery is not significantly related to outcomes. This is relevant to discussion of military service members because they sometimes undergo short periods of time during special missions when dietary intakes may be less than the MDRIs, but these short-term deficits apparently do not affect their health status or performance. Based on the Department of Defense (DoD) testimony, the committee assumed that the nutrition status of active-duty military personnel is similar to that of the general population of the United States. Even with the presumption that their nutrition status is adequate, there may still be opportunities to target intake of specific nutrients having the potential to maximize resilience to an injury such as TBI.

The question of how to maximize the use of nutrition to optimize resilience to TBI should address the overall nutritional status of military personnel, but it should also identify particular nutrients that may be more important than others in a generally well-nourished population. In order to plan menus and rations to ensure adequate diets for military personnel, military nutrition standards and menu-planning procedures have been established and implemented. In the future, these standards and procedures might consider specific nutrition approaches if there is evidence that they would benefit those at higher risk of experiencing TBI.

MILITARY NUTRITION STANDARDS

Historically, the military has reviewed the nutrition standards (DRIs) for the general U.S. population and determined whether adjustments were necessary for military personnel, specifically for those experiencing situations unique to the military, such as being deployed in extreme environments and under high levels of physical and mental stress. Previous reports concluded that service members may have nutritional requirements that differ from those of the general U.S. population. Previous committees of the Institute of Medicine (IOM) also have recognized that the dietary intake of military personnel might be different from that of the general U.S. population and have recommended evaluation of nutritional status throughout the military services (e.g., IOM, 2006, *Mineral Requirements for Military Personnel*). The MDRIs were last updated in 2001 in a tri-service regulation (Baker-Fulco et al., 2001; U.S. Departments of the Army, 2001). This regulation established nutritional standards for military feeding as well as nutritional standards for operational rations (NSORs). The Army, the lead agency, is tasked with the responsibility to "establish nutritional standards of meals served to military personnel subsisting under normal operating conditions and while under simulated or actual combat conditions" and "establish nutritional standards for operational rations and restricted rations." Each military service is responsible for ensuring there are mechanisms in place to meet nutritional standards in menus, including compliance requirements in contracts with food service operations. The current MDRIs, shown in Table 5-1, were adapted from the 1989 Recommended Dietary Allowances (RDA, 10th revised edition) and thereafter from the DRIs for the following nutrients: calcium, phosphorus, magnesium, vitamin D, fluoride, thiamine, riboflavin, niacin, vitamin B_6, folate, vitamin B_{12}, pantothenic acid, biotin, choline, vitamin C, vitamin E, selenium, and carotenoids (Baker-Fulco et al., 2001). The regulation acknowledged that DRIs for some nutrients (i.e., vitamins A and K,

TABLE 5-1 Comparison of Current MDRIs[a] with DRIs

		Men[b]		Women[b]	
	Unit	MDRI	RDA, AI[c]	MDRI	RDA, AI[c]
Energy,[d] general/ routine	Kcal/d	3,250	Based on weight, height, and activity levels	2,300	Based on weight, height, and activity levels
Light activity	Kcal/d	3,000	See above	2,200	See above
Moderate activity	Kcal/d	3,250	See above	2,300	See above
Heavy activity	Kcal/d	3,950	See above	2,700	See above
Exceptionally heavy activity	Kcal/d	4,600	See above	3,150	See above
Protein[e]	g/d	91 (63–119)	56	72 (50–93)	46
Vitamin A	µg RE/d	1,000	900	800	700
Vitamin D	µg/d	5	15	5	15
Vitamin E	mg/d	15	15	15	15
Vitamin K	µg/d	80	120[c]	65	90[c]
Vitamin C	mg/d	90	90	75	75
Choline	mg/d	–	550	–	425
Thiamin	mg/d	1.2	1.2	1.1	1.1
Riboflavin	mg/d	1.3	1.3	1.1	1.1
Niacin[f]	mg NE/d	16	16	14	14
Vitamin B$_6$	mg/d	1.3	1.3	1.3	1.3
Folate[g]	mg DFE/d	400	400	400	400
Vitamin B$_{12}$	µg/d	2.4	2.4	2.4	2.4
Calcium	mg/d	1,000	1,000	1,000	1,000
Phosphorus[a]	mg/d	700	700	700	700
Magnesium	mg/d	420	400–420	320	310–320
Iron	mg/d	10	8	15	18
Zinc	mg/d	15	11	12	8
Sodium	mg/d	5,000 (4,550–5,525)	1,500[c]	3,600 (3,220–3,910)	1,500[c]
Iodine	µg/d	150	150	150	150
Selenium	µg/d	55	55	55	55
Fluoride	mg/d	4.0	4[c]	3.1	3[c]
Potassium	mg/d	3,200	4,700[c]	2,500	4,700[c]

[a] Values for energy, protein, and associated nutrients are expressed as average daily nutrient intakes and based on moderate activity levels and reference body weights of 79 kg (174 lb) for military men and 62 kg (136 lb) for military women.

[b] RDA values represent those for adults ages 19–50 years old.

[c] AI = Adequate Intake. Data were insufficient to determine an RDA.

AMDR = Acceptable Macronutrient Distribution Range. This is the percentage of energy intake that is associated with reduced risk of chronic disease and provides adequate amounts of essential nutrients.

[d] Energy recommendations for various activity levels are estimates only and vary among individuals. The general values are for moderate levels of activity and are appropriate for most personnel in garrison. Values are rounded up to the nearest 50 kcal.

[e] The RDA for protein is based on 0.8 g/kg/day; the MDRI for protein was based on 0.8–1.5 g/kg/day.

[f] Expressed as mg/day as niacin equivalents (NE). 1 mg of niacin = 60 mg of tryptophan.

[g] Expressed as µg/day as dietary folate equivalents (DFEs). 1 DFE = 1 µg food folate = 0.6 µg of folic acid from fortified food or as a supplement consumed with food = 0.5 µg of folic acid from a supplement taken on an empty stomach.

SOURCES: IOM, 2006a, 2010; U.S. Departments of the Army, Navy, and Air Force, 2001.

chromium, copper, iodine, iron, manganese, molybdenum, and zinc) were published after the MDRIs were established, and that interim guidance would be necessary to update the regulation as new DRI reports were published (U.S. Departments of the Army, Navy, and Air Force, 2001).

The MDRIs are currently under revision, and increases from the previous MDRIs are being considered for three nutrients (vitamin K, iron [for women], and potassium), while decreases are being considered for four nutrients (vitamin A, iron [for men], sodium, and fluoride).

In addition to the MDRIs, there are also NSORs for rations that are intended for use under limited circumstances. Operational rations include meals, ready-to-eat (MREs) and group feeding rations (Unitized B ration, and Unitized Group rations); these are also designed to be nutritionally adequate, and menus, when averaged, will meet the NSORs. Restricted rations (e.g., survival rations; meals, cold weather; long-range patrol rations) are intended for special purposes and for short-term use (i.e., less than 10 days) and are not required to be nutritionally adequate. The MDRIs consider military circumstances that affect nutrient requirements, such as the need for higher intake of energy and some minerals when performing intensely demanding physical tasks in a variety of environments (e.g., extremes of altitude or temperature). The military also has considered adding to the rations components that improve cognitive functions essential for the performance of military duties, like attentiveness or the ability to make rapid decisions. One such example that was reviewed and later introduced into rations is caffeine. As new challenges emerge, such as TBI in all its forms, military diets will need to be reconsidered and readjusted.

DEVELOPMENT OF MENUS

The committee was asked to assume that both predeployment and postdeployment nutritional intakes are similar to the diets of the general U.S. population as evaluated in the National Health and Nutrition Examination Survey (NHANES) and Dietary Guidelines Advisory Committee reports.[1,2] While in theater, many deployed service members are provided food comparable to meals in a garrison dining facility. The in-theater menus are developed at Fort Lee by the Joint Culinary Center of Excellence (JCCoE) in accordance with the Army and DoD nutritional standards (AR 40-25) and the Army menu standards (AR 30-22 and DA PAM 30-22). AR 40-25 provides the nutritional foundation of the menu while AR 30-22/DA PAM 30-22 describes the procedures used to meet the nutrition standards through menu patterns and food choices. As prescribed in AR 40-25, 2-1f, menus are required to meet the MDRIs over a 5- to 10-day period.

Oversight of menus prepared by JCCoE is provided by the Food Service Management Board (FSMB). Briefly, the FSMB consists of the food program manager/food advisor, a dietitian, a supply representative, representatives from all supported major subordinate commands, prime vendor representatives, a preventive medicine representative, and a veterinary services member. One of the primary functions of the FSMB is to review the menu and incorporate new products based on their nutritional value, sensory appeal, and customer and regional preferences. Changes made to the JCCoE menus at the local installation level are reviewed by the dietitian, a voting member of the FSMB, who provides feedback on nutritional adequacy of menus. Nutrient analysis is not routinely conducted when planned menu items are replaced with other items because of local food preferences or other causes. The

---

[1] Available online: http://www.cdc.gov/nchs/nhanes.htm (accessed December 23, 2010).
[2] Available online: http://www.cnpp.usda.gov/DGAs2010-DGACReport.htm (accessed January 14, 2010).

dietitian's designated role at the FSMB is to recommend specific changes in levels of nutrients when necessary to preserve the health of the troops, to review the menus and compare them with standards, to advise the board on the nutritional aspects of revised menus, to educate and advise the board on nutritional topics such as the nutritive value of each product sample and current nutrition trends, and to discuss the availability of more healthful products with the prime vendor for the local installation.

The performance of contract services that provide food for the dining facilities in theater is reviewed by a Quality Assurance Evaluator. Although evaluators complete the Food Service Contract Management (FSCM) course and other training for the Contracting Officer Representative/Quality Assurance Evaluator, they are not required to have nutrition knowledge. Evaluators assess whether the menus in dining facilities meet the standards in regulations AR 30-22 and DA PAM 30-22 for providing the components of meals, but they do not conduct nutritional analyses of menus.

DIETS OF MILITARY PERSONNEL

As explained above, menus offered in contract dining facilities in theater are intended to meet the MDRIs, but each service member's actual nutrient intake is of course dependent on the individual's knowledge, preferences, and habits. Although a one-hour block of nutrition education is included during basic training, it isn't clear whether this is sufficient to ensure adequate understanding of the importance of general nutrition in overall performance. An Army nutrition education initiative called Go for Green that color-codes menu items according to nutrition characteristics may provide additional valuable information to help support more healthful choices by soldiers. The Go for Green nutrition education program allows incorporation of additional nutritional criteria when the science becomes strong enough. The outcomes of this initiative have not been measured yet. Similar nutrition education in other services may also be appropriate, as well as nutrition education targeted to particular military situations or concerns, e.g., specific to TBI when the likelihood of this type of injury is high. The Soldier Fueling Initiative provides additional concrete examples of how to use menu-planning items when menu standards are modified (e.g., the inclusion of more foods high in specific nutrients).[3]

Although it could be argued that the dietary intake of those with access to dining facilities mirrors that of the general U.S. population, data documenting current dietary intake while in theater are not available. Other service members consume a variety of operational rations while on patrols in remote areas, which should also be considered when attempting to provide nutrition support for resilience to TBI. Service members do not normally subsist solely on operational rations (e.g., MREs) for longer than 21 days, but unfortunately there is only limited data available for intake under these circumstances. The proportion of deployed service members consuming each of the various rations[4] is not known. Likewise, information on the intake of these rations by military personnel is also not available. There are further variations in the components of the rations based on availability, and the logistics of transporting food in theater will have a significant effect on what is actually served.

Informal reports from deployed military dietitians indicate that some military members lose significant weight (either intentionally or unintentionally) while deployed, while others, given constant access to dining facilities, gain weight. It is acknowledged that in longer

---

[3] Available online: http://www.quartermaster.army.mil/jccoe/Operations_Directorate/QUAD/Nutrition/nutrition_main.html (accessed December 23, 2010).

[4] A rations that include fresh, frozen, and canned foods; B rations consisting of only canned and dried foods (e.g., unitized rations); and operational rations such as MREs or other specific operational rations.

deployments individuals can respond in different ways: from using the time away to actively seek optimal health by restricting calories to lose weight accompanied with working out to increase physical fitness, to eating unrestrictedly because a variety of food is available throughout the day. In addition other factors may affect dietary intake such as the risk of going outside to dining facilities or the reluctance to don the appropriate protective gear for the short interval needed for mealtime (Col. George Dilly, personal communication, July 2010). For these reasons, the committee was not persuaded that it is appropriate to use dietary intake data on the general U.S. population as a surrogate measure for military intake in theater, and concluded that it would be more prudent to assess military diets.

Ascertaining the actual preinjury intake of specific nutrients of interest from the variety of rations as well as dietary supplements in both types of military environments (i.e., eating in dining facilities or a predominantly ration diet) is critical to determining the policies and procedures most likely to ensure that military personnel receive optimal nutrition to promote resilience to TBI. Previous reports (e.g., IOM, 2008) identified the need for ongoing monitoring of usual dietary intake that included both food and dietary supplements to serve as the basis of nutrition policies, and this report likewise identifies that as a critical gap in knowledge.

Table 5-2 summarizes the NHANES data on dietary intakes for comparable U.S. populations and is provided for illustration. Although NHANES does include dietary supplements, there are only limited data available on their use. The data below should be interpreted in the context that approximately one-third of military personnel regularly use multivitamins, multiminerals, or both as dietary supplements.

NHANES data can be reviewed to estimate nutrition status of military personnel, assuming that the military dietary intake is similar to that of the general U.S. population. These data indicate that for a relatively high proportion of the general U.S. population, dietary intakes are less (e.g., vitamin A, magnesium, vitamin E, and zinc) than the Estimated Average Requirements. Other nutrients (e.g., choline, eicosapentaenoic or docosahexaenoic acids) are not specifically addressed in these datasets. Researchers have concluded that choline intake is likely to be low, but this is difficult to ascertain due to genetic polymorphisms that seem to modulate requirements. Databases providing the choline content of foods were not available until recently. Using the 2003–2004 NHANES data, researchers have estimated that only 10 percent of the U.S. population has choline intakes that meet or exceed the Adequate Intake level (Zeisel and da Costa, 2009).

Some dietary components or bioactives of particular interest to the military in the past because of their high frequency of use, potential for adverse effects, or both (the reader is referred to the 2008 IOM review of dietary supplement use by military personnel) are also important in the context of this study because of their possible influence on brain function and neurological outcome. Owing to the unique demands of military operations, intake of 100–600 mg/day of caffeine has been recommended for military personnel to maintain cognitive performance in situations of sleep deprivation and to enhance physical endurance, especially when affected by high altitude (IOM, 2001). It should be noted, however, that chronic frequent use of caffeine can lead to tolerance and reduce these benefits. As noted in the 2008 IOM report, not all aspects of cognitive and neurobehavioral functions may be affected by caffeine, and it may compromise physical performance in certain environments because of its physiological effects at high dosages, sustained intake, or both, such as heat retention and dieresis.

Besides coffee, which remains the primary source of caffeine among the U.S. population, soft drinks, tea, and energy drinks are substantial contributors to caffeine consumption. Within the military, tolerance caused by the increase in caffeine intake via widespread

TABLE 5-2 Current Status in U.S. Diet Compared to DRI

	Percent Less Than EAR	
	Male, Aged 19+ y	Female, Aged 19+ y
Vitamin A	57	48
Vitamin E	89	97
Thiamin	4	10
Riboflavin	< 3	< 3
Niacin	< 3	< 3
Vitamin B$_6$	7	28
Folate	6	16
Vitamin B$_{12}$	< 3 for ages 19–50	< 3 for ages 19–50
Vitamin C	40	38
Phosphorus	< 3	< 3
NHANES 05–06	< 3	3 (0.7)
Magnesium	64	67
NHANES 05–06	53	56
Iron	< 3	10
Zinc	11	17
Copper	< 3	10
Selenium	< 3	< 3
	Percent Less Than Adequate Intake	
Vitamin K	80	59
Potassium	94	> 97
Dietary fiber	> 97	92
Linoleic acid 18:2	47	44
Linolenic acid 18:3	47	39

SOURCES: Adapted from Moshfegh et al., 2005, 2009.

consumption of beverages and dietary supplements or medications may reduce caffeine's cognitive and physical performance–enhancing benefits. Furthermore, beverages like energy drinks often contain other methylxanthines and caffeine analogues, such as guarana, in addition to other herbal compounds, like ginseng; the mechanisms of action, potential benefits, and safety concerns of these substances remain unclear.

Emerging evidence suggests that caffeine exerts a neuroprotective effect in animal models of TBI, stroke, and Parkinson's disease (Sachse et al., 2008). A retrospective study of caffeine concentration measured in cerebrospinal fluid of patients with severe TBI also found an association between caffeine concentration and favorable Glasgow Outcome Scale scores (Sachse et al., 2008). However, the evidence, depending on the dose, model, and timing, is conflicting, and warrants further investigation.

The combination of caffeine and alcohol has been found to be beneficial in experimental TBI and stroke models (Dash et al., 2004). Even on its own, alcohol has also been associated with improved outcomes in patients with moderate to severe TBI (Berry et al., 2010; Opreanu et al., 2010). Despite a possible neuroprotective role of alcohol, it is important to emphasize that alcohol intoxication is a leading factor in civilian cases of TBI, especially among individuals with a history of substance abuse. At the same time, TBI is a noted risk factor for substance abuse (Graham and Cardon, 2008). Excessive and chronic consumption of alcohol has also been associated with negative interactions with certain nutrients, such as impaired absorption (zinc), depletion (magnesium), and depressed fatty-acid oxidation (polyunsaturated fatty acids) (IOM, 2006b).

DIETARY SUPPLEMENT USE BY THE MILITARY

Even assuming that the eating habits of deployed military personnel are not significantly different from those of the general U.S. population, total nutrient intake may still vary because of dietary supplement use. In a representative sample of active-duty U.S. Army soldiers (n = 990), Lieberman and colleagues (2010) found that 53 percent of participants reported taking any dietary supplement one or more times per week during the preceding six months. The most commonly used dietary supplements were multivitamins, multiminerals, or both (37.5 percent), protein and amino acids (18.7 percent), and individual vitamins and minerals (17.9 percent). Deployment status appeared to be associated with patterns of dietary supplement use. Soldiers in Iraq were less likely than those stationed in the continental United States to report using any dietary supplements (48.8 versus 54.2 percent) or multivitamin and multimineral supplements (27.7 versus 39.1 percent), but more likely to report using protein and amino acids (25.6 versus 18.7 percent). Older age, greater educational attainment, higher body mass index, strength training, or being officers or members of the Special Forces were further associated with greater likelihood of dietary supplement use (Lieberman et al., 2010).

Overall military dietary supplement use was similar to that of the U.S. general population. In NHANES 2003–2006, 53.4 percent of participants reported use of any dietary supplement in the preceding month (Bailey et al., 2010), compared to 53 percent of soldiers (Lieberman et al., 2010); the prevalence rates were 52 percent in NHANES 1999–2000 and 40 percent in NHANES III (1988–1994) (Ervin et al., 2004; Radimer et al., 2004; Rock, 2007). Prevalence rates of multivitamin and multimineral use were slightly higher in soldiers (37.5 percent reported use of such supplements one or more times per week) than in civilians (35 percent during the preceding month, based on NHANES 1999–2000) (Radimer et al., 2004). However, there were substantial differences in the use of dietary supplements other than vitamins and minerals, especially protein and amino acid supplements. Among soldiers, 18.7 percent reported using protein and amino acid supplements one or more times per week (Lieberman et al., 2010); based on a representative sample of the noninstitutionalized U.S. population, only 4 percent of men and no women aged 18–44 used creatine (Kaufman et al., 2002), which is the most commonly used amino acid supplement in the United States. In another national survey that included 2,743 noninstitutionalized adults aged 18 and over, 3.4 percent of participants reported using any amino acid supplements in the previous 12 months (Timbo et al., 2006). A 2008 IOM report on dietary supplement use in the military recommended establishing an oversight process to coordinate the evaluation of dietary intake, adverse event surveillance, and educational components to preclude the risk of adverse effects from dietary supplement use.

CONCLUSIONS AND RECOMMENDATIONS

The military recognizes the importance of nutrition in achievement and maintenance of optimal performance during military tasks. Proof of this is the development of MDRIs specific to this population, the development of rations that meet the needs of those performing particular tasks, and various educational efforts, among many other initiatives. Conducting studies on the nutrition status and nutrient and dietary supplement intake within the military is not only costly, as in the civilian population, but also logistically challenging. These types of nutrition assessments are not typically conducted among active-duty military personnel. A comprehensive survey of dietary supplement intake by military personnel (Lieberman et al., 2010) conducted in 2010 helps provide a clearer picture of nutrition in the military, but such a study does not answer questions about intake of essential nutrients. There is no military equivalent of NHANES data (i.e., health and nutritional data on adults and children in the United States) on food consumption and nutrient intakes in theater to enable meaningful recommendations for preventive nutrition prior to the occurrence of TBI. A clear picture of the nutrient and food intake characterizing the nutritional profile accompanying various severities and stages of TBI is likewise necessary to make nutrition recommendations for TBI recovery. This committee believes that knowing the nutrition status of a TBI patient will be essential to determine whether supplementation of specific nutrients would improve health outcomes. In addition, information about nutrition status of TBI patients will help elucidate whether a particular nutrient, dietary supplement, or diet taken prior to the injury is associated with outcomes of TBI. It is also important to collect data on the consumption of other substances that might interact with these nutrients, such as caffeine, alcohol, nicotine, and medications, in conjunction with the assessment of essential nutrient intake.

RECOMMENDATION 5-1. DoD should conduct dietary intake assessments in different military settings (e.g., when eating in military dining facilities or when subsisting on a predominantly ration-based diet) both predeployment and during deployment to determine the nutritional status of soldiers as a basis for recommending increases in intake of specific nutrients that may provide resilience to TBI.

RECOMMENDATION 5-2. Routine dietary intake assessments of TBI patients in medical treatment facilities should be undertaken as soon after hospitalization as possible to estimate preinjury nutrition status as well as to provide optimal nutritional intake throughout the various stages of treatment.

RECOMMENDATION 5-3. In individuals with TBI, DoD should estimate preinjury and postinjury dietary intake or status for those nutrients, dietary supplements, and diets that might show a relationship to TBI outcome. For example, based on the current evidence, the committee recommends collecting those estimates for creatine, n-3 fatty acids, choline, and vitamin D. The data could be used to investigate potential relationships between preinjury nutritional intake or status and recovery progress. Such data also would show possible synergistic effects between nutrients and dietary supplements.

REFERENCES

Bailey, R. L., K. W. Dodd, J. A. Goldman, J. J. Gahche, J. T. Dwyer, A. J. Moshfegh, C. T. Sempos, and M. F. Picciano. 2010. Estimation of total usual calcium and vitamin D intakes in the United States. *Journal of Nutrition* 140(4):817–822.

Baker-Fulco, C. J., G. P. Bathalon, M. E. Bovill, and H. R. Lieberman. 2001. *Military Dietary Reference Intakes: Rationales for tabled values.* Technical Note TN-00/10. Natick, MA: U.S. Army Research Insitute of Environmental Medicine.

Berry, C., A. Salim, R. Alban, J. Mirocha, D. R. Margulies, and E. J. Ley. 2010. Serum ethanol levels in patients with moderate to severe traumatic brain injury influence outcomes: A surprising finding. *American Surgeon* 76(10):1067–1070.

Dash, P. K., A. N. Moore, M. R. Moody, R. Treadwell, J. L. Felix, and G. L. Clifton. 2004. Post-trauma administration of caffeine plus ethanol reduces contusion volume and improves working memory in rats. *Journal of Neurotrauma* 21(11):1573–1583.

Ervin, R. B., J. D. Wright, and D. Reed-Gillette. 2004. Prevalence of leading types of dietary supplements used in the Third National Health and Nutrition Examination Survey, 1988–94. *Advance Data* (349):1–7.

Garrouste-Orgeas, M., G. Troche, E. Azoulay, A. Caubel, A. de Lassence, C. Cheval, L. Montesino, M. Thuong, F. Vincent, Y. Cohen, and J. F. Timsit. 2004. Body mass index—An additional prognostic factor in ICU patients. *Intensive Care Medicine* 30(3):437–443.

Graham, D. P., and A. L. Cardon. 2008. An update on substance use and treatment following traumatic brain injury. *Annals of the New York Academy of Sciences* 1141:148–162.

IOM (Institute of Medicine). 2001. *Caffeine for the sustainment of mental task performance*. Washington, DC: National Academy Press.

IOM. 2006a. *Dietary Reference Intakes: The essential guide to nutrient requirements*. Washington, DC: The National Academies Press.

IOM. 2006b. *Nutrient composition of rations for short-term, high-intensity combat operations*. Washington, DC: The National Academies Press.

IOM. 2008. *Use of dietary supplements by military personnel*. Washington, DC: The National Academies Press.

IOM. 2010. *Dietary Reference Intakes for calcium and vitamin D*. Washington, DC: The National Academies Press.

Kaufman, D. W., J. P. Kelly, L. Rosenberg, T. E. Anderson, and A. A. Mitchell. 2002. Recent patterns of medication use in the ambulatory adult population of the United States—The Slone survey. *The Journal of the American Medical Association* 287(3):337–344.

Lieberman, H. R., T. B. Stavinoha, S. M. McGraw, A. White, L. S. Hadden, and B. P. Marriott. 2010. Use of dietary supplements among active-duty U.S. Army soldiers. *American Journal of Clinical Nutrition* 92(4):985–995.

Moshfegh, A., J. Goldman, and L. Cleveland. 2005. *What we eat in America, NHANES 2001–2002: Usual nutrient intakes from food compared to Dietary Reference Intakes*: U.S. Department of Agriculture; Agricultural Research Service.

Moshfegh, A., J. Goldman, J. Ahuja, D. Rhodes, and R. LaComb. 2009. *What We Eat in America, NHANES 2005–2006: Usual nutrient intakes from food and water compared to 1997 Dietary Reference Intakes for vitamin D, calcium, phosphorus, and magnesium*: U.S. Department of Agriculture; Agricultural Research Service.

O'Brien, J. M., G. S. Phillips, N. A. Ali, M. Lucarelli, C. B. Marsh, and S. Lemeshow. 2006. Body mass index is independently associated with hospital mortality in mechanically ventilated adults with acute lung injury. *Critical Care Medicine* 34(3):738–744.

Opreanu, R. C., D. Kuhn, and M. D. Basson. 2010. Influence of alcohol on mortality in traumatic brain injury. *Journal of the American College of Surgeons* 210(6):997–1007.

Radimer, K., B. Bindewald, J. Hughes, B. Ervin, C. Swanson, and M. F. Picciano. 2004. Dietary supplement use by U.S. adults: Data from the National Health and Nutrition Examination Survey, 1999–2000. *American Journal of Epidemiology* 160(4):339–349.

Rock, C. L. 2007. Multivitamin-multimineral supplements: Who uses them? *American Journal of Clinical Nutrition* 85(1):277S–279S.

Sachse, K. T., E. K. Jackson, S. R. Wisniewski, D. G. Gillespie, A. M. Puccio, R. S. B. Clark, C. E. Dixon, and P. M. Kochanek. 2008. Increases in cerebrospinal fluid caffeine concentration are associated with favorable outcome after severe traumatic brain injury in humans. *Journal of Cerebral Blood Flow and Metabolism* 28(2):395–401.

Timbo, B. B., M. P. Ross, P. V. McCarthy, and C. T. J. Lin. 2006. Dietary supplements in a national survey: Prevalence of use and reports of adverse events. *Journal of the American Dietetic Association* 106(12):1966–1974.

Tremblay, A., and V. Bandi. 2003. Impact of body mass index on outcomes following critical care. *Chest* 123(4):1202–1207.

U.S. Departments of the Army, Navy, and Air Force. 2001. *Nutrition standards and education*. AR 40-25/BUMEDINST 10110.6/AFI 44-141. Washington, DC: U.S. Department of Defense.

Zeisel, S. H., and K. A. da Costa. 2009. Choline: An essential nutrient for public health. *Nutrition Reviews* 67(11):615–623.

6

Energy and Protein Needs During Early
Feeding Following Traumatic Brain Injury

Several Cochrane reviews have established a reasonable basis for early and adequate feeding following traumatic brain injury (TBI), although the number and size of the trials supporting this recommendation are limited (Perel et al., 2006; Yanagawa et al., 2002). Improvements in mortality and neurological outcome have been suggested, with a relative risk for mortality of 0.67 (0.41–1.07) for early feeding compared to not feeding and of 0.75 (0.50–1.11) for death and disability (Perel et al., 2006). In a meta-analysis of studies of nutritional support in critical illness, including studies in TBI requiring admission to an intensive care unit (ICU), and using an intent-to-treat analysis, total parenteral nutrition (TPN) was found superior to enteral nutrition in reducing mortality, although it significantly increased the risk of infection (Doig et al., 2008). However, this improvement in mortality was related to the early and adequate feeding, because of patients who were fed adequately plus early by either enteral nutrition or TPN both did better than those receiving late enteral feeding (Doig et al., 2008). Although there are other meta-analyses that did not demonstrate any difference in mortality between parenteral and enteral feeding in the critically ill (Gramlich et al., 2004; Koretz et al., 2007; Mazaki and Ebisawa, 2008; Peter et al., 2005), only Doig et al. (2008) evaluated exclusively patients in the ICU. Certainly patients with TBI are among the most critically ill in terms of degree of catabolic stress; eliminating those with less serious conditions, such as post-operative patients, when conducting meta-analyses would seem appropriate. Early feeding is generally defined as beginning within the first 24 hours after injury (Doig et al., 2009), but the definition of adequacy is still somewhat uncertain. An analysis of prospective data on the outcome of TBI related to feeding in 797 patients in 22 centers gathered by the Brain Trauma Foundation in 2008 found that mortality was significantly improved by each 10 kcal/kg increase in intake, with the curve becoming asymptotic at about 25 kcal/kg (Hartl et al., 2008). The majority of patients (62 percent) did not reach 25 kcal/kg/day within seven days. The likelihood of death for patients with TBI who were not fed within five days of injury was double that of patients who were fed, and those not fed within seven days had four times greater likelihood of death (Hartl et al., 2008). Interestingly, the benefits of early feeding were most prominent in those with elevated intracranial pressure, suggesting that nutrition was most effective in those likely to have the greatest injury response, with attenuation of that response a potential mechanism (Hartl et al., 2008). These findings should be contrasted with the earlier general recommendations of the Brain Trauma Foundation regarding nutrition in TBI that suggested full feeding to metabolic expenditure, which might approach 50 kcal/kg by seven days postinjury (Bratton et al., 2007), with the goal of maintaining lean tissue.

Traditionally, total daily energy expenditure has been considered to be composed of basal energy expenditure, often estimated by the Harris-Benedict equations; activity energy expenditure, which is generally quite limited in hospitalized, critically ill patients; and a small component due to the thermal effect of feeding, representing about 10 percent of the total. The Harris-Benedict equations estimate energy expenditure based on height, weight, sex, and age. A rough estimate of basal energy expenditure for most patients who are not severely malnourished and who are in the same age group is approximately 22–24 kcal/kg/day. Basal energy expenditure increases with injury in proportion to the degree of systemic inflammatory response, ranging usually from 0–100 percent increases from basal expenditure (Duke et al., 1970), with a similar range in TBI (McEvoy et al., 2009). It is likely that all military personnel experiencing TBI will be of normal body composition without malnutrition or obesity. In normal subjects, total energy intake must meet energy expenditure, and provision of adequate protein (0.8 g/kg) and other essential micronutrients is needed to maintain the protein content of the body, the lean body mass. However, for the critically ill, permissive underfeeding (i.e., the modest restriction of nutrient intake, specifically in critically ill patients, over a short term) is recommended. A recent study concluded that, for critically ill patients, permissive underfeeding (60–70 percent of calculated requirement) may be associated with lower mortality rates than underfeeding (90–100 percent of calculated requirement) (Arabi et al., 2011). With severe injury such as TBI, energy intakes in the range of 25–30 kcal/kg/day are generally recommended (Cerra et al., 1997; McClave et al., 2009). Harris-Benedict values are similar at 22–24 kcal/kg, but their calculation includes the additional factors of height, sex, and age. Both values are likely to be underestimates of total energy expenditure, and less likely to promote hyperglycemia for the first two weeks of injury. It should be noted that this concept of permissive underfeeding is different from the concept of underfeeding. Underfeeding is defined as a cumulative total caloric deficit of greater than 10,000 kcal (Bartlett et al., 1982) or a caloric intake of less than nine kcal/kg/day in the first seven days postinjury (Krishnan et al., 2003); both of these situations are associated with higher mortality rates. Furthermore, with the grossly inadequate caloric intake in underfeeding, protein intakes are often even more severely limited. For instance, in the trial of intensive insulin therapy in medical patients, while the caloric intakes were in the range of 1,500 kcal/day, protein intakes were less than 15 g/day in the first three days (Van den Berghe et al., 2006). For reasonable retention of lean tissue with injury, both energy sufficient to meet at least basal energy expenditure and a greater amount of protein (up to 1.5 g/kg/day) are required (Bistrian and Babineau, 1998); even then, total sparing of lean tissue is often impossible in the acute phase of injury, due to the impact of the systemic inflammatory response on the protein catabolic rate (Jensen et al., 2010; Ling et al., 1997). The maximal amount of protein that can be utilized for protein synthesis (i.e., about 1.5 g/kg/day when accompanied by these modest energy intakes) was determined by isotope studies in severely burned individuals (Wolfe et al., 1983) and sophisticated measures of body composition change using in vivo neutron activation analysis (Ishibashi et al., 1998). A second and very important aspect of the relationship between nutrient intake and body composition during injury, including TBI, is that increasing energy intake adversely affects glucose homeostasis. When glucose intakes as TPN exceed 30 kcal/kg (or about 5 mg/kg/min, representing 500 g of glucose per day for a 70 kg individual), the majority of hospitalized patients will have blood glucose levels greater than 200 mg/dL (Rosmarin et al., 1996). Because most patients suffering TBI, particularly military service members, are well nourished at the outset, serious protein-calorie malnutrition does not occur in the first seven days. However, because early plus adequate feeding in the critically ill can still improve outcome, the concept of permissive underfeeding (see above) has been developed (Burke et al., 2010; McCowen et al., 2000). A retrospective analysis of energy intakes and morbidity and mortality in the critically ill suggests that the middle tertile of intakes, 9–18 kcal/kg/day, provides the optimal outcome, with greater or lesser intakes associated with poorer outcomes (Krishnan et al., 2003). This strongly suggests that the mechanism for outcome improvement resulting from feeding early in the first week may be related to something other than optimal retention of lean body mass, such as providing sufficient glucose energy to meet the needs of key tissues including the brain, kidney, heart, and immune system, while maintaining protein synthetic rates for new protein synthesis, including for the immune system and tissue repair. Furthermore, permissive underfeeding may be beneficial by reducing the intensity of the systemic inflammatory response from a given level of injury (Burke et al., 2010). There is some support for this possibility in TBI, where patients receiving enhanced enteral nutrition showed lower levels of C-reactive protein than those receiving standard enteral nutrition during the first week after injury (Taylor et al., 1999). The greater likelihood of glucose homeostasis achieved with lower energy intakes may additionally reduce the known adverse impacts of hyperglycemia on morbidity and mortality outcomes in the critically ill (Fahy et al., 2009; McCowen et al., 2001; Pasquel et al., 2010). Most critically ill patients receive their invasive nutritional support by enteral nutrition rather than through TPN for a variety of reasons, including concerns about the relative safety and ease of administration of the two modes of feeding. However, enteral intakes are often limited by intestinal tolerance and temporary discontinuation for other procedures. Thus, although intakes of 25–30 kcal/kg/day are generally recommended in the critically ill (Cerra et al., 1997; McClave et al., 2009) to meet total energy expenditure and maintain lean tissue, intakes are usually substantially less than this, and generally less than 50 percent of goal (Krishnan et al., 2003), including in TBI (Hartl et al., 2008) during its initial phase. A small randomized trial of enhanced enteral feeding versus standard enteral feeding in TBI showed a significant reduction in infections and complications, with a suggestion of improved neurologic outcome (Taylor et al., 1999). Providing energy intake of at least 50 percent of energy needs up to 25–30 kcal/kg/day is likely appropriate for both the brain injury and for any associated critical injury. A corollary of this concept of permissive underfeeding is the interrelationship of energy and protein intake. When energy intakes are limited, supplying greater amounts of protein, up to 1.5 g/kg/day, will improve the preservation of lean body mass and improve protein synthetic rates (Hoffer et al., 1984; Ishibashi et al., 1998). Thus, it is beneficial to increase protein intakes when energy intake is less than energy expenditure. Because those enteral formulas generally employed have fixed compositions, either protein supplementation of present formulas or the development of new formula compositions incorporating these principles will need to be developed to test this hypothesis. Alternatively, enhanced enteral feeding techniques (Taylor et al., 1999) may need to be widely adopted. Beyond the initial two-week period, when the intensity of the systemic inflammatory response to TBI has generally remitted to some degree, attempting to provide sufficient energy to meet total energy expenditure in order to optimize protein metabolism is a reasonable goal. Estimating total energy expenditure by various formulas—including adding stress factors to the Harris-Benedict estimates—is inadequately sensitive, perhaps in part because nonseptic patients in medical ICU have less pronounced hypercatabolism than burn or trauma patients (Dickerson,

2011). Under these conditions, and particularly for patients with ventilatory support or that remain critically ill, measuring energy expenditure by indirect calorimetry is the gold standard. In patients who are recuperating well, careful assessment of energy and protein intake to meet estimated needs while monitoring weight changes at weekly intervals should suffice.

In summary, permissive underfeeding (initially 50 percent of energy needs, progressing up to 25–30 kcal/kg/day in the first 2 weeks) is probably an appropriate feeding regimen to be initiated within the first 24 hours. A protein intake higher than that recommended (approximately 1.5 g/kg/day) for the general population also will be appropriate for TBI patients in order to improve synthesis of protein and preserve lean body mass. The optimal nutritional goals beyond two weeks postinjury are not yet determined, but an attempt to meet total energy needs along with continued provision of 1.5 g of protein kg/day seems appropriate.

GLUCOSE HOMEOSTASIS

There is extensive literature documenting the substantial association of hyperglycemia with poorer outcomes in the critically ill (Fahy et al., 2009; McCowen et al., 2001). Whether this reflects the severity of the illness or an actual impact of hyperglycemia on pathophysiological processes is not certain and there is evidence for both factors to happen (Aljada et al., 2006; Ling et al., 2007; McCowen et al., 2001). Hyperglycemia has also been shown to have an adverse impact in TBI (Salim et al., 2009); however, because neurons are an obligate consumer of glucose, the risks presented by hypoglycemia in injured brain tissue are substantially greater than for other tissues (Oddo et al., 2008). A retrospective analysis of outcome in 380 TBI patients found increased mortality with a blood glucose < 60 mg/dL and > 160 mg/dL, unrelated to the severity of injury (Liu-DeRyke et al., 2009). Similarly, using cerebral microdialysis glucose levels, a brain energy crisis associated with much higher mortality rates was seen with tight glucose control of 80–120 mg/dL versus intermediate levels of 121–180 mg/dL (Oddo et al., 2008). Intensive insulin therapy to treat hyperglycemia has certainly been shown to reduce the intensity of the systemic inflammatory response and improve outcome (Hansen et al., 2003; Van den Berghe et al., 2001). In 2001, Van den Berghe and colleagues examined the effect of intensive insulin therapy to maintain a goal glucose level of 80–110 mg/dL in surgical patients in the ICU and showed a dramatic reduction in morbidity and mortality. This landmark article changed critical care practice significantly over the ensuing decade. The majority of patients in this study received TPN, and all received 200 g parenteral glucose per day at initiation. The most common diagnosis was cardiac surgery, which is known to particularly benefit from glucose administration. Hyperglycemia that develops with TPN correlates with morbidity and mortality (Lin et al., 2007). A subsequent study in medical ICU patients by the same group did not show improved mortality, but morbidity was improved with intensive insulin therapy (Van den Berghe et al., 2006). In this later study, patients received only enteral nutrition, had much lower energy and protein intakes, and hypoglycemia was substantially more common in the intensive insulin therapy group than in the first study (Van den Berghe et al., 2001, 2006). Subsequent large, randomized, clinical trials conducted in multiple centers were unable to confirm similar benefits using these glucose goals. The Glucontrol Study (Preiser et al., 2009), a large multi-center randomized clinical trial of intensive insulin therapy of tight (80–110 mg/dL) versus intermediate control, was discontinued prematurely beause of the high level of protocol violation (Preiser et al., 2009). Even so, there was significantly more hypoglycemia, without difference in mortality, in the tight control group in this underpowered study. The Nice/Sugar Study compared tight glucose control of 81–108 mg/dL to an intermediate level of below 180 mg/dL, and also found a significantly higher risk of hypoglycemia and increased mortality in the intensive insulin therapy group (Finfer et al., 2009). There were methodological differences between the original Van den Berghe study (2001) and succeeding versions, including different target ranges for blood glucose, different accuracies of glucometers, and varying levels of expertise of the participating institutional staff (Van den Berghe et al., 2009). All randomized trials following the initial Van den Berghe study also principally used enteral nutrition rather than TPN. Subsequent trials had tighter glucose control in the control group than in the original Van den Berghe study, where the control group received insulin only when blood glucose exceeded 200 mg/dL. Recent trials have thus been comparing very tight control accompanied by a high risk of hypoglycemia, to less severe control (to about the 150 mg/dL level) having much less risk of hypoglycemia but still substantially better glucose control than in previous years. Enteral nutrition may be an important factor in the development of hypoglycemia, as intestinal absorption is frequently impaired in the critically ill, and tube feeding is often interrupted for various clinical procedures while insulin continues to be administered. Additionally, TPN at full feeding levels may provide from 300–400 g of glucose per day, which elicits much higher insulin levels than enteral nutrition with the same amount of nutrient intake (Wene et al., 1975). Insulin resistance that occurs with hyperinsulinemia may therefore be partially protective against the development of insulin-induced hypoglycemia. In the critically ill, 400–500 g of glucose per day, provided into arterial circulation by TPN, should meet cerebral metabolic needs despite maximal suppression of gluconeogenesis by insulin levels of 100–200 µU/mL elicited by TPN (Bistrian, 2011). Although hypoglycemia might sometimes arise through insulin-mediated glucose uptake in insulin-responsive tissues when assessed by venous access, this would reflect the presence of an arterial-venous glucose difference that can arise in those that are fully fed. Even though hypoglycemia might sometimes be detected in venous blood or even by capillary determinations, neuroglycopenia should be unlikely when TPN provides more than 300 g of glucose in 24 hours. This interpretation is supported by the recent reevaluation of the impact of enteral and parenteral nutrition by Van den Berghe and colleagues, combining data from both their medical and surgical studies (Bistrian, 2010; Meyfroidt and Van den Berghe, 2010). They found that glucose variability was significantly greater in enterally fed patients, and hypoglycemia 2.2 times more common than in patients receiving TPN (Meyfroidt and Van den Berghe, 2010).

The important issues concerning glucose homeostasis to be determined in TBI are whether intensive insulin therapy should be employed, and if so, what the goal level for glucose should be? It is likely that if enteral nutrition is to remain the principal mode of support, and levels of nutritional support are increased by such means as nursing algorithms, acceptance of higher residuals, and maintaining flow rates and new formulas, then mild hyperglycemia greater than 160 mg/dL will probably become more common. This situation may thus benefit from intense insulin therapy with an intermediate goal for blood glucose. Several trials of intensive insulin therapy in TBI have been conducted. One small study that sought very tight control of 80–110 mg/dL showed no short- or long-term improvement with intensive insulin therapy, with much greater incidence of hypoglycemia (82.1 percent versus 17.5 percent) (Coester et al., 2010). A second study with similar blood glucose goals also found significantly more hypoglycemia events (a median of 7 versus 15) than with less-stringent glucose control, and no change in Glasgow Outcome Score (Bilotta et al., 2008). Finally, a study in TBI patients in a Neonatal Intensive Care Unit (NICU) found improved Glasgow Outcome Scores at six months in the intensively treated group, with shorter NICU stays and significantly reduced infections (Yang et al., 2009). Goals for levels of nutritional support and for blood glucose homeostasis therefore still remain to be firmly established.

CONCLUSIONS AND RECOMMENDATIONS

Several reviews and guidelines have established regimens for early feeding after severe trauma, including severe TBI. The use of generic critical illness guidelines for ICU patients with polytrauma is prevalent; however, development of specific sections that identify unique concerns relative to TBI may be warranted. Although further research in TBI populations is required, the committee concluded that the existing evidence on TBI raises questions about the appropriateness of the following three areas of current generic clinical practice guidelines: (1) the targets for early and adequate feeding, (2) the target range of serum glucose for tight glucose control, and (3) the type of feeding regimen for intense insulin therapy.

Current generic guidelines for critically ill patients indicate feeding to meet energy needs by day 7; however, it may be more appropriate to focus on the energy consumption within 72 hours and not 7 days. There is sufficient evidence to indicate the importance of feeding trauma patients shortly after injury. For example, in a retrospective multi-center study of TBI patients, lower mortality rates were found when patients were fed during the first five to seven days after a TBI. Such a study, however, does not provide evidence to develop best feeding practices, because feeding regimens were not uniform across centers. Although patients with severe TBI will remain in intensive care for variable amounts of time, it would be appropriate to develop best feeding practices for both the period initially following TBI, when the systemic inflammatory response is likely to be at its height, and in the later period (commencing at about two weeks), when concern about lean tissue maintenance and repletion assumes greater importance and tolerance to feeding is likely to be improved.

Critical care guidance for TBI recommends increasing the amount of calories provided beyond actual energy expenditure. The committee concluded that, although increasing the amount of calories beyond expenditure might better improve lean tissue preservation, this feeding regimen increases the risk for hyperglycemia or gastrointestinal intolerance, depending on the feeding regimen employed (parenteral nutrition or enteral nutrition, respectively). The target, therefore, may not be meeting energy needs, but rather a specified level of permissive underfeeding (i.e., the modest restriction of nutrient intake).

Maintenance of glucose above 60 mg/dL and below 150–160 mg/dL probably improves TBI outcome. Intense insulin therapy makes this achievable, but if enteral feeding is used, there is also substantial risk of hypoglycemia due to normal feeding interruptions occurring in conjunction with constant levels of insulin, variations in the rate of food absorption from the gut, and delivery of food to the liver before the systemic circulation when maintaining a narrow range of glucose (80–110 mg/dL). Because of these risks, the goal for glucose in enteral feeding with intense insulin therapy should be higher, probably 150 or 160 mg/dL. The amounts of 300–400 g/day of parenteral glucose, usually provided with the direct infusion of glucose into the systemic circulation through TPN, exceed the maximal rate of hepatic glucose production in the critically ill in the postabsorptive state. Since insulin works to lower serum glucose primarily by inhibiting hepatic glucose production and all the glucose required is already provided with TPN, hypoglycemia is unlikely under these circumstances. However, there may occasionally be much lower venous glucose levels, reflecting insulin's effect to increase uptake of glucose in insulin-sensitive tissue. This effect is not systemic, and therefore would not be an issue unless one is concerned only with venous glucose levels. Current generic guidelines have not established whether tight control of serum glucose at 80–110 mg/dL or a slightly higher range (e.g., less than 150 mg/dL) is more appropriate for critical illness, particularly TBI where the potential for hypoglycemia is more damaging. Thus, there may be rationale for considering a slightly higher range (e.g., less than 150 mg/dL) while factoring for variation of the range depending on the feeding regimen (i.e., enteral or parenteral). This higher level may be more consistent with clinical practice guidelines for immediate post-stroke treatment as a model of brain injury.

RECOMMENDATION 6-1. The committee recommends that evidence-based guidelines include the provision of early (within 24 hours after injury) nutrition (more than 50 percent of total energy expenditure and 1–1.5 g/kg protein) for the first two weeks after injury. This intervention is critical to limit the intensity of the inflammatory response to TBI, and to improve outcome.

RECOMMENDATION 6-2. DoD should conduct human trials to determine appropriate levels of blood glucose following TBI to minimize morbidity and mortality. These should be clinical trials of early feeding using intensive insulin therapy to maintain blood glucose concentrations at less than 150–160 mg/dL versus current usual care of severe TBI in ICU settings for the first two weeks.

RECOMMENDATION 6-3. DoD should conduct clinical trials of the benefits of insulin therapy for care of acute TBI in inpatient settings with TPN alone (or plus enteral feeding) versus enteral feeding alone. The goals for blood glucose in the TPN group should be lower (e.g., less than 120 mg/dL) than in the enteral group (e.g., less than 150–160 mg/dL). Variables to measure include clinical outcomes and incidence of hypoglycemia.

RECOMMENDATION 6-4. DoD should conduct studies to determine the optimal goals for nutrition (e.g., when to begin meeting total energy expenditure for optimal lean tissue maintenance or repletion) after the first two weeks following severe injury.

REFERENCES

Aljada, A., J. Friedman, H. Ghanim, P. Mohanty, D. Hofmeyer, A. Chaudhuri, and P. Dandona. 2006. Glucose ingestion induces an increase in intranuclear nuclear factor kappaB, a fall in cellular inhibitor kappaB, and an increase in tumor necrosis factor alpha messenger RNA by mononuclear cells in healthy human subjects. *Metabolism: Clinical and Experimental* 55(9):1177–1185.

Arabi, Y. M., H. M. Tamim, G. S. Dhar, A. Al-Dawood, M. Al-Sultan, M. H. Sakkijha, S. H. Kahoul, and R. Brits. 2011. Permissive underfeeding and intensive insulin therapy in critically ill patients: A randomized controlled trial. *American Journal of Clinical Nutrition* 93(3):569–577.

Bartlett, R. H., R. E. Dechert, J. R. Mault, S. K. Ferguson, A. M. Kaiser, and E. E. Erlandson. 1982. Measurement of metabolism in multiple organ failure. *Surgery* 92(4):771–779.

Bilotta, F., R. Caramia, I. Cernak, F. P. Paoloni, A. Doronzio, V. Cuzzone, A. Santoro, and G. Rosa. 2008. Intensive insulin therapy after severe traumatic brain injury: A randomized clinical trial. *Neurocritical Care* 9(2):159–166.

Bistrian, B. R. 2010. Parenteral feeding and intensive insulin therapy. *Critical Care Medicine* 38(9):1922; author reply 1922–1923.

Bistrian, B. R. 2011. Is total parenteral nutrition protective against hypoglycemia during intense insulin therapy? A hypothesis. *Critical Care Medicine* (Published electronically February 10, 2011).

Bistrian, B. R., and T. Babineau. 1998. Optimal protein intake in critical illness? *Critical Care Medicine* 26(9):1476–1477.

Bratton, S. L., R. M. Chestnut, J. Ghajar, F. F. McConnell Hammond, O. A. Harris, R. Hartl, G. T. Manley, A. Nemecek, D. W. Newell, G. Rosenthal, J. Schouten, L. Shutter, S. D. Timmons, J. S. Ullman, W. Videtta, J. E. Wilberger, and D. W. Wright. 2007. Guidelines for the management of severe traumatic brain injury. XII. Nutrition. *Journal of Neurotrauma* 24(Suppl 1.):S77–S82.

Burke, P. A., L. S. Young, and B. R. Bistrian. 2010. Metabolic vs nutrition support: A hypothesis. *Journal of Parenteral and Enteral Nutrition* 34(5):546–548.

Cerra, F. B., M. R. Benitez, G. L. Blackburn, R. S. Irwin, K. Jeejeebhoy, D. P. Katz, S. K. Pingleton, J. Pomposelli, J. L. Rombeau, E. Shronts, R. R. Wolfe, and G. P. Zaloga. 1997. Applied nutrition in ICU patients. A consensus statement of the American College of Chest Physicians. *Chest* 111(3):769–778.

Coester, A., C. R. Neumann, and M. I. Schmidt. 2010. Intensive insulin therapy in severe traumatic brain injury: A randomized trial. *Journal of Trauma* 68(4):904–911.

Dickerson, R. N. 2011. Optimal caloric intake for critically ill patients: First, do no harm. *Nutrition in Clinical Practice* 26(1):48–54.

Doig, G. S., F. Simpson, S. Finfer, A. Delaney, A. R. Davies, I. Mitchell, and G. Dobb. 2008. Effect of evidence-based feeding guidelines on mortality of critically ill adults: A cluster randomized controlled trial. *The Journal of the American Medical Association* 300(23):2731–2741.

Doig, G. S., P. T. Heighes, F. Simpson, E. A. Sweetman, and A. R. Davies. 2009. Early enteral nutrition, provided within 24 h of injury or intensive care unit admission, significantly reduces mortality in critically ill patients: A meta-analysis of randomised controlled trials. *Intensive Care Medicine* 35(12):2018–2027.

Duke, J. H., Jr., S. B. Jorgensen, J. R. Broell, C. L. Long, and J. M. Kinney. 1970. Contribution of protein to caloric expenditure following injury. *Surgery* 68(1):168–174.

Fahy, B. G., A. M. Sheehy, and D. B. Coursin. 2009. Glucose control in the intensive care unit. *Critical Care Medicine* 37(5):1769–1776.

Finfer, S., D. R. Chittock, S. Y. Su, D. Blair, D. Foster, V. Dhingra, R. Bellomo, D. Cook, P. Dodek, W. R. Henderson, P. C. Hebert, S. Heritier, D. K. Heyland, C. McArthur, E. McDonald, I. Mitchell, J. A. Myburgh, R. Norton, J. Potter, B. G. Robinson, and J. J. Ronco. 2009. Intensive versus conventional glucose control in critically ill patients. *The New England Journal of Medicine* 360(13):1283–1297.

Gramlich, L., K. Kichian, J. Pinilla, N. J. Rodych, R. Dhaliwal, and D. K. Heyland. 2004. Does enteral nutrition compared to parenteral nutrition result in better outcomes in critically ill adult patients? A systematic review of the literature. *Nutrition* 20(10):843–848.

Hansen, T. K., S. Thiel, P. J. Wouters, J. S. Christiansen, and G. Van den Berghe. 2003. Intensive insulin therapy exerts antiinflammatory effects in critically ill patients and counteracts the adverse effect of low mannose-binding lectin levels. *Journal of Clinical Endocrinology and Metabolism* 88(3):1082–1088.

Hartl, R., L. M. Gerber, Q. Ni, and J. Ghajar. 2008. Effect of early nutrition on deaths due to severe traumatic brain injury. *Journal of Neurosurgery* 109(1):50–56.

Hoffer, L. J., B. R. Bistrian, V. R. Young, G. L. Blackburn, and D. E. Matthews. 1984. Metabolic effects of very low calorie weight reduction diets. *Journal of Clinical Investigation* 73(3):750–758.

Ishibashi, N., L. D. Plank, K. Sando, and G. L. Hill. 1998. Optimal protein requirements during the first 2 weeks after the onset of critical illness. *Critical Care Medicine* 26(9):1529–1535.

Jensen, G. L., J. Mirtallo, C. Compher, R. Dhaliwal, A. Forbes, R. F. Grijalba, G. Hardy, J. Kondrup, D. Labadarios, I. Nyulasi, J. C. Castillo Pineda, and D. Waitzberg. 2010. Adult starvation and disease-related malnutrition: A proposal for etiology-based diagnosis in the clinical practice setting from the international consensus guideline committee. *Journal of Parenteral and Enteral Nutrition* 34(2):156–159.

Koretz, R. L., A. Avenell, T. O. Lipman, C. L. Braunschweig, and A. C. Milne. 2007. Does enteral nutrition affect clinical outcome? A systematic review of the randomized trials. *American Journal of Gastroenterology* 102(2):412–429; quiz 468.

Krishnan, J. A., P. B. Parce, A. Martinez, G. B. Diette, and R. G. Brower. 2003. Caloric intake in medical ICU patients: Consistency of care with guidelines and relationship to clinical outcomes. *Chest* 124(1):297–305.

Lin, L. Y., H. C. Lin, P. C. Lee, W. Y. Ma, and H. D. Lin. 2007. Hyperglycemia correlates with outcomes in patients receiving total parenteral nutrition. *American Journal of the Medical Sciences* 333(5):261–265.

Ling, P. R., J. H. Schwartz, and B. R. Bistrian. 1997. Mechanisms of host wasting induced by administration of cytokines in rats. *American Journal of Physiology* 272(3 Pt 1):E333–339.

Ling, P. R., R. J. Smith, and B. R. Bistrian. 2007. Acute effects of hyperglycemia and hyperinsulinemia on hepatic oxidative stress and the systemic inflammatory response in rats. *Critical Care Medicine* 35(2):555–560.

Liu-DeRyke, X., D. S. Collingridge, J. Orme, D. Roller, J. Zurasky, and D. H. Rhoney. 2009. Clinical impact of early hyperglycemia during acute phase of traumatic brain injury. *Neurocritical Care* 11(2):151–157.

Mazaki, T., and K. Ebisawa. 2008. Enteral versus parenteral nutrition after gastrointestinal surgery: A systematic review and meta-analysis of randomized controlled trials in the English literature. *Journal of Gastrointestinal Surgery* 12(4):739–755.

McClave, S. A., R. G. Martindale, V. W. Vanek, M. McCarthy, P. Roberts, B. Taylor, J. B. Ochoa, L. Napolitano, and G. Cresci. 2009. Guidelines for the provision and assessment of nutrition support therapy in the adult critically ill patient: Society of Critical Care Medicine (SCCM) and American Society for Parenteral and Enteral Nutrition (ASPEN). *Journal of Parenteral and Enteral Nutrition* 33(3):277–316.

McCowen, K. C., C. Friel, J. Sternberg, S. Chan, R. A. Forse, P. A. Burke, and B. R. Bistrian. 2000. Hypocaloric total parenteral nutrition: Effectiveness in prevention of hyperglycemia and infectious complications—a randomized clinical trial. *Critical Care Medicine* 28(11):3606–3611.

McCowen, K. C., A. Malhotra, and B. R. Bistrian. 2001. Stress-induced hyperglycemia. *Critical Care Clinics* 17(1):107–124.

McEvoy, C. T., G. W. Cran, S. R. Cooke, and I. S. Young. 2009. Resting energy expenditure in non-ventilated, non-sedated patients recovering from serious traumatic brain injury: Comparison of prediction equations with indirect calorimetry values. *Clinical Nutrition* 28(5):526–532.

Meyfroidt, G., and G. Van den Berghe. 2010. The authors reply. *Critical Care Medicine September* 38(9).

Oddo, M., J. M. Schmidt, E. Carrera, N. Badjatia, E. S. Connolly, M. Presciutti, N. D. Ostapkovich, J. M. Levine, P. Le Roux, and S. A. Mayer. 2008. Impact of tight glycemic control on cerebral glucose metabolism after severe brain injury: A microdialysis study. *Critical Care Medicine* 36(12):3233–3238.

Pasquel, F. J., R. Spiegelman, M. McCauley, D. Smiley, D. Umpierrez, R. Johnson, M. Rhee, C. Gatcliffe, E. Lin, E. Umpierrez, L. Peng, and G. E. Umpierrez. 2010. Hyperglycemia during total parenteral nutrition: An important marker of poor outcome and mortality in hospitalized patients. *Diabetes Care* 33(4):739–741.

Perel, P., T. Yanagawa, F. Bunn, I. Roberts, R. Wentz, and A. Pierro. 2006. Nutritional support for head-injured patients. *Cochrane Database of Systematic Reviews* (4):CD001530.

Peter, J. V., J. L. Moran, and J. Phillips-Hughes. 2005. A metaanalysis of treatment outcomes of early enteral versus early parenteral nutrition in hospitalized patients. *Critical Care Medicine* 33(1):213–220; discussion 260–211.

Preiser, J. C., P. Devos, S. Ruiz-Santana, C. Melot, D. Annane, J. Groeneveld, G. Iapichino, X. Leverve, G. Nitenberg, P. Singer, J. Wernerman, M. Joannidis, A. Stecher, and R. Chiolero. 2009. A prospective randomised multi-centre controlled trial on tight glucose control by intensive insulin therapy in adult intensive care units: The Glucontrol study. *Intensive Care Medicine* 35(10):1738–1748.

Rosmarin, D. K., G. M. Wardlaw, and J. Mirtallo. 1996. Hyperglycemia associated with high, continuous infusion rates of total parenteral nutrition dextrose. *Nutrition in Clinical Practice* 11(4):151–156.

Salim, A., P. Hadjizacharia, J. Dubose, C. Brown, K. Inaba, L. S. Chan, and D. Margulies. 2009. Persistent hyperglycemia in severe traumatic brain injury: An independent predictor of outcome. *American Surgeon* 75(1):25–29.

Taylor, S. J., S. B. Fettes, C. Jewkes, and R. J. Nelson. 1999. Prospective, randomized, controlled trial to determine the effect of early enhanced enteral nutrition on clinical outcome in mechanically ventilated patients suffering head injury. *Critical Care Medicine* 27(11):2525–2531.

Van den Berghe, G., P. Wouters, F. Weekers, C. Verwaest, F. Bruyninckx, M. Schetz, D. Vlasselaers, P. Ferdinande, P. Lauwers, and R. Bouillon. 2001. Intensive insulin therapy in the critically ill patients. *The New England Journal of Medicine* 345(19):1359–1367.

Van den Berghe, G., A. Wilmer, G. Hermans, W. Meersseman, P. J. Wouters, I. Milants, E. Van Wijngaerden, H. Bobbaers, and R. Bouillon. 2006. Intensive insulin therapy in the medical ICU. *The New England Journal of Medicine* 354(5):449–461.

Van den Berghe, G., M. Schetz, D. Vlasselaers, G. Hermans, A. Wilmer, R. Bouillon, and D. Mesotten. 2009. Clinical review: Intensive insulin therapy in critically ill patients: Nice-sugar or leuven blood glucose target? *Journal of Clinical Endocrinology and Metabolism* 94(9):3163–3170.

Wene, J. D., W. E. Connor, and L. DenBesten. 1975. The development of essential fatty acid deficiency in healthy men fed fat-free diets intravenously and orally. *Journal of Clinical Investigation* 56(1):127–134.

Wolfe, R. R., R. D. Goodenough, J. F. Burke, and M. H. Wolfe. 1983. Response of protein and urea kinetics in burn patients to different levels of protein intake. *Annals of Surgery* 197(2):163–171.

Yanagawa, T., F. Bunn, I. Roberts, R. Wentz, and A. Pierro. 2002. Nutritional support for head-injured patients. *Cochrane Database of Systematic Reviews* (3):CD001530.

Yang, M., Q. Guo, X. Zhang, S. Sun, Y. Wang, L. Zhao, E. Hu, and C. Li. 2009. Intensive insulin therapy on infection rate, days in NICU, in-hospital mortality and neurological outcome in severe traumatic brain injury patients: A randomized controlled trial. *International Journal of Nursing Studies* 46(6):753–758.

7

Antioxidants

Oxidative stress has been implicated as a central pathogenic mechanism in traumatic brain injury (TBI) because the brain is especially vulnerable to such stress, compared to other tissues (Floyd, 1999; Floyd and Carney, 1992). Overproduction of reactive oxygen species (ROS), that is, chemically reactive molecules containing oxygen, can trigger many of the harmful biological events associated with TBI such as DNA (deoxyribonucleic acid) damage, brain-derived neurotrophic factor (BDNF) dysfunction, and disruption of the membrane phospholipid architecture, and has therefore been suggested as a principal culprit in both acute and long-term events of TBI (Eghwrudjakpor and Allison, 2010; Hall et al., 2010). The effects of antioxidants on TBI have not yet been examined in human studies; however, several clinical trials have investigated whether antioxidant supplementation could reduce the risk of developing other forms of trauma (e.g., stroke and epilepsy) or protect against developing adverse health outcomes after injury. This chapter offers the current evidence to support further exploration of the role of antioxidants as neuroprotectants for TBI.

There are many compounds having antioxidant properties, some of which are essential nutrients. As evidence became available, it was observed that effectiveness in animals or excellent antioxidant activity observed in vitro does not necessarily translate into effectiveness to prevent human diseases associated with oxidative stress. Initial expectations of these compounds to prevent chronic diseases associated with oxidative stress have been disappointed. It has nevertheless become clear that oxidative stress after TBI triggers many of its outcomes, and antioxidant compounds should be considered to ameliorate these outcomes. It would not be feasible for this committee to do a review of all the many compounds that have been identified as having antioxidant activity. Vitamins E and C were selected as examples of antioxidant nutrients for this review because their potential to prevent chronic diseases has been studied extensively. Some non-essential food components with reported antioxidant properties also are reviewed in this chapter. Finally, based on the fact that antioxidants seem to act synergistically, the possibility that a combination of antioxidants might be more effective that a single one is also considered. The intention of this chapter is not to review every combination of antioxidants that might have been tested, but to give a flavor of the potential benefits of this class of compounds when used in combination.

VITAMIN E (ALPHA-TOCOPHEROL)

Introduction

Vitamin E is a family of fat-soluble α-, β-, γ-, and δ-tocopherols and corresponding four tocotrienols. The α-tocopherol has been the most studied, as it is the form preferentially absorbed and transported to tissues in humans. For example, the U.S. dietary requirements have been developed considering mainly this form. Although vitamin E is an antioxidant that stops the production of ROS formed when fat undergoes oxidation, its in vivo roles are not well understood. The level of alpha-tocopherol is high in the brain, and its concentration is normally regulated (Spector and Johanson, 2007).

The consumption of vitamin E beyond the requirement levels cited in the Dietary Reference Intakes (DRIs) has been studied extensively from 1990 through 2010. Early observational studies and animal studies suggested that vitamin E's antioxidant properties would protect the body against devastating chronic diseases having oxidative stress as part of their pathobiology, such as cardiovascular diseases and cancer; however, results from observational studies are mixed, and have not resulted in a clear association between intake of vitamin E and reduction of chronic disease (Hirvonen et al., 2000; Mezzetti et al., 2001; Watkins et al., 2000; Yochum et al., 2000). Large human trials conducted since 2000 have also failed to demonstrate such benefits. The reader is referred to the numerous discussions that can be found on this topic and on the potential reasons for the disappointing findings (Fletcher and Fairfield, 2002; Huang et al., 2006; Lichtenstein, 2009; Pryor, 2000; Steinberg, 2000). Table 7-1 lists large human trials that have evaluated the association of vitamin E with cardiovascular diseases, as well as a recent study on TBI presented at a conference (Razmkon et al., 2010). The occurrence or absence of adverse effects in humans is included if reported by the authors. The 2006 IOM report *Nutrient Composition of Rations for Short-term, High-Intensity Combat Operations* reviewed vitamin E in the context of preventing oxidative damage from exhausting physical exercise in the military. That report showed no clear benefit either in reducing muscle injury due to exercise or in improving performance, and therefore no recommendation was offered to increase intake of vitamin E (IOM, 2006). That report did not review evidence on vitamin E and potential benefits for TBI.

Uses and Safety

The Recommended Dietary Allowance (RDA) for vitamin E (as alpha-tocopherol) is set at 15 mg for men 19–50 years of age. This requirement was based on maintaining plasma tocopherol concentration at a level that limited hemolysis in red blood cells resulting from peroxide exposure to less than 12 percent.

A comparison of U.S. dietary intake from National Health and Nutrition Examination Survey (NHANES) 2001–2002 data with the Estimated Average Requirements (EARs) of alpha-tocopherol (see Table 5-2 in Chapter 5) suggests that 89 percent of males and 97 percent of females older than 19 years of age consume far less vitamin E than the recommended EAR. However, overt signs of vitamin E deficiency occur very rarely in humans and have not been reported as a result of low dietary intakes, except in conjunction with moderate to severe malnutrition.

The Tolerable Upper Intake Level (UL) of vitamin E was established at 1,000 mg, based

TABLE 7-1 Relevant Data Identified for Vitamin E (alpha-tocopherol, alpha-tocotrienol)

Reference	Type of Injury/ Insult	Type of Study and Subjects	Treatment	Findings/Results
Tier 1: Clinical trials				
Razmkon et al., 2010	TBI (Glasgow Coma Scale scores of 8 or less and radiologic diagnoses of diffuse axonal injury)	Multi-center, randomized, double-blind, placebo-controlled trial, n^d=100 (83 male)	Postinjury, vitamin E (intravenous at 400 IU/day for 7 days) Postinjury, vitamin C (500 mg/day for seven days or 10 g on the day of admission and 4 days later), or placebo	Vitamin E significantly decreased in-hospital mortality following TBI by 8% (p=0.01). The vitamin E group had significantly better Glasgow Outcome Scale scores at discharge and at 2 and 6 months of follow up (p=0.04). No adverse effects were observed.
Schürks et al., 2010	Stroke	Meta-analysis of 9 randomized, controlled trials	Vitamin E supplementation	Vitamin E supplementation did not reduce the risk for total stroke, but it was associated with increased risk for hemorrhagic stroke (pooled RR^b=1.22; 95% CI^c: 1.00, 1.48, p=0.045). And vitamin E was associated with decreased risk for ischemic stroke (pooled RR=0.90; 95% CI: 0.82, 0.99, p < 0.02). There was no evidence of heterogeneity (I^{2d}=0.0%) or small study effect for either variable. Data on adverse bleeding from vitamin E treatment is unclear: fatal bleeding among two individuals in the treatment group was reported in one trial, while another trial reported non-fatal bleedings among both the treatment and placebo groups. A third trial found no overall increased rate of bleeding, but observed a small significantly increased risk for epistaxis among the treatment group.
Milman et al., 2008	Cardiovascular events (i.e, myocardial infarction [MI], stroke, or cardiovascular death) in patients with type 2 diabetes mellitus (DM)	Randomized, prospective, double-blind trial n=1,434 DM individuals aged 55 years or older with Hp 2-2 genotype	Vitamin E (400 IU/day) or placebo	Analysis of composite cardiovascular disease events (CVD death, non-fatal MI, and stroke) show that subjects in vitamin E group had significantly fewer events than control group (2.2% in vitamin E vs. 4.7% in placebo; HR^e=0.47, 95% CI: 0.27–0.82; p=0.01 by Log-Rank). This significance can largely be attributed to vitamin E treatment effect on MI (1.0% in vitamin E vs. 2.4% in placebo; p=0.04). Perceived side effects caused 11 individuals (5 in vitamin E group and 6 in placebo group) to discontinue their participation in the study.

TABLE 7-1 Continued

Reference	Type of Injury/ Insult	Type of Study and Subjects	Treatment	Findings/Results
Sesso et al., 2008	Cardiovascular events (MI, stroke, or CVD death)	Randomized, double-blind, placebo-controlled trial (Physicians' Health Study II) n=14,641 U.S. male physicians, aged 50 years or older	Vitamin E (400 IU α-tocopherol) or placebo every other day for mean 8 years	The cumulative incidence rate of major cardiovascular events per year for vitamin E and placebo were similar. Vitamin E also had no effect on the incidence of MI, stroke, or congestive heart failure. However, among the men who were diagnosed with stroke during the study period, risk of hemorrhagic stroke was significantly higher in those in vitamin E group, compared to placebo group (HR=1.74, 95% CI: 1.04–2.91; p=0.04). Vitamin E also had no preventive effect on non-fatal cardiovascular events, CVD mortality, or total mortality. No interaction with vitamin C was found for any of the cardiovascular events. Compared to placebo, vitamin E had no significant adverse effects.
Cook et al., 2007	Cardiovascular events (MI, stroke, coronary revascularization, or CVD death)	Randomized, double-blind, placebo-controlled trial (Women's Antioxidant Cardiovascular Study) n=8,171 female health professionals, aged 40 years or older; mean follow-up years=9.4	Vitamin E (600 IU d-α-tocopherol acetate) every other day	After excluding noncompliant subjects from analysis, vitamin E had significant effect reducing overall CVD morbidity and mortality (RR=0.87, 95% CI: 0.76–0.99; p=0.04), stroke (RR=0.73, 95% CI: 0.54–0.98; p=0.04), and combination MI, stroke, and CVD death (RR=0.77, 95% CI: 0.64–0.92; p=0.005). And in those with previous CVD events at baseline, fewer CVD events were observed during the study period in the vitamin E group (RR=0.89, 95% CI: 0.79–1.00; p=0.04). Subjects taking both vitamins C and E had significantly fewer strokes than those taking placebos for both vitamins (RR=0.69, 95% CI: 0.49–0.98; p=0.04), suggesting an interaction (p for interaction=0.02). No statistically significant adverse effects were observed.

continued

TABLE 7-1   Continued

Reference	Type of Injury/Insult	Type of Study and Subjects	Treatment	Findings/Results
Buring, 2006a Lee et al., 2005	Cardiovascular events (MI, stroke, or CVD death) and cancer	Randomized, placebo-controlled trial (Women's Health Study) n=39,876 female health professionals	Aspirin (100 mg) or placebo vs. vitamin E (600 IU) or placebo every other day	Vitamin E had no significant effect on major CVD events, total stroke, all stroke subtypes, total MI, all MI events, or all-cause death. But vitamin E did reduce CVD death by 24% (RR=0.76, p=0.03). In women > 65 years old, vitamin E reduced total CVD events (RR=0.74, p=0.009), MI (RR=0.66, p=0.04), and CVD death (RR=0.51, p < 0.001). Vitamin E had no effect at all on cancer. The only significant adverse effect of vitamin E was 6% increased risk of epistaxis (RR=1.06, p=0.02). No interaction between aspirin and vitamin E was noted.
Eidelman et al., 2004	Cardiovascular events (MI, stroke, or CVD death)	Meta-analysis and overview of 7 randomized trials from 1990 to present on effectiveness of vitamin E in the treatment and prevention of CVD total n=106,625	Natural and synthetic vitamin E, 30–800 mg	Meta-analysis of the 7 trials showed that compared to placebo, vitamin E treatment was not significant in preventing CVD events. 4,832 major CVD events occurred in patients receiving vitamin E treatment, and 4,895 events occurred in placebo-treated patients (OR^f=0.98, 95% CI: 0.94–1.03). Vitamin E also had no effect on CVD death (OR=1.00, 95% CI: 0.94–1.05), non-fatal MI (OR=1.00, 95% CI: 0.92–1.00), non-fatal stroke (OR=1.03, 95% CI: 0.93–1.14), ischemic stroke (OR=1.01; 95% CI: 0.90–1.14), or hemorrhagic stroke (OR=1.24, 95% CI: 0.96–1.59). No adverse effects were mentioned.

TABLE 7-1   Continued

Reference	Type of Injury/ Insult	Type of Study and Subjects	Treatment	Findings/Results
Heart Protection Study Collaborative Group, 2002	Cardiovascular events (MI, stroke, or CVD death)	Randomized, placebo-controlled trial (Heart Protection Study) n=20,536 UK adults, aged 40–80 years at high risk for coronary disease due to previous medical history	Antioxidant vitamin supplementation (600 mg [synthetic] vitamin E, 250 mg vitamin C, and 20 mg β-carotene), daily, mean 5-yr follow up	Compliance to treatment was high and equal in both groups (83% for both). Analysis of blood assays showed that subjects taking vitamins had higher levels of plasma α-tocopherol, vitamin C, and β-carotene. Vitamins had no effect on mortality due to composite CVD events, any CVD subevents, or any non-CVD events. No significant effects were noted for vitamins in incidence of: stroke, of all types and severity; any major CVD events, regardless of whether subjects had CVD in the past or not; cancers; neuropsychiatric disorders; respiratory diseases; or fractures. Vitamin treatment group had increase of 0.15 mmol of total cholesterol, 0.08 mmol of low-density lipoprotein cholesterol, and 0.21 mmol of triglycerides (p < 0.05 for all). Over 5 years of vitamin use, the incidence of major adverse events (e.g., heart attacks, strokes, cancers) did not substantially increase.
Collaborative Group of the Primary Prevention Project, 2001	Cardiovascular events (MI, stroke, or CVD death)	Randomized, placebo-controlled, open-label trial (Primary Prevention Project) n=4,495 aged 50 years or older, with at least one of the major recognized cardiovascular risk factors	2X2 factorial design: vitamin E (100 mg synthetic α-tocopherol) daily and aspirin (100 mg enteric-coated aspirin a day) for mean 3.6 years	Vitamin E had no significant effect on combined endpoints (CVD death, non-fatal MI, and non-fatal stroke) or most individual events (CVD and non-CVD death, all MI, all stroke, angina pectoris, transient ischemic attack, and revascularization). Vitamin E significantly reduced risk of peripheral-artery disease (RR=0.54, 95% CI: 0.30–0.99; p=0.043). No significant adverse effect was observed for vitamin E.

continued

TABLE 7-1 Continued

Reference	Type of Injury/ Insult	Type of Study and Subjects	Treatment	Findings/Results
Leppala et al., 2000	Stroke	Randomized, double-blind, placebo-controlled trial (Alpha-Tocopherol, Beta-Carotene Cancer Prevention Study [ATBC Study]) n=28,519 Finnish, male, cigarette smokers aged 50 to 69 years without history of stroke	2X2 factorial design: 50 mg α-tocopherol or placebo daily; and 20 mg β-carotene or placebo daily for 6 years	Compared to those taking only β-carotene or placebo, subjects taking α-tocopherol had a non-significantly higher incidence of subarachnoid hemorrhage and a significantly lower incidence of cerebral infarction (RR=0.86, 95% CI: 0.75–0.99; p=0.03). α-tocopherol had no effect on incidence of intracranial hemorrhage or total stroke. There was no interaction between α-tocopherol and β-carotene. No adverse effects were mentioned.
Yusuf et al., 2000	Cardiovascular events (MI, stroke, or CVD death)	Randomized, placebo-controlled trial n=9,541, aged 55 years or older at high risk because they had CVD or diabetes in addition to one other risk factor average follow-up period=4.5 years	Natural vitamin E (400 IU/day) or matching placebo plus either an angiotensin-converting-enzyme inhibitor (ramipril) or matching placebo	Other than a 17% increase in risk of heart failure (RR=1.17, 95% CI: 1.03–1.32, p=0.02), vitamin E had no effect on total CVD incidence, total CVD death, MI, stroke, all-cause mortality rate, hospitalization for unstable angina or heart failure, revascularization or limb amputation, new onset or worsening angina, or diabetes complications. There was still no effect after stratification by age, sex, history of CVD and diabetes, and smoking. No interaction between vitamin E and ramipril was noted. No significant adverse effects of vitamin E were observed.

TABLE 7-1 Continued

Reference	Type of Injury/ Insult	Type of Study and Subjects	Treatment	Findings/Results
Daga et al., 1997	Acute ischemic stroke	Randomized, placebo-controlled trial n=50	Vitamin E (300 mg/day) or placebo; patients evaluated at day 1, day 15, and 6 weeks	At day 15, vitamin E group had plasma lipid peroxidation level that was 1.67 mmol/mL lower than the placebo group ($p < 0.01$). Plasma α-tocopherol level in the vitamin E group was 4.52 mmol/mL higher than that of the placebo group ($p < 0.01$). There was no difference between the two groups regarding plasma β-carotene level.

Neurological condition was measured using Matthew scale from days 1–15 and Barthel Index (BI) from day 15–6 weeks. Neither group experienced change in their Matthew scale between day 1 and day 15; there was also no significant difference between groups. However, vitamin E group achieved greater improvement at 6 weeks with an increase of 246 points on their BI ($p < 0.05$); the placebo group had an increase of 136.8 points.

No adverse effects were mentioned. |
| Raju et al., 1994 | Refractory epilepsy | Randomized, double-blind, placebo-controlled, cross-over trial n=43 | d-α-tocopherol (600 IU/day) or placebo as add-on therapy to antiepileptic drugs | Compared to baseline, all patients had a significant reduction in seizure frequency ($p < 0.001$) with no significant difference between the vitamin E arm and the placebo arm. In those who had > 50% reduction, vitamin E also had no effect. Patients with primary generalized seizures had significantly reduced seizure frequency during treatment period compared to baseline ($p < 0.05$) but the reduction achieved during the vitamin E arm was similar to the placebo arm. In all patients, order of vitamin E treatment made no difference ($p > 0.1$).

No significant side effects were observed for vitamin E. |

Tier 2: Observational studies

None found

continued

TABLE 7-1   Continued

Reference	Type of Injury/ Insult	Type of Study and Subjects	Treatment	Findings/Results
Tier 3: Animal studies				
Wu et al., 2010	Mild TBI (mTBI), mild fluid percussion injury	Male Sprague-Dawley rats	Preinjury, regular diet (containing 40 IU/kg of vitamin E) or supplemented diet (with 500 IU/kg of vitamin E) beginning 4 weeks prior to injury	Compared to injured rats on regular diet, injured rats on supplemented diet had better performance in the Morris water maze ($p < 0.05$).
				Level of oxidative stress in injured rats was 39% higher than that of sham-injured rats ($p < 0.01$), but vitamin E supplementation decreased the level of oxidative stress to 44% of the level observed in sham-injured rats ($p < 0.01$ vs. injured, regular diet rats and sham rats).
				Vitamin E supplementation significantly restored levels of brain-derived neurotrophic factors after injury.
				Compared to rats on regular diet, rats on vitamin E supplemented diet had higher levels of synapsin I ($p < 0.05$) and CREB ($p < 0.05$).
				Vitamin E also restored the level of CaMKII to 96% of the sham-injured rats, the level of superoxide dismutase to 92% of sham-injured rats, and the level of Sir2 to 95% of sham-injured rats.
Conte et al., 2004	Repetitive concussive brain injury (RCBI, two injuries, 24 hours apart) and modified controlled cortical impact model	Tg2576 female mice	Preinjury: regular diet or diet supplemented with 2 IU/g of vitamin E 4 weeks before injury Postinjury: regular diet or diet supplemented with 2 IU/g of vitamin E fed for up to preinjury 8 weeks postinjury	Vitamin E supplementation increased the level of brain vitamin E ($p < 0.01$) and decreased the level of $8,12\text{-iso-iPF}_{2\alpha}\text{-VI}$ ($p < 0.01$) in injured mice. There was no difference in brain vitamin E level between sham-injured and untreated mice, but untreated, injure mice had significantly higher level of $8,12\text{-iso-iPF}_{2\alpha}\text{-VI}$ compared to sham-injured mice ($p < 0.05$).
				Mice on vitamin E supplemented diet had improved cognitive function than mice on regular diet ($p < 0.01$).
				Mice on regular diet had increased levels of $A\beta 1\text{-}40$ and $A\beta 1\text{-}42$ compared to sham-injured mice ($p < 0.05$), and significantly higher level of $A\beta 1\text{-}42$ in the cortex and hippocampus compared to mice on vitamin E supplementation ($p < 0.01$).

TABLE 7-1 Continued

Reference	Type of Injury/ Insult	Type of Study and Subjects	Treatment	Findings/Results
Inci et al., 1998	Mild (200 g × cm) and severe (1,000 g × cm) TBI	Guinea pigs, aged 3–4 months	Preinjury, α-tocopherol injection (100 mg/kg) 8 hours before injury	Compared to uninjured controls, all injured guinea pigs had higher levels of lipid peroxides. Highest level of lipid peroxide was observed in untreated guinea pigs that underwent severe TBI. Levels of lipid peroxide increased over time in guinea pigs with severe TBI regardless of treatment. And lipid peroxide levels decreased over time in guinea pigs with mild TBI, regardless of treatment.

[a] n: sample size.
[b] RR: relative risk.
[c] CI: confidence interval.
[d] I^2: degree of heterogeneity.
[e] HR: hazard ratio.
[f] OR: odds ratio.

on hemorrhagic effects. However, there are concerns about increasing mortality if doses larger than 400 IU (400 mg of all-rac-alpha-tocopheryl acetate) are given (Miller et al., 2005). Although the data are mixed, a 2007 review of the adverse-event data for high doses of vitamin E revealed that those papers categorized as having high methodological quality were more likely to report increased mortality than studies with low methodological quality (Bjelakovic et al., 2007).

Evidence Indicating Effect on Resilience

Human Studies

Except for one recent study reported at a conference, there has been no human study conducted to test the potential effects of vitamin E on providing resilience to TBI. Some additional indication of this possibility comes from data on vitamin E and cardiovascular diseases, where vitamin E was shown to decrease oxidation of low-density lipoproteins. For risk of cardiovascular diseases, this chapter presents only the larger randomized controlled studies on vitamin E.

Contrary to preliminary studies, results from clinical trials do not support a protective effect of vitamin E supplementation on the risk of cardiovascular diseases (CVD) (Eidelman et al., 2004; Lichtenstein, 2009; Steinberg, 2000). In a double-blind clinical trial including 1,434 individuals aged 55 years or older with both Type 2 diabetes and the haptoglobin 2-2 genotype (which is associated with a high level of oxidative stress), participants were randomized to vitamin E (400 IU/day) or placebo (Milman et al., 2008). After 18 months of follow-up, vitamin E treatment was not significantly associated with a lower incidence of stroke than the placebo. In another randomized, placebo-controlled trial including 9,541 adults (aged 55 or older) with CVD or diabetes in addition to one other risk factor of CVD, treatment with vitamin E (400 IU/day) for an average 4.5 years did not significantly decrease the risk of major cardiovascular events (occurrence of myocardial infarction [MI], stroke, or cardiovascular death) or stroke, compared with the placebo group (Yusuf et al., 2000). Vitamin E supplementation similarly failed to show protective effects against the risk of stroke in the Women's Health study (n = 39,873, 600 IU/day of vitamin E for 10 years) (Buring, 2006; Lee et al., 2005), the Women's Antioxidant Cardiovascular study (n = 8,171, 600 IU/day of vitamin E every other day for 9.4 years) (Cook et al., 2007), and the Physicians' Health study-II (n = 14,641, 400 IU/day of vitamin E every other day for 8 years) (Sesso et al., 2008). A trial including 28,519 male cigarette smokers who were free of stroke at baseline found that vitamin E supplementation (50 mg/day) for approximately six years significantly increased the risk of developing fatal hemorrhagic strokes, but prevented cerebral infarction (Leppala et al., 2000).

In a 2010 meta-analysis including nine randomized controlled trials, vitamin E supplementation was not associated with total stroke. However, when stroke subtypes were analyzed, use of vitamin E increased risk for hemorrhagic stroke but decreased risk for ischemic stroke, which is much more common in the United States (Schürks et al., 2010).

Animal Studies

Three animal studies on the effects of vitamin E on TBI were identified. In a 2010 study (Wu et al., 2010), male rats (weighing 200–240 g) were fed a regular diet with or without α-tocopherol (500 IU/kg) for four weeks (n = 6–8 within each group) prior to administration of a mild fluid percussion injury (FPI). When assessed one week after brain injury, vitamin E supplementation was associated with a favorable brain status of oxidized proteins, brain-derived neurotrophic factor (BDNF), calcium/calmodulin dependent kinase II (CaMKII), synapsin I, cAMP-response element-binding protein, superoxide dismutase, and Sir2. Rats treated with vitamin E also had better cognitive function, as assessed by a Morris water maze (MWM) test starting at day 5 after TBI, than untreated rats. Protective effects of vitamin E on cognitive impairment due to TBI were further supported by another study using Tg2576 mice (female, aged 11 months), a mouse model of Alzheimer's disease (AD) brain amyloidosis. Conte and colleagues (2004) found that mice with preinjury supplementation of vitamin E (2 IU/g, n = 9) had a significant decrease in brain lipid peroxidation levels and a better cognitive performance in the MWM test compared with untreated mice (n = 13), although the two groups had similar levels of amyloid deposition. In another animal study including 65 guinea pigs (aged 3–4 months), alpha-tocopherol (100 mg/kg) administered intraperitoneally before brain injury was also associated with lower lipid peroxide levels in traumatized brain tissues, independent of severity of injury (Inci et al., 1998).

Evidence Indicating Effect on Treatment

Human Studies

There has been no human study conducted to test the potential effectiveness of vitamin E for treating TBI. Clinical trials examining whether vitamin E exerts neuroprotective effects among participants with various other forms of brain trauma have generated mixed results. Raju and colleagues (1994) conducted a double-blind, crossover trial of vitamin E among 43 patients with uncontrolled epilepsy, and observed no significant difference in seizure frequency between the group receiving vitamin E and the placebo group. Another small trial including 30 patients with acute ischemic stroke found that vitamin E supplementation had no significant effect on early neurological outcomes or on the level of plasma lipid peroxides after acute ischemic stroke, but it led to a significant improvement in subsequent recovery and rehabilitation (Daga et al., 1997). In a trial (n = 11,324 patients in the GISSI-Prevenzione trial) including 72 ischemic stroke patients, the use of antioxidants (300 mg of α-tocopherol daily) was not associated with a lower risk of mortality, but after a year of follow-up there was a trend to lower mortality in those groups treated with polyunsaturated fatty acids (850–882 mg eicosapentaenoic or docosahexaenoic acid [EPA/DHA] [ratio EPA/DHA 1:2] daily, either alone or in conjunction with 300 mg of α-tocopherol) (Garbagnati et al., 2009; GISSI-Prevenzione Investigators, 1999). Recently, a small (100 patients, 83 male), randomized, clinical controlled study showed that in patients with TBI (Glasgow Coma Scale scores of 8 or less and radiologic diagnoses of diffuse axonal injury), in-hospital mortality was significantly lower in those receiving high doses of vitamin E (intravenous at 400 IU daily for 7 days) than in those receiving low (500 mg daily for 7 days) or high (10 g on the day of admission and 4 days later) doses of vitamin C or placebo (Razmkon et al., 2010).

VITAMIN C (ASCORBIC ACID)

Introduction

Vitamin C (L-ascorbic acid or L-ascorbate) is an essential nutrient that protects the body against oxidative stress. The biological function of vitamin C comes from its ability to donate reducing equivalents to reactions, including reduction of reactive oxygen that damages cells. It is a cofactor in at least eight enzymatic reactions, and is required for metabolic reactions. Vitamin C is the electron donor for eight enzymes involved in collagen hydroxylation, carnitine biosynthesis, and hormone and amino acid biosynthesis. Vitamin C deficiency is characterized by impairments in connective tissue, specifically impairment of collagen synthesis. Vitamin C has also been shown to affect components of the immune response (IOM, 2000). The IOM considered levels higher than the Military Dietary Reference Intakes (MDRIs) for prevention of oxidative damage and muscle injury associated with high-intensity exercise (IOM, 2006) or for acute oxidative stress (IOM, 1999), but found insufficient evidence to make such recommendations. Those reports did not review evidence on vitamin C and potential benefits for TBI.

The brain has particularly high levels of vitamin C, approximately 100 times higher than levels in most other tissues in the body (Grunewald, 1993; Rice, 2000). Vitamin C is pumped into the central nervous system by the sodium-dependent vitamin C transporter-2 systems in series in the epithelial and neuronal cell membranes, but there is no sound evidence for a carrier-mediated transport (Spector, 2009). A study to assess antioxidant depletion in patients additionally showed that those with intracranial hemorrhage and head trauma had lower plasma levels of vitamin C than controls, and that its levels were significantly inversely correlated with the several outcomes of the disease (i.e., severity of the neurological impairment and diameter of the lesion). However, to the committee's best knowledge, there are no human or animal studies to examine the potential neuroprotective effects of vitamin C on TBI, except for the study by Razmkon described above presented at a 2010 conference. The committee identified five human studies regarding vitamin C supplementation and stroke or subarachnoid hemorrhage. Table 7-2 lists those studies, plus the study on TBI presented at a conference. As with Table 7-1, the occurrence or absence of adverse effects is included if reported.

TABLE 7-2 Relevant Data Identified for Vitamin C

Reference	Type of Injury/ Insult	Type of Study and Subjects	Treatment	Findings/Results
Tier 1: Clinical trials				
Razmkon et al., 2010	TBI (Glasgow Coma Scale scores of 8 or less and radiologic diagnoses of diffuse axonal injury)	Multi-center, randomized, double-blind, placebo-controlled trial n=100 (83 male)	Postinjury, vitamin E (intravenously at 400 IU daily for 7 days) Postinjury, vitamin C (500 mg daily for 7 days or 10 g on the day of admission and 4 days later), or placebo	The high dose of vitamin C stabilized or reduced the diameter of peri-lesional edema/infarct in 68% of patients (p=0.01). No adverse effects were observed.
Sesso et al., 2008	Cardiovascular events (MI, stroke, or CVD death)	Randomized, double-blind, placebo-controlled trial (Physicians' Health Study II) n=14,641 U.S. male physicians, aged 50 years or older 8-year follow-up	500 mg/day of vitamin C or placebo	The cumulative incidence rate of major cardiovascular events per year for vitamin E and placebo were similar. Vitamin C had no significant treatment or preventive effect on the individual incidence of MI, stroke, or total mortality. Vitamin C treatment did not benefit men with previous cardiovascular diseases at baseline. No interaction with vitamin E was found for any of the cardiovascular events. Compared to placebo, no significant adverse effects of vitamin C were observed.
Cook et al., 2007	Cardiovascular events (MI, stroke, coronary revascularization, or CVD death)	Randomized, double-blind, placebo-controlled trial (Women's Antioxidant Cardiovascular Study) n=8,171 female health professionals, aged 40 years or older mean follow-up=9.4 years	Vitamin C (500 mg/day), vitamin E (600 IU d-α tocopherol acetate every other day), or beta carotene (50 mg every other day)	Vitamin C had no significant effect on major CVD morbidity and mortality (RR=1.02). There was no significant difference in cumulative incidence rate of CVD events between subjects taking vitamin C and those taking placebo. Subjects taking both vitamins C and E had significantly fewer strokes than those taking placebos for both vitamins (RR=0.69, 95% CI: 0.49–0.98; p=0.04), suggesting an interaction (p for interaction=0.02). No statistically significant adverse effects were observed.

TABLE 7-2 Continued

Reference	Type of Injury/ Insult	Type of Study and Subjects	Treatment	Findings/Results
Polidori et al., 2005	Ischemic stroke	Randomized, open-label trial n=59	Postinjury, vitamin C (200 mg/day) + aspirin (300 mg/ day) or aspirin only	Barthel Index (BI): There was no difference between treatment group and control group at baseline or after 3 months. But BI of subjects in both groups increased over the study period (p < 0.05).
				Plasma vitamin C: Levels were higher in the vitamin C plus aspirin group compared to control group, both in the first week (p < 0.02) and over the entire study period (p < 0.01).
				Plasma 8,12-isoprostane $F_{2\alpha}$-VI: Levels decreased in both groups over the study period. But vitamin C plus aspirin group had significantly lower levels than control group from day 1 to day 7 (p=0.01); the difference between the two groups from day 1 to day 90 was not significant. There was no correlation between plasma vitamin C level and levels of 8,12-isoprostane $F_{2\alpha}$-VI.
				No adverse effects were observed.
Tier 2: Observational studies				
Kodama et al., 2000	Subarachnoid hemorrhage with a significant risk for symptomatic vasospasm (Fisher CT group 3 and CT number > 60)	n=217	Cisternal irrigation therapy with urokinase (120 IU/mL) and ascorbic acid (4 mg/mL)	The clinical outcomes of 80.6% of patients (n=175) were rated as "excellent" or "good" at hospital discharge, while the morbidity (those rated as "fair" or "poor") rate was 16.6% (n=36), the mortality rate was 2.8% (n=6), and 2.8% of patients developed vasospasm (n=6). None of the deaths were caused by vasospasm.
				Mean total drained blood volume was 113.7±12.0 mL; volume from red blood cell count was 96.5±9.6 mL, and from cell-free Hb count was 17.2±2.4 mL. Average total drainage from subjects who developed vasospasm during the study was 46.0 mL.
				Ascorbic acid absorption was determined by reduction in value of oxy-hemoglobin (Oxy-Hb) peak. Compared to patients who only had cisternal drainage, those who had cisternal irrigation had decreased Oxy-Hb value.
				Complications from irrigation include seizure (0.9%, n=2), meningitis infection (0.9%, n=2), and intracranial hemorrhage (1.9%, n=4).

continued

TABLE 7-2 Continued

Reference	Type of Injury/Insult	Type of Study and Subjects	Treatment	Findings/Results
Rabadi and Kristal, 2007	Ischemic stroke	Retrospective, matched, case-control trial n=46, aged 49–89 years	Postinjury, 1,000 mg of vitamin C per day Control group did not take vitamin C	There was no significant difference between the two groups in terms of changes in total functional independence measure score, functional independence measure-cognition score, or functional independence measure–motor score. There was no difference in length of stay and whether patient was discharged to home or a long-term care facility. No adverse effects were mentioned.

Tier 3: Animal studies

None
found

Uses and Safety

The EAR for vitamin C was based on maintaining near-maximal neutrophil concentrations with minimal urinary loss, and was set at 75 mg/day for men and 60 mg for women. A comparison of U.S. dietary intake from NHANES 2001–2002 data with the EAR of vitamin C (Table 5-2) suggests that 40 percent of males and 38 percent of females older than 19 years of age consume less vitamin C than the recommended EAR. The UL for vitamin C is 2 g/day based on gastrointestinal disturbance, but there are concerns that vitamin C could act as a prooxidant, depending on the dose (Childs et al., 2001).

Evidence Indicating Effect on Resilience

Human Studies

Effects of vitamin C supplementation on risk of stroke were examined in the Women's Antioxidant Cardiovascular Study (n = 8,171, 500 mg/day for 9.4 years) (Cook et al., 2007) and the Physicians' Health Study II (n = 14,641, 500 mg/day for 8 years) (Sesso et al., 2008). No protective effects were observed in these trials, either for total, or for different subtypes of stroke (Cook et al., 2007; Sesso et al., 2008).

Evidence Indicating Effect on Treatment

Human Studies

Polidori and colleagues (2005) reported that treatment with vitamin C (200 mg/day) in combination with aspirin therapy in 59 patients with ischemic stroke of recent onset (< 24 hours) was associated with significantly lower lipid peroxidation, as assessed by plasma 8,12-iPF2α-VI concentrations, than a control group receiving only aspirin. Kodama and colleagues (2000) also showed that subarachnoid hemorrhage patients (n = 217) who were treated with urokinase and vitamin C recovered without neurological deficits. (It should be noted, however, that this study lacked a control group.) In another trial including 46 ischemic stroke patients, 1,000 mg/day of vitamin C had no impact on motor recovery (Rabadi and Kristal, 2007).

The small randomized, clinical controlled study described above that showed benefits associated with high doses of vitamin E following TBI did not find vitamin C to be associated with positive neurologic outcomes, but the high doses of the vitamin (10 g on the day of admission and 4 days later) slowed the progression of perilesional edema (Razmkon et al., 2010).

COMBINATION OF ANTIOXIDANTS

Evidence Indicating Effect on Resilience

Human Studies

Results from observational studies are mixed and have not resulted in any clear association between chronic diseases and intake of antioxidants (Hirvonen et al., 2000; Mezzetti et al., 2001; Voko et al., 2003; Watkins et al., 2000; Yochum et al., 2000). Although the committee's literature reviews did not include cancer as a disease outcome because its pathology and etiology is dissimilar to that of TBI, one study is presented here to illustrate how a combination of antioxidants showed benefits where single nutrients did not. A randomized controlled trial was conducted in a region of China where esophageal and gastric cancers are prevalent and low intake of micronutrients has also been observed. Mortality and cancer incidence were ascertained for 29,584 adults who were assigned to take daily vitamin and mineral supplementation of (1) retinol and zinc; (2) riboflavin and niacin; (3) vitamin C and molybdenum; and (4) beta-carotene, vitamin E, and selenium. Those in the group taking beta-carotene, vitamin E, and selenium had lower mortality than controls, mainly because of lower cancer rates (Blot et al., 1993).

There are other studies showing that supplementation with both vitamin C and vitamin E (compared to vitamins C or E alone) is more effective in protecting from oxidative stress because vitamin E is regenerated by vitamin C. There were 8,171 women recruited for the Women's Antioxidant Cardiovascular Study, designed to test the effects of ascorbic acid (500 mg/day), vitamin E (600 IU every other day), and beta-carotene (50 mg every other day) on cardiovascular disease in a $2 \times 2 \times 2$ factorial design. Participants were 40 years of age or older, postmenopausal or had no intention of becoming pregnant, and had a self-reported history of CVD or at least three cardiac risk factors (Cook et al., 2007). During 9.4 years of follow-up, those in the active groups for both vitamin E and ascorbic acid had a lower risk of developing stroke relative to those in the placebo group for both agents. However, other two- or three-way interactions among these three antioxidants were not significant for stroke (Cook et al., 2007). In contrast, the Physicians' Health Study II Randomized Controlled Trial, a 2×2 factorial design to test the effect of ascorbic acid (500 mg/day) and vitamin E (400 IU every other day) in 14,641 U.S. men aged 50 years or older, failed to find any significant protective effects of these agents or their combination on stroke risk during a mean follow-up of eight years (Sesso et al., 2008). Another large, randomized controlled study that observed vascular disease, cancer, and other adverse outcomes in which participants (20,536 adults aged 40–80) were randomly allocated to receive antioxidant vitamin supplementation (600 mg vitamin E, 250 mg vitamin C, and 20 mg beta-carotene daily) or matching placebo showed no significant effects on cancer incidence or on hospitalization for any other nonvascular cause (Heart Protection Study Collaborative, 2002).

In another randomized controlled trial in Finland that included 28,519 male cigarette smokers free of stroke at baseline, the incidence of stroke in those who received both acti-vated vitamin E (50 mg/day) and beta-carotene (20 mg/day) (258 out of 7118) was similar, during mean six years of follow-up, to the incidence in those who received placebos (252 out of 7153). However, the significance of difference of stroke risk between these two groups was not reported (Leppala et al., 2000).

Evidence Indicating Effect on Treatment

Human Studies

In a randomized, double-blind and placebo-controlled trial, 200 patients in intensive care (113 with organ failure after complicated cardiac surgery, 66 with major trauma, and 21 with subarachnoid hemorrhage) were provided intravenous antioxidant supplements (vitamin C, vitamin E, selenium, zinc, and vitamin B_1) for 5 days, starting within 24 hours of admission. There was a reduction of early organ dysfunction and significantly reduced serum C-reactive protein concentrations relative to the control group (Berger et al., 2008). The difference did not, however, reach a significant level in individual subgroups (e.g., trauma patients or patients with subarachnoid hemorrhage) (Berger et al., 2008). A study including 96 acute ischemic stroke patients found that use of antioxidants (800 IU vitamin E and 500 mg vitamin C) within 12 hours of symptom onset enhanced antioxidant capacity, mitigated oxidative damage, and may have had an anti-inflammatory effect, as assessed by serum C-reactive protein concentrations (Ullegaddi et al., 2006).

There has been one ongoing clinical trial identified that will contribute to the strength of the evidence about whether antioxidants may be beneficial in improving outcomes of TBI. The trial will examine whether providing high doses of glutamine and antioxidants (i.e., selenium, zinc, beta carotene, vitamin E and vitamin C) to critically ill patients will be associated with improved survival. Although patients with severe acquired brain injury are excluded from the study, the critically ill might also experience other less severe brain injuries; hence, the results of this study will contribute to our knowledge about this potential combination of antioxidants.

CONCLUSIONS AND RECOMMENDATIONS

The use of single antioxidant supplements to treat a variety of chronic diseases, includ-ing coronary heart disease, cancer, and ocular and skin diseases, has been disappointing. These apparently conflicting results may be due to the fact that all the trials with individual antioxidants reported here were conducted with α-tocopherol. The interactions of a diet high in α-tocopherol with other forms of vitamin E (e.g., γ-tocopherol, the form most abun-dant in the American diet) are not known. Other reasons for this discrepancy are possible, such as interactions with other food components and the existence of confounders such as diet and lifestyle patterns. For example, individuals who report using nutrient supplements are also more likely to have overall more healthful lifestyles. In the context of TBI, several conclusions can be derived from the review of the evidence of potential benefits of specific antioxidants. Although oxidative stress is a substantial risk factor for adverse events fol-lowing TBI, there is minimal evidence at this time to support recommendations to either supplement the diet with these nutrients beyond the dietary requirements or provide them after injury. For example, while the results from animal trials with vitamin E are encouraging, the human trials do not support the concept that vitamin E could have beneficial effects for TBI. There is one recent study with encouraging results for treating TBI patients with vitamin E. However, the committee concluded that, as with the study on cancer, a combination of various antioxidants including vitamins E, C, and carotenoids might be more efficacious. There is sufficient literature from animal and human trials with other acute injuries associated with oxidative stress to warrant a carefully designed trial with TBI patients using an array of antioxidants. Any trials that may be undertaken should ensure that dose levels of antioxidants do not approach levels that might cause adverse events, such as higher risk of mortality (Miller et al., 2005). The committee recommends that DoD track the findings of the current trial using a combination of antioxidants in the critically ill and any similar future human trials that may follow.

RECOMMENDATION 7-1. Based on the literature from animal and human trials concerning stroke and epilepsy, DoD should consider a clinical trial with TBI patients using an array of antioxidants in combination (e.g., vitamins E and C, selenium, beta-carotene).

REFERENCES

Berger, M. M., L. Soguel, A. Shenkin, J. P. Revelly, C. Pinget, M. Baines, and R. L. Chiolero. 2008. Influence of early antioxidant supplements on clinical evolution and organ function in critically ill cardiac surgery, major trauma, and subarachnoid hemorrhage patients. *Critical Care* 12(4):R101.

Bjelakovic, G., D. Nikolova, L. L. Gluud, R. G. Simonetti, and C. Gluud. 2007. Mortality in randomized trials of antioxidant supplements for primary and secondary prevention. *The Journal of the American Medical Association* 297(8):842–857.

Blot, W. J., J.-Y. Li, P. R. Taylor, W. Guo, S. Dawsey, G.-Q. Wang, C. S. Yang, S.-F. Zheng, M. Gail, G.-Y. Li, Y. Yu, B.-q. Liu, J. Tangrea, Y.-h. Sun, F. Liu, J. F. Fraumeni, Y.-H. Zhang, and B. Li. 1993. Nutrition intervention trials in Linxian, China: Supplementation with specific vitamin/mineral combinations, cancer incidence, and disease-specific mortality in the general population. *Journal of the National Cancer Institute* 85(18):1483–1491.

Buring, J. E. 2006. Aspirin prevents stroke but not MI in women; vitamin E has no effect on CV disease or cancer. *Cleveland Clinic Journal of Medicine* 73(9):863–870.

Childs, A., C. Jacobs, T. Kaminski, B. Halliwell, and C. Leeuwenburgh. 2001. Supplementation with vitamin C and n-acetyl-cysteine increases oxidative stress in humans after an acute muscle injury induced by eccentric exercise. *Free Radical Biology and Medicine* 31(6):745–753.

Collaborative Group of the Primary Prevention Project. 2001. Low-dose aspirin and vitamin E in people at cardiovascular risk: A randomised trial in general practice. Collaborative group of the primary prevention project. *Lancet* 357(9250):89–95.

Conte, V., K. Uryu, S. Fujimoto, Y. Yao, J. Rokach, L. Longhi, J. Q. Trojanowski, V. M. Lee, T. K. McIntosh, and D. Pratico. 2004. Vitamin E reduces amyloidosis and improves cognitive function in Tg2576 mice following repetitive concussive brain injury. *Journal of Neurochemistry* 90(3):758–764.

Cook, N. R., C. M. Albert, J. M. Gaziano, E. Zaharris, J. MacFadyen, E. Danielson, J. E. Buring, and J. E. Manson. 2007. A randomized factorial trial of vitamins C and E and beta carotene in the secondary prevention of cardiovascular events in women—results from the women's antioxidant cardiovascular study. *Archives of Internal Medicine* 167(15):1610–1618.

Daga, M. K., Madhuchhanda, T. K. Mishra, and A. Mohan. 1997. Lipid peroxide, beta-carotene and alpha-tocopherol in ischaemic stroke and effect of exogenous vitamin E supplementation on outcome. *Journal of the Association of Physicians of India* 45(11):843–846.

Eghwrudjakpor, P. O., and A. B. Allison. 2010. Oxidative stress following traumatic brain injury: Enhancement of endogenous antioxidant defense systems and the promise of improved outcome. *Nigerian Journal of Medicine* 19(1):14–21.

Eidelman, R. S., D. Hollar, P. R. Hebert, G. A. Lamas, and C. H. Hennekens. 2004. Randomized trials of vitamin E in the treatment and prevention of cardiovascular disease. *Archives of Internal Medicine* 164(14):1552–1556.

Fletcher, R. H., and K. M. Fairfield. 2002. Vitamins for chronic disease prevention in adults. *The Journal of the American Medical Association* 287(23):3127–3129.

Floyd, R. A. 1999. Antioxidants, oxidative stress, and degenerative neurological disorders. *Proceedings of the Society for Experimental Biology and Medicine* 222(3):236–245.

Floyd, R. A., and J. M. Carney. 1992. Free radical damage to protein and DNA: Mechanisms involved and relevant observations on brain undergoing oxidative stress. *Annals of Neurology* 32(Suppl.):S22–S27.

Garbagnati, F., G. Cairella, A. De Martino, M. Multari, U. Scognamiglio, V. Venturiero, and S. Paolucci. 2009. Is antioxidant and n-3 supplementation able to improve functional status in poststroke patients? Results from the Nutristroke Trial. *Cerebrovascular Diseases* 27(4):375–383.

GISSI (Gruppo Italiano per lo Studio della Sopravvivenza nell'Infarto miocardico)-Prevenzione Investigators. 1999. Dietary supplementation with n-3 polyunsaturated fatty acids and vitamin E after myocardial infarction: Results of the GISSI-Prevenzione trial. *Lancet* 354(9177):447–455.

Grunewald, R. A. 1993. Ascorbic acid in the brain. *Brain Research. Brain Research Reviews* 18(1):123–133.

Hall, E. D., R. A. Vaishnav, and A. G. Mustafa. 2010. Antioxidant therapies for traumatic brain injury. *Neurotherapeutics* 7(1):51–61.

Heart Protection Study Collaborative Group. 2002. MRC/BHF Heart Protection Study of antioxidant vitamin supplementation in 20,536 high-risk individuals: A randomised placebo-controlled trial. *Lancet* 360(9326):23–33.

Hirvonen, T., J. Virtamo, P. Korhonen, D. Albanes, and P. Pietinen. 2000. Intake of flavonoids, carotenoids, vitamins C and E, and risk of stroke in male smokers. *Stroke* 31(10):2301–2306.

Huang, H.-Y., B. Caballero, S. Chang, A. J. Alberg, R. D. Semba, C. R. Schneyer, R. F. Wilson, T.-Y. Cheng, J. Vassy, G. Prokopowicz, G. J. Barnes, and E. B. Bass. 2006. The efficacy and safety of multivitamin and mineral supplement use to prevent cancer and chronic disease in adults: A systematic review for a National Institutes of Health state-of-the-science conference. *Annals of Internal Medicine* 145(5):372–385.

Inci, S., O. E. Ozcan, and K. Kilinc. 1998. Time-level relationship for lipid peroxidation and the protective effect of alpha-tocopherol in experimental mild and severe brain injury. *Neurosurgery* 43(2):330–335; discussion 335–336.

IOM (Institute of Medicine). 1999. *Military strategies for sustainment of nutrition and immune function in the field*. Washington, DC: National Academy Press.

IOM. 2000. *Dietary Reference Intakes for vitamin C, vitamin E, selenium, and carotenoids*. Washington, DC: National Academy Press.

IOM. 2006. *Nutrient composition of rations for short-term, high-intensity combat operations*. Washington, DC: The National Academies Press.

Kodama, N., T. Sasaki, M. Kawakami, M. Sato, and J. Asari. 2000. Cisternal irrigation therapy with urokinase and ascorbic acid for prevention of vasospasm after aneurysmal subarachnoid hemorrhage. Outcome in 217 patients. *Surgical Neurology* 53(2):110–117; discussion 117–118.

Lee, I. M., N. R. Cook, J. M. Gaziano, D. Gordon, P. M. Ridker, J. E. Manson, C. H. Hennekens, and J. E. Buring. 2005. Vitamin E in the primary prevention of cardiovascular disease and cancer—the Women's Health Study: A randomized controlled trial. *The Journal of the American Medical Association* 294(1):56–65.

Leppala, J. M., J. Virtamo, R. Fogelholm, J. K. Huttunen, D. Albanes, P. R. Taylor, and O. P. Heinonen. 2000. Controlled trial of alpha-tocopherol and beta-carotene supplements on stroke incidence and mortality in male smokers. *Arteriosclerosis, Thrombosis, and Vascular Biology* 20(1):230–235.

Lichtenstein, A. H. 2009. Nutrient supplements and cardiovascular disease: A heartbreaking story. *Journal of Lipid Research* 50(Suppl.):S429–S433.

Mezzetti, A., G. Zuliani, F. Romano, F. Costantini, S. D. Pierdomenico, F. Cuccurullo, R. Fellin, and S. Associazione Medica. 2001. Vitamin E and lipid peroxide plasma levels predict the risk of cardiovascular events in a group of healthy very old people. *Journal of the American Geriatrics Society* 49(5):533–537.

Miller, E. R., 3rd, R. Pastor-Barriuso, D. Dalal, R. A. Riemersma, L. J. Appel, and E. Guallar. 2005. Meta-analysis: High-dosage vitamin E supplementation may increase all-cause mortality. *Annals of Internal Medicine* 142(1):37–46.

Milman, U., S. Blum, C. Shapira, D. Aronson, R. Miller-Lotan, Y. Anbinder, J. Alshiek, L. Bennett, M. Kostenko, M. Landau, S. Keidar, Y. Levy, A. Khemlin, A. Radan, and A. P. Levy. 2008. Vitamin E supplementation reduces cardiovascular events in a subgroup of middle-aged individuals with both type 2 diabetes mellitus and the haptoglobin 2-2 genotype: A prospective double-blinded clinical trial. *Arteriosclerosis, Thrombosis & Vascular Biology* 28(2):341–347.

Polidori, M. C., D. Pratico, T. Ingegni, E. Mariani, L. Spazzafumo, P. Del Sindaco, R. Cecchetti, Y. Yao, S. Ricci, A. Cherubini, W. Stahl, H. Sies, U. Senin, and P. Mecocci. 2005. Effects of vitamin C and aspirin in ischemic stroke-related lipid peroxidation: Results of the AVASAS (Aspirin Versus Ascorbic acid plus Aspirin in Stroke) Study. *Biofactors* 24(1–4):265–274.

Pryor, W. A. 2000. Vitamin E and heart disease: Basic science to clinical intervention trials. *Free Radical Biology and Medicine* 28(1):141–164.

Rabadi, M. H., and B. S. Kristal. 2007. Effect of vitamin C supplementation on stroke recovery: A case-control study. *Clinical Interventions in Aging* 2(1):147–151.

Raju, G. B., M. Behari, K. Prasad, and G. K. Ahuja. 1994. Randomized, double-blind, placebo-controlled, clinical trial of D-alpha-tocopherol (vitamin E) as add-on therapy in uncontrolled epilepsy. *Epilepsia* 35(2):368–372.

Razmkon, A., A. Sadidi, E. Sherafat-Kazemzadeh, A. Mehrafshan, and A. Bakhtazad. 2010. *Beneficial effects of vitamin C and vitamin E administration in severe head injury: A randomized double-blind control trial.* Paper presented at Congress of Neurological Surgeons Annual Meeting, San Francisco, CA.

Rice, M. E. 2000. Ascorbate regulation and its neuroprotective role in the brain. *Trends in Neurosciences* 23(5):209–216.

Schürks, M., R. J. Glynn, P. M. Rist, C. Tzourio, and T. Kurth. 2010. Effects of vitamin E on stroke subtypes: Meta-analysis of randomised controlled trials. *British Medical Journal* 341:c5702.

Sesso, H. D., J. E. Buring, W. G. Christen, T. Kurth, C. Belanger, J. MacFadyen, V. Bubes, J. E. Manson, R. J. Glynn, and J. M. Gaziano. 2008. Vitamins E and C in the prevention of cardiovascular disease in men the Physicians' Health Study II randomized controlled trial. *Journal of the American Medical Association* 300(18):2123–2133.

Spector, R. 2009. Nutrient transport systems in brain: 40 years of progress. *Journal of Neurochemistry* 111(2):315–320.

Spector, R., and C. E. Johanson. 2007. Vitamin transport and homeostasis in mammalian brain: Focus on vitamins B and E. *Journal of Neurochemistry* 103(2):425–438.

Steinberg, D. 2000. Is there a potential therapeutic role for vitamin E or other antioxidants in atherosclerosis? *Current Opinion in Lipidology* 11(6):603–607.

Ullegaddi, R., H. J. Powers, and S. E. Gariballa. 2006. Antioxidant supplementation with or without B-group vitamins after acute ischemic stroke: A randomized controlled trial. *Journal of Parenteral and Enteral Nutrition* 30(2):108–114.

Voko, Z., M. Hollander, A. Hofman, P. J. Koudstaal, and M. M. B. Breteler. 2003. Dietary antioxidants and the risk of ischemic stroke: The Rotterdam Study. *Neurology* 61(9):1273–1275.

Watkins, M. L., J. D. Erickson, M. J. Thun, J. Mulinare, and C. W. Heath, Jr. 2000. Multivitamin use and mortality in a large prospective study. *American Journal of Epidemiology* 152(2):149–162.

Wu, A. G., Z. Ying, and F. Gomez-Pinilla. 2010. Vitamin E protects against oxidative damage and learning disability after mild traumatic brain injury in rats. *Neurorehabilitation and Neural Repair* 24(3):290–298.

Yochum, L. A., A. R. Folsom, and L. H. Kushi. 2000. Intake of antioxidant vitamins and risk of death from stroke in postmenopausal women. *American Journal of Clinical Nutrition* 72(2):476–483.

Yusuf, S., G. Dagenais, J. Pogue, J. Bosch, and P. Sleight. 2000. Vitamin E supplementation and cardiovascular events in high-risk patients. The heart outcomes prevention evaluation study investigators. *The New England Journal of Medicine* 342(3):154–160.

8

Branched-Chain Amino Acids

The branched-chain amino acids (BCAAs) (leucine, isoleucine, and valine) are nutritionally essential in that they cannot be synthesized endogenously by humans and must be supplied by diet. They differ from other essential amino acids in that the liver lacks the enzymes necessary for their catabolism.

In addition to their function as structural components of proteins, BCAAs also seem to exert regulatory control of protein metabolism. In rodent tissue in vitro, increased concentrations of BCAAs stimulate protein synthesis and inhibit protein catabolism, whereas other amino acid mixtures lacking BCAAs have no such influence. In humans, BCAAs inhibit protein catabolism, but have little effect on synthesis (see Matthews, 2005, for review).

BRANCHED-CHAIN AMINO ACIDS AND THE BRAIN

In the brain, BCAAs have two important influences on the production of neurotransmitters. As nitrogen donors, they contribute to the synthesis of excitatory glutamate and inhibitory gamma-aminobutyric acid (GABA) (Yudkoff et al., 2005). They also compete for transport across the blood-brain barrier (BBB) with tryptophan (the precursor to serotonin), as well as tyrosine and phenylalanine (precursors for catecholamines) (Fernstrom, 2005). Ingestion of BCAAs therefore causes rapid elevation of the plasma concentrations and increases uptake of BCAAs to the brain, but diminishes tryptophan, tyrosine, and phenylalanine uptake. The decrease in these aromatic amino acids directly affects the synthesis and release of serotonin and catecholamines. The reader is referred to Fernstrom (2005) for a review of the biochemistry of BCAA transportation to the brain. Oral BCAAs have been examined as treatment for neurological diseases such as mania, motor malfunction, amyotrophic lateral sclerosis, and spinocerebral degeneration. Excitotoxicity as a result of excessive stimulation by neurotransmitters such as glutamate results in cellular damage after traumatic brain injury (TBI). However, because BCAAs also contribute to the synthesis of inhibitory neurotransmitters, it is unclear to what extent the role of BCAAs in synthesis of both excitatory and inhibitory neurotransmitters might contribute to their potential effects in outcomes of TBI.

A list of human studies (years 1990 and beyond) evaluating the effectiveness of BCAAs in providing resilience or treating TBI or related diseases or conditions (i.e., subarachnoid hemorrhage, intracranial aneurysm, stroke, anoxic or hypoxic ischemia, epilepsy) in the acute phase is presented in Table 8-1; this also includes supporting evidence from animal models of TBI. The occurrence or absence of adverse effects in humans is included if reported by the authors.

USES AND SAFETY

The Estimated Average Requirements (EARs) for leucine, isoleucine, and valine are 34, 15, and 19 mg/kg/day, respectively (IOM, 2005). Using the recommended intake for a 70 kg individual as a reference, the actual mean daily intake in the United States for each of the BCAAs is approximately threefold higher for men and approximately twofold higher for women (IOM, 2005). BCAA-enriched protein or amino acid mixtures or BCAAs alone have been used in a variety of metabolic disorders, such as chronic liver disease, encephalopathy, sepsis, and others, usually in an effort to reduce the uptake of aromatic amino acids by the brain and to raise low circulating levels. BCAA supplements are marketed to healthy individuals with claims that they enhance muscle mass, reduce soreness after exercise, and reduce central fatigue, although peer-reviewed research data rarely support these claims (Wagenmakers, 1999). A previous Institute of Medicine (IOM) committee considered the addition of higher amounts of specific amino acids, including BCAAs, to rations used during short-term, high-intensity combat operations. That committee found no evidence to recommend the addition of specific amino acids to those rations (IOM, 2006). As a result of claims for fitness benefits, athletes and military personnel striving to enhance physical performance may have BCAA intakes even higher than those of the general public. A survey by Lieberman et al. (2010) found that 23 percent of military personnel involved in combat arms and 47 percent of those in Special Forces were taking protein or amino acid supplements.

A 2005 IOM report found no studies of adverse events associated with normal diets containing BCAAs or with infused supplemental doses up to 9.75 g, but there was no Tolerable Upper Intake Level (UL) determined because of the lack of dose-response data. Studies of acute or chronic oral administration of BCAAs have reported no adverse effects, even at a high single dose of 60 grams (Fernstrom, 2005). The outcomes of interest measured in these studies were related to physical performance, phenylketonuria, hepatic cirrhosis, and neurological and psychiatric diseases. It is, however, difficult to assess whether some of the outcomes that were not regarded as adverse effects would present a concern in a military setting. As an example, after examining one of the studies reporting no adverse effects, the committee concluded that excessive intake of BCAAs may be deleterious; in that study, oral doses of 10, 30, and 60 grams of BCAAs caused small increases in spatial recognition memory latency in healthy human subjects, but no changes in visual information processing or pattern recognition (Gijsman et al., 2002). The authors attributed the increased latency to a reduced ratio of (tyrosine+phenylalanine) to BCAAs, resulting in reduced transport of tyrosine and phenylalanine across the BBB, and hence reduced dopamine synthesis.

TABLE 8-1 Relevant Data Identified for BCAA

Reference	Type of Injury/Insult	Type of Study and Subjects	Treatment	Findings/Results
Tier 1: Clinical trials				
Aquilani et al., 2008	TBI	Randomized, placebo-controlled trial n^a=41 rehabilitation patients with a posttraumatic vegetative or minimally conscious state, 47±24 days postinjury	Postinjury, short-term parenteral supplementation of BCAAs (500 mL of 4% mixture of amino acids solution; provided 19.6 g of BCAAs and 1.6 g arginine) for 15 days	Disability Rating Scores (DRS) improved significantly for treated patients (p < 0.001; geometric mean of DRS decreased, from 23.17 to 19.68), while the score in placebo recipients remained virtually unchanged. 68% of treated patients achieved DRS scores that allowed them to exit the vegetative or minimally conscious state. From day 15 to discharge from rehabilitation center, further significant brain function improvement was detected in patients in treatment group (p < 0.03); no improvement was detected in placebo group. No adverse effects were mentioned.
Aquilani et al., 2005	Severe TBI	Randomized, placebo-controlled trial n=60 men with TBI	Postinjury, 15 days of intravenous BCAA supplementation (19.6 g/day)	After 15 days, DRS for both treatment and placebo groups improved significantly (p < 0.02) compared to baseline. But improvement in treatment group was significantly greater than placebo group (p < 0.004). After 15 days, significant increase in total BCAA was seen only in treated group (p < 0.01). Plasma tyrosine level increased in the treated group (p < 0.01), while tryptophan increased in the placebo group (p < 0.01). No adverse effects were mentioned.

TABLE 8-1 Continued

Reference	Type of Injury/Insult	Type of Study and Subjects	Treatment	Findings/Results
Evangeliou et al., 2009	Refractory epilepsy	Pilot, prospective trial n=17 children, aged 2 to 7 years	Ketogenic diet, supplemented by powdered mixture of BCAA (45.5 g leucine, 30 g isoleucine, and 24.5 g valine) Fat-to-protein ratio with addition of BCAA changed from 4:1 to around 2:5:1	Adding BCAA to ketogenic diet resulted in a 100% seizure reduction in 3 patients who had experienced seizure reduction on ketogenic diet alone. Four patients who already had > 50% reduction on ketogenic diet alone achieved an additional 20–30% reduction. One patient, who had 20% reduction on ketogenic diet alone, achieved 50% reduction after adding BCAA. Addition of BCAA did not reduce seizure in patients who didn't already experience seizure reduction on ketogenic diet only. No reduction in ketosis was found with the addition of BCAA. A slight increase in heart rate was reported at treatment initiation in 3 patients, but returned to normal without a reduction in the dose of BCAA. No other adverse effects were observed.

Tier 2: Observational studies

None found

Tier 3: Animal studies

| Cole et al., 2010 | TBI, lateral fluid percussion brain injury (LFPI) | Adult male C57BL/ J6 mice

5–7 weeks old, 20–25 g | Postinjury, dietary consumption of BCAAs (100 μM leucine, isoleucine, and valine) starting 2 days after LFPI and continuing until 7 days after injury

Hippocampal slices incubated with BCAA (100 μM) | After being treated with BCAA for 5 days after injury, BCAA level in injured mice is not significantly different from sham mice.

In behavioral assessments, treated mice behaved no differently from control mice ($p < 0.05$).

In vitro analysis showed that hippocampal slices from injured mice incubated with BCAA fully restored synaptic function ($p < 0.05$). |

[a] n: sample size.

EVIDENCE INDICATING EFFECT ON RESILIENCE

Human Studies

There have been no clinical trials to test the effects of BCAAs on resilience for TBI or related diseases or conditions (i.e., subarachnoid hemorrhage, intracranial aneurysm, stroke, anoxic or hypoxic ischemia, epilepsy).

Animal Studies

There have been no animal studies addressing increased resilience for TBI. One study has examined the possibility of a negative influence of BCAAs at high concentrations. Contrusciere and colleagues (2010) noticed a high risk for amyotrophic lateral sclerosis among professional soccer players, and hypothesized that it could be due to excess consumption of sports beverages containing BCAAs. These beverages typically contain 1–3 grams of total BCAAs per 12-ounce serving. To test their hypothesis, the authors incubated rat neuronal cultures with 2.5–25 mM concentrations of BCAAs, and found that these extremely high doses induced toxicity. Note that normal BCAA concentrations in human cerebrospinal fluid are several orders of magnitude lower, ranging from ~5–15 μM (Garseth et al., 2001).

A review of the literature was also conducted for outcomes related to the TBI disease process (i.e., subarachnoid hemorrhage, intracranial aneurysm, stroke, anoxic or hypoxic ischemia, epilepsy). A search on the effects of BCAAs and epilepsy revealed several studies that examined their impact in either the latency to a seizure or the duration of a seizure. Two studies used different animal models (pentylenetetrazol- or picrotoxin-induced seizures), but reported similar results: leucine and isoleucine increased the latency of the seizures (an indication of seizure threshold) compared to a controlled, balanced amino acid solution (Dufour et al., 1999; Skeie et al., 1994). The studies did differ, however, on the impact of valine in latency; while Skeie and colleagues (1994) found that valine at 300 mg/kg increased the mean latency time to onset of seizures, the study by Dufour found no such effect for valine.

EVIDENCE INDICATING EFFECT ON TREATMENT

Human Studies

Only one prospective randomized clinical study has investigated the efficacy of BCAAs as an acute treatment for TBI (Ott et al., 1988). Starting on the first day of hospitalization, 20 brain-injured patients were randomized to either a standard intravenous amino acid formula or one containing higher percentages of leucine (154 percent of the standard formula), isoleucine (153 percent), and valine (174 percent). The formulas had equivalent total calories and protein. Those patients on the BCAA-enriched formula exhibited positive nitrogen balance (+1.8%), whereas those on the standard formula were in negative balance (–8.0 percent) (Ott et al., 1988).

Two small, randomized, placebo-controlled trials have been published reporting that BCAA supplementation enhanced cognitive recovery by patients with TBI (Aquilani et al., 2005, 2008). However, these studies began administering BCAAs anywhere from 19 to 140 days after injury, and therefore did not address the efficacy of BCAAs in treating the primary or secondary effects of neurotrauma.

Seven additional studies have addressed BCAA supplementation in other forms of trauma (reviewed in De Bandt and Cynober, 2006). Of these, four reported no beneficial effect on nitrogen balance, whereas three found positive results. The number of patients in each study tended to be small (ranging from 5 to 101, mean = 31) and the patients were heterogeneous in terms of type and severity of trauma.

A prospective, randomized controlled study of patients undergoing curative hepatic resection found that perioperative oral nutrition including BCAAs resulted in higher serum erythropoietin concentrations than a control diet (for patients who did not have hepatitis). The authors suggested that higher erythropoietin concentrations might provide protection from ischemic injury (Ishikawa et al., 2010).

When BCAAs were added as additional therapy to the ketogenic diet of children with refractory epilepsy, 13 out of 17 benefited, with a 50–100 percent seizure reduction compared to the ketogenic diet alone (Evangeliou et al., 2009). The authors suggested that BCAAs may not only increase the effectiveness of the ketogenic diet, but that the diet could be more easily tolerated by the patients because of the change in the ratio of fat to protein.

Animal Studies

Cole and colleagues reported that brain-injured mice exhibited cognitive improvement when treated with BCAA-supplemented drinking water (each BCAA at a concentration of 100 mM), beginning two days after injury (Cole et al., 2010). The injury was a 20 millisecond pressure pulse of saline to the dura, and hippocampal-dependent cognition was assessed using a conditioned fear response. Responses diminished by approximately 50% in the injured mice compared to sham controls, whereas injured mice drinking BCAA-supplemented water behaved no differently from controls. In addition to behavioral assessments, Cole et al. (2010) analyzed synaptic function in vitro. The excitatory postsynaptic potentials generated in hippocampal slices from injured mice were diminished compared to sham controls, but incubating the slices with BCAAs at concentrations of 100 μM fully restored synaptic function (Cole et al., 2010).

CONCLUSIONS AND RECOMMENDATIONS

Leucine and other essential amino acids are necessary, and their benefit in increasing protein synthesis and lean body mass is well documented. However, there are not yet compelling data to support a recommendation to supplement rations with BCAAs to ameliorate or treat TBI. There is some indication from a pilot study that BCAAs might act synergistically with a ketogenic diet in epilepsy, one of the many possible sequelae of TBI.

The only randomized clinical trial (Ott et al., 1988) suggests that intravenous infusion of BCAAs may be beneficial for maintaining positive nitrogen balance following TBI, but the influence of BCAAs on morbidity and mortality was not reported. There is one encouraging animal study in which mice supplemented with BCAAs (dissolved in water at 100 mM) showed improvements in cognition and diminished excitatory potentials in hippocampal slices (Cole et al., 2010). Taken altogether, however, there is not enough evidence from animal studies to support initiating research in humans.

Because a large percentage of military personnel take BCAAs as supplements to their diets, BCAAs should be included in the dietary intake assessments of TBI patients in medical treatment facilities to identify preinjury nutritional intake and status, as well as nutritional intake during the various stages of treatment. The data could be used to establish potential relationships between preinjury nutritional intake/status and recovery progress.

RECOMMENDATION 8-1. DoD should continue to monitor the literature on the effects of nutrients, dietary supplements, and diets on TBI, particularly those reviewed in this report but also others that may emerge as potentially effective in the future. For example, although the evidence was not sufficiently compelling to recommend that research be conducted on BCAAs, DoD should monitor the scientific literature for relevant research.

REFERENCES

Aquilani, R., P. Iadarola, A. Contardi, M. Boselli, M. Verri, O. Pastoris, F. Boschi, P. Arcidiaco, and S. Viglio. 2005. Branched-chain amino acids enhance the cognitive recovery of patients with severe traumatic brain injury. *Archives of Physical Medicine and Rehabilitation* 86(9):1729–1735.

Aquilani, R., M. Boselli, F. Boschi, S. Viglio, P. Iadarola, M. Dossena, O. Pastoris, and M. Verri. 2008. Branched-chain amino acids may improve recovery from a vegetative or minimally conscious state in patients with traumatic brain injury: A pilot study. *Archives of Physical Medicine and Rehabilitation* 89(9):1642–1647.

Cole, J. T., C. M. Mitala, S. Kundu, A. Verma, J. A. Elkind, I. Nissim, and A. S. Cohen. 2010. Dietary branched chain amino acids ameliorate injury-induced cognitive impairment. *Proceedings of the National Academy of Sciences of the United States of America* 107(1):366–371.

Contrusciere, V., S. Paradisi, A. Matteucci, and F. Malchiodi-Albedi. 2010. Branched-chain amino acids induce neurotoxicity in rat cortical cultures. *Neurotoxicity Research* 17:392–397.

De Bandt, J.-P., and L. Cynober. 2006. Therapeutic use of branched-chain amino acids in burn, trauma and sepsis. *Journal of Nutrition* 136:308S–313S.

Dufour, F., K. A. Nalecz, M. J. Nalecz, and A. Nehlig. 1999. Modulation of pentylenetetrazol-induced seizure activity by branched-chain amino acids and [alpha]-ketoisocaproate. *Brain Research* 815(2):400–404.

Evangeliou, A., M. Spilioti, V. Doulioglou, P. Kalaidopoulou, A. Ilias, A. Skarpalezou, I. Katsanika, S. Kalamitsou, K. Vasilaki, I. Chatziioanidis, K. Garganis, E. Pavlou, S. Varlamis, and N. Nikolaidis. 2009. Branched chain amino acids as adjunctive therapy to ketogenic diet in epilepsy: Pilot study and hypothesis. *Journal of Child Neurology* 24(10):1268–1272.

Fernstrom, J. D. 2005. Branched-chain amino acids and brain function. *Journal of Nutrition* 135(6 Suppl.):1539S–1546S.

Garseth, M., L. R. White, and J. Aasly. 2001. Little change in cerebrospinal fluid amino acids in subtypes of multiple sclerosis compared with acute polyradiculoneuropathy. *Neurochemistry International* 39(2):111–115.

Gijsman, H. J., A. Scarna, C. J. Harmer, S. F. B. McTavish, J. Odontiadis, P. J. Cowen, and G. M. Goodwin. 2002. A dose-finding study on the effects of branch chain amino acids on surrogate markers of brain dopamine function. *Psychopharmacology* 160(2):192–197.

IOM (Institute of Medicine). 2005. *Dietary Reference Intakes for energy, carbohydrate, fiber, fat, fatty acids, cholesterol, protein, and amino acids.* Washington, DC: The National Academies Press.

IOM. 2006. *Nutrient composition of rations for short-term, high-intensity combat operations.* Washington, DC: The National Academies Press.

Ishikawa, Y., H. Yoshida, Y. Mamada, N. Taniai, S. Matsumoto, K. Bando, Y. Mizuguchi, D. Kakinuma, T. Kanda, and T. Tajiri. 2010. Prospective randomized controlled study of short-term perioperative oral nutrition with branched chain amino acids in patients undergoing liver surgery. *Hepato-Gastroenterology* 57(99–100):583–590.

Lieberman, H. R., T. B. Stavinoha, S. M. McGraw, A. White, L. S. Hadden, and B. P. Marriott. 2010. Use of dietary supplements among active-duty U.S. Army soldiers. *American Journal of Clinical Nutrition* 92(4):985–995.

Matthews, D. E. 2005. Observations of branched-chain amino acid administration in humans. *Journal of Nutrition* 135(6 Suppl.):1580S–1584S.

Ott, L. G., J. J. Schmidt, A. B. Young, D. L. Twyman, R. P. Rapp, P. A. Tibbs, R. J. Dempsey, and C. J. McClain. 1988. Comparison of administration of two standard intravenous amino acid formulas to severely brain-injured patients. *Drug Intelligence and Clinical Pharmacy* 22(10):763–768.

Skeie, B., A. J. Petersen, T. Manner, J. Askanazi, and P. A. Steen. 1994. Effects of valine, leucine, isoleucine, and a balanced amino acid solution on the seizure threshold to picrotoxin in rats. *Pharmacology Biochemistry and Behavior* 48(1):101–103.

Wagenmakers, A. J. M. 1999. Amino acid supplements to improve athletic performance. *Current Opinion in Clinical Nutrition and Metabolic Care* 2:539–544.

Yudkoff, M., Y. Daikhin, I. Nissim, O. Horyn, B. Lyhovyy, A. Lazarow, and N. I. Nissim. 2005. Brain amino acid requirements and toxicity: The example of leucine. *Journal of Nutrition* 135(6 Suppl.):1531S–1538S.

9

Choline

Choline has multiple roles as an essential nutrient. A major dietary component found in eggs and liver, its absorption in the intestine is mediated by choline transporters. The majority of choline is used to synthesize phosphatidylcholine, the predominant lipid in cell membranes. As well as being essential in the synthesis of membrane components, choline accelerates the synthesis and release of acetylcholine, an important neurotransmitter involved in memory storage and muscle control. Choline is an essential element in neurodevelopment. As a major dietary source of methyl groups, choline also participates in the biosynthesis of lipids, regulation of metabolic pathways, and detoxification in the body.

Health outcomes associated with choline involve memory, heart disease, and inflammation, which also explain the consideration of choline as a plausible intervention in traumatic brain injury (TBI). Although there are no human studies examining the effect of supplementation during pregnancy on enhanced memory of the newborn, there are animal studies showing that choline supplementation provided during hippocampal development has an effect on maintaining memory in older age. This effect appears to involve changes in gene expression via gene methylation. Changes in homocysteine due to choline supplementation are also hypothesized to reduce cardiovascular disease (CVD) risk. In the Framingham Offspring Study, combined dietary intakes of choline and betaine were associated with lower concentrations of homocysteine, a marker for inflammation. During the ATTICA study, a cross-sectional survey (1,514 men and 1,528 women with no history of CVD) of health and nutrition being carried out in the region of Attica, Greece, the association between inflammatory markers and choline intakes was measured. Participants who consumed higher levels of choline (> 310 vs. < 250 mg/day) had lower concentrations of C-reactive protein, interleukin-6, and tumor necrosis factor-alpha (Detopoulou et al., 2008). For an overview of the metabolism, functions, and health effects of choline, the reader is referred to previous reviews (IOM, 1998; Zeisel, 2006; Zeisel and da Costa, 2009; Zeisel et al., 1991).

Because of its undesirable organoleptic characteristics when administered in doses that exceed the capacity of the small intestine to absorb it, choline is not readily accepted by patients. The most common form of choline in the diet is phosphatidylcholine, an ester of choline that is not used as a substrate by gut bacteria and does not result in fishy body odor (Zeisel et al., 1983). Most studies reviewed in this chapter used an intermediary in the synthesis of phosphatidylcholine, CDP-choline. CDP-choline is composed of cytidine and choline and is hydrolyzed in the small intestine before absorption as citidine and choline. After absorption, citidine and choline are rephosphorylated and then CDP-choline is resynthesized again. CDP-choline also serves as a donor of choline in the synthesis of acetylcholine. This chapter includes evidence for the potential use of CDP-choline in TBI.

CHOLINE AND THE BRAIN

Choline has a critical role in neurotransmitter function because of its impact on acetylcholine and dopaminergic function. Studies in animals suggest that CDP-choline supplements increase dopamine receptor densities and can ameliorate memory impairment. In Parkinson's disease, for example, CDP-choline may increase the availability of dopamine. A Cochrane review of randomized trials testing the efficacy of CDP-choline in the treatment of cognitive, emotional, and behavioral deficits associated with chronic cerebral disorders in the elderly revealed no evidence of a beneficial effect on attention, but some evidence of benefit on memory function and behavior (Fioravanti and Yanagi, 2005). The brains of those with Alzheimer's disease have decreased phosphatidylcholine and phosphatidylethanolamine, and it has been suggested that CDP-choline may provide benefit by repairing cell membrane damage and enhancing acetylcholine synthesis. Both sphingomyelin and phosphatidylcholine, major constituents of brain membranes, are synthesized from the precursor choline (Zeisel, 2005). The role of choline in regulating the synthesis of phospholipids (e.g., phosphatidylcholine, phosphatidylethanolamine, phosphatidylinositol, and sphingomyelin) as constituents of cell membranes is reviewed in Saver (2008). This review also includes a discussion of the evidence showing that choline promotes rapid repair of injured cell surfaces and mitochondrial membranes as well as maintenance of cell integrity and bioenergetic capacity. Increases in biomarkers representative of CDP-choline activity, such as phosphodiesters, were observed on proton magnetic resonance spectroscopy and were associated with improvements in verbal memory in humans (Babb et al., 2002; Fioravanti and Yanagi, 2005).

It is hypothesized that CDP-choline may exert neuroprotective effects in an injured brain through its ability to improve phosphatidylcholine synthesis (Adibhatla and Hatcher, 2002). In addition to its neuroprotective capability, CDP-choline potentiates neurorecovery, which has led to its evaluation as treatment for both stroke and TBI in animal models and in human clinical trials (Cohadon et al., 1982; Levin, 1991; Warach et al., 2000). The positive effects seen in models of ischemia and hypoxia may be explained by increased Bcl-2 expression, decreased apoptosis, and reduced expression of pro-caspase. Inhibiting caspase activity may decrease apoptotic activity and calcium-mediated cell death. Supporting these ideas, in vitro studies have also revealed that choline deficiency induces apoptosis in the liver by mechanisms independent of protein 53, which likely involve abnormal mitochondrial membrane phosphatidylcholine, leakage of oxygen radicals, and activation of caspases (Albright and Zeisel, 1997; Albright et al., 1996, 1998, 1999a, 199b, 2003; Chen et al., 2010). In humans, a choline-deficient diet also causes DNA damage and apoptosis (da Costa et al., 2006).

In addition, CDP-choline is hypothesized to attenuate the loss of phospholipid and increase in fatty acids after global and focal cerebral ischemia by preventing activation of phospholipase A2. CDP-choline may also act to protect against oxidative stress since it has been shown to increase total glutathione levels, glutathione reductase activity, decreased oxidized glutathione, and glutathione oxidation ratio (Adibhatla and Hatcher, 2005).

In rat models, the availability of choline to the fetus influences neurogenesis in the fetal brain (Craciunescu et al., 2003), and choline status in early life influences neurogenesis rates in the adult hippocampus (Glenn et al., 2007), an area of the brain that is often dysfunctional in TBI. Additionally suggesting choline mechanisms of action relevant to TBI are the fact that in rodents, choline deficiency is associated with lipid peroxidation in liver (Ghoshal et al., 1984, 1990) and that deletion of a choline metabolism gene results in mitochondrial dysfunction in the liver, sperm, testis, heart, and kidney (Johnson et al., 2010). A list of human studies (years 1990 and beyond) evaluating the effectiveness of CDP-choline in providing resilience or treating TBI or related diseases or conditions (i.e., subarachnoid hemorrhage, intracranial aneurysm, stroke, anoxic or hypoxic ischemia, epilepsy) in the acute phase in humans is presented in Table 9-1; this also includes supporting evidence from animal models of TBI. The table includes the occurrence or absence of adverse effects in humans.

USES AND SAFETY

In 1998, the Institute of Medicine (IOM) recognized choline as an essential nutrient (IOM, 1998; Zeisel and da Costa, 2009) and set the Adequate Intake (AI) for choline at 550 mg/day and 425 mg/day for men and women 19 years of age and older, respectively. These levels were set based on the dietary intakes of the U.S. population, and on the development of liver damage seen with lower intake. The Tolerable Upper Intake Level (UL) for choline is 3.5 g/day for adults 19 years of age or older, based on fishy body odor and hypotension (IOM, 1998).

Choline is found in a variety of foods including eggs and liver. Deficiency has been clearly linked to atherosclerosis, neurodevelopmental diseases, and liver disease (Penry and Manore, 2008). The human body is unable to synthesize sufficient choline via direct methylation of phosphatidylethanolamine to phosphatidylcholine, so choline must also be acquired via the diet. Analysis of choline intake has suggested a high level of deficiency in the U.S. population (Fischer et al., 2005; Jensen et al., 2007). Choline deficiency has been linked to a variety of secondary disease processes, such as liver disease; cardiac, neurodegenerative and neurodevelopmental problems; and breast cancer (Li and Vance, 2008; Zeisel, 2006). In addition, it is estimated that up to 50 percent of the population carries genetic variations that require increased choline intake (Zeisel and da Costa, 2009).

Direct choline therapy, when administered in doses higher than the intestine can absorb, often leads to malodor that is unacceptable to participants. The use of forms of choline that are efficiently absorbed and avoid this problem is desirable. All the studies reported by the committee have used CDP-choline, an endogenous compound and intermediary of the synthesis of phosphatidylcholine. CDP-choline was originally identified as the key intermediary in the biosynthesis of phosphatidylcholine by Kennedy in 1956 (2003), and is now also sold as a dietary supplement. However, there is no evidence that CDP-choline is the most effective form, and other forms of choline could be tested in future TBI studies.

CDP-choline has been used in the treatment of cerebrovascular disorders for many years, under a variety of protocols and to ameliorate various conditions. In several European countries, for example, CDP-choline is frequently prescribed for cognitive impairment and in the treatment of Parkinson's disease.

CDP-choline is generally considered safe; the side effect most noted in clinical trials has been mild diarrhea, with leg edema, back pain with headache, tinnitus, insomnia, vision

TABLE 9-1   Relevant Data Identified for Citicoline/CDP-Choline

Reference	Type of Injury/Insult	Type of Study and Subjects	Treatment	Findings/Results
Tier 1: Clinical trials				
Zafonte et al., 2009	Mild, moderate, and severe TBI	Randomized, double-blind, placebo-controlled, multi-center trial n^a=1,292	Postinjury, 90 days treatment of citicoline (1,000 mg twice a day), administered enterally or orally	Trial in progress
Saver, 2008	Stroke	Meta-analysis; 10 trials n=2,279	CDP-choline	Mortality and disability rates are lower in CDP-choline-treated patients than in placebo patients (OR^b=0.64, 95% CI^c: 0.54–.077, p < 0.00001; p for heterogeneity=0.01, χ^{2d}=21.40).
				Due to large amount of scatter in smaller studies, another analysis of the 4 largest studies (n > 100) was conducted; treatment effect on mortality and disability was still significant (OR=0.70, 95% CI: 0.58–0.85; p=0.0003).
				In patients with NIHSS (National Institutes of Health Stroke Scale) ≥ 8, overall recovery occurred more often in CDP-choline-treated patients (OR=1.30, 95% CI: 1.1–1.6; p < 0.004). More CDP-choline patients (25.2%) achieved NIHSS of 0–1, Barthel Index of ≥ 95, and modified Rankin Score of 0–1 than placebo patients (20.2%).
				There were no adverse effects observed due to the treatments.
Davalos et al., 2002	Moderate to severe stroke	Pooled data analysis; randomized, placebo-controlled, double-blind clinical trials n=1,372 (583=placebo; 789=treatment)	Postinjury; oral CDP-choline (500 mg, 1,000 mg, and 2,000 mg) vs. placebo; treatment within 24 hours after injury	Global recovery after 3 months was seen in 25.2% of CDP-choline-treated patients and 20.2% of placebo-treated patients (OR=1.33; 95% CI: 1.10–1.62; p=0.0034). Greatest improvement was seen in 2000 mg group, 27.9% (OR=1.38, 95% CI: 1.10–1.72, p=0.0043). Compared to placebo-group, CDP-choline-treated group saw an increase of 29% on Barthel Index score (95% CI: 3–62), 42% in modified Rankin Score (95% CI: 8–88), and 28% on NIHSS (95% CI: –1 to 65).
				There is no significant mortality rate and overall frequency of adverse events between treated and placebo groups. Significantly higher events were found in the treatment group for anxiety and leg edema (p=0.036 and 0.032, respectively).

TABLE 9-1 Continued

Reference	Type of Injury/Insult	Type of Study and Subjects	Treatment	Findings/Results
Clark et al., 2001	Acute ischemic stroke, NIHSS ≥ 8	118-center, randomized, double-blind, efficacy trial n=899	Postinjury; CDP-choline (2,000 mg per day); 6-week treatment, 6-week follow-up	At week 12, about the same proportion of patients in placebo (51%) and treatment (52%) groups showed a 7-point improvement on their NIHSS scores. Although the treatment group did significantly better (27% vs. 21%; p=0.04) than placebo group on the Barthel Index at week 6, it lost that advantage at week 12. There was no significant difference in mortality rate or other serious adverse events (e.g., cardiovascular events, central nervous system events) between the treatment and placebo groups.
Leon-Carrion et al., 2000	TBI	**Exp 1:** Non-randomized trial n=7 patients with severe memory disorders who were discharged > 6 months prior to study **Exp 2:** Randomized trial n=10 patients with severe memory deficits (including the 7 patients from Exp 1)	**Exp 1:** 1 g of CDP-choline **Exp 2:** 1 g/day of CDP-choline or placebo administered with patients' neuropsychological treatment	**Exp1:** Patients showed a hypoperfusion of the inferior left temporal lobe at resting state, but hypoperfusion disappeared after taking CDP-choline. Cerebral blood flow increased in the left temporal areas and decreased in right frontal lobe. **Exp2:** While the CPD-choline group improved in all 5 measures of the neuropsychological treatment, only improvements in verbal fluency and Luria Memory Words were significant (p < 0.05). There were no side effects reported for patients in Exp 1. There were no observed side effects in Exp 2.

continued

TABLE 9-1 Continued

Reference	Type of Injury/Insult	Type of Study and Subjects	Treatment	Findings/Results
Warach et al., 2000	Acute ischemic stroke and lesions of 1–120 cc in cerebral gray matter	Randomized, double-blind, placebo-controlled trial n=100, onset 24 hrs or less	Post-injury, CDP-choline (500 mg/day) or placebo administered orally for 6 weeks, follow-up for 12 weeks	From baseline to week 12, the distribution of changes in ischemic lesion volume was not significantly different between placebo group and CDP-choline-treat group. However, CDP-choline group showed significantly greater reduction ($p < 0.01$) in analysis of week 1 to week 12 change. Significant ($p \leq 0.0001$) covariates of change in lesion volume are: size of baseline perfusion abnormality, baseline NIHSS score, and presence of arterial lesion seen on MRA. Patients' improvement of NIHSS ≥ 7 points showed greater lesion volume reduction ($p \leq 0.001$). The difference in mortality rate between the treatment and placebo group was not significant. Edema of the extremities and back pain were significantly higher in the CDP-choline group than in the placebo group ($p \leq 0.05$ for both).
Clark et al., 1999	Acute ischemic stroke, NIHSS ≥ 5	Randomized, double-blind, efficacy trial at 31 centers n=394 (127=placebo, 267=CDP-choline)	Postinjury, oral CDP-choline (500 mg/day); 6 weeks of treatment, 6 weeks of follow-up	Post hoc analyses found that among patients with baseline NIHSS ≥ 8, CDP-choline-treated patients were overall more likely to have a full recovery (OR=1.9, $p=0.04$). No treatment effect was seen in patients with baseline NIHSS < 8. CDP-choline-treated patients were significantly ($p=0.01$) more likely to achieve a 7-point improvement in NIHSS score than placebo-treated patients. There was no significant difference in mortality rate or other serious adverse events between the treatment and placebo groups.

TABLE 9-1 Continued

Reference	Type of Injury/Insult	Type of Study and Subjects	Treatment	Findings/Results
Clark et al., 1997	Acute ischemic stroke, NIHSS ≥ 5	Randomized, double-blind, placebo-controlled trial at 21 centers n=259	6 weeks of CDP-choline (50 mg, 1,000 mg, or 2,000 mg daily) or placebo	Primary analysis using NIHSS as a covariate showed that, overall, CDP-choline had treatment effect compared to placebo (p ≤ 0.05). The 500-mg group (OR=2.0) and the 20,00-mg group (OR=2.1) achieved a significantly (p < 0.05) higher Barthel Index score at week 12. Overall, CDP-choline treatment at week 12 was associated with full recovery, as defined by Barthel Index of ≥ 95 (p=0.011); specifically, the 500-mg group had a significant (p=0.03) improvement compared to placebo group. The 500-mg group also significantly (p=0.03) improved on Rankin Scale score. Treatment effect on cognitive function (MMSE ≥ 25) at 12 weeks was seen in 500-mg group (OR=2.6, p=0.02) and the 2,000-mg group (OR=2.4, p=0.03). There was no significant difference in mortality rate or other serious adverse events between the treatment and placebo groups. Adverse events that were significantly higher in the treatment groups than in the placebo group were dizziness and accidental injury (p ≤ 0.05).
Levin, 1991	Mild to moderate closed head injury	Randomized, double-blind, placebo-controlled trial n=14 men	Postinjury, oral CDP-choline (1 g) or placebo	Patients treated with CDP-choline had greater improvement (100%) on tests recalling designs than placebo-treated patients (29%, p < 0.02). While placebo-treated patients have higher absolute score on tests to create unique designs than CDP-choline treated patients (p < 0.05) during the 1-month follow-up, the change in scores from baseline was not significantly different between the two groups. Although CDP-choline was well tolerated, there were more complaints about gastrointestinal distress from patients in the treatment group.

continued

TABLE 9-1 Continued

Reference	Type of Injury/Insult	Type of Study and Subjects	Treatment	Findings/Results
Maldonado et al., 1991	Severe and moderate closed TBI, GCS (Glasgow Coma Score) between 5 and 10	Randomized, single-blind trial n=216	Conventional treatment vs. CDP-choline added to conventional treatment; follow-up after 3 months	Patients treated with CDP-choline had shorter hospital stays than control patients ($p < 0.05$). CDP-choline group showed overall improvement in all initial symptoms, but only the improvement in character was significant ($p < 0.05$). CDP-choline patients also showed significantly better results on GOS (Glasgow Outcome Score) (p=0.05). There was no significant difference between groups in terms of mortality. There were no adverse effects reported.

Tier 2: Observational studies

None found

Tier 3: Animal studies

| Dempsey and Raghavendra Rao, 2003 | Moderate-grade TBI, controlled cortical impact (CCI) | Adult, male Sprague-Dawley rats | Postinjury, intraperitoneal injections of CDP-choline (100, 200, or 400 mg/kg body weight) or saline $\leq$ 3 minutes postinjury and 6 hours postinjury | Compared to sham-injured rats, injured rats treated with saline and 100 mg/kg of CDP-choline had greater neuron loss in the CA2 and CA3 regions of the hippocampus ($p < 0.05$ for both). However, treatment with 200 mg/kg and 400 mg/kg of CDP-choline reduce the loss in the same regions ($p < 0.05$ vs. injured, saline-treated rats).

Treatment with 200 mg/kg and 400 mg/kg of CDP-choline also reduced the volume of cortical contusion by 21 mm^3 ($p < 0.05$).

Rats treated with 200 or 400 mg/kg of CDP-choline significantly recovered their neurological function by day 7 to 88% of their preinjury level ($p < 0.05$). |
| Baskaya et al., 2000 | TBI, CCI | Adult, male Sprague-Dawley rats | Postinjury, intraperitoneal injections of saline or CDP-choline (50, 100, or 400 mg/kg body weight) administered 5 minutes and 4–6 hours after injury | 100 mg/kg CDP-choline significantly reduced edema in the cortex ($p < 0.05$ vs. saline treatment), while 400 mg/kg CDP-choline significantly reduced edema in both the cortex and the ipsilateral hippocampus ($p < 0.05$ vs. saline treatment).

Doses of 100 and 400 mg/kg body weight CDP-choline significantly ($p < 0.05$) reduced blood-brain barrier breakdown in both the injured cortex and ipsilateral hippocampus. |

TABLE 9-1 Continued

Reference	Type of Injury/Insult	Type of Study and Subjects	Treatment	Findings/Results
Dixon et al., 1997	TBI, lateral CCI	Adult, male Sprague-Dawley rats	Postinjury, daily intraperitoneal injection of CDP-choline (100 mg/kg) for 18 days, beginning 1 day postinjury	Compared to injured, saline-treated rats, CDP-choline-treated rats had greater latency on beam balancing task (p < 0.01) and shorter latency beam walking task (p < 0.05) at day 1. The difference between two groups in both tasks was minimized by day 4. CDP-choline treated rats also had shorter latency in completing the Morris water maze than saline-treated rats (p < 0.005). Acetylcholine outflow was significantly increased in the dorsal hippocampus (p < 0.014) and neocortex (p < 0.036) after treatment with CDP-choline.

[a] n: sample size.
[b] OR: odds ratio.
[c] CI: confidence interval.
[d] $\chi 2$: chi-square.

problems, and dizziness reported much less frequently (Adibhatla and Hatcher, 2002; Clark et al., 1997; Levin, 1991). There were no adverse events reported even with doses as high as 4,000 mg/day (Calatayud Maldonado et al., 1991). It is notable that in a study by Clark and colleagues (2001), a dose of 2,000 mg/day by enteral administration did not induce severe adverse events at a rate any higher than placebo in the 899 patients.

EVIDENCE INDICATING EFFECT ON RESILIENCE

The committee found no clinical or animal trials that have tested the potential benefits of choline or CDP-choline in TBI or in other diseases or conditions included in the reviews of the literature (subarachnoid hemorrhage, intracranial aneurysm, stroke, anoxic or hypoxic ischemia, epilepsy).

EVIDENCE INDICATING EFFECT ON TREATMENT

Human Studies

In human studies, patients who were administered CDP-choline early in the postischemia recovery process demonstrated improved levels of consciousness (Tazaki et al., 1988) as well as improvements in the modified Rankin scale (a measure of function after stroke) (Clark et al., 2001). Consistent with this observation, magnetic resonance imaging data show a decrease in lesion volume with CDP-choline compared to placebo in a preliminary trial (Warach et al., 2000). A meta-analysis was conducted of four randomized clinical trials of CDP-choline in stroke in the United States (Davalos et al., 2002). Although the conclusion from pooling the data in the meta-analysis was positive and the authors concluded that oral CDP-choline increases the probability of recovery, the results of the individual studies are ambiguous. CDP-choline improved functional outcome and reduced neurological deficit in one of those studies (Clark et al., 1997); however, two subsequent studies failed to demonstrate improvement, although a post hoc analysis showed improvements in moderate to severe stroke cases (Clark et al., 1999, 2001). One of the studies (Clark et al., 2001) showed a beneficial effect of CDP-choline as measured by the Rankin scale, a secondary outcome metric in these trials. A separate meta-analysis of acute and subacute stroke, published in abstract form only, suggested a positive treatment effect of CDP-choline precursors on rates of death and disability (Saver et al., 2002).

In early randomized clinical trials of CDP-choline in TBI, it was associated with faster recovery from focal motor deficits in patients with severe TBI (Cohadon et al., 1982); improved recall design (a measure of memory) (Levin, 1991); a reduction of postconcussion symptoms following mild TBI (Levin, 1991); and reduced inpatient hospital stay and requirement for outpatient follow-up (Calatayud Maldonado et al., 1991). CDP-choline has also been shown to enhance cerebral blood flow. Among patients with TBI and very severe memory deficits, hypoperfusion of the inferior left temporal lobe normalized after administration of CDP-choline (Leon-Carrion et al., 2000).

Clinical trials of CDP-choline in TBI have demonstrated efficacy in secondary outcome measures but not in primary measures. These ambiguous results of some of the human trials in the United States may be due to a combination of causes. Many of the trials used doses substantially lower than may be optimal for highest efficacy (Agut et al., 1983; Clark et al., 1997). Also, this failure may have been due to substantial weaknesses in study designs, such as insufficient sample size (Calatayud Maldonado et al., 1991; Cohadon et al., 1982; Tazaki et al., 1988) or lack of sensitivity of the chosen outcomes measure (Glasgow Outcome Scale) (Clark et al., 2001). For example, Clark's study of patients with stroke did not show a significant difference in the primary outcome measure (an improvement of total score by > 7 in the National Institutes of Health Stroke Scale), but post hoc analysis using a standard of "excellent recovery" showed a possible treatment effect. In this study, the primary outcome measure may have been too stringent (Clark et al., 2001). Differences in outcomes also may have been due to the route of administration of CDP-choline. Although bioavailability data suggest that enteral and intravenous routes are similar, brain uptake of CDP-choline may vary depending on the route of administration (Adibhatla and Hatcher, 2002; Grotta, 2002; Secades and Frontera, 1995). Theoretically, it is possible that intravenous administration may yield higher brain delivery (Agut et al., 1983; Secades and Frontera, 1995).

Animal Studies

In animal models, CDP-choline has been demonstrated to exert acute neuroprotection, as well as positive effects in chronic brain injury and stroke and in epilepsy.

A major mechanism of secondary injury in TBI is the formation of reactive oxygen species and lipid peroxidases, which cause significant tissue damage. Animal models of TBI support a key role for oxidative stress (Ikeda and Long, 1990; Kontos et al., 1992). The exogenous administration of CDP-choline or its precursors significantly increased levels of glutathione (Adibhatla et al., 2001; Barrachina et al., 2003; De la Cruz et al., 2000), a powerful endogenous antioxidant. CDP-choline also attenuates release of arachidonic acid, cardiolipin, and sphingomyelin (Adibhatla and Hatcher, 2002). Studies in animal models of ischemia and hypoxia also found that CDP-choline treatment improves concentration of free fatty acids, decreases neurological deficits, and improves behavioral performance on learning and memory (Rao et al., 2001). Increased expression of B-cell lymphoma 2, a regulator of apoptosis; decreased apoptosis; and reduced expression of both pro-caspase (Krupinski et al., 2002) and cleaved caspase-3 (Mir et al., 2003) also may explain the functional findings. Inhibiting caspase activity may decrease apoptotic activity and calcium-mediated cell death.

CDP-choline was found to be neuroprotective in an animal model of uninterrupted occlusion of the basilar artery after subarachnoid hemorrhage (Alkan et al., 2001). CDP-choline was associated with greater arterial pressure, smaller infarct volumes, and lower mortality than controls. These results also suggest that CDP-choline provides significant neuroprotection during cerebral ischemia.

Dietary choline may promote functional recovery from status epilepticus (Holmes et al., 2002; Wong-Goodrich et al., 2010). Following the status epilepticus, rats given a choline-supplemented diet for four weeks performed better on the Morris water maze test than rats receiving a control diet (Holmes et al., 2002).

Animal studies (Baskaya et al., 2000; Dempsey and Raghavendra Rao, 2003; Dixon et al., 1997) demonstrated the neuroprotective effect of CDP-choline in TBI. The studies showed that CDP-choline had a significant preventive effect on TBI-induced neuronal loss in the hippocampus, decreased cortical contusion volume, and improved neurological recovery. Additionally, there was a dose-dependent attenuation of chronic deficits in motor and spatial performance following CDP-choline administration. Extracellular levels of acetylcholine, a key mediator of memory processes, were increased (Dixon et al., 1997), suggesting that CDP-choline enhances cholinergic transmission and may ameliorate chronic functional deficits. A second mechanism that may explain why CDP-choline improves function in chronically injured animals focuses on observed decreases in dopamine following injury (Yan et al., 2001). In such models, CDP-choline increased dopamine levels (Secades and Frontera, 1995; Yan et al., 2001), which enhanced neurorecovery (Kline et al., 2004).

CONCLUSIONS AND RECOMMENDATIONS

Since 2000, several neuroprotective trials for TBI have failed to show efficacy in any of the interventions tested. One reason may be that many of these agents have targeted one portion of the cascade of injury that occurs after TBI. Such agents have a time-limited opportunity to prevent the secondary brain injury and are rarely involved in the restorative process. An ideal agent would provide both neuroprotection and a means to facilitate the recovery process.

Although clinical trials in stroke and trauma have suggested efficacy in secondary outcome measures related to functional outcome and cognition, design weaknesses in these studies may have affected findings in the primary outcome. Design limitations include insufficient sample size (Tazaki et al., 1988), low dosage (Clark et al., 1997, 1999), variations derived from intravenous versus enteral delivery (Calatayud Maldonado et al., 1991; Clark et al., 2001), and in some cases inadequate outcome measures (Clark et al., 2001).

Preliminary animal data suggest that CDP-choline works via numerous mechanisms to limit the acute secondary injury cascade after ischemic and traumatic injury. In the more chronic setting, CDP-choline appears responsible for an upregulation in acetylcholine synthesis. The diversity of CDP-choline's mechanisms of action suggests that it may offer neuroprotection and neurofacilitation to patients with TBI through multiple avenues, thereby increasing the possibility of that treatment improving outcome. The optimal clinical dose and duration of treatment of CDP-choline for injured patients is yet unclear.

There is one ongoing human trial on the effect of CDP-choline (Citicoline Brain Injury Treatment [COBRIT] trial) on cognition and functional measures on severe, moderate, and complicated mild TBI being led by a member of the committee (Zafonte et al., 2009). The committee recognizes the significance of this trial in that the findings will reveal more insights about the potential for this nutrient in the treatment of TBI. It was the consensus of the committee to emphasize the importance of monitoring the results of this trial before conducting more human studies. If ongoing trials with CDP-choline and TBI patients show positive results, further studies are warranted to confirm the optimal duration of treatment and clinical dose of choline for injured patients. Likewise, if those studies reveal that choline is a promising intervention, the effect of choline supplementation prior to injury to improve resilience could be explored by conducting animal studies. The impact on neurologic outcome of the choline deficiency observed in the population needs to be explored. Although there are no data regarding supplementation to enhance resilience, choline's critical role in the maintenance of health suggests that individuals should be cautioned to avoid deficiency. Based on findings from animal studies, it would be prudent to consider potential gender differences in the metabolism of choline when designing studies (Fischer et al., 2007; Resseguie et al., 2007, 2011).

RECOMMENDATION 9-1. DoD should monitor the results of the COBRIT trial, a human experimental trial examining the effect of CDP-choline and genomic factors on cognition and functional measures in severe, moderate, and complicated mild TBI. If the results of that trial are positive, then DoD should conduct animal studies to define the optimal clinical dose and duration of treatment for choline (CDP-choline) following TBI, as well as to explore choline's potential to promote resilience to TBI when used as a preinjury supplement.

REFERENCES

Adibhatla, R. M., and J. F. Hatcher. 2002. Citicoline mechanisms and clinical efficacy in cerebral ischemia. *Journal of Neuroscience Research* 70(2):133–139.

Adibhatla, R. M., and J. F. Hatcher. 2005. Cytidine 5′-diphosphocholine (CDP-choline) in stroke and other CNS disorders. *Neurochemical Research* 30(1):15–23.

Adibhatla, R. M., J. F. Hatcher, and R. J. Dempsey. 2001. Effects of citicoline on phospholipid and glutathione levels in transient cerebral ischemia. *Stroke* 32(10):2376–2381.

Agut, J., E. Font, A. Sacristan, and J. A. Ortiz. 1983. Bioavailability of methyl-14c CDP-choline by oral route. *Arzneimittelforschung* 33(7A):1045–1047.

Albright, C. D., and S. H. Zeisel. 1997. Choline deficiency causes increased localization of transforming growth factor-beta1 signaling proteins and apoptosis in rat liver. *Pathobiology* 65(5):264–270.

Albright, C. D., R. Lui, T. C. Bethea, K.-A. da Costa, R. I. Salganik, and S. H. Zeisel. 1996. Choline deficiency induces apoptosis in SV40-immortalized CWSV-1 rat hepatocytes in culture. *The Federation of American Societies for Experimental Biology Journal* 10(4):510–516.

Albright, C. D., R. I. Salganik, W. K. Kaufmann, A. S. Vrablic, and S. H. Zeisel. 1998. A p53-dependent G1 checkpoint function is not required for induction of apoptosis by acute choline deficiency in immortalized rat hepatocytes in culture. *The Journal of Nutritional Biochemistry* 9(8):476–481.

Albright, C. D., C. B. Friedrich, E. C. Brown, M. H. Mar, and S. H. Zeisel. 1999a. Maternal dietary choline availability alters mitosis, apoptosis and the localization of TOAD-64 protein in the developing fetal rat septum. *Brain Research* 115(2):123–129.

Albright, C. D., A. Y. Tsai, C. B. Friedrich, M. H. Mar, and S. H. Zeisel. 1999b. Choline availability alters embryonic development of the hippocampus and septum in the rat. *Brain Research* 113(1–2):13–20.

Albright, C. D., R. I. Salganik, C. N. Craciunescu, M. H. Mar, and S. H. Zeisel. 2003. Mitochondrial and microsomal derived reactive oxygen species mediate apoptosis induced by transforming growth factor-beta1 in immortalized rat hepatocytes. *Journal of Cellular Biochemistry* 89(2):254–261.

Alkan, T., N. Kahveci, B. Goren, E. Korfali, and K. Ozluk. 2001. Ischemic brain injury caused by interrupted versus uninterrupted occlusion in hypotensive rats with subarachnoid hemorrhage: Neuroprotective effects of citicoline. *Archives of Physiology and Biochemistry* 109(2):161–167.

Babb, S. M., L. L. Wald, B. M. Cohen, R. A. Villafuerte, S. A. Gruber, D. A. Yurgelun-Todd, and P. F. Renshaw. 2002. Chronic citicoline increases phosphodiesters in the brains of healthy older subjects: An in vivo phosphorus magnetic resonance spectroscopy study. *Psychopharmacology* 161(3):248–254.

Barrachina, M., I. Dominguez, S. Ambrosio, J. Secades, R. Lozano, and I. Ferrer. 2003. Neuroprotective effect of citicoline in 6-hydroxydopamine-lesioned rats and in 6-hydroxydopamine-treated SH-SY5Y human neuro-blastoma cells. *Journal of the Neurological Sciences* 215(1–2):105–110.

Baskaya, M. K., A. Dogan, A. M. Rao, and R. J. Dempsey. 2000. Neuroprotective effects of citicoline on brain edema and blood-brain barrier breakdown after traumatic brain injury. *Journal of Neurosurgery* 92(3):448–452.

Calatayud Maldonado, V., J. B. Calatayud Perez, and J. Aso Escario. 1991. Effects of CDP-choline on the recovery of patients with head injury. *Journal of the Neurological Sciences* 103(Suppl.):S15–S18.

Chen, M., L. Peyrin-Biroulet, A. George, F. Coste, A. Bressenot, C. Bossenmeyer-Pourie, J. M. Alberto, B. Xia, B. Namour, and J. L. Gueant. 2010. Methyl deficient diet aggravates experimental colitis in rats. *Journal of Cellular and Molecular Medicine*. Published electronically December 29, 2010. doi: 10.1111/j.1582-4934.2010.01252.x.

Clark, W., B. Williams, K. Selzer, R. Zweifler, L. Sabounjian, and R. Gammans. 1999. A randomized efficacy trial of citicoline in patients with acute ischemic stroke. *Stroke* 30(12):2592–2597.

Clark, W. M., S. J. Warach, L. C. Pettigrew, R. E. Gammans, and L. A. Sabounjian. 1997. A randomized dose-response trial of citicoline in acute ischemic stroke patients. *Neurology* 49(3):671–678.

Clark, W. M., L. R. Wechsler, L. A. Sabounjian, and U. E. Schwiderski. 2001. A phase III randomized efficacy trial of 2000 mg citicoline in acute ischemic stroke patients. *Neurology* 57(9):1595–1602.

Cohadon, F., E. Richer, and B. Poletto. 1982. A metabolic precursor of phospholipids in severe traumatic comas. *Neurochirurgie* 28(4):287–290.

Craciunescu, C. N., C. D. Albright, M. H. Mar, J. Song, and S. H. Zeisel. 2003. Choline availability during embryonic development alters progenitor cell mitosis in developing mouse hippocampus. *The Journal of Nutrition* 133(11):3614–3618.

da Costa, K. A., M. D. Niculescu, C. N. Craciunescu, L. M. Fischer, and S. H. Zeisel. 2006. Choline deficiency increases lymphocyte apoptosis and DNA damage in humans. *American Journal of Clinical Nutrition* 84(1):88–94.

Davalos, A., J. Castillo, J. Alvarez-Sabin, J. Secades, J. Mercadal, S. Lopez, E. Cobo, S. Warach, D. Sherman, W. Clark, and R. Lozano. 2002. Oral citicoline in acute ischemic stroke: An individual patient data pooling analysis of clinical trials. *Stroke* 33(12):2850–2857.

De la Cruz, J. P., J. Pavia, J. A. Gonzalez-Correa, P. Ortiz, and F. S. de la Cuesta. 2000. Effects of chronic administration of s-adenosyl-l-methionine on brain oxidative stress in rats. *Naunyn-Schmiedebergs Archives of Pharmacology* 361(1):47–52.

Dempsey, R. J., and V. L. Raghavendra Rao. 2003. Cytidinediphosphocholine treatment to decrease traumatic brain injury-induced hippocampal neuronal death, cortical contusion volume, and neurological dysfunction in rats. *Journal of Neurosurgery* 98(4):867–873.

Detopoulou, P., D. B. Panagiotakos, S. Antonopoulou, C. Pitsavos, and C. Stefanadis. 2008. Dietary choline and betaine intakes in relation to concentrations of inflammatory markers in healthy adults: The ATTICA Study. *American Journal of Clinical Nutrition* 87(2):424–430.

Dixon, C. E., X. Ma, and D. W. Marion. 1997. Effects of CDP-choline treatment on neurobehavioral deficits after TBI and on hippocampal and neocortical acetylcholine release. *Journal of Neurotrauma* 14(3):161–169.

Fioravanti, M., and M. Yanagi. 2005. Cytidinediphosphocholine (CDP-choline) for cognitive and behavioural disturbances associated with chronic cerebral disorders in the elderly. *Cochrane Database of Systematic Reviews* (2):CD000269.

Fischer, L. M., J. A. Scearce, M. H. Mar, J. R. Patel, R. T. Blanchard, B. A. Macintosh, M. G. Busby, and S. H. Zeisel. 2005. Ad libitum choline intake in healthy individuals meets or exceeds the proposed adequate intake level. *The Journal of Nutrition* 135(4):826–829.

Fischer, L. M., K. daCosta, L. Kwock, P. Stewart, T.-S. Lu, S. Stabler, R. Allen, and S. Zeisel. 2007. Sex and menopausal status influence human dietary requirements for the nutrient choline. *American Journal of Clinical Nutrition* 85(5):1275–1285.

Ghoshal, A. K., T. Rushmore, Y. Lim, and E. Farber. 1984. Early detection of lipid peroxidation in the hepatic nuclei of rats fed a diet deficient in choline and methionine. *Proceedings of the American Association for Cancer Research* 25:94.

Ghoshal, A. K., T. H. Rushmore, C. P. Buc, M. Roberfroid, and E. Farber. 1990. Prevention by free radical scavenger AD5 of prooxidant effects of choline deficiency. *Free Radical Biology and Medicine* 8(1):3–7.

Glenn, M. J., E. M. Gibson, E. D. Kirby, T. J. Mellott, J. K. Blusztajn, and C. L. Williams. 2007. Prenatal choline availability modulates hippocampal neurogenesis and neurogenic responses to enriching experiences in adult female rats. *European Journal of Neuroscience* 25(8):2473–2482.

Grotta, J. 2002. Neuroprotection is unlikely to be effective in humans using current trial designs. *Stroke* 33(1):306–307.

Holmes, G. L., Y. Yang, Z. Liu, J. M. Cermak, M. R. Sarkisian, C. E. Stafstrom, J. C. Neill, and J. K. Blusztajn. 2002. Seizure-induced memory impairment is reduced by choline supplementation before or after status epilepticus. *Epilepsy Research* 48(1–2):3–13.

Ikeda, Y., and D. M. Long. 1990. The molecular-basis of brain injury and brain edema—the role of oxygen free-radicals. *Neurosurgery* 27(1):1–11.

IOM (Institute of Medicine). 1998. *Dietary reference intakes for thiamin, riboflavin, niacin, vitamin B6, folate, vitamin B12, pantothenic acid, biotin, and choline.* Washington, DC: National Academy Press.

Jensen, H. H., S. P. Batres-Marquez, A. Carriquiry, and K. L. Schalinske. 2007. Choline in the diets of the U.S. population: NHANES, 2003–2004. *The Federation of American Societies for Experimental Biology Journal* 21:lb219.

Johnson, A. R., C. N. Craciunescu, Z. Guo, Y. W. Teng, R. J. Thresher, J. K. Blusztajn, and S. H. Zeisel. 2010. Deletion of murine choline dehydrogenase results in diminished sperm motility. *The Federation of American Societies for Experimental Biology Journal* 24(8):2752–2761.

Kennedy, J. E., P. F. Clement, and G. Curtiss. 2003. WAIS-III processing speed index scores after TBI: The influence of working memory, psychomotor speed and perceptual processing. *Clinical Neuropsychologist* 17(3):303–307.

Kline, A. E., J. L. Massucci, X. C. Ma, R. D. Zafonte, and C. E. Dixon. 2004. Bromocriptine reduces lipid peroxidation and enhances spatial learning and hippocampal neuron survival in a rodent model of focal brain trauma. *Journal of Neurotrauma* 21(12):1712–1722.

Kontos, C. D., E. P. Wei, J. I. Williams, H. A. Kontos, and J. T. Povlishock. 1992. Cytochemical detection of superoxide in cerebral inflammation and ischemia invivo. *American Journal of Physiology* 263(4):H1234–H1242.

Krupinski, J., I. Ferrer, M. Barrachina, J. J. Secades, J. Mercadal, and R. Lozano. 2002. CDP-choline reduces pro-caspase and cleaved caspase-3 expression, nuclear DNA fragmentation, and specific PARP-cleaved products of caspase activation following middle cerebral artery occlusion in the rat. *Neuropharmacology* 42(6):846–854.

Leon-Carrion, J., J. M. Dominguez-Roldan, F. Murillo-Cabezas, M. D. Dominguez-Morales, and M. A. Munoz-Sanchez. 2000. The role of citicholine in neuropsychological training after traumatic brain injury. *Neurorehabilitation* 14(1):33–40.

Levin, H. S. 1991. Treatment of postconcussional symptoms with CDP-choline. *Journal of the Neurological Sciences* 103(Suppl.):S39–S42.

Li, Z., and D. E. Vance. 2008. Phosphatidylcholine and choline homeostasis. *Journal of Lipid Research* 49(6):1187–1194.

Maldonado, V., J. B. Perez, and J. Escario. 1991. Effects of CDP-choline on the recovery of patients with head injury. *Journal of the Neurological Sciences* 103(Suppl.):S15–18.

Mir, C., J. Clotet, R. Aledo, N. Durany, J. Argemi, R. Lozano, J. Cervos-Navarro, and N. Casals. 2003. CDP-choline prevents glutamate-mediated cell death in cerebellar granule neurons. *Journal of Molecular Neuroscience* 20(1):53–59.

Penry, J. T., and M. M. Manore. 2008. Choline: An important micronutrient for maximal endurance-exercise performance? *International Journal of Sport Nutrition and Exercise Metabolism* 18(2):191–203.

Rao, A. M., J. F. Hatcher, and R. J. Dempsey. 2001. Does CDP-choline modulate phospholipase activities after transient forebrain ischemia? *Brain Research* 893(1–2):268–272.

Resseguie, M., J. Song, M. D. Niculescu, K. A. da Costa, T. A. Randall, and S. H. Zeisel. 2007. Phosphatidylethanolamine N-methyltransferase (PEMT) gene expression is induced by estrogen in human and mouse primary hepatocytes. *The Federation of American Societies for Experimental Biology Journal* 21(10):2622–2632.

Resseguie, M. E., K. A. da Costa, J. A. Galanko, M. Patel, I. J. Davis, and S. H. Zeisel. 2011. Aberrant estrogen regulation of PEMT results in choline deficiency-associated liver dysfunction. *The Journal of Biological Chemistry* 286(2):1649–1658.

Saver, J. L. 2008. Citicoline: Update on a promising and widely available agent for neuroprotection and neurorepair. *Reviews in Neurological Diseases* 5(4):167–177.

Saver, J. L., C. S. Kidwell, M. C. Leary, B. Ovbiagele, M. F. Tremwel, M. Eckstein, K. N. Ferguson, K. J. Gough, J. N. Llanes, E. M. Eraklis, R. Masamed, and S. Starkman. 2002. Results of the field administration of stroke treatment—Magnesium (FAST-MAG) pilot trial: A study of prehospital neuroprotective therapy. *Stroke* 33(1):66.

Secades, J. J., and G. Frontera. 1995. CDP-choline—Pharmacological and clinical review. *Methods and Findings in Experimental and Clinical Pharmacology* 17(Suppl. B):1–54.

Tazaki, Y., F. Sakai, E. Otomo, T. Kutsuzawa, M. Kameyama, T. Omae, M. Fujishima, and A. Sakuma. 1988. Treatment of acute cerebral infarction with a choline precursor in a multicenter double-blind placebo-controlled study. *Stroke* 19(2):211–216.

Warach, S., L. C. Pettigrew, J. F. Dashe, P. Pullicino, D. M. Lefkowitz, L. Sabounjian, K. Harnett, U. Schwiderski, R. Gammans, and I. Citicoline. 2000. Effect of citicoline on ischemic lesions as measured by diffusion-weighted magnetic resonance imaging. *Annals of Neurology* 48(5):713–722.

Wong-Goodrich, S. J., M. J. Glenn, T. J. Mellott, Y. B. Liu, J. K. Blusztajn, and C. L. Williams. 2010. Water maze experience and prenatal choline supplementation differentially promote long-term hippocampal recovery from seizures in adulthood. *Hippocampus*. Published electronically March 15, 2010. doi: 10.1002/hipo.20783

Yan, H. Q., A. E. Kline, X. C. Ma, E. L. Hooghe-Peters, D. W. Marion, and C. E. Dixon. 2001. Tyrosine hydroxylase, but not dopamine beta-hydroxylase, is increased in rat frontal cortex after traumatic brain injury. *Neuroreport* 12(11):2323–2327.

Zafonte, R., W. T. Friedewald, S. M. Lee, B. Levin, R. Diaz-Arrastia, B. Ansel, H. Eisenberg, S. D. Timmons, N. Temkin, T. Novack, J. Ricker, R. Merchant, and J. Jallo. 2009. The citicoline brain injury treatment (COBRIT) trial: Design and methods. *Journal of Neurotrauma* 26(12):2207–2216.

Zeisel, S. H. 2005. Choline: Critical role during fetal development and dietary requirements in adults. *Annual Review of Nutrition* 26:229–250.

Zeisel, S. H. 2006. Choline: Critical role during fetal development and dietary requirements in adults. *Annual Review of Nutrition* 26:229–250.

Zeisel, S. H., and K. A. da Costa. 2009. Choline: An essential nutrient for public health. *Nutrition Reviews* 67(11):615–623.

Zeisel, S. H., J. S. Wishnok, and J. K. Blusztajn. 1983. Formation of methylamines from ingested choline and lecithin. *The Journal of Pharmacology and Experimental Therapeutics* 225(2):320–324.

Zeisel, S. H., K. A. Dacosta, P. D. Franklin, E. A. Alexander, J. T. Lamont, N. F. Sheard, and A. Beiser. 1991. Choline, an essential nutrient for humans. *The Federation of American Societies for Experimental Biology Journal* 5(7):2093–2098.

10

Creatine

Creatine (N-[aminoiminomethyl]-N-methyl glycine) is an amino acid–like compound that is produced endogenously in the liver, kidney, pancreas, and possibly the brain from the biosynthesis of the essential amino acids methionine, glycine, and arginine, or obtained from dietary sources. The primary dietary sources are high-protein foods including meat, fish, and poultry. Once synthesized or ingested, creatine is transferred from the plasma through the intestinal wall into other tissues by specific creatine transporters located in skeletal muscles, the kidney, heart, liver, and brain.

Creatine and the creatine kinase/phosphocreatine system play an important role as re-served sources of energy in tissues with high and fluctuating energy requirements (e.g., muscle and brain). Creatine's role in energy metabolism involves the transfer of N-phosphoryl groups from phosphorylcreatine to adenosine diphosphate (ADP) to regenerate adenosine triphosphate (ATP) through a reversible reaction catalyzed by phosphorylcreatine kinase (Andres et al., 2008; Brosnan and Brosnan, 2007).

Both creatine and phosphocreatine are broken down spontaneously to creatinine, which is removed from the body in urine. The rate of loss is approximately 1.7 percent of the total body pool of creatine per day. Because more than 90 percent of creatine and phosphocre-atine is located in skeletal muscle, creatine losses and creatine excretion vary as a function of differences in muscle mass resulting from age, gender, and levels of daily activity. Creatinine excretion is greatest in young men between 18 and 29 years of age—the typical age of most military personnel in combat (Brosnan and Brosnan, 2007).

CREATINE AND THE BRAIN

Although the brain represents only 2 percent of total body weight, it uses approximately 20 percent of the body's energy. As the brain requires significant ATP turnover to maintain membrane potentials and signaling capacity, creatine metabolism and the creatine kinase/phosphocreatine system are important for normal brain function, and may be compromised in diseases of the central nervous system (Andres et al., 2008) (see also papers by Sullivan and by Hall in Appendix C).

Evidence of the importance of the creatine system for brain function comes from animal studies using creatine kinase knockout mice, which display significant reductions in hippocampal functioning and impairments in both learning and memory compared to non-genetically modified mice. Learning is further compromised in mice given a drug that competitively inhibits the creatine transporter and results in reductions of creatine pools in muscle and brain (Andres et al., 2008). In contrast, mice fed a diet supplemented with 1 percent creatine live longer, have less reactive oxygen species in their brains, and show better memory function than nonsupplemented littermates (Bender et al., 2008).

In humans, individuals born with errors in creatine synthesis or x-linked creatine transporter defects suffer from mental retardation, autistic behavior, severe language and speech impairments, epilepsy, and brain atrophy. In some individuals, the cognitive deficits resulting from these congenital errors can be improved, though not totally reversed, with chronic administration of large doses of creatine (Andres et al., 2008; Gualano et al., 2010).

Studies using nuclear magnetic resonance spectroscopy have shown that creatine supplementation increases brain levels of both creatine and phosphocreatine (Dechent et al., 1999; Pan and Takahashi, 2007). These increases in brain creatine may translate into improvements in cognitive behavior, particularly under stressful or compromised conditions. For example, young men given creatine supplements prior to experiencing 36 hours of sleep deprivation did better on a test of executive functioning than nonsupplemented individuals (McMorris et al., 2006). Creatine supplements have additionally been shown to enhance working memory in vegetarians, who typically have lower levels of creatine than omnivores (Rae et al., 2003), and to improve performance on tests of verbal and spatial memory in elderly individuals (McMorris et al., 2007).

There is growing evidence that creatine may be of value in the treatment of a number of neurological conditions, including congenital creatine deficiency syndromes, age-related cognitive decline (e.g., Alzheimer's disease), and neurodegenerative diseases (e.g., Parkinson's disease, Huntington's disease, amyotrophic lateral sclerosis), all of which are linked to dysfunctional energy metabolism (Andres et al., 2008; Gualano et al., 2010). Creatine supplementation is also beginning to attract attention as a complementary strategy in the treatment of psychiatric disorders (e.g., depression, posttraumatic stress disorder, and schizophrenia) (Allen et al., 2010; Amital et al., 2006b; Roitman et al., 2007).

As described in Chapter 3, damage following traumatic brain injury (TBI) can be categorized as primary, secondary, and long-term. Although understanding of the mechanisms underlying secondary injury is yet in its early stage, data indicate that impairments of mitochondrial function play a role in mediating the delayed consequences of TBI (Andres et al., 2008; Scheff and Dhillon, 2004; Sullivan et al., 2000; Zhu et al., 2004). It has been hypothesized that creatine's neuroprotective effects following TBI may involve creatine-induced maintenance of mitochondrial bioenergetics (Sullivan et al., 2000). Supporting this hypothesis is the finding by Sullivan and colleagues (2000) that rats fed a diet containing one percent creatine for four weeks displayed significantly higher mitochondrial membrane potentials and maintained levels of ATP better than nonsupplemented rats following controlled cortical contusion. Other indications of improved mitochondrial function in creatine-treated rats included decreased levels of reactive oxidative intermediaries and intramitochondrial calcium.

Brain levels of both lactate and free fatty acids increase following focal brain injury. These increases are believed to be a consequence of secondary brain damage resulting from the accumulation of excitotoxic levels of the neurotransmitter glutamate. Scheff and Dhillon

(2004) demonstrated that cortical and hippocampal levels of lactate and free fatty acids are lower in rats fed creatine than in nonsupplemented rats (Scheff and Dhillon, 2004). These results provide support for the hypothesis that creatine's neuroprotective effects are at least partly due to a reduction in the processes associated with secondary brain damage.

It also has been proposed that the neuroprotective effects of creatine may reflect its ability to improve cerebrovascular function (Prass et al., 2007). Support for this proposal comes from a recent study demonstrating that feeding creatine to mice subjected to middle artery occlusion resulted in reductions in infarct volumes. Although there were no changes in brain creatine, phosphocreatine, ATP, ADP, or adenosine monophosphate (AMP), such supplementation did improve cerebral blood flow in these animals, suggesting that creatine may have beneficial effects on cerebrovascular functioning.

A list of human studies (years 1990 and beyond) evaluating the effectiveness of creatine in providing resilience or treating TBI or related diseases or conditions (i.e., subarachnoid hemorrhage, intracranial aneurysm, stroke, anoxic or hypoxic ischemia, epilepsy) in humans is presented in Table 10-1. This also includes supporting evidence from animal models of TBI. Although this report does not generally include studies on the effectiveness of nutrition interventions on long-term effects of TBI effects, depression as an effect of TBI has been included in this chapter. The occurrence or absence of adverse effects in human studies is included if reported by the authors.

USES AND SAFETY

Creatine is one of the most widely used dietary supplements. Athletes, body builders, and military personnel use creatine to enhance muscle mass and increase strength. Creatine is also used as an ergogenic aid to improve performance of high-intensity exercise of short duration (Bemben and Lamont, 2005; Branch, 2003; IOM, 2008). Creatine's popularity as a dietary supplement was further increased by a 2006 study demonstrating its positive effect on cognitive and psychomotor performance (McMorris et al., 2006).

Because it can be synthesized in the body, there is no Recommended Dietary Allowance for creatine; however, as a result of daily losses, creatine stores need to be maintained either by diet or synthesis. Research indicates that creatine supplementation increases the creatine and phosphocreatine pools in muscle, particularly in younger individuals who are engaging in vigorous physical activity, and in vegetarians, who may have a less than optimal pool of phosphocreatine (Brosnan and Brosnan, 2007; Burke et al., 2003; Rawson et al., 2002).

Experiments among athletes and military personnel indicate that creatine taken at levels commonly available in supplements produces minimal, if any, side effects (IOM, 2008; Shao and Hathcock, 2006). Using evidence from well-designed, randomized controlled human clinical trials of creatine, Shao and Hathcock (2006) concluded that chronic intake of 5 g/day of creatine was safe and posed no significant health risks.

EVIDENCE INDICATING EFFECT ON RESILIENCE

Human Studies

As with other nutrients or food components, the committee found no human studies testing the potential benefits of creatine in TBI or other related diseases or conditions included in the reviewed of the literature (subarachnoid hemorrhage, intracranial aneurysm, stroke, anoxic or hypoxic ischemia, epilepsy).

TABLE 10-1 Relevant Data Identified for Creatine

Reference	Type of Injury/Insult	Type of Study and Subjects	Treatment	Findings/Results
Tier 1: Clinical trials				
Sakellaris et al., 2008	TBI	Prospective, randomized, comparative, open-labeled pilot study n^a=39 TBI patients ages 1–18 years, Glasgow Coma Scale (GCS) score between 3 and 9	Postinjury, creatine (0.4 g/kg) oral suspension form daily for 6 months or nothing; follow-up at 6 months	In short-term assessments, patients treated with creatine were less likely to experience post-traumatic amnesia (p=0.019). At 6 months, creatine-treated patients were less likely to experience headaches (χ^{2b}= 23.139; df^c=1; p < 0.001), dizziness (χ^2=7.886, df=1; p=0.005), and fatigue (χ^2=17.881, df=1; p < 0.001). No side effects due to creatine administration were observed.
Sakellaris et al., 2006	TBI	Prospective, randomized, comparative, open-labeled pilot study n=39 TBI patients ages 1–18 years, GCS between 3 and 9	Postinjury, creatine (0.4 g/kg) oral suspension form daily for 6 months, or nothing; follow-up at 3 and 6 months	Short-term assessment showed that patients treated with creatine were less likely to experience posttraumatic amnesia (p=0.019). Long-term analysis at 3 months showed that patients in the creatine group had better overall outcomes than the control group (χ^2=21.099, df=7; p=0.004). Specifically, creatine group performed better in neurophysical parameters (χ^2=14.269, df=4; p=0.006), cognitive parameters (χ^2=18.453, df=4; p=0.001), personality/behavioral outcomes (χ^2=19.595, df=4; p=0.001), and sociability measures (χ^2 = 20.562, df=4; p < 0.001). However, no significant differences were observed regarding locomotion, self care, and communication. At 6 months, creatine patients were more likely to achieve "good recovery" as measured using GOS (Glasgow Outcome Scores)-8 than control group (χ^2=29.231; df=5; p < 0.001). Creatine group showed greater improvement on cognitive (χ^2=29.262, df=4; p < 0.001) and personality/behavioral measures (χ^2=29.262, df=4; p < 0.001), as well as self care (χ^2=9.050, df=3; p=0.029) and communication (χ^2=8.011, df=2; p=0.029). No significant difference was observed on neurophysical, social, and locomotion measures after 6 months. No side effects due to creatine administration were observed.
Tier 2: Observational studies				
None found				

continued

TABLE 10-1   Continued

Reference	Type of Injury/Insult	Type of Study and Subjects	Treatment	Findings/Results
Tier 3: Animal studies				
Scheff and Dhillon, 2004	Moderate TBI	Adult, male Sprague-Dawley rats n=85	Preinjury, 0.5% or 1% creatine-supplemented diet (0.5% or 1%) or regular rodent diet fed for 2 weeks before TBI; some rats were killed 30 minutes or 6 hours after injury, while others were killed 7 days after injury	Lactate level: In the ipsilateral cortex, levels of lactate were higher 6 hours postinjury than 30 minutes after injury ($p < 0.002$). TBI rats had higher levels than sham-injured rats at both times ($p < 0.05$). At 30 minutes, rats on regular diet had higher lactate levels than rats on 1% creatine diet ($p < 0.05$). At 6 hours, lactate levels of regular diet group was higher than both creatine groups ($p < 0.05$).

In the penumbra of the ipsilateral cortex, all injured groups had higher lactate levels than sham-injured rats at 30 minutes ($p < 0.05$), with regular diet group at higher levels than 1% creatine rats ($p < 0.05$). At 6 hours, regular diet-fed rats had higher lactate levels than sham-injured rats and both creatine groups ($p < 0.05$), but creatine groups were not different from sham-injured rats.

In the ipsilateral hippocampus, regular diet group and 0.5% creatine group had higher levels than sham injury rats ($p < 0.05$) at 30 minutes. Levels in 1% creatine rats were not different from sham group. Lactate levels at 6 hours were greater than at 30 minutes ($p < 0.02$), with all TBI groups at higher levels than sham group ($p < 0.05$), and regular diet group at higher levels than 1% creatine group.

Free fatty acid (FFA) level: In the ipsilateral cortex, at 30 minutes, TBI rats had higher FFA levels than sham-injured rats ($p < 0.05$) and creatine-fed rats had lower levels of all FFAs than regular diet rats ($p < 0.05$). At 6 hours, only regular diet group and 0.5% creatine group had higher levels than sham controls ($p < 0.05$). Compared to regular diet rats, palmitic and stearic acids were lower in both creatine groups, and arachidonic was lower in 1% creatine group ($p < 0.05$).

In the penumbra, at 30 minutes, both creatine groups were lower than regular diet group ($p < 0.05$) but were not different from sham group. However, at 6 hours, all injured rats had higher levels than sham group ($p < 0.05$). Creatine-fed rats had lower FFA levels than regular diet rats, specifically in the levels of palmitic and stearic acids ($p < 0.05$).

In the ipsilateral hippocampus, at 30 minutes, regular diet group and 0.5% creatine group had higher levels than sham group ($p < 0.05$), while 1% creatine group was not significantly different from sham group. 1% creatine group had lower levels of palmitic, stearic, and arachidonic acids than regular diet group ($p < 0.05$). No significant FFA differences were observed among any group at 6 hours. |

TABLE 10-1 Continued

Reference	Type of Injury/Insult	Type of Study and Subjects	Treatment	Findings/Results
Sullivan et al., 2000	TBI (controlled cortical contusion)	Sprague-Dawley rats (n=24) and ICR mice (n=40)	Mice: injection of creatine monohydrate suspended in olive oil or vehicle 1, 3, or 5 days before injury; killed 7 days after injury Rats: fed normal diet or diet enriched with 1% creatine for 4 weeks 12 rats (6 on creatine diet and 6 on normal diet) were killed 1 hour after injury Remaining 12 rats were fed diets for additional 1 week after injury, then killed preinjury	Mice: There was a significant difference in cortical damage between creatine and vehicle groups (F[5,34]=4.16; p < 0.01). Although creatine showed no significant benefit for rats treated for 1 day, significant protection was observed in rats treated for 3 days (p < 0.05) and for 5 days (p < 0.01). Rats: Cortical damage was significantly smaller in rats fed with creatine-enriched diet before TBI (p < 0.01) than in rats fed with normal diet; all 12 rats were killed 7 days after TBI. In rats that were killed 1 hour postinjury, mitochondrial potential was significantly lower in rats fed with normal diet (t[4]=4.02; p < 0.05). Creatine-fed rats showed significantly lower reactive oxygen intermediate levels (t[4]=−7.63; p < 0.05) and Ca^{2+} levels (t[4]=−2.79; p < 0.05), but higher ATP levels (t[4]=5.54; p < 0.01).

[a] n: sample size.
[b] χ2: chi-square.
[c] df: degree of freedom.

Animal Studies

Animal studies provide a way to determine the effects of creatine supplementation on the biochemical and physiological as well as the behavioral consequences of TBI. The majority of studies assessing the neuroprotective effects of creatine have used mild cortical contusions as a model of TBI. These contusions result in significant reductions in cortical tissue, disruption of the blood-brain barrier, loss of hippocampal neurons, and severe behavioral deficits. Using this model, Sullivan and colleagues (2000) demonstrated dose-related reductions in cortical damage following contusions in mice that had been given intraperitoneal injections of creatine for 1, 3, or 5 days before the induction of brain damage. Similarly, rats fed a standard rodent diet supplemented with 1 percent creatine for four weeks before the induction of TBI demonstrated 50 percent less cortical damage than nonsupplemented rats. Further evidence of the potentially neuroprotective effects of creatine comes from a study by Scheff and Dhillon (2004), who found that rats fed a diet containing 1 percent creatine before experiencing controlled cortical contusions had significantly more sparing of cortical tissue than rats not given creatine.

These positive findings are supported by studies conducted on other brain injury models. For example, Prass and colleagues (2007) reported that mice fed diets containing 1 or 2 percent creatine for three weeks preceding middle cerebral artery occlusion, a model of ischemia, suffered significantly less brain damage than mice not given creatine. In this study, however, the neuroprotective effects of creatine were not observed when a large dose of creatine was given immediately following the onset of ischemia, or when a smaller dose was fed for 12 months.

EVIDENCE INDICATING EFFECT ON TREATMENT

Human Studies

There have been no studies to examine the effects on TBI of creatine supplementation in adults. Results of preliminary studies by Sakellaris and colleagues (2006; 2008) suggest that creatine supplementation may be useful in the treatment of the secondary and long-term symptoms of TBI that are not the immediate consequences of the trauma, but develop within minutes, hours, or days after the injury. The statement of task for this study did not include a systematic review of the effectiveness of nutrition interventions on long-term effects of TBI. Studies on creatine and long-term effects such as depression are included here as a prelude to a review that the committee believes should be conducted in the future. In the first study, the neuroprotective effects of an oral suspension of 0.4 g/kg of creatine given first within 4 hours from the time of injury and then once a day for 6 months were examined in TBI patients between the ages of 1 and 18. Children and adolescents given creatine spent less time in an intensive care unit and required tube feeding for a shorter period of time than controls not given creatine. When examined three and six months after injury, individuals who had received creatine supplementation displayed greater improvements in cognitive functioning, self-care, sociability, and communication skills than controls (Sakellaris et al., 2006). In a second part of the study with the same patient population and using the same creatine dosage regimen, the proportion of children with headaches, dizziness, and fatigue during a six-month observation period was significantly lower in the creatine-supplemented group than in the control group (Sakellaris et al., 2008). There were no side effects reported from creatine supplementation.

Depression is a noted long-term effect of TBI. There is growing evidence that impairments in cellular resilience, neural plasticity, and bioenergetic function within the brain are associated with the pathogenesis of depression. It has been hypothesized that by reversing these impairments, creatine could be useful in preventing or treating depression. Results of a number of studies indicate a relationship between depression, a frequent concomitant of TBI (Bombardier et al., 2010; Jorge and Starkstein, 2005; Masel and DeWitt, 2010), and creatine, and suggest that creatine may be of value in the treatment of the depressive symptoms observed in patients with TBI. The first evidence of a role for creatine in depression came from studies demonstrating a significant negative correlation between creatine metabolites and self-reported suicidal ideation in patients suffering from major depressive disorders (Agren and Niklasson, 1988). Studies performed since 2000 also found that levels of brain creatine are inversely related to the severity of a depressive episode (Dager et al., 2004; Segal et al., 2007). Support for the potential usefulness of creatine in the treatment of depression comes from open-labeled studies demonstrating that daily oral intake of three to five grams of creatine elevated mood in depressed patients resistant to antidepressant drugs and in patients with comorbid posttraumatic stress disorder (Amital et al., 2006b; Roitman et al., 2007).

Patients with fibromyalgia often suffer from chronic pain, fatigue, difficulty sleeping, and depression, symptoms also common following brain injury; a strong overlap has been reported between fibromyalgia and posttraumatic stress disorder (Amital et al., 2006a). In an eight-week, open-labeled study of creatine, significant improvements were observed in quality of life, sleep patterns, and pain in patients with fibromyalgia. These improvements deteriorated four weeks after stopping creatine therapy. In all of the preceding studies, adverse reactions to creatine supplementation, if any, were mild (e.g., nausea) and decreased over time.

Although the results of the preceding studies suggest promise for the possible use of creatine in the treatment of TBI, they are limited by their small number of participants and lack of double-blind procedures.

Animal Studies

Creatine supplementation also can reduce a number of detrimental consequences of cerebral ischemia. Following middle cerebral artery occlusion, mice fed a diet supplemented with two percent creatine for one month displayed significantly better neurologic function and significantly less brain damage than controls not receiving creatine. Creatine also significantly reduced ischemia-mediated depletion of ATP as well as caspase-3-activation and cytochrome *c* release, indicators of cell damage (Zhu et al., 2004).

As noted above, depression is one of the most common symptoms of TBI. In support of human studies on creatine and depression, chronic intake of diets supplemented with one or two percent creatine decreased depressive-like behavior in a dose-dependent manner in female rats in the forced swim test, an animal model of depression. In male rats, however, intake of the creatine-supplemented diets failed to reduce depressive behavior (Allen et al., 2010). The observation of sex-specific effects of creatine are interesting, given the fact that depression is more commonly diagnosed in women than in men.

CONCLUSIONS AND RECOMMENDATIONS

Based on results of both animal and human studies, creatine represents a promising nutritional supplement for increasing resilience to and treating TBI. Taken together, the results of the studies presented indicate that the neuroprotection resulting from intake of creatine-supplemented diets is due, at least in part, to a suppression of secondary brain injury. Although more research is needed in both animal and human populations, these findings suggest that prophylactic creatine treatment could be useful for people with an elevated potential to incur TBI; however, there are a number of issues that need to be addressed prior to initiating creatine use in military populations.

The question of how to experimentally assess the prophylactic effects of creatine on resilience remains unanswered. Researchers could give creatine to a group of high-risk individuals (e.g., individuals with a high risk of stroke, or a higher than normal risk of head injury) and compare brain functioning and behavior in those who ultimately experience brain injury with that of individuals in similar groups who were not given creatine. There are, however, challenges to conducting such a study. First, obtaining a statistically adequate number of participants for a long-term prospective study might be difficult. An additional problem is the current lack of definitive guidelines on how much creatine should be given or for how long it should be provided. Indeed, animal studies suggest that long-term feeding of creatine may reduce its ability to protect against the consequences of brain injury (Prass et al., 2007). These challenges to the feasibility of prospective studies will be common to any nutrient or food component of interest. To overcome these challenges, the committee recommends in Chapter 5 that a study be conducted on preinjury and postinjury dietary intake status (e.g., dietary supplement use) in individuals with TBI in order to determine any relationship to TBI outcome, including an analysis of the possible synergistic effects between nutrients, food components, and dietary supplements. Creatine should be included as part of that study.

With respect to treatment, preliminary studies by Sakellaris and colleagues (2006, 2008) provide evidence of the potentially positive therapeutic effects of creatine on brain function and behavior after brain injury. These positive effects should be confirmed in the adult population.

RECOMMENDATION 10-1. Based on the evidence supporting the effects of creatine on brain function and behavior after brain injury in children and adolescents, DoD should initiate studies in adults to assess the value of creatine for treating TBI patients.

REFERENCES

Agren, H., and F. Niklasson. 1988. Creatinine and creatine in CSF—indexes of brain energy-metabolism in depression. *Journal of Neural Transmission* 74(1):55–59.

Allen, P. J., K. E. D'Anci, R. B. Kanarek, and P. F. Renshaw. 2010. Chronic creatine supplementation alters depression-like behavior in rodents in a sex-dependent manner. *Neuropsychopharmacology* 35(2):534–546.

Amital, D., L. Fostick, M. L. Polliack, S. Segev, J. Zohar, A. Rubinow, and H. Amital. 2006a. Posttraumatic stress disorder, tenderness, and fibromyalgia syndrome: Are they different entities? *Journal of Psychosomatic Research* 61(5):663–669.

Amital, D., T. Vishne, S. Roitman, M. Kotler, and J. Levine. 2006b. Open study of creatine monohydrate in treatment-resistant posttraumatic stress disorder. *Journal of Clinical Psychiatry* 67(5):836–837.

Andres, R. H., A. D. Ducray, U. Schlattner, T. Wallimann, and H. R. Widmer. 2008. Functions and effects of creatine in the central nervous system. *Brain Research Bulletin* 76(4):329–343.

Bemben, M. G., and H. S. Lamont. 2005. Creatine supplementation and exercise performance—recent findings. *Sports Medicine* 35(2):107–125.

Bender, A., J. Beckers, I. Schneider, S. M. Holter, T. Haack, T. Ruthsatz, D. M. Vogt-Weisenhorn, L. Becker, J. Genius, D. Rujescu, M. Irmler, T. Mijalski, M. Mader, L. Quintanilla-Martinez, H. Fuchs, V. Gailus-Dumer, M. H. de Angelis, W. Wurst, J. Schmid, and T. Klopstock. 2008. Creatine improves health and survival of mice. *Neurobiology of Aging* 29(9):1404–1411.

Bombardier, C. H., J. R. Fann, N. R. Temkin, P. C. Esselman, J. Barber, and S. S. Dikmen. 2010. Rates of major depressive disorder and clinical outcomes following traumatic brain injury. *Journal of the American Medical Association* 303(19):1938–1945.

Branch, J. D. 2003. Effect of creatine supplementation on body composition and performance: A meta-analysis. *International Journal of Sport Nutrition and Exercise Metabolism* 13(2):198–226.

Brosnan, J. T., and M. E. Brosnan. 2007. Creatine: Endogenous metabolite, dietary, and therapeutic supplement. *Annual Review of Nutrition* 27:241–261.

Burke, D. G., P. D. Chilibeck, G. Parise, D. G. Candow, D. Mahoney, and M. Tarnopolsky. 2003. Effect of creatine and weight training on muscle creatine and performance in vegetarians. *Medicine and Science in Sports and Exercise* 35(11):1946–1955.

Dager, S. R., S. D. Friedman, A. Parow, C. Demopulos, A. L. Stoll, K. Lyoo, D. L. Dunner, and P. F. Renshaw. 2004. Brain metabolic alterations in medication-free patients with bipolar disorder. *Archives of General Psychiatry* 61(5):450–458.

Dechent, P., P. J. Pouwels, B. Wilken, F. Hanefeld, and J. Frahm. 1999. Increase of total creatine in human brain after oral supplementation of creatine-monohydrate. *American Journal of Physiology* 277(3 Pt 2):R698–704.

Gualano, B., G. G. Artioli, J. R. Poortmans, and A. H. Lancha. 2010. Exploring the therapeutic role of creatine supplementation. *Amino Acids* 38(1):31–44.

IOM (Institute of Medicine). 2008. *Use of dietary supplements by military personnel.* Washington, DC: The National Academies Press.

Jorge, R. E., and S. E. Starkstein. 2005. Pathophysiologic aspects of major depression following traumatic brain injury. *Journal of Head Trauma Rehabilitation* 20(6):475–487.

Masel, B. E., and D. S. DeWitt. 2010. Traumatic brain injury: A disease process, not an event. *Journal of Neurotrauma* 27(8):1529–1540.

McMorris, T., R. C. Harris, J. Swain, J. Corbett, K. Collard, R. J. Dyson, L. Dye, C. Hodgson, and N. Draper. 2006. Effect of creatine supplementation and sleep deprivation, with mild exercise, on cognitive and psychomotor performance, mood state, and plasma concentrations of catecholamines and cortisol. *Psychopharmacology* 185(1):93–103.

McMorris, T., R. C. Harris, A. N. Howard, G. Langridge, B. Hall, J. Corbett, M. Dicks, and C. Hodgson. 2007. Creatine supplementation, sleep deprivation, cortisol, melatonin and behavior. *Physiology and Behavior* 90(1):21–28.

Pan, J. W., and K. Takahashi. 2007. Cerebral energetic effects of creatine supplementation in humans. *American Journal of Physiology-Regulatory Integrative and Comparative Physiology* 292(4):R1745–R1750.

Prass, K., G. Royl, U. Lindauer, D. Freyer, D. Megow, U. Dirnagl, G. Stockler-Ipsiroglu, T. Wallimann, and J. Priller. 2007. Improved reperfusion and neuroprotection by creatine in a mouse model of stroke. *Journal of Cerebral Blood Flow and Metabolism* 27(3):452–459.

Rae, C., A. L. Digney, S. R. McEwan, and T. C. Bates. 2003. Oral creatine monohydrate supplementation improves brain performance: A double-blind, placebo-controlled, cross-over trial. *Proceedings of the Royal Society of London Series B-Biological Sciences* 270(1529):2147–2150.

Rawson, E. S., P. M. Clarkson, T. B. Price, and M. P. Miles. 2002. Differential response of muscle phosphocreatine to creatine supplementation in young and old subjects. *Acta Physiologica Scandinavica* 174(1):57–65.

Roitman, S., T. Green, Y. Osher, N. Karni, and J. Levine. 2007. Creatine monohydrate in resistant depression: A preliminary study. *Bipolar Disorders* 9:754–758.

Sakellaris, G., M. Kotsiou, M. Tamiolaki, G. Kalostos, E. Tsapaki, M. Spanaki, M. Spilioti, G. Charissis, and A. Evangeliou. 2006. Prevention of complications related to traumatic brain injury in children and adolescents with creatine administration: An open label randomized pilot study. *Journal of Trauma-Injury Infection & Critical Care* 61(2):322–329.

Sakellaris, G., G. Nasis, M. Kotsiou, M. Tamiolaki, G. Charissis, and A. Evangeliou. 2008. Prevention of traumatic headache, dizziness and fatigue with creatine administration. A pilot study. *Acta Paediatrica* 97(1):31–34.

Scheff, S. W., and H. S. Dhillon. 2004. Creatine-enhanced diet alters levels of lactate and free fatty acids after experimental brain injury. *Neurochemical Research* 29(2):469–479.

Segal, M., A. Avital, M. Drobot, A. Lukanin, A. Derevenski, S. Sandbank, and A. Weizman. 2007. Serum creatine kinase level in unmedicated nonpsychotic, psychotic, bipolar and schizoaffective depressed patients. *European Neuropsychopharmacology* 17(3):194–198.

Shao, A., and J. N. Hathcock. 2006. Risk assessment for creatine monohydrate. *Regulatory Toxicology and Pharmacology* 45(3):242–251.

Sullivan, P. G., J. D. Geiger, M. P. Mattson, and S. W. Scheff. 2000. Dietary supplement creatine protects against traumatic brain injury. *Annals of Neurology* 48(5):723–729.

Zhu, S., M. W. Li, B. E. Figueroa, A. J. Liu, I. G. Stavrovskaya, P. Pasinelli, M. F. Beal, R. H. Brown, B. S. Kristal, R. J. Ferrante, and R. M. Friedlander. 2004. Prophylactic creatine administration mediates neuroprotection in cerebral ischemia in mice. *Journal of Neuroscience* 24(26):5909–5912.

11

Ketogenic Diet

Originally developed to mimic biochemical changes associated with starvation or periods of limited food availability, the ketogenic diet is composed of 80–90 percent fat and provides adequate protein but limited carbohydrates (Gasior et al., 2006). In normal metabolism, carbohydrates contained in food are converted into glucose, which is the body's preferred substrate for energy production. Under some circumstances, like fasting, glucose is not available because the diet contains insufficient amounts of carbohydrates to meet metabolic needs. Consequently, fatty acid oxidation becomes favored, and the liver converts fat into fatty acids and ketone bodies that serve as an efficient alternative fuel for brain cells. The conversion leads to the synthesis of three ketone bodies in particular: β-hydroxybutyrate, acetoacetate, and acetone. Although fatty acids cannot cross the blood-brain barrier, these three ketone bodies can enter the brain and serve as an energy source.

KETOGENIC DIET AND THE BRAIN

Since their development to treat epileptic children in 1921, ketogenic diets have been most studied in the context of pediatric epilepsy syndromes (Kossoff et al., 2009), but the ketogenic diet has been further shown to be neuroprotective in animal models of several central nervous system (CNS) disorders, including Alzheimer's disease (AD), Parkinson's disease, hypoxia, glutamate toxicity, ischemia, and traumatic brain injury (TBI) (see Prins, 2008, for a review). Neurodegenerative disorders and other CNS injuries share some common pathophysiological events with the metabolic injury cascade that follows TBI, such as the increased production of reactive oxygen species (ROS) and mitochondrial dysfunction. Despite evidence of efficacy and a track record of clinical use and animal research on the ketogenic diet's antiepileptic action, the mechanisms by which the ketogenic diet confers neuroprotection are still poorly understood.

The effect of the ketogenic diet on energy metabolism is believed to be a key contributor to the diet's neuroprotective action, possibly by increasing resistance to metabolic stress and resilience to neuronal loss through the upregulation of energy metabolism genes, stimulation of mitochondrial biogenesis, and enhancement of alternative energy substrates (Bough, 2008; Bough et al., 2006; Davis et al., 2008; Gasior et al., 2006). The ketogenic diet is also hypothesized to promote neuroinhibitory actions. One aspect of this hypothesis is an associated modification of the tricarboxylic acid cycle to increase the synthesis of the neurotransmitter gamma-aminobutyric acid (GABA), leading to neuronal hyperpolarization (Bough and Rho, 2007). GABA is the primary inhibitor of neurotransmission, making a neuron more refractory to abnormal firing due to hyperpolarization. Seizures can be decreased by effects on GABA such as increasing its synthesis or decreasing its metabolism and breakdown. For this reason, GABA effects are an important target for some anticonvulsant drugs. Polyunsaturated fatty acid (PUFA) levels are likewise increased in patients on the ketogenic diet, and consequently induce the expression of neuronal uncoupling proteins (UCPs) (Fraser et al., 2003; Freeman et al., 2006). In one experimental study, mice fed a ketogenic diet were found to have increased UCPs, thus limiting the generation of ROS (Sullivan et al., 2004). Other mechanisms that possibly contribute to neuroprotection and enhanced mitochondrial function include, but are not limited to, promoting synthesis of adenosine triphosphate (ATP), interfering with glutamate toxicity, and bypassing the inhibition of complex I in the mitochondrial respiratory chain (Gasior et al., 2006; Prins, 2008; Zhao et al., 2006). Premature electron leakage occurs at complex I; moreover, it is one of the main sites of production of harmful superoxide and resultant apoptosis. Bypassing complex I can therefore reduce production of ROS and nonlytic cell death.

There have been two studies demonstrating evidence of neuroprotection against glutamate excitotoxicity, reduced mitochondrial ROS production, chronic hypoglycemia, and oxygen-glucose deprivation with in vitro exposure to beta-hydroxybutyrate of rat brain hippocampal slice cultures that were subsequently subjected to chronic hypoglycemia, oxygen-glucose deprivation, and N-methyl-D-aspartate-induced excitotoxicity (Maalouf et al., 2009; Samoilova et al., 2010).

USES AND SAFETY

Because ketone bodies are typically developed as an alternative energy source during intervals of fasting or starvation, they are not considered an essential nutrient nor has their absence been considered a nutritional deficiency. The traditional ketogenic diet consists of four parts fat to one part protein, with the fat components derived primarily from long-chain fatty acids. Modifications to the ketogenic diet have included a change of ratio to three parts fat to one part protein, the use of medium-chain triglycerides (MCT) for the fat component, and substitution of a modified Atkins diet or low-glycemic-index diet.

The most well-known clinical application of the ketogenic diet is in pediatric epilepsy syndromes, whose patients generally tolerate the special diet well with only mild side effects. Long-term use in the pediatric population has sometimes been associated with growth retardation, kidney stones, bone fractures due to osteopenia, and hypercholesterolemia; short-term side effects include low-grade acidosis, constipation, dehydration, vomiting or nausea, and hypoglycemia (if there is an initial fasting period) (Prins, 2008).

Consideration of adverse effects should take into account complications that may arise from the associated state of starvation or fasting that may lead to formation of ketone bodies. Such starvation is typically designed to provide 80–90 percent of the estimated caloric needs, based on age and weight (Kossoff et al., 2009). When diet is the primary means of achieving ketosis, there may be a need to consider an intermittent timing schedule. There have been some studies utilizing exogenous administration of ketone body precursors such as 1,3-butanediol or MCT, but there have been reports of adverse gastrointestinal symptoms such as diarrhea from one such exogenous ketogenic agent (Henderson et al., 2009). At least one prospective study among patients with refractory epilepsy also noted that patients had difficulty adhering to the specialized diet and experienced a considerable (albeit reversible) increase of cholesterol levels, thus indicating possible impediments to long-term implementation of the ketogenic diet as a therapeutic agent (Mosek et al., 2009).

EVIDENCE INDICATING EFFECT ON RESILIENCE

There are no human clinical studies or animal studies that have specifically evaluated associations between the use of ketogenic diet and resilience prior to CNS injury.

EVIDENCE INDICATING EFFECT ON TREATMENT

A relevant selection of animal studies (years 1990 and beyond) illustrating the effectiveness of the ketogenic diet in treating TBI in the acute phase of injury is presented in Table 11-1. This table also includes supporting evidence from human studies from the same time frame that evaluate the treatment efficacy of the ketogenic diet for other CNS injuries or disorders, such as epilepsy, hypoxia, and ischemic stroke. Some evidence of the effectiveness of the ketogenic diet on neurodegenerative disorders, like amyotrophic lateral sclerosis (ALS), AD, and Parkinson's disease, is also included in the following discussion and Table 11-1, even though this report, in general, does not review the efficacy of nutritional interventions on long-term effects of TBI. There were frequent tolerability side effects in humans, which are listed along with other side effects if mentioned by the authors.

Human Studies

There are no known human clinical trials evaluating the role of ketogenic diet in TBI; however, ketogenic diets have been shown to be effective in difficult-to-treat childhood epilepsy syndromes in many cohort studies and two recent clinical trials. The classic 4:1 ketogenic diet, as well as modified ketogenic diets like the MCT diet, demonstrated similar efficacy in symptomatic generalized epilepsy syndromes and partial epilepsy syndromes, with the majority of cohort studies indicating greater than 50 percent reduction in seizures (Beniczky et al., 2010; Coppola et al., 2010; Nathan et al., 2009; Porta et al., 2009; Sharma et al., 2009; Villeneuve et al., 2009). A combined analysis of outcome data from eleven cohort studies published since 1970 estimated that 15.8 percent of patients became free of seizures, 32 percent experienced greater than 90 percent reduction in seizure frequency, and nearly 56 percent of the patients had greater than 50 percent reduction of seizures (Cross and Neal, 2008). Similar results were found in a systematic review of 14 studies (Keene, 2006); however, the 2003 Cochrane review on the ketogenic diet for epilepsy concluded that although the diet is a treatment option for patients with difficult epilepsy (those taking multiple antiepileptic drugs), there is no reliable evidence from randomized control trials to support the diet's general use in people with epilepsy (Levy and Cooper, 2003).

When the first multi-center, randomized control trial was reported in 2008 (Neal et al., 2008), the results at three months showed a significant effect in achieving seizure control, with a greater than one-third reduction in seizure frequency in the diet group compared to controls. This study found no significant differences in efficacy at 3, 6, and 12 months between classical ketogenic diets that contained long-chain fatty acids, and a modified ketogenic diet with MCTs (Neal et al., 2009). A clinical trial of children with intractable Lennox-Gastaut syndrome investigated the efficacy of the ketogenic diet in conjunction with

TABLE 11-1   Relevant Data Identified for Ketogenic Diet

Reference	Type of Injury/ Insult	Type of Study and Subjects	Treatment	Findings/Results
Tier 1: Clinical trials				
Freeman, 2009; Freeman et al., 2009	Intractable Lennox-Gastaut syndrome	Randomized, double-blind, crossover study n^d=20 children, (days 1–2: all patients fast; day 3: treatment began; days 6–7: fasting; day 8: patients change treatment groups, treatment began; day 11: treatment ends)	In addition to a classic ketogenic diet, patients were given 60 g/day of saccharin or glucose (which negates ketosis and therefore serves as placebo) solutions; 24-hour EEGs were taken on days 1, 6, and 11	There was no significant difference in the number of parent-reported seizures between saccharin and glucose groups, and there was no difference in EEG-identified events. The sequence of treatment did not affect the number of seizures identified by EEG. At day 6, there was a reduction in both EEG-identified events (p=0.03) and parent-reported events (p=0.001). At day 12, frequency of seizures was significantly reduced from baseline (p=0.003). Finally, although serum β-hydroxyburate (BOH) levels were significantly lower in glucose groups when compared to saccharin groups (p < 0.001), glucose group still had some levels of serum BOH (Freeman et al., 2009). Additionally, fasting appeared to effect seizure frequency regardless of treatment assignment. At day 6, EEG-identified events reduced by a median of 22.5 seizure per day (p=1.03), and parent-reported events reduced by 14.5 seizures per day (p=0.001) (Freeman, 2009).
Neal et al., 2009	Intractable epilepsy	Randomized, double-blinded trial n=94 children aged 2–16 years, followed up at 3, 6, and 12 months	Classic, long-chain triglycerides ketogenic diet or medium-chain triglycerides ketogenic diet (MCT)	There was no significant difference in mean seizure frequency reduction between the two groups at 3, 6, or 12 months. The type of ketogenic diet also had no significant effect on the number of children achieving > 50% or > 90% seizure reduction. The classical ketogenic diet group had a significantly higher mean acetoacetate level than the MCT group at 3, 6, and 12 months (p < 0.005 at all three periods) and higher BOH level at 3 and 6 months (p ≤ 0.001 for both). Seizure reduction was correlated with acetoacetate level (r^b=-0.238, p < 0.036) and BOH level (r=-0.312, p < 0.01) at 3 months. There was no significant difference in tolerability to the two diet types, but the classical group reported lack of energy at 3 months and vomiting at 12 months more frequently (p < 0.05) than the MCT group.

continued

TABLE 11-1　Continued

Reference	Type of Injury/ Insult	Type of Study and Subjects	Treatment	Findings/Results
Neal et al., 2008	Intractable epilepsy	Randomized, controlled trial n=145 children aged 2–16 years, (n=103 included in final analysis)	Diet group (n=73) received ketogenic diet; control group (n=73) had no change to their diet	At 3 months, the diet group had a 38% reduction in average seizure frequency, whereas the control group had a 37% increase; the difference between the two groups was 76.6% (95% CI[c]: 44.4–108.9; p < 0.0001). The treatment had no significant effect on the type of seizure (generalized vs. focal) experienced by patients in either group.
Levy and Cooper, 2003	Epilepsy (all seizure types and syndromes)	Meta-analysis of randomized control trials	Ketogenic diet (mainly classic and MCT) vs. placebo or other antiepileptic treatment	No randomized controlled trials were found in the search of the literature; therefore, risk of bias and treatment effect could not be determined.

Tier 2: Observational studies

Reference	Type of Injury/ Insult	Type of Study and Subjects	Treatment	Findings/Results
Beniczky et al., 2010	Severe pharmacoresistant epilepsy	Retrospective study n=50	Ketogenic diet	After 3 months, 33 of the 50 patients had reduced seizure frequency of ≥ 50%. Of these 33 patients (responders), 18 had a > 90% reduction. Patients who had < 50% reduction had significantly greater epileptiform discharge (p=0.03) compared to responders. A multivariate analysis showed that epileptiform discharge was an independent predictor of treatment failure (OR[d]=5; 95% CI: 1.2–20). The difference in incidence of epileptiform discharge between responders with > 90% reduction and non-responders was significant (p=0.04).

TABLE 11-1 Continued

Reference	Type of Injury/ Insult	Type of Study and Subjects	Treatment	Findings/Results
Coppola et al., 2010	Refractory epilepsy encephalopathies	n=38 children, aged 3 months to 5 years, affected by drug-resistant symptomatic partial epilepsy and cryptogenic-symptomatic epileptic encephalopathies	For 29 children, at least 80% of their daily caloric intake came from ketocal milk during the study; 9 patients were fed with classic ketogenic diet because of poor compliance with ketocal milk Average time on diet was 10.3±7.4 months	A seizure frequency reduction of 50% was seen in 76% of children at 1 month, 77% at 3 months, and 100% at 6, 9, and 12 months. Response to treatment was not significantly associated with epileptic syndrome, age, sex, or etiology type. BMI also was not associated with efficacy of ketogenic diet. Adverse side effects were recorded in 65.8% of the children.
Patel et al., 2010	Intractable epilepsy	Questionnaires n=101; median age at the time of survey was 13 years (range 2–26 years) median ketogenic diet treatment duration was 1.4 years (range 0.2–8 years); median time since treatment stopped was 6 years (range 0.8–14 years)	Ketogenic diet	A significantly greater (p=0.0001) number of children had a > 50% seizure reduction at the time of the survey (79%) than at the time of ketogenic diet discontinuation (52%). While 96% of survey responders would recommend ketogenic diet treatment to others, only 54% would try said diet prior to anticonvulsants if given the choice again. The effect of ketogenic diet on growth in children younger than 18 years was measured using z-scores. The mean z-score for height was −1.3 (SEM^e=0.2) and for weight was −0.8 (SEM=0.2). BMI was used for patients older than 18; average BMI was 22.2. A few survey responders reported adverse effects such as cardiovascular diseases, kidney stones, bone fractures, and increased illnesses.

continued

TABLE 11-1 Continued

Reference	Type of Injury/ Insult	Type of Study and Subjects	Treatment	Findings/Results
Evangeliou et al., 2009	Refractory epilepsy	Pilot, prospective study n=17 children, aged 2 to 7 years	Ketogenic diet supplemented by powdered mixture of branched-chain amino acids (BCAA) (45.5 g leucine, 30 g isoleucine, and 24.5 g valine) Fat-to-protein ratio with addition of BCAA changed from 4:1 to around 2:5:1	Adding BCAA to ketogenic diet resulted in a 100% seizure reduction in 3 patients who had previously experienced seizure reduction on ketogenic diet alone. 4 patients who already had > 50% reduction on ketogenic diet alone achieved an additional 20–30% reduction. One patient, who had 20% reduction on ketogenic diet alone, achieved 50% reduction after adding BCAA. Addition of BCAA did not reduce seizure in patients who didn't already experience seizure reduction on ketogenic diet only. No reduction in ketosis was found with the addition of BCAA. No side effects were observed except 3 patients with slight increase in heart rate at initiation, which returned to normal.
Mosek et al., 2009	Refractory epilepsy	Prospective, pilot study n=8 patients, aged 18 to 45 years with at least two monthly focal seizures documented by 8-week follow-up	Classic ketogenic diet treatment (90% fat) for 12 weeks	Only 2 patients were on the diet for the full 12 weeks; they had more than a 50% reduction in the frequency of seizures. Compared to baseline, patients on ketogenic diet for 4–7 weeks experienced a 26% increase in cholesterol ($p < 0.02$) and 32% increase in LDL ($p < 0.03$). Those on ketogenic diet for 11–12 weeks had a 33% increase in cholesterol ($p < 0.002$) and 54% increase in LDL ($p < 0.0001$). No significant changes in HDL or triglycerides were recorded. Improvement in quality of life was reported in only 3 patients.
Nathan et al., 2009	Uncontrolled epilepsy	Prospective, non-blinded study n=105 children, aged 4 months to 18 years; average follow-up duration was 25.7±20.3 months	Ketogenic diet consisting of typical Indian foods	72% of patients had > 50% reduction in frequency of seizures ($p < 0.05$) compared to baseline. Of the two major types of seizure, there was a greater reduction in epileptic encephalopathies than in localization-related seizure ($p < 0.05$). The average number of anti-epileptic drugs (AEDs) was significantly reduced by the end of the study ($p < 0.005$) from 3.67 to 1.95. 11 patients completely stopped taking AEDs, while 70 patients took fewer drugs, and 23 patients took the same number of drugs ($p < 0.005$). Minor and temporary adverse effects were recorded such as gastrointestinal disturbances.

TABLE 11-1 Continued

Reference	Type of Injury/ Insult	Type of Study and Subjects	Treatment	Findings/Results
Nikanorova et al., 2009	Encephalopathy with continuous spikes and waves during slow sleep (CSWS)	n=5 children between 8 and 13 years old (1 patient withdrew from treatment at 9 months); follow-up period was 2 years after starting ketogenic diet	Conventional antiepileptic drugs and steroids supplemented with ketogenic diet	At 12 months, a slight reduction (< 85%) in spike-wave index was seen in only patients 1 and 2; patients 3 and 5 had an increase from baseline. At 24 months, patient 1 experienced an increase in spike-wave index, patient 2 remain the same, patient 3 decreased to normal level (CSWS ceased), and patient 5 experienced a decrease. The changes in spike-wave index were correlated with IQ scores—an increase in spike-wave index was associated with lowered IQ score, and a decrease was associated with improvement or maintenance of IQ score. The diet was well tolerated, and no adverse effects were mentioned.
Porta et al., 2009	Intractable epilepsy	Retrospective study n=27 children; follow up at 1, 3, 6, and 12 months	Ketogenic diet or modified Atkins diet	After 1 month, there was no significant difference in the number of responders (i.e., children with > 50% seizure reduction) between the two groups; 59% in ketogenic group, 50% in modified Atkins group. After 3 months, ketogenic group had significantly more responders than modified Atkins group (p=0.03); 64% vs. 20%. However, the significance disappeared after 6 months; 41% vs. 20%. Median frequency of status epilepticus in both diet groups was significantly lowered from 1 at baseline to 0 (p=0.005). Children's serum fatty acid levels were tested. After 1 month, responders had higher levels of serum palmitoleic acid and lower levels of arachidonic acid (p < 0.05). And after 3 months, responders had lower levels of arachidonic acid and docosahexaenoic acid (p < 0.05).

continued

TABLE 11-1   Continued

Reference	Type of Injury/ Insult	Type of Study and Subjects	Treatment	Findings/Results
Sharma et al., 2009	Refractory epilepsy	Prospective, uncontrolled study n=27 children, aged 6 months to 5 years, with at least 1 seizure/day (or at least 7 seizures/week); follow-up at 1, 3, 6, and 12 months	Ketogenic diet	At 3 months, 24 of the 27 children were on the diet, but 3 discontinued the diet. Of the 24, 66.7% of them achieved a > 50% reduction in seizure frequency, with 12.5% completely seizure-free. 15 children were on the diet at 6 months. Among these, 86.7% had > 50% reduction. At 12 months, only 10 children were still on the diet, and all of these children had > 50% reduction. Biochemical analysis show that, over the study period, the children had a significant decrease in serum albumin (p=0.05) and a significant increase in spot urinary calcium-creatinine ratio (p=0.03) compared to baseline. Lipid profiles showed no significant change over the study period. Digestive disorder was the most common side effect, experienced by 74% of patients.
Spulber et al., 2009	Pharmotherapy-resistant epilepsy	Prospective study n=22 children (median age of 5.5 years); height, height velocity, weight, BMI, and insulin-like growth factor I (IGF-I) level were taken 1 year before diet, just before starting diet, and 1 year after diet	Ketogenic diet for 12 months	14 patients had > 50% reduction in seizure frequency. Standard deviation scores (SDSs) of children's weight, height, and BMI decreased significantly after 1 year of ketogenic diet (p < 0.05); the median height SDS decreased 0.12 from 1 year before to just before starting the ketogenic diet, and it decreased 0.37 from just before to 1 year after starting the ketogenic diet. In the same intervals, weight SDS decreased 0.17, then 0.52; and BMI SDS decreased 0.33, then 0.5. The difference between the SDSs of these measurements 1 year before and just before starting ketogenic diet was not significant. Height velocity, calculated at just before the start of ketogenic diet and 1 year after, was significantly lower after ketogenic diet (p < 0.05); it decreased by 3.5. IGF-I also decreased 2.21 (p < 0.05). Height velocity correlated negatively with β-hydroxybutyric acid level during ketogenic diet (r=−0.48, p < 0.05) and positively with serum IGF-I both before (r=0.52, p < 0.05) and during (r=0.41, p < 0.05) the diet. No adverse effects were mentioned.

TABLE 11-1 Continued

Reference	Type of Injury/ Insult	Type of Study and Subjects	Treatment	Findings/Results
Villeneuve et al., 2009	Pharmacoresistant focal epilepsy, with recent worsening of seizure frequency (100% frequency increase within past month)	Retrospective study n=22 children, aged 5 months to 18.5 years, with focal epilepsy; of these, 10 had recent worsening of seizures	Ketogenic diet	At 1 month, 10 children had > 50% reduction in seizure frequency. Children with recent worsening of seizure frequency before ketogenic diet were more likely to be responders than children who did not experience a recent increase in seizures (70% vs. 25%, p=0.046). 7 children who were responders at 1 month continued their response to the diet after 6 months. 10 children experienced no side effects on the diet, but 4 patients experienced severe vomiting and 1 patient, severe anorexia. The remaining patients reported minor adverse effects.
You et al., 2009	West syndrome (infantile spasms)	n=98 children, monitored for 3 years	Ketogenic diet (n=33), antiepileptic drugs (n=31), hormonal therapy (n=60), epileptic surgery (n=3), and either no treatment or herbal medication (n=4)	During the study, 48 children's West syndrome (49%) evolved into Lennox-Gastaut syndrome, which has a worse prognosis. Bivariate logistic regression analysis showed that children who were treated with ketogenic diet, hormone therapy (prednisolone or adrenocorticotropic), or a combination of the two had a lower risk of West syndrome evolving to Lennox-Gastaut syndrome (p < 0.05). No other adverse effects were mentioned.
Hemingway et al., 2001	Epilepsy	Follow-up to prospective study n=150 children with difficult-to-control seizures	Classical ketogenic diet	At the follow-up for the current study (3–6 years after the original study), 20 children were seizure free, 21 had 90–99% seizure reduction, 24 had 50–90% reduction, and 18 had < 50% reduction. 83 of the 150 children were still on the diet at 12 months; of these, 11 were seizure free, 41 had > 90% reduction in seizure frequency, and 74 had > 50% reduction. 28 children were not taking any medication, and 45 were taking ≥ 1 medication at follow-up. 135 of the 150 children had discontinued the diet at follow-up. Of these, 27 discontinued because of improvement in seizure control, 49 because of ineffectiveness of the diet, 27 found the diet too restrictiveness, 28 stopped because of illness, and the remaining 4 were lost to follow-up. 4 children died and 9 children underwent cortical resection surgery.

continued

TABLE 11-1 Continued

Reference	Type of Injury/ Insult	Type of Study and Subjects	Treatment	Findings/Results
Tier 3: Animal studies				
Appelberg et al., 2009	TBI, controlled cortical impact (CCI)	Male, Sprague-Dawley rats (35 days and 75 days old)	Postinjury, ketogenic diet or standard diet for 7 days	Ketogenic diet had no effect on the weight of the older rats. But younger rats on ketogenic diet weighed less than rats of the same age on standard diet (p < 0.05).
				The older rats' performance on beam walking test was not affected by injury or diet. However, injured 35-day-old rats on standard diet had significantly worse performance than all other groups of the same age (p < 0.05).
				Among older rats, footslips were more frequent in injured than uninjured rats (p < 0.05) on all days; specifically, injured rats on ketogenic diet had the most number of footslips. Among younger rats, footslips were most frequent in injured, untreated rats than all other groups (p < 0.05); injured rats on ketogenic diet had fewer footslips than sham-injured rats (p < 0.05).
				Injured 75-day-old rats had worse performance than sham-injured rats (p < 0.05), and ketogenic diet did not improve performance. In 35-day-old rats, injured, untreated rats performed worse than injured, treated rats and sham-injured rats (p < 0.05); performance of treated rats were not different from sham-injured rats. Swim speed was not affected by age, injury, or diet.
Hu et al., 2009b	TBI, Feeney's weight-drop model	Male, juvenile Sprague-Dawley rats	Postinjury, ketogenic or normal diet	While injury increased brain edema (p < 0.01 vs. sham), ketogenic diet after injury reduced edema (p < 0.01 vs. injured rats on normal diet).
				Compared to injured rats on normal diet, injured rats fed with ketogenic diet had decreased cytosolic cytochrome c level (p < 0.01) and increased cytochrome c immunoreactivity (p < 0.05). Injured rats had greater apoptosis and increased caspase-3 expression compared to uninjured rats (p < 0.01 for both), but treatment with ketogenic diet significantly reduced apoptosis and caspase-3 expression (p < 0.01 vs. injured, untreated rats).

TABLE 11-1 Continued

Reference	Type of Injury/ Insult	Type of Study and Subjects	Treatment	Findings/Results
Hu et al., 2009a	TBI, Feeney's weight-drop model	Male, juvenile Sprague-Dawley rats	Postinjury, ketogenic or normal diet	Bax mRNA and protein levels were increased significantly by TBI ($p < 0.01$ vs. sham-injured rats) and decreased by ketogenic diet ($p < 0.01$ vs. rats on normal diet). Bcl-2 mRNA and protein levels were not affected by injury or diet. Apoptosis in the penumbra area was increased after TBI ($p < 0.05$ vs. sham-injured rats), but was decreased with ketogenic diet ($p < 0.01$ vs. rats on normal diet).
Jarrett et al., 2008	Epilepsy	Adolescent, male Sprague-Dawley rats (P28)	Ketogenic or control diet for 3 weeks	After 3 weeks, rats on ketogenic diet had higher serum β-hydroxybutyric levels ($p < 0.0001$) and lower glucose levels ($p < 0.01$). Assessment of hippocampal mitochondria showed significantly higher GSH levels ($p < 0.01$), but not GSSG levels. Rats on the ketogenic diet also had increased GSH-GSSG ratio ($p < 0.05$) and reduced GSH/GSSG redox potential compared to control rats (-246.6 mV vs. -230.0 mV; $p < 0.05$).
				Measurements of the two GSH biosynthetic enzymes, GCL and GS, showed 1.3 times increased activity in GCL ($p < 0.05$), but none in GS. Compared to control rats, subunit GCLM showed a 1.6-fold increase ($p < 0.05$) and GCLC showed a 1.9-fold increase ($p < 0.01$).
				To confirm the results from measurements of GSH and GSSG, a second redox couple was measured, CoASH/CoASSG. Compared to control rats, hippocampal mitochondria in rats on Ketogenic diet showed significantly increased levels of CoASH ($p < 0.05$), but not CoASSG, and an increased CoASH/CoASSG ratio ($p < 0.05$).
				Levels of lapoic acid were increased in the hippocampus of ketogenic diet rats, but not in the frontal cortex ($p < 0.05$).
				H_2O_2 production in isolated mitochondria was significantly decreased in ketogenic diet rats ($p < 0.05$), while no difference between the groups was observed in H_2O_2 production in hippocampal homogenate. When exposed to exogenous H_2O_2, control rats exhibited significant mtDNA damage that increased with time ($p < 0.0001$).

continued

TABLE 11-1   Continued

Reference	Type of Injury/ Insult	Type of Study and Subjects	Treatment	Findings/Results
Prins et al., 2005	TBI, controlled cortical impact	Male, Sprague-Dawley rats aged 17, 35, 45, and 65 days	Postinjury, ketogenic diet	Ketogenic diet had no effect on contusion volume of 17-and 65-day-old rats, but it decreased contusion volume of 35- (by 58%, F=0.019, p < 0.001) and 45-day-old (by 39%, F=0.074, p < 0.05) rats.
				Glucose level was increased in all age groups on ketogenic diet at 24 hours (p < 0.05) compared to rats on normal diet. Additionally, 35-day-old rats showed increased glucose at 1 hour as well as 7 days, and 45- and 65-day-old rats had increased glucose at 7 days.
				17- and 35-day-old rats had decreased lactate level at 7 days (p < 0.05), while 45- and 65-day-old rats on ketogenic diet had decreased lactate level at 24 hours (p < 0.05).
				β-hydroxybutrate level was decreased in rats on ketogenic giet across all age groups at 24 hours and 7 days (p < 0.01 vs. rats on normal diet).

[a] n: sample size.
[b] r: correlation coefficient.
[c] CI: confidence interval.
[d] OR: odds ratio.
[e] SEM: standard error of mean.

a solution of either glucose or saccharin (60 g/day) to negate ketosis after a 36-hour fasting period, and found a similar significant decrease in seizures (Freeman et al., 2009).

Long-term beneficial outcomes to 24 months have been demonstrated with the ketogenic diet in certain childhood epilepsy syndromes (Kossoff and Rho, 2009). These studies have led to even more recent understandings regarding the mechanism of action, such as recent evidence that suggests the ketogenic diet mechanism is related to its increasing extracellular adenosine and the actions of adenosine at the A1 receptor, which include inhibiting glutamergic effects (Masino et al., 2009).

Studies show that the percentage of patients remaining on a ketogenic diet beyond 24 months decreases over time. Hemingway and colleagues (2001) found that 39 percent of patients remained on the diet at two years, 20 percent at three years, and 12 percent at four years. The main reason given for discontinuing the ketogenic diet beyond 24 months was the patient being seizure-free or having a significant seizure reduction. Although there are no human short- or long-term studies evaluating the ketogenic diet for TBI, these data suggest that use of the ketogenic diet should be most strongly considered during the initial rehabilitation interval associated with the greatest gains.

As mentioned earlier, several observational studies have investigated the use of ketogenic diets modified in an effort to improve tolerability. In 2009, Evangeliou and colleagues examined the role of branched-chain amino acids (BCAAs) as a supplemental therapeutic agent to the ketogenic diet in children with intractable epilepsy, based on evidence of antiepileptic action in animal models (for further discussion on the role of BCAAs in TBI and other CNS injuries, see Chapters 4 and 8). Although the fat-to-protein ratio was altered from the classic 4:1 to 2.5:1, there was no observed effect on ketosis. Furthermore, 47 percent (n = 17) of the patients who had already achieved a reduction of seizures on the ketogenic diet saw an even greater reduction after the BCAA supplementation, with three patients experiencing a complete cessation of seizures (Evangeliou et al., 2009). Further studies are needed to examine this particular combination; however, the results of this prospective pilot suggest a possible synergistic action between the ketogenic diet and BCAAs.

Pharmacological research on dementia has used a cognitive assessment instrument known as the Alzheimer's disease (AD) Assessment Scale-Cognitive subscale (ADAS-Cog), which provides quantification of cognitive domains such as memory and attention in order to assess outcomes. There is some evidence that administering a form of MCTs in patients with a normal diet increased the serum level of the ketone body gamma hydroxybutyrate and increased ADAS-Cog scores in a population of patients with mild to moderate AD compared to placebo in the same population (Henderson et al., 2009; Reger et al., 2004). Given that multiple studies have shown a decreased risk of developing AD in those consuming foods high in essential fatty acids, it is also possible that the ketogenic diet may confer greater neuroprotection in people with AD than normal or high-carbohydrate diets (Gasior et al., 2006; Henderson, 2004; Morris et al., 2003a, 2003b).

Animal Studies

Studies with a rat model of TBI have suggested reduction in volume of damage and improved recovery with use of the ketogenic diet (Prins, 2008). One study demonstrated increased protection against oxidative stress and deoxyribonucleic acid damage because of increased redox status in the hippocampus (Jarrett et al., 2008). Several investigators have identified an age-dependent effect in rat TBI models, with greater levels of reduction of edema, cytochrome c release, and cellular apoptosis being observed in younger rats (Appelberg et al., 2009; Hu et al., 2009a).

Evidence of neuroprotection has been demonstrated with 24-hour fasting in rodent models of controlled cortical impact injury following moderate but not severe injury. Fasting for 48 hours demonstrated no significant benefit (Davis et al., 2008).

As mentioned earlier, animal studies have evaluated the ketogenic diet in stroke, another form of acquired brain injury, as well as in neurodegenerative disorders such as AD, Parkinson's disease, and ALS (Gasior et al., 2006; Prins, 2008; Zhao et al., 2006). The majority of experimental studies in other models of CNS injury support the evidence suggesting beneficial effects of the ketogenic diet. It is also important to note that age-related differences in ketogenesis and cerebral utilization of ketones have been observed in animal models, and suggest the developing brain has a greater capacity to generate, transport, and utilize ketone bodies as an energy substrate (Appelberg et al., 2009; Prins, 2008; Prins et al., 2005).

Because the only TBI data available has been from rodent models, there are significant limitations (as stated in Chapter 3) in correlating the results from animal studies to humans (e.g., rodents tend to eat immediately after injury, which is not typical human behavior). An additional limitation encountered when conducting energy metabolism studies with rodents is that they have lesser energy reserves than humans and a higher metabolic rate; prolonged fasting also can be more devastating to rodents than to humans. Fasting rodents for longer than a few days will likely result in their death, while uninjured humans can fast for five to six weeks without mortality. However, feeding rats a fat-only diet has been demonstrated to prolong survival (Moldawer et al., 1981) and should be investigated as a possible model to measure the efficacy of compounds that alter energy metabolism.

CONCLUSIONS AND RECOMMENDATIONS

Based on the evidence presented, the ketogenic diet does hold some promise of effectiveness in improving the outcomes of TBI. There are indications that ketones may provide an alternative and readily usable energy source for the brain that might reduce its dependence on glucose metabolism, which may be impaired immediately following TBI. However, important knowledge gaps must be addressed before either the classic or modified ketogenic diet can be recommended as a treatment for TBI. Although it would not be feasible to prescribe ketogenic diets to improve resilience against TBI, identifying dietary compounds that are precursors of ketones, such as medium-chain triglycerides, and evaluating whether they have positive effects when administered after the injury is warranted.

There is a general need for demonstration of the benefit of ketone bodies and ketogenic diets in human TBI, including the use of exogenous agents to enhance the production and utilization of ketone bodies. Several questions relate to that broad gap in knowledge. None of the animal models previously used has incorporated blast injury as a mechanism for TBI. An appropriate animal model for following TBI recovery is also necessary to evaluate the efficacy and applicability of a ketogenic diet. This nutritional strategy utilizes an alternative metabolic pathway, and there is limited data on issues such as dosing and duration of either diet-controlled ketosis or exogenous administration of agents that enhance ketone production. As with other interventions considered in this report, there is an absence of information on which forms of TBI—mild/concussion, moderate, severe, and penetrating—might benefit from such therapy. Another consideration is the feasibility of prescribing such a strict diet when treating nonhospitalized patients. Although ensuring compliance with any nutrition intervention may present a challenge, this is especially true when the whole diet needs to be altered. Because of the diversity of nutritional needs and metabolic demands of military service, diet-induced ketosis also may not be practical for treatment of military injuries, especially in the context of polytrauma and the need to balance other nutritional recommendations following injury.

RECOMMENDATION 11-1. DoD should conduct animal studies to examine the specific effects of ketogenic diets, other modified diets (e.g., structured lipids, low-glycemic-index carbohydrates, fructose), or precursors of ketone bodies that affect energetics and have potential value against TBI. These animal studies should specifically consider dose, time, and clinical correlates with injury as variables. Results from these studies should be used to design human studies with these various diets to determine if they improve outcome against severe TBI. These studies should include time as a variable to determine whether there is an optimal initiation point and length of use.

RECOMMENDATION 11-2. If these studies show benefits, then DoD should further investigate whether the potential beneficial effect of such ketogenic or modified diets or precursors to ketone bodies applies to concussion/mild and moderate TBI. Before conducting these studies, DoD should consider the feasibility (i.e., how to ensure compliance with a modified diet) of using diets that affect the metabolic energy available, such as ketogenic diets, for the treatment of TBI.

REFERENCES

Appelberg, K. S., D. A. Hovda, and M. L. Prins. 2009. The effects of a ketogenic diet on behavioral outcome after controlled cortical impact injury in the juvenile and adult rat. *Journal of Neurotrauma* 26(4):497–506.

Beniczky, S., M. Jose Miranda, J. Alving, J. Heber Povlsen, and P. Wolf. 2010. Effectiveness of the ketogenic diet in a broad range of seizure types and EEG features for severe childhood epilepsies. *Acta Neurologica Scandinavica* 121(1):58–62.

Bough, K. 2008. Energy metabolism as part of the anticonvulsant mechanism of the ketogenic diet. *Epilepsia* 49(Suppl. 8):91–93.

Bough, K. J., and J. M. Rho. 2007. Anticonvulsant mechanisms of the ketogenic diet. *Epilepsia* 48(1):43–58.

Bough, K. J., J. Wetherington, B. Hassel, J. F. Pare, J. W. Gawryluk, J. G. Greene, R. Shaw, Y. Smith, J. D. Geiger, and R. J. Dingledine. 2006. Mitochondrial biogenesis in the anticonvulsant mechanism of the ketogenic diet. *Annals of Neurology* 60(2):223–235.

Coppola, G., A. Verrotti, E. Ammendola, F. F. Operto, R. della Corte, G. Signoriello, and A. Pascotto. 2010. Ketogenic diet for the treatment of catastrophic epileptic encephalopathies in childhood. *European Journal of Paediatric Neurology* 14(3):229–234.

Cross, J. H., and E. G. Neal. 2008. The ketogenic diet—update on recent clinical trials. *Epilepsia* 49(Suppl. 8):6–10.

Davis, L. M., J. R. Pauly, R. D. Readnower, J. M. Rho, and P. G. Sullivan. 2008. Fasting is neuroprotective following traumatic brain injury. *Journal of Neuroscience Research* 86(8):1812–1822.

Evangeliou, A., M. Spilioti, V. Doulioglou, P. Kalaidopoulou, A. Ilias, A. Skarpalezou, I. Katsanika, S. Kalamitsou, K. Vasilaki, I. Chatziioanidis, K. Garganis, E. Pavlou, S. Varlamis, and N. Nikolaidis. 2009. Branched chain amino acids as adjunctive therapy to ketogenic diet in epilepsy: Pilot study and hypothesis. *Journal of Child Neurology* 24(10):1268–1272.

Fraser, D. D., S. Whiting, R. D. Andrew, E. A. Macdonald, K. Musa-Veloso, and S. C. Cunnane. 2003. Elevated polyunsaturated fatty acids in blood serum obtained from children on the ketogenic diet. *Neurology* 60(6):1026–1029.

Freeman, J., P. Veggiotti, G. Lanzi, A. Tagliabue, and E. Perucca. 2006. The ketogenic diet: From molecular mechanisms to clinical effects. *Epilepsy Research* 68(2):145–180.

Freeman, J. M. 2009. The ketogenic diet: Additional information from a crossover study. *Journal of Child Neurology* 24(4):509–512.

Freeman, J. M., E. P. G. Vining, E. H. Kossoff, P. L. Pyzik, X. Ye, and S. N. Goodman. 2009. A blinded, crossover study of the efficacy of the ketogenic diet. *Epilepsia* 50(2):322–325.

Gasior, M., M. A. Rogawski, and A. L. Hartman. 2006. Neuroprotective and disease-modifying effects of the ketogenic diet. *Behavioural Pharmacology* 17(5–6):431–439.

Hemingway, C., J. M. Freeman, D. J. Pillas, and P. L. Pyzik. 2001. The ketogenic diet: A 3- to 6-year follow-up of 150 children enrolled prospectively. *Pediatrics* 108(4):898–905.

Henderson, S. T. 2004. High carbohydrate diets and Alzheimer's disease. *Medical Hypotheses* 62(5):689–700.

Henderson, S. T., J. L. Vogel, L. J. Barr, F. Garvin, J. J. Jones, and L. C. Costantini. 2009. Study of the ketogenic agent AC-1202 in mild to moderate Alzheimer's disease: A randomized, double-blind, placebo-controlled, multicenter trial. *Nutrition and Metabolism* 6:31.

Hu, Z.-G., H.-D. Wang, L. Qiao, W. Yan, Q.-F. Tan, and H.-X. Yin. 2009a. The protective effect of the ketogenic diet on traumatic brain injury-induced cell death in juvenile rats. *Brain Injury* 23(5):459–465.

Hu, Z. G., H. D. Wang, W. Jin, and H. X. Yin. 2009b. Ketogenic diet reduces cytochrome c release and cellular apoptosis following traumatic brain injury in juvenile rats. *Annals of Clinical and Laboratory Science* 39(1):76–83.

Jarrett, S. G., J. B. Milder, L. P. Liang, and M. Patel. 2008. The ketogenic diet increases mitochondrial glutathione levels. *Journal of Neurochemistry* 106(3):1044–1051.

Keene, D. L. 2006. A systematic review of the use of the ketogenic diet in childhood epilepsy. *Pediatric Neurology* 35(1):1–5.

Kossoff, E. H., and J. M. Rho. 2009. Ketogenic diets: Evidence for short- and long-term efficacy. *Neurotherapeutics* 6(2):406–414.

Kossoff, E. H., B. A. Zupec-Kania, P. E. Amark, K. R. Ballaban-Gil, A. G. Christina Bergqvist, R. Blackford, J. R. Buchhalter, R. H. Caraballo, J. Helen Cross, M. G. Dahlin, E. J. Donner, J. Klepper, R. S. Jehle, H. D. Kim, Y. M. Christiana Liu, J. Nation, D. R. Nordli, Jr., H. H. Pfeifer, J. M. Rho, C. E. Stafstrom, E. A. Thiele, Z. Turner, E. C. Wirrell, J. W. Wheless, P. Veggiotti, E. P. G. Vining, Charlie Foundation, Practice Committee of the Child Neurology Society, Practice Committee of the Child Neurology Society, and International Ketogenic Diet Study Group. 2009. Optimal clinical management of children receiving the ketogenic diet: Recommendations of the International Ketogenic Diet Study Group. *Epilepsia* 50(2):304–317.

Levy, R., and P. Cooper. 2003. Ketogenic diet for epilepsy. *Cochrane Database of Systematic Reviews* (3):CD001903.

Maalouf, M., J. M. Rho, and M. P. Mattson. 2009. The neuroprotective properties of calorie restriction, the ketogenic diet, and ketone bodies. *Brain Research Reviews* 59(2):293–315.

Masino, S. A., M. Kawamura, C. A. Wasser, L. T. Pomeroy, and D. N. Ruskin. 2009. Adenosine, ketogenic diet and epilepsy: The emerging therapeutic relationship between metabolism and brain activity. *Current Neuropharmacology* 7(3):257–268.

Moldawer, L. L., B. R. Bistrian, and G. L. Blackburn. 1981. Factors determining the preservation of protein status during dietary-protein deprivation. *Journal of Nutrition* 111(7):1287–1296.

Morris, M. C., D. A. Evans, J. L. Bienias, C. C. Tangney, D. A. Bennett, N. Aggarwal, J. Schneider, and R. S. Wilson. 2003a. Dietary fats and the risk of incident Alzheimer disease. *Archives of Neurology* 60(2):194–200.

Morris, M. C., D. A. Evans, J. L. Bienias, C. C. Tangney, D. A. Bennett, R. S. Wilson, N. Aggarwal, and J. Schneider. 2003b. Consumption of fish and n-3 fatty acids and risk of incident Alzheimer disease. *Archives of Neurology* 60(7):940–946.

Mosek, A., H. Natour, M. Y. Neufeld, Y. Shiff, and N. Vaisman. 2009. Ketogenic diet treatment in adults with refractory epilepsy: A prospective pilot study. *Seizure* 18(1):30–33.

Nathan, J. K., A. S. Purandare, Z. B. Parekh, and H. V. Manohar. 2009. Ketogenic diet in Indian children with uncontrolled epilepsy. *Indian Pediatrics* 46(8):669–673.

Neal, E. G., H. Chaffe, R. H. Schwartz, M. S. Lawson, N. Edwards, G. Fitzsimmons, A. Whitney, and J. H. Cross. 2008. The ketogenic diet for the treatment of childhood epilepsy: A randomised controlled trial. *Lancet Neurology* 7(6):500–506.

Neal, E. G., H. Chaffe, R. H. Schwartz, M. S. Lawson, N. Edwards, G. Fitzsimmons, A. Whitney, and J. H. Cross. 2009. A randomized trial of classical and medium-chain triglyceride ketogenic diets in the treatment of childhood epilepsy. *Epilepsia* 50(5):1109–1117.

Nikanorova, M., M. J. Miranda, M. Atkins, and L. Sahlholdt. 2009. Ketogenic diet in the treatment of refractory continuous spikes and waves during slow sleep. *Epilepsia* 50(5):1127–1131.

Patel, A., P. L. Pyzik, Z. Turner, J. E. Rubenstein, and E. H. Kossoff. 2010. Long-term outcomes of children treated with the ketogenic diet in the past. *Epilepsia* 51(7):1277–1282.

Porta, N., L. Vallee, E. Boutry, M. Fontaine, A.-F. Dessein, S. Joriot, J.-M. Cuisset, J.-C. Cuvellier, and S. Auvin. 2009. Comparison of seizure reduction and serum fatty acid levels after receiving the ketogenic and modified Atkins diet. *Seizure* 18(5):359–364.

Prins, M. L. 2008. Cerebral metabolic adaptation and ketone metabolism after brain injury. *Journal of Cerebral Blood Flow and Metabolism* 28(1):1–16.

Prins, M. L., L. S. Fujima, and D. A. Hovda. 2005. Age-dependent reduction of cortical contusion volume by ketones after traumatic brain injury. *Journal of Neuroscience Research* 82(3):413–420.

Reger, M. A., S. T. Henderson, C. Hale, B. Cholerton, L. D. Baker, G. S. Watson, K. Hyde, D. Chapman, and S. Craft. 2004. Effects of beta-hydroxybutyrate on cognition in memory-impaired adults. *Neurobiology of Aging* 25(3):311–314.

Samoilova, M., M. Weisspapir, P. Abdelmalik, A. A. Velumian, and P. L. Carlen. 2010. Chronic in vitro ketosis is neuroprotective but not anti-convulsant. *Journal of Neurochemistry* 113(4):826–835.

Sharma, S., S. Gulati, V. Kalra, A. Agarwala, and M. Kabra. 2009. Seizure control and biochemical profile on the ketogenic diet in young children with refractory epilepsy—Indian experience. *Seizure* 18(6):446–449.

Spulber, G., S. Spulber, L. Hagenas, P. Amark, and M. Dahlin. 2009. Growth dependence on insulin-like growth factor-1 during the ketogenic diet. *Epilepsia* 50(2):297–303.

Sullivan, P. G., N. A. Rippy, K. Dorenbos, R. C. Concepcion, A. K. Agarwal, and J. M. Rho. 2004. The ketogenic diet increases mitochondrial uncoupling protein levels and activity. *Annals of Neurology* 55(4):576–580.

Villeneuve, N., F. Pinton, N. Bahi-Buisson, O. Dulac, C. Chiron, and R. Nabbout. 2009. The ketogenic diet improves recently worsened focal epilepsy. *Developmental Medicine and Child Neurology* 51(4):276–281.

You, S. J., H. D. Kim, and H.-C. Kang. 2009. Factors influencing the evolution of West syndrome to Lennox-Gastaut syndrome. *Pediatric Neurology* 41(2):111–113.

Zhao, Z., D. J. Lange, A. Voustianiouk, D. MacGrogan, L. Ho, J. Suh, N. Humala, M. Thiyagarajan, J. Wang, and G. M. Pasinetti. 2006. A ketogenic diet as a potential novel therapeutic intervention in amyotrophic lateral sclerosis. *BMC Neuroscience* 7:29.

12

Magnesium

Magnesium is an essential nutrient that serves as a cofactor for more than 300 enzymes involved in biological reactions important for cellular energy metabolism, protein synthesis, maintenance of cardiovascular health, regulation of blood glucose levels, and normal nervous system functioning. Approximately 50 percent of the magnesium in the body is found in bone, while the other 50 percent is found predominantly in soft tissue (Fleet and Cashman, 2001; Shils, 1999). Magnesium levels in the body are tightly regulated by absorption and excretion of the mineral. Increasing dietary magnesium intake leads to reductions in magnesium absorption and increases in urinary output. Conversely, reductions in magnesium intake are compensated by more efficient gastrointestinal absorption and renal reabsorption (Shils, 1999).

MAGNESIUM AND THE BRAIN

Magnesium, which is transported to the brain by an active mechanism, plays an important role in brain functioning. Under normal conditions, magnesium inhibits the actions of the excitatory neurotransmitter glutamate. More specifically, magnesium blocks the calcium channel of the N-methyl-D-aspartate (NMDA) glutamate receptor, and thereby regulates calcium entry into the postsynaptic neuron. Magnesium also relaxes vascular smooth muscle, resulting in vasodilation and increased cerebral blood flow.

Moreover, magnesium plays an important role in the homeostatic regulation of the pathways involved in the secondary phase of brain injury (Sen and Gulati, 2010). Following traumatic brain injury (TBI), reduction in magnesium levels in the brain is associated with an influx of glutamate and calcium into the postsynaptic neuron. The entry of these compounds into the brain is considered to be the predominant contributor to neuronal degeneration and cell death, secondary to the original insult (Bullock et al., 1998; Faden et al., 1989; Fleet and Cashman, 2001; McKee et al., 2005a; Sen and Gulati, 2010). Magnesium has also been linked to antidepressant effects in experimental studies because it affects the functioning of monoaminergic and serotonergic neurotransmitter systems, which are disrupted as part of the secondary injury cascade following TBI, and alters the activity of the hypothalamic-pituitary-adrenocortical system (Fromm et al., 2004).

A relevant selection of human and animal studies (years 1990 and later) examining the effectiveness of magnesium intake in providing resilience or treating TBI in the acute phase of injury is presented in Table 12-1. This table elaborates on the treatment methodology and includes review articles on magnesium intake in humans for other central nervous system (CNS) injuries such as subarachnoid hemorrhage, stroke, and hypoxia in the case of human studies. The occurrence or absence of adverse effects in humans is included if reported by the authors.

USES AND SAFETY

The Recommended Dietary Allowance (RDA) for magnesium ranges from 80 mg/day in children between the ages of one and three, to 420 mg/day in males over the age of 30 and 320 mg/day in females over the age of 30. Recommendations for military personnel in garrison training are the same as those for adults over 30 years of age (IOM, 2006). Good dietary sources of magnesium include green leafy vegetables, beans, nuts, seeds, and unrefined whole grains.

According to 2005–2006 data from the National Health and Nutrition Examination Survey (NHANES), just more than half (56 percent) of all individuals aged one year and older had inadequate intakes of magnesium.[1] The percentage below the Estimated Average Requirement (EAR) was greatest among 14- to 18-year-olds and adults aged 71 years and over. Two small research studies assessing dietary intake of Army Rangers and Special Forces soldiers in garrison found that approximately 40 percent of these individuals were not meeting the EAR for magnesium, and about 60 percent were not meeting the RDA (IOM, 2006). Although a 2006 analysis found that First Strike Rations and Meals, Ready-to-Eat (MREs) contained sufficient magnesium (IOM, 2006), the Institute of Medicine Committee on Mineral Requirements for Cognitive and Physical Performance of Military Personnel concluded that the information on magnesium status of military personnel in various types of training was too limited to provide evidence of magnesium sufficiency (IOM, 2006).

Magnesium toxicity is not a problem in the context of normal dietary intake. However, intake of magnesium supplements can lead to decreased blood pressure, abdominal cramping, and nausea. These adverse effects have been observed primarily with pharmacological uses of magnesium, rather than intake from food and water. Derived from studies on excessive intake from nonfood sources, the Tolerable Upper Intake Level (UL) of 350 mg/day for individuals nine years of age and over is based on diarrhea as the critical endpoint (IOM, 1997). The risk of magnesium-induced diarrhea mediates against the use of high-dose magnesium supplements. Symptoms of magnesium toxicity are more likely to occur in individuals suffering from renal failure, when the kidney loses its ability to remove excess magnesium (Fleet and Cashman, 2001; IOM, 1997).[2]

EVIDENCE INDICATING EFFECT ON RESILIENCE

Human Studies

The committee's review of the literature found no clinical trials investigating the effects of magnesium on resilience for TBI or related diseases or conditions (i.e., subarachnoid hemorrhage, intracranial aneurysm, stroke, anoxic or hypoxic ischemia, or epilepsy). An

---

[1] Available online at http://www.cdc.gov/nchs/nhanes.htm (accessed December 22, 2010).
[2] Available online at http://ods.od.nih.gov/factsheets/magnesium/ (accessed December 22, 2010).

TABLE 12-1 Relevant Data Identified for Magnesium

Reference	Type of Injury/ Insult	Type of Study and Subjects	Treatment	Findings/Results
Tier 1: Clinical trials				
Kidwell et al., 2009	Acute ischemic stroke	Multicenter, randomized, double-blind, placebo-controlled clinical trial (substudy of IMAGES trial) n^a=104 patients with diffusion-weighted imaging (DWI) lesion volume of ≥ 3 mL	Magnesium sulfate ($MgSO_4$) solution (bolus dose of 16 mmol infused over 15 minutes, then 65 mmol/day) or matching amount of saline)	For all patients, baseline lesion volume measured by DWI (r^b=0.654, p < 0.001) and perfusion-weighted imaging (r=0.805, p < 0.001) correlated with final infarct size. At day 90, there was no significant difference between the $MgSO_4$ group and placebo group in lesion growth, clinical outcome, or mortality rate. However, patients with poor clinical outcome tended to have greater percentage infarct growth (p=0.015) and absolute infarct growth (p=0.004). Although baseline serum glucose level correlated with infarct growth (p ≤ 0.028) in the $MgSO_4$ group, higher glucose level was not detected in patients with growth of > 0% compared to those with growth of ≤ 0%. Serum glucose level was not significantly correlated with infarct growth in placebo patients. No adverse effects were mentioned.
Wong et al., 2009	Aneurysmal subarachnoid hemorrhage (SAH)	Multi-center, randomized, placebo-controlled trial n=22 patients who were simultaneously participating in an intravenous $MgSO_4$ after aneurysmal SAH trial	$MgSO_4$ infusion (80mmol/day) or normal saline for 10–14 days	Throughout the study, the treatment group had a higher plasma magnesium level than the control group (p < 0.001). The average plasma magnesium level in the treatment group was between 1.59–1.84 mmol/L, while the average in the control group ranged from 0.85–1.02 mmol/L. Although the treatment group had higher levels of cerebrospinal fluid magnesium overall, the difference was significant only on day 2 and days 5–8 (p ≤ 0.035). The average levels of cerebrospinal fluid magnesium ranged from 1.22–1.278 mmol/L in the treatment group, and from 1.09–1.10 mmol/L in the control group; the increase ranged from 10.5–21.3%. The treatment group also had significantly higher 24-hour urine levels of magnesium (p ≤ 0.005); the group's average ranged from 47.9–77.3 mmol, while the control group's average ranged from 2.7–3.5 mmol. No adverse effects were mentioned.

continued

TABLE 12-1   Continued

Reference	Type of Injury/ Insult	Type of Study and Subjects	Treatment	Findings/Results
Dhandapani et al., 2008	Closed TBI	Randomized trial n=60	Postinjury, standard care or supplementation with $MgSO_4$ (initiation of 4 g intravenously [i.v.] and 5 g intramuscularly [i.m.], then continuation of 5 g every 4 hours for 24 hours)	At 3 months, 73.3% of the patients on $MgSO_4$ supplementation had good to moderate outcome compared to just 40% of the standard care group (OR^c=4.13, 95% CI^d: 1.39–12.27, p=0.009). Specifically, 46.7% of patients in $MgSO_4$ group had good recovery compared to 20% of the patients in standard care group (OR=3.5, 95% CI: 1.11–11.02, p=0.028). Significantly greater number of patients in the control group (73.3%) experienced intra-operative brain swelling during surgical decompression than patients in the $MgSO_4$ group (29.4%, OR=0.15, 95% CI: 0.03–0.71, p=0.01). At 1 month, mortality rate was higher in control group (43.3%) than $MgSO_4$ group (13.3%, OR=0.2, 95% CI: 0.06–0.72, p=0.01). Logistic regression analysis showed that favorable outcome was associated with patients' early entry into trial (< 8 hours, OR=8.2, p=0.008), CT finding of uneffaced cisterns (OR=4.67, p=0.04), and assignment to $MgSO_4$ treatment (OR=0.038). No significant adverse effects were observed.

TABLE 12-1 Continued

Reference	Type of Injury/ Insult	Type of Study and Subjects	Treatment	Findings/Results
van den Bergh et al., 2008	SAH	Randomized, placebo-controlled trial n=167	I.v. MgSO$_4$ (64 mmol/day) vs. placebo (saline) for up to 20 days	Regression analysis showed that serum magnesium level is inversely associated with ionized serum calcium level (B^e=–0.09; 95% CI: –0.12 to –0.06). This relationship remained the same even after adjusting for parathyroid hormone (PTH) and calcitriol levels (B=–0.11; 95% CI: –0.12 to 0.06). Further, the analysis showed no relationship between serum magnesium and PTH (B=–0.37; 95% CI: –3.44 to 2.70) or calcitriol (B=50.4; 95% CI: –11.7 to 112.4).
				Increased level of serum PTH heightened the risk of poor outcome, defined by having a modified Rankin Scale score of 4 or worse (OR=5.4; 95% CI: 1.6–8.9), but not the risk of developing delayed cerebral ischemia. PTH's effect on risk of poor outcome increased after adjusting for age and gender (OR=16.3; 95% CI: 2.2–119.2).
				No other adverse effects were mentioned.

continued

TABLE 12-1   Continued

Reference	Type of Injury/ Insult	Type of Study and Subjects	Treatment	Findings/Results
Dorhout Mees et al., 2007	SAH	Randomized, placebo-controlled trial n=155	MgSO₄ therapy (64 mmol/day) vs. placebo for up to 20 days	Over the course of the study, 17% of the patients developed delayed cerebral ischemia (DCI) (median day of onset was day 8), and 26% had poor outcome, defined by modified Rankin score of ≥ 4. During treatment, the average serum magnesium level of patients with poor outcome was 0.22 mmol/L higher than patients with no poor outcome (95% CI: 0.09–0.36 mmol/L). The serum magnesium level measured at day 8 (the median day of onset of DCI) was 0.42 mmol/L higher in patients with poor outcome than in those with no poor outcome (95% CI: 0.14–0.69 mmol/L). Patient with serum magnesium levels of > 1.28 mmol/L at day 8 (categorized as quartiles 2nd–4th) had lower risk (adjusted OR=0.2; 95% CI: lower limit 0.0–0.1, upper limit 0.8–0.9) of developing DCI than patients whose serum magnesium was between 1.10–1.28 mmol/L at day 8 (1st quartile). Compared to the 1st quartile, patients in 2nd (1.28–1.40 mmol/L) and 4th (> 1.62 mmol/L) quartiles tended to have higher risk developing poor outcome (adjusted OR=1.8, 95% CI: 0.5–7.0; adjusted OR=4.9, 95% CI: 1.2–19.7, respectively). The risk was not higher for patients in the 3rd quartile (1.40–1.62 mmol/L). No other adverse effects were mentioned.
Natale et al., 2007	Severe TBI	Randomized, double-blind, placebo-controlled, multi-center trial n=6 pediatric (3 months to 18 yrs) patients with severe TBI	Postinjury, saline vs. MgSO₄ (50 mg/kg bolus followed by 8.3 mg/kg/hr infusion for 24 hours)	Mean arterial pressure, at 14–24 hour period of the infusion, showed significant change from baseline with an 11 mmHg increase. The other 4 variables used to determine hemodynamic effects of MgSO₄—heart rate, corrected quartile interval, intracranial pressure, and cerebral perfusion pressure—showed no significant changes during the administration of MgSO₄ bolus or 24-hour infusion when compared to baseline. MgSO₄ had no adverse effect on cerebral blood flow velocity, and no other adverse effects were mentioned.

TABLE 12-1 Continued

Reference	Type of Injury/ Insult	Type of Study and Subjects	Treatment	Findings/Results
Temkin et al., 2007	Moderate and severe TBI	Single center, randomized, double-blind, parallel group trial n=499 patients with moderate or severe TBI, with Glasgow Coma Score (GCS) between 3–12	Postinjury, i.v. $MgSO_4$ (low target group: loading dose of 0.30 mmol/ kg over 15 minutes within 8 hours of injury, followed by a continuous infusion of 0.05 mmol/ kg/hour; high target group: loading dose of 0.425 mmol/kg, followed by an infusion of 0.10 mmol/kg/hour for 5 days) or placebo	$MgSO_4$ treatment at the higher target level had no effect on the composite outcome measure (variables include survival, seizure occurrence, and neurobehavioral functioning). But, at the lower target level, patients treated with $MgSO_4$ had worse outcomes than those treated with placebo (p=0.007). Analysis of the characteristics of patients in the low target group showed that $MgSO_4$ was associated with worse outcomes if patients were ≤ 40 years old (p=0.02), male (p=0.007), an ethnic minority (p=0.01), had severe injury (p=0.001), had no emergent intracranial surgery (p=0.02), and/or began their loading dose > 4 hours from injury (p=0.03). Analysis of individual outcomes showed that mortality rate was higher with $MgSO_4$ treatment than with placebo (p=0.05) at the high target level and functional status at 6 months was worse with $MgSO_4$ than placebo at the low target group (p=0.05). No other adverse effects were mentioned.
Van de Water et al., 2007	SAH	Randomized, placebo-controlled trial n=137	Postinjury, i.v. magnesium (64 mmol/day; n=70) or normal saline (50 mL/ day; n=67)	There was an inverse relationship between serum magnesium and serum calcium (B=–0.27; 95% CI: –0.33 to 0.20; p < 0.001). Patients with low calcium levels (< 2.0 mmol/L) were more likely to develop delayed cerebral ischemia than patients with normal calcium level (HR^f=2.1; 95% CI: 1.0–4.3). Hypocalcaemic patients also had significantly higher risk of poor outcome after 3 months (OR=2.9; 95% CI: 1.4–6.4); however the risk was not significantly higher when multivariable analysis was used to adjust for age, World Federation of Neurological Surgeons (WFNS) score, and ventricular blood (OR=1.9; 95% CI: 0.8–4.7). No other adverse effects were mentioned.

continued

TABLE 12-1 Continued

Reference	Type of Injury/ Insult	Type of Study and Subjects	Treatment	Findings/Results
Arango and Bainbridge, 2006	Acute TBI	Meta-analysis of 3 randomized controlled trials	Magnesium vs. no magnesium or placebo	Analysis of mortality showed that magnesium treatment increased mortality (RR[g]=1.48, 95% CI: 1.00–2.19, overall effect: z^h=1.96, p=0.05). However, there was evidence of heterogeneity among the studies.
				Analysis of functional outcome showed that magnesium had no significant effect on Glasgow Outcome Scale (GOS) at 6 months. There was also evidence of heterogeneity.
				No differences in medical complications were observed.
Schmid-Elsaesser et al., 2006	Aneurysmal SAH	Pilot study, randomized trial n=104	I.v. $MgSO_4$ (loading 10 mg/kg followed by continuous infusion of 30 mg/kg daily) or nimodipine (48 mg/day)	Although there was no significant difference of mean maximum neuronal markers level between $MgSO_4$ and nimodipine groups, there was a significant difference when comparing patients with different severity of neurological outcome.
				Patients with worse neurological outcome (WFNS grades 4–5) in both $MgSO_4$ and nimodipine groups had significantly higher levels of S-100 in serum (p < 0.05). Patients with WFNS grades 4–5 in $MgSO_4$ group also had a higher level of S-100 in cerebrospinal fluid, as well as higher levels of neuron-specific enolase in both serum and cerebrospinal fluid (p < 0.05). There was no significant difference in blood flow velocity and incidence of vasospasm between $MgSO_4$ and nimodipine groups.
				Among patients who experienced vasospasm, incidence of cerebral infarction was approximately equal regardless of treatment. There was no difference in outcomes after 1 year between the two treatment groups; 55% of patients in each group had GOS scores of 4–5.
				No adverse effects were mentioned.

TABLE 12-1 Continued

Reference	Type of Injury/ Insult	Type of Study and Subjects	Treatment	Findings/Results
Gorelick and Ruland, 2004; IMAGES Study Investigators, 2004	Acute ischemic stroke	Multicenter, randomized, placebo-controlled, double-blind trial n=2,386 stroke patients ≥ 18 years old	MgSO$_4$ solution (bolus dose of 16 mmol infused over 15 minutes, then 65 mmol/day) or matching amount of saline	At day 90, magnesium had no effect on death or disability (common OR=0.95, 95% CI: 0.80–1.12; p=0.53). The magnesium group was not significantly different from the placebo group in terms of risk of death (OR=1.22, 95% CI: 0.98–1.53; p=0.073); when time to death was examined with Kaplan-Meier analysis, HR for death was 1.18 (95% CI: 0.97–1.42; p=0.098).
				The length of time between injury and treatment and the type of stroke (ischemic vs. intracerebral hemorrhage) had no effect on outcome. However, patients without cortical ischemic stroke had significantly fewer poor outcomes if treated with magnesium (OR=0.75, 95% CI: 0.58–0.97; p=0.026); analysis showed a significant interaction between magnesium treatment and the group of patients with non-cortical syndromes (p=0.011).
				Post hoc analysis showed that there were also fewer poor outcomes in magnesium-treated patients with lacunar syndromes (OR=0.70, 95% CI: 0.53–0.92) and with mean arterial pressure > 108.3 mmHg (OR=0.78, 95% CI: 0.61–0.99); there was significant interaction with both subgroups of patients (p=0.0046, p=0.019, respectively).
				Compared to placebo group, blood pressure was lower in magnesium group (p ≤ 0.0001) up to 24 hours after starting treatment, but it was not different at 48 hours. Heart rate of magnesium-treated patients was lower after 12 hours of treatment, but not at other times.
				No other adverse effects were mentioned.

continued

TABLE 12-1 Continued

Reference	Type of Injury/ Insult	Type of Study and Subjects	Treatment	Findings/Results
Saver et al., 2004	Acute stroke	Non-randomized, open-label, phase II feasibility trial n=20, aged 44–92	A loading dose of 2.5 g $MgSO_4$ during transport to hospital, then another 1.5 g $MgSO_4$ in the ER, was followed by maintenance infusion of 16 g/day $MgSO_4$. Time to treatment of study subjects was compared to control group, which consisted of patients participating in other neuroprotective trials at UCLA	The average time between paramedics' arrival on scene and initiation of treatment was significantly shorter in FAST-MAG patients (26 minutes, 95% CI: 21.8–30.2; range 15–61) than in control patients (139 minutes, 95% CI: 111–167; range 66–300; $p < 0.0001$). Duration of transport to hospital was not significantly different between the two groups. Paramedics completed Paramedic Global Impression Change Form and rated the condition of 4 patients as improved, 15 as unchanged, and 1 as worsened. At day 90, 60% of patients had a modified Rankin score of ≤ 2, and 40% had ≤ 1. No significant adverse events were associated with treatment.
Chia et al., 2002	Aneurismal SAH	Non-randomized, pilot study n=23	Nimodipine (20 µg/kg/hr) alone vs. nimodipine supplemented by 1.0–1.5 mmol/L/ hr of $MgSO_4$	No adverse event was associated with magnesium treatment. 70% of patients treated with nimodipine alone developed cerebral vasospasm compared to 15% of magnesium-supplemented patients ($p < 0.008$).

TABLE 12-1 Continued

Reference	Type of Injury/ Insult	Type of Study and Subjects	Treatment	Findings/Results
Lampl et al., 2001	Acute stroke	Randomized, placebo-controlled, double-blind trial n=44	Magnesium (i.v. loading dose of 4 g over 15 minutes and a continuous infusion of 35 g/ day for 5 days) or placebo	Compared to patients treated with placebo, those treated with magnesium had significantly higher Orgogozo score beginning on day 3 (p=0.0173) that continued into day 30 (p=0.0002). Magnesium-treated patients also had higher Matthew score beginning on day 8 (p=0.044) that continued into day 30 (p=0.0087).
				Although both groups of patients recovered in the first month (p for time < 0.001), as demonstrated by improvement in Orgogozo score, magnesium-treated patients recovered at a faster rate than placebo-treated patients (p=0.007). However, magnesium had no significant effect on recovery as measured by Matthew score, Rankin disability score, and Barthel Index.
				The magnesium group also had greater percentage of patients with improvement of > 20 points on the Orgogozo scale (p=0.0003) and the Matthew scale (p=0.003).
				No adverse effects were mentioned.

Tier 2: Observational studies

Reference	Type of Injury/ Insult	Type of Study and Subjects	Treatment	Findings/Results
Bayir et al., 2009	Acute ischemic or hemorrhagic stroke	Case-control study, n=60 (n=20 healthy controls, n=20 ischemic stroke patients, n=20 hemorrhagic stroke patients); stroke patients arrived at ER within 3 hours of symptom onset)		Serum Mg^{2+} levels of both groups of stroke patients were not significantly different from controls. No significant relationship was observed between serum Mg^{2+} level and either GCS or cerebral spinal fluid (CSF) Mg^{2+} level. However, mean CSF Mg^{2+} levels were significantly lower in ischemic stroke patients (0.6±0.4) when compared to controls (0.9±0.1) and hemorrhagic stroke patients (0.8±0.2; p=0.006).
				There was a correlation between CSF Mg^{2+} level and GCS for ischemic stroke patients (r=55; p=0.031), with CSF Mg^{2+} level decreasing as GCS decreased. Ischemic patients with GCS ≤ 8 had the lowest CSF Mg^{2+} level compared to all other cases and was significantly lower than controls (p < 0.05).
				Ischemic stroke patients who died 7 days after stroke onset had significantly lower Mg^{2+} levels than controls (p=0.002), while the CSF Mg^{2+} level of hemorrhagic stroke patients was not significantly different from controls.

continued

TABLE 12-1 Continued

Reference	Type of Injury/ Insult	Type of Study and Subjects	Treatment	Findings/Results
Kerz et al., 2008	DCI after SAH	Retrospective, single-center observational case control study n=100 SAH patients	Simvastatin (20 mg for 3 days, then 40 mg/day for 11 days) and 80 mmol/day of magnesium, solely simvastatin, or control	There was no significant difference between the groups in terms of proportions of patients who developed DCI and proportions of patients who died during the 14-day hospital stay. Initial neurological condition, as measured by GCS score, is strongly associated with mortality during the 14-day hospital stay (p < 0.001); patients with lower GCS were more likely to die. No other adverse effects were mentioned.
Larsson et al., 2008	Stroke	Cohort study n=26,556 Finnish male smokers, aged 50 to 69 years, who were free from stroke at baseline		Increase of magnesium intake was associated with decrease in risk of cerebral infarction (p=0.003) but not other stroke types. Compared to subjects with the lowest intake, those with highest intake were less likely to have cerebral infarction (RR=0.85, 95% CI: 0.75–0.96). This relationship remained even after adjusting for cardiovascular risk factors (RR=0.85, 95% CI: 0.76–0.97). Multivariate analysis of both potassium and magnesium comparing highest to lowest intake produced a RR=0.86 for magnesium and RR=1.02 for potassium. Subjects taking the highest amount of both minerals were less likely to develop cerebral infarction than those taking the least amount of both minerals (RR=0.87, 95% CI: 0.76–1.00). Further multivariable analysis of highest and lowest magnesium intake showed that higher intake in men younger than 60 was associated with lower risk of cerebral infarction (RR=0.67, 95% CI: 0.64–0.89) compared to men older than 60. The different RRs demonstrated modification by age (p=0.02). No adverse effects were mentioned.

TABLE 12-1 Continued

Reference	Type of Injury/ Insult	Type of Study and Subjects	Treatment	Findings/Results
Stippler et al., 2007	Severe TBI	Retrospective cohort study (1996–2006) n=216 TBI patients with GCS ≤ 8	None, but MgSO$_4$ was given to hypomagnesemia (≤ 1.2 mEq/L) patients as part of routine care	Patients with low initial serum Mg^{2+} levels (< 1.3mEq/L) had a greater risk of having low GCS score (OR=2.37, 95% CI: 1.18–4.78; p=0.016), although there was no association between serum Mg^{2+} level and GCS score. 26% of patients with low initial serum Mg^{2+} level were treated with MgSO$_4$ within 24 hours of admission; however, these patients had significantly higher risk of developing worse outcomes at 6 months (OR=11.03, 95% CI: 1.87–68.14; p=0.008) than low Mg^{2+} level patients not treated within 24 hours. Data on CSF Mg^{2+} levels were available for 44 patients. Analysis of these data showed that patients with low serum Mg^{2+} and those with GCS 1–3 had higher level of CSF Mg^{2+} (r=0.572; p=0.013). Patients with high CSF Mg^{2+} were more likely to develop poor outcomes (OR=7.63, p=0.05). High CSF Mg^{2+} was associated with high CSF glucose (p=0.027) and low brain tissue oxygen pressure (p=0.029). No adverse effects were mentioned.
McKee et al., 2005b	Acute brain injury resulting in intracranial hypertension requiring ventriculostomy and CSF drainage	Prospective study n=30 patients ≥ 18years old	Postinjury, i.v. MgSO$_4$ (bolus of 20 mmol over 30 minutes, then infusion of 8 mmol/hr for 24 hours)	Compared to baseline, there was a significant increase of mean total and ionized Mg^{2+} in serum and in CSF throughout the study period (p < 0.008). Total CSF Mg^{2+} increased a maximum value of 1.43±0.13 mmol/L after 12 hours and 1.40±0.16 mmol/L after 24 hours; both represented 15% increases from baseline. Ionized CSF Mg^{2+} increased to 0.89±0.12 mmol/L after 12 hours, and 0.88±0.11 mmol/L after 24 hours; both represented 11% increases from baseline. There was no relationship between serum Mg^{2+} and CSF Mg^{2+}. But CSF Mg^{2+} values at 24 hours were inversely associated with GOS (r=-0.44, p=0.03). No adverse effects were mentioned.

continued

TABLE 12-1 Continued

Reference	Type of Injury/ Insult	Type of Study and Subjects	Treatment	Findings/Results
Song et al., 2005	Cardiovascular diseases (CVD)	Randomized, placebo-controlled, double-blind trial n=35,601 women with no coronary heart disease (CHD) at randomization Median follow-up: 10 years	Magnesium intake	Magnesium intake, in both dietary and supplement forms, was not associated with risk of CVD, CHD, non-fatal myocardial infarction (MI), CVD death, total stroke, or any stroke subtypes. Still no significant association was found when the analysis was restricted to just dietary intake. No adverse effects were mentioned.
Begum et al., 2001	Eclampsia (convulsions)	Prospective study, n=65 patients with antepartum or postpartum eclampsia	$MgSO_4$: loading dose of 4 g i.v. and 2.5 g i.m. over 15 minutes, then 2.5 g i.m. every 4 hours for 24 hours after administration of first dose	All patients had normal respiratory rate (16–25 breaths/min). The average serum Mg^{2+} level in patients was 3.34 ± 0.27mg/dL (range 1.08–6 mg/dL). However, 5 patients had decreased knee jerks; the average Mg^{2+} level of those 5 patients was 3.32 ± 0.78 mg/dL (range 3.0–3.8 mg/dL). 76% of patients regained consciousness 12 hours after first dose, and 100% after 20 hours. No adverse effects were mentioned and serum levels of Mg^{2+} remain lower than those producing toxicity.
Iso et al., 1999	Stroke	Prospective cohort study (part of Nurses' Health Study) n=86,368 women with no history of stroke, cancer, CVD, myocardial infarction, or angina; follow-up=14 years	Dietary and supplementary magnesium intake	No significant association was observed between dietary or supplementary magnesium intake and risk of total or ischemic stroke in women. No other adverse effects were mentioned.

TABLE 12-1 Continued

Reference	Type of Injury/ Insult	Type of Study and Subjects	Treatment	Findings/Results
Ascherio et al., 1998	Stroke	Prospective cohort study (the Health Professional Follow-up Study) n=43,738 men with no history of MI, stroke, angina, coronary artery surgery, peripheral arterial disease, or diabetes	Dietary magnesium intake	Dietary magnesium intake was inversely associated with risk of total stroke (χ for trend=−2.21), and men with the highest intake (452 mg/day) had 30% reduced risk compared to men with the lowest intake (243 mg/day, RR=0.70, 95% CI: 0.49–1.01, p=0.027). Further analysis showed that the association was significant in hypertensive men (RR=0.53, p for trend=0.006) but not in non-hypertensive men. Magnesium intake was correlated with intake of potassium (r=0.65) and fiber (r=0.62). Reduced risk of total or ischemic stroke was not associated with intake of magnesium supplements. No adverse effects were mentioned.

Tier 3: Animal studies

Reference	Type of Injury/ Insult	Type of Study and Subjects	Treatment	Findings/Results
Ghabriel et al., 2006	Diffused TBI, impact-acceleration model of diffuse TBI	Male Sprague-Dawley rats	Postinjury, i.v. $MgSO_4$ (30 mg/kg) administered 30 minutes after injury	All injured rats had increased immunolabeling for AQP4 in neuropil and inner and outer glia limitans and decreased micro-vessel labeling. However, compared to untreated rats, $MgSO_4$-treated rats had decreased AQP4 activity and increased labeling of micro-vessels. Labeling in treated rats was restored to the level of sham-injured controls and uninjured rats. Electron microscopy showed immunolabeling for AQP1 around brain vessels circumference in sham-injured rats and $MgSO_4$-treated rats but not untreated rats.

continued

TABLE 12-1 Continued

Reference	Type of Injury/ Insult	Type of Study and Subjects	Treatment	Findings/Results
Enomoto et al., 2005	Lateral fluid-percussion injury (LFPI)	Male Wistar rats n=68	Preinjury, i.v. $MgCl_2$ (150 µmol) or saline administered from 20 to 5 minutes before injury	Brain tissue samples were taken from some rats from both injury groups at 10, 30, 60, and 120 minutes after injury.
				Compared to sham-injured rats, LFPI-injured rats had higher levels of phospho-ERK in their ipsilateral hippocampus at all times ($p < 0.05$ at 120 minutes; $p < 0.01$ at all other times). Significantly higher levels of phospho-ERK was observed in LFPI rats after 10 minutes ($p < 0.01$) but not other times.
				Compared to LFPI rats treated with saline, Mg^{2+} treatment had no effect on ERK level in FP rats at 10 minutes. But significantly lower levels of ERK were seen in the ipsilateral hippocampus of Mg^{2+}-treated LFPI rats at 60 minutes ($p < 0.05$); this change was not seen in their contralateral hippocampus.
				Compared to sham-injured rats, LFPI rats had a larger amount of neuronal loss in the ipsilateral CA3 region of the hippocampus ($p < 0.01$) but not in the contralateral CA3 region. However, compared to saline-treated rats, Mg^{2+}-treated rats had smaller amount of neuronal loss ($p < 0.05$).
				The rats' memories were tested using a radial arm maze 2 weeks after injury. LFPI rats had significantly impaired working and reference memory compared to sham-injured rats ($p < 0.0001$), but Mg^{2+} significantly reduced impairment of both working ($p < 0.0001$) and reference ($p < 0.05$) memory.
Browne et al., 2004	TBI (fluid percussion model)	Adult, male Sprague-Dawley rats	Postinjury, $MgSO_4$ (15 minutes after), NPS 1506 (15 minutes and 4 hours after), or saline (15 minutes after); sham-injured rats were treated with saline 90 minutes after	Cognitive functions tested using Morris water maze showed that all injured rats spent more time than sham-injured rats completing the task ($p < 0.001$). However, performance was not significantly different between the treatment groups among injured rats.
				Evaluation of tissue loss in the hippocampus showed that rats treated with $MgSO_4$ had significantly reduced loss (14%) compared to rats treated with NPS 1506 (38%) or saline (34%, $p < 0.001$). Loss in the ipsilateral cortex was not significantly different between the treatment groups.

TABLE 12-1 Continued

Reference	Type of Injury/ Insult	Type of Study and Subjects	Treatment	Findings/Results
Fromm et al., 2004	Diffuse TBI, impact-acceleration model	Adult, male Sprague-Dawley rats n=32	Postinjury, i.v. MgSO$_4$ (250 μmol/kg) 30 minutes after injury or no treatment	At day 7, MgSO$_4$-treated rats had higher scores on the Open Field Test than untreated controls (p < 0.05). Compared to their preinjury scores, control rats were 69% lower (p < 0.001), whereas the MgSO$_4$-treated rats were only 28% lower.
				At day 28, scores for MgSO$_4$-treated rats were better than controls (p < 0.05) and not significantly different from preinjury values. At day 42, MgSO$_4$-treated rats were performing better than control rats (p < 0.01) and were at 76% of preinjury level.
				Depression over the 42-day study period was noted in 68% of control rats and 34% of MgSO$_4$-treated rats. At day 42, incidence of depression was significantly greater in control rats (90%) than MgSO$_4$-treated rats (30%, p < 0.05).
Park and Hyun, 2004	Weight-drop induced moderate diffuse axonal injury	Adult, male Sprague-Dawley rats	Postinjury, MgSO$_4$ (750 μmol/kg) or saline at 30 minutes after injury	Although serum Mg^{2+} level was reduced immediately after injury (p < 0.05), it returned to preinjury levels after 12 hours. Postinjury total Mg^{2+} levels were not significantly different from preinjury levels.
				Compared to preinjury values, postinjury serum calcium to serum Mg^{2+} ratio (calcium level relative to serum Mg^{2+} level) was significantly higher between hours 1–3 (p < 0.05); it was not different from preinjury level after 6 hours.
				MgSO$_4$ treatment had no effect on arterial blood pressure. Apoptotic Index was higher in untreated rats at 12 and 24 hours postinjury compared to treated rats (p < 0.05), but there was no difference after 48 hours.
Turner et al., 2004	TBI, impact-acceleration model of diffuse TBI	Adult, male Sprague-Dawley rats	Postinjury, 250 μmol/kg of MgSO$_4$, magnesium gluconate, or saline administered 30 minutes after injury	Rats treated with MgSO$_4$ and magnesium gluconate had improved motor performance (p < 0.01) and faster cognitive recovery (p < 0.05) compared to saline-treated rats.
				MgSO$_4$ and magnesium gluconate treatment also resulted in lesser degree of cell stress in the cortex and hippocampus than saline treatment (p < 0.05). There was no significant difference between the two magnesium treatments in any of the three variables.

continued

TABLE 12-1 Continued

Reference	Type of Injury/ Insult	Type of Study and Subjects	Treatment	Findings/Results
Esen et al., 2003	TBI, closed injury model	Adult, male Sprague-Dawley rats n=68	Postinjury, intraperitoneal bolus of $MgSO_4$ (750 μm/kg) or saline 30 minutes after injury	Compared to injured, saline-treated controls, injured, $MgSO_4$-treated rats had significantly reduced brain water content ($p < 0.05$) and increased brain tissue specific gravity ($p < 0.05$) in both hemispheres. Blood-brain barrier integrity was significantly reduced in injured rats, compared to sham-injured rats ($p < 0.05$). But $MgSO_4$ treatment increased integrity to a level that was greater than injured controls ($p < 0.05$) and that was not significantly different from uninjured controls.
Hoane et al., 2003	TBI, bilateral anterior medial cortex lesions (bAMC)	Male Sprague-Dawley rats	Postinjury, $MgCl_2$ (at 1 mmol/kg or 2 mmol/kg) or saline administered 15 minutes, 24 hours, and 72 hours after injury	Treatment with 1 mmol or 2 mmol of $MgCl_2$ had no effect on memory acquisition. Working memory was improved with 2 mmol of $MgCl_2$ on days 1 ($p < 0.03$) and 2 ($p < 0.01$), while 1 mmol of $MgCl_2$ resulted in improvement on day 2 ($p < 0.03$). Delayed match-to-sample test showed that rats treated with 2 mmol $MgCl_2$ completed the test faster than injured, saline-treated rats ($p < 0.009$); treatment with 1 mmol $MgCl_2$ made no significant difference. In bilateral tactile removal test, performance was improved by 2 mmol of $MgCl_2$ on days 1–3 ($p < 0.04$) and by 1 mmol of $MgCl_2$ on day 1 ($p < 0.01$). Lesion size was not significantly affected by $MgCl_2$.
Vink et al., 2003	Diffuse TBI	Male Sprague-Dawley rats	Postinjury, i.v. $MgSO_4$ (250 μmol/kg) or saline	At 28 days after injury, $MgSO_4$-treated rats had better sensorimotor abilities, as measured by Rotarod scores, than saline-treated rats ($p < 0.05$). Although injury significantly lowered performance on the Open Field Test ($p < 0.001$), magnesium treatment restored the rats' performance to the level of sham-injured rats. On the Barnes Maze testing spatial learning abilities, saline-treated rats showed significantly slower improvement in performance than sham-injured rats ($p < 0.05$), improving at a rate of 11% of sham-injured rats. However, magnesium-treated rats were performing at 62% of sham-injured rats.

TABLE 12-1 Continued

Reference	Type of Injury/ Insult	Type of Study and Subjects	Treatment	Findings/Results
Hoane and Barth, 2002	TBI, focal injury model	Male, Wistar rats	Postinjury, $MgCl_2$ (initial injection of 1.0 mmol/kg at 15 minutes, 8 hours, or 24 hours following injury, then subsequent injections at 24 hour and 72 hours after first injection) or saline (injected at 15 minutes after injury, then 24 hours and 48 hours after first injection)	All rats recovered from an initial decline following injury in performance in the vibrissae-forelimb placing, forelimb-forelimb placing, and foot-fault tests ($p < 0.0001$ for all three tests). But rats treated with $MgCl_2$ performed better ($p < 0.0001$ for all three tests) and recovered faster ($p < 0.02$ for all three tests) than saline-treated rats. $MgCl_2$-treated rats had better performance and recovery rate on the vibrissae-forelimb placing and forelimb-forelimb placing tests regardless of the time of the initial injection ($p < 0.002$), and there was no significant difference between rats receiving the initial injection at different times. In the foot-fault test, $MgCl_2$ injection at 15 minutes and 8 hours postinjury led to significantly better performance and faster recovery ($p < 0.05$), but $MgCl_2$ at 24 hours postinjury did not lead to better results. $MgCl_2$ had no effect on lesion volume. Compared to saline treatment, $MgCl_2$ at 15 minutes postinjury was associated with less thalamic cell loss ($p < 0.001$). $MgCl_2$ at other times were not significantly different from saline treatment or from each other.
Heath and Vink, 2001	TBI, closed head injury model of diffused brain injury	Male Sprague-Dawley rats	Postinjury, i.v. $MgSO_4$ (250 μmol/kg) or saline at 30 minutes after injury	58% of the rats had subdural hematoma 1 week after injury; 23% were treated with $MgSO_4$, and 35% were treated with saline. Rotarod scores were higher in $MgSO_4$-treated rats without hematoma compared to all saline-treated rats (both with and without hematoma, $p < 0.05$). All injured rats had decreased free magnesium concentration immediately after injury. But only $MgSO_4$-treated rats without hematoma recovered to preinjury level ($p < 0.05$); all other rats remained at depressed level.

continued

TABLE 12-1   Continued

Reference	Type of Injury/ Insult	Type of Study and Subjects	Treatment	Findings/Results
Saatman et al., 2001	TBI, lateral fluid percussion brain injury	Adult, male Sprague-Dawley rats, n=40	Preinjury: magnesium-deficient diet vs. normal diet Postinjury: rats fed a normal diet before injury were administered MgCl$_2$ (15 minute infusion of 125 μmol) or saline at 10 minutes after injury; rats fed a magnesium-deficient diet were administered saline	Among the injured rats, mortality rate was not affected by preinjury diet or postinjury treatment. Lesion size in the cortex was greater in rats fed magnesium-deficient diet than in rats fed with normal diet and treated with saline at both −3.3 mm ($p < 0.05$) and −5.3 mm ($p < 0.01$) Bregma. In injured rats, cortical lesion was smaller in MgCl$_2$-treated rats than in saline-treated rats at −3.3 mm and −5.3 mm Bregma ($p < 0.05$ for both). Lesion size at the ipsilateral CA3 region was the same in all injured rats. At −3.3 mm Bregma, MgCl$_2$-treated rats had smaller spectrin breakdown area in the cortex than rats fed with magnesium-deficient diet ($p < 0.05$). At −5.3 mm Bregma, MgCl$_2$-treated rats had smaller spectrin breakdown area in the cortex than the rats on magnesium-deficient diets ($p < 0.005$) and injured, saline-treated rats ($p < 0.05$). In the CA3 region, MgCl$_2$-treated rats had smaller spectrin breakdown area than saline-treated rats ($p < 0.05$). Rats fed with magnesium-deficient diet had greater loss of microtubule-associated protein-2 (MAP-2) in the dentate hilus than sham-injured rats ($p < 0.001$). Magnesium-deficient rats also had greater MAP-2 loss in the CA3 region than MgCl$_2$-treated rats ($p < 0.05$).

TABLE 12-1 Continued

Reference	Type of Injury/ Insult	Type of Study and Subjects	Treatment	Findings/Results
Bareyre et al., 1999	TBI, LFPI	Male Sprague-Dawley rats	Postinjury, $MgCl_2$ (125 µmol) or saline administered 1 hour after injury	Ionized, free Mg^{2+} level in serum in injured rats treated with saline was decreased compared to uninjured controls ($p < 0.01$) and was lower than injured rats treated with $MgCl_2$ throughout the 24-hour period ($p < 0.05$).
				Mean total Mg^{2+} level was unchanged in all saline-treated rats. It was increased in injured rats treated with $MgCl_2$ at 2 hours ($p < 0.001$), but it returned to normal level after 24 hours.
				At days 14 and 15, learning deficit was smaller in uninjured rats than injured rats ($p < 0.001$) and was not affected by $MgCl_2$ treatment. $MgCl_2$ treatment did not affect neurologic motor function in injured rats in the first 48 hours after injury, but it improved motor function after 1 week ($p < 0.01$) and 2 weeks ($p < 0.001$).
				Ionized, free Mg^{2+} level at 24 hours was correlated with neurologic motor function at week 1 ($r=0.51$, $p < 0.05$) and week 2 ($r=0.81$, $p < 0.001$).
Heath and Vink, 1999a	Closed head model of diffused axonal injury	Male, Sprague-Dawley rats	Postinjury, i.m. $MgSO_4$ (bolus of 750 µmol/kg 30 minutes, 8 hours, 12 hours, or 24 hours after injury, or initial dose at 30 minutes postinjury, then additional doses every 12 hours after injury) or no treatment	TBI led to significant reduction in Rotarod scores in untreated rats ($p < 0.001$), but $MgSO_4$ 30 minutes after injury significantly improved the scores ($p < 0.01$). Rats treated at 8, 12, and 24 hours postinjury also had significantly improved scores ($p < 0.05$) compared to saline-treated rats, but the rate of their improvement was slower than rats treated at 30 minutes.
				For up to 2 days after injury, blood free-Mg^{2+} level was significantly lower in untreated rats ($p < 0.05$), but administration of $MgSO_4$ at 30 minutes after injury increased and sustained blood free-Mg^{2+} to above preinjury level for up to 12 hours.
				Although rats that had repeated injection of $MgSO_4$ at 12-hour intervals for 1 week after injury had better neurological motor performance than untreated rats, their performance was not significantly different from rats treated with a single bolus of $MgSO_4$.

continued

TABLE 12-1   Continued

Reference	Type of Injury/ Insult	Type of Study and Subjects	Treatment	Findings/Results
Heath and Vink, 1999b	Severe, diffuse closed TBI	Male, Sprague-Dawley rats	Postinjury, i.v. or i.m. bolus of $MgSO_4$ or $MgCl_2$ (both at doses of 100, 250, 500, 750, 1,000, or 1,250 µmol/kg) 30 minutes after injury	Compared to untreated, injured controls, performance on Rotarod test was better in rats treated with i.m. $MgSO_4$ at 250–1,000 µmol/kg, i.v. $MgSO_4$ at 250–500 µmol/kg, i.m. $MgCl_2$ at 750 µmol/kg, and i.v. $MgCl_2$ at 100–250 µmol/kg ($p < 0.05$ for all).
				Metabolic outcome was analyzed using phosphorus magnetic resonance spectroscopy with i.m. $MgSO_4$ at 750 µmol/kg. Injury did not change the brain intracellular pH level or ATP concentration. Free magnesium in both control and treated rats declined significantly ($p < 0.01$) from preinjury level; however, the $MgSO_4$ group experienced an increase that was significantly higher than controls ($p < 0.05$) but not significantly different from preinjury level. Brain bioenergetic status declined after injury in both control and $MgSO_4$ groups ($p < 0.05$). Bioenergetic status of rats with $MgSO_4$ treatment was increased to preinjury level and was higher than controls ($p < 0.05$).
				Rotarod scores were highly correlated with free magnesium concentration ($r=0.92$, $p < 0.001$) and bioenergetic status ($r=0.94$, $p < 0.001$).

TABLE 12-1 Continued

Reference	Type of Injury/ Insult	Type of Study and Subjects	Treatment	Findings/Results
Hoane et al., 1998	TBI, electrolytic lesion model of cortical injury	Male Wistar rats, 11–12 weeks old n=24	Preinjury daily intraperitoneal injections of $MgCl_2$ (1 mmol/ kg) or saline (1 mL/kg) starting at 5 or 2 days before injury; last injection at 24 hours before injury	In both the vibrissae-forelimb placing test and forelimb-forelimb placing test, rats treated for 5 or 2 days showed significantly less impairment for up to 3 weeks after surgery ($p < 0.0001$ for vibrissae-forelimb placing and $p < 0.02$ for forelimb-forelimb placing) compared to saline-treated rats, but the difference was minimized after 3 weeks, showing that the number of days after injury has significant effect on impairment reduction (on both tests: $p < 0.0001$ for effect of number of days). Analysis of recovery rate showed that rats treated for 5 or 2 days recovered significantly faster than saline-treated rats (treatment/days interactions for vibrissae-forelimb test: $p < 0.0001$; for forelimb-forelimb: $p < 0.009$). In vibrissae-forelimb test, both 5-day and 2-day group recovered significantly faster than saline group ($p < 0.0001$ for both groups). But in forelimb-forelimb test, only 2-day group recovered faster than saline group ($p < 0.0004$). In both tests, difference in recovery rate of 5-day and 2-day groups was not significantly different. In the foot-fault test, 5-day and 2-day rats made fewer mistakes than saline-treated rats ($p < 0.0002$), but that difference disappeared after 7 days, suggesting that number of days has an effect on test performance test ($p < 0.0001$). $MgCl_2$-treated rats also recovered faster than saline-treated rats ($p < 0.0002$ for both 2-day and 5-day vs. saline comparisons). There was a difference in recovery rate between 5-day group and 2-day group ($p < .005$). Comparison of striatal atrophy between 5-day group and saline group showed that saline group had significantly greater reduction in ipsilateral striatum volume ($p < 0.05$), with 20% reduction in saline rats and almost no reduction in 5-day treated rats.

continued

TABLE 12-1 Continued

Reference	Type of Injury/ Insult	Type of Study and Subjects	Treatment	Findings/Results
Feldman et al., 1996	TBI, closed head injury	Male, Sprague-Dawley rats	Postinjury, $MgSO_4$ (600 mg/kg 1 hour after injury) or no treatment	At both 18 and 48 hours after injury, injured rats treated with $MgSO_4$ had significantly improved neurological severity score than untreated rats ($p < 0.05$ for both times).
				TBI led to brain edema in injured rats compared to sham-injured rats ($p < 0.05$). Rats treated for 48 hours had reduced edema compared to untreated rats ($p < 0.05$). However 18 hours of $MgSO_4$ treatment had no effect on edema size.
				Brain Mg^{2+} level in rats treated with $MgSO_4$ for 48 hours was significantly higher when compared to sham-injured, untreated rats ($p < 0.01$), but not when compared to injured, untreated rats.
				Serum osmolality was not significantly different from baseline after $MgSO_4$ treatment.

[a] n: sample size.
[b] r: correlation coefficient.
[c] OR: odds ratio.
[d] CI: confidence interval.
[e] B: regression coefficient.
[f] HR: hazard ratio.
[g] RR: relative risk.
[h] z: z-score.

observational study by Larsson and colleagues (2008) examined the relationship between dietary magnesium intake and the risk of stroke among the Alpha-Tocopherol, Beta-Carotene Cancer Prevention Study cohort of more than 26,000 male Finnish smokers. The subjects were 50 to 69 years of age and free from stroke at baseline. After adjusting for age and cardiovascular risk factor, magnesium intake was significantly inversely associated with risk of cerebral infarction, but not intracerebral or subarachnoid hemorrhage. This association was found to be strongest in men younger than 60 years of age. A similar inverse association was observed in the Health Professionals Follow-up Study of more than 43,000 U.S. men. Specifically, magnesium intake was significantly inversely associated with risk of total stroke, most strongly among hypertensive subjects (Ascherio et al., 1998). Other cohort studies did not find a significant association between magnesium intake and risk of stroke (Iso et al., 1999; Song et al., 2005).

Animal Studies

The majority of recent animal studies of magnesium therapy for TBI have investigated its effectiveness as a treatment for physiological events that occur during the secondary injury process. However, early animal head-injury models involving magnesium examined its prophylactic use to determine whether an intervention before injury would improve neurological outcome and decrease mortality by attenuating the postinjury decline of intracellular magnesium concentration (McIntosh et al., 1988; Vink and McIntosh, 1990; Vink et al., 1988). The prevention of such postinjury decline of intracellular magnesium levels was associated with enhanced neurological recovery following intravenous magnesium sulfate administration 15 minutes before fluid percussion brain injury (McIntosh et al., 1988). Rats receiving prophylactic administration of magnesium chloride prior to electrolytic lesions of the somatic sensorimotor cortex also had more improved sensorimotor recovery than control rats (Hoane et al., 1998). Enomoto and colleagues reported in 2005 that intravenous administration of magnesium 5 to 20 minutes before the induction of traumatic brain damage by a lateral fluid percussion brain injury model prevented injury-induced neuronal loss in the hippocampus, as well as injury-induced impairments in working and reference memory on the Morris water maze, a test of spatial memory.

Experimental studies have also examined the effect of preinjury magnesium deficiency on postinjury outcomes. When compared to controls fed a normal diet, rats fed a magnesium-deficient diet for two weeks prior to lateral fluid percussion brain injury responded with significantly greater neurological impairment that persisted for four weeks postinjury, as well as increased mortality (McIntosh et al., 1988).

EVIDENCE INDICATING EFFECT ON TREATMENT

Human Studies

Based on studies demonstrating negative correlations between serum magnesium levels and the severity of neurological deficits following brain trauma as well as the neuroprotective effects of magnesium observed in experimental animals, a number of clinical studies have assessed the contribution of magnesium to recovery following stroke. Overall, the results of these studies indicate that intravenous administration of magnesium sulfate raises cerebrospinal fluid and brain extracellular levels of magnesium. Magnesium administration also appears to be well tolerated, with few side effects reported (Dorhout Mees et al., 2007; McKee et al., 2005a; Meloni et al., 2006).

The results of studies examining the neuroprotective effects of magnesium have been mixed. On the positive side, Dhandapani and colleagues (2008) reported that patients given parenteral magnesium sulfate within 12 hours after closed head injury displayed less brain swelling and lower mortality than patients not given magnesium. Further evidence of beneficial effects of magnesium comes from work demonstrating that patients given magnesium sulfate within the first 24 hours after a stroke displayed more functional independence one month after the stroke than patients given a placebo (Lampl et al., 2001). Patients given magnesium within 4 days of suffering a subarachnoid hemorrhage, and then for the subsequent 20 days, also reportedly had less risk of delayed cerebral ischemia than patients given a placebo. However, the authors did note that a high concentration of serum magnesium could have a negative effect on clinical outcome (Dorhout Mees et al., 2007).

Although the results of some clinical studies indicate a neuroprotective role for magnesium, results of other studies have been less positive (Kidwell et al., 2009; McKee et al.,

2005a; Stippler et al., 2007; Temkin et al., 2007). In a double-blind trial, Temkin and colleagues (2007) evaluated the effects of intravenous administration of two doses of magnesium sulfate or placebo given within eight hours of traumatic brain injury and continuing for five days in 499 patients. Magnesium had no significant positive effects on survival, seizure occurrence, or neurobehavioral functioning. Similarly, the Intravenous Magnesium Efficacy in Stroke (IMAGES) trial failed to demonstrate a survival benefit in more than 2,500 patients with acute ischemic stroke who received either magnesium sulfate or placebo within 12 hours of stroke onset (IMAGES Study Investigators, 2004). Moreover, in a subsequent report of a substudy within the IMAGES trial using magnetic resonance imaging, there were no differences in infarct growth observed between patients who had received magnesium and those who had not (Kidwell et al., 2009). In an analysis of three randomized control trials, a Cochrane review concluded that magnesium therapy in patients with acute brain injury is not currently supported by the evidence (Arango and Mejia-Mantilla, 2006).

Animal Studies

More than 20 years ago, Vink and colleagues (Heath and Vink, 1998; Vink et al., 1988) reported that TBI in laboratory rodents was associated with a decline in intracellular free magnesium and further noted that the greater the reduction in magnesium, the more severe the trauma-induced neurological deficits. In subsequent work, these investigators demonstrated that magnesium deficiency exacerbated the physiological and behavioral outcomes of traumatic brain injury, while pretreatment with magnesium improved them (McIntosh et al., 1988, 1989). More specifically, they found that rats receiving a magnesium-deficient diet for 14 days before a fluid percussion injury displayed more profound neurological impairments and higher mortality rates than rats fed a standard laboratory diet. In comparison, rats given intravenous infusions of magnesium sulfate 15 minutes before injury demonstrated improved cellular bioenergetics and neurological functioning relative to rats fed the standard diet (McIntosh et al., 1988).

Since 1990, a variety of animal models of TBI that included fluid percussion injury, impact-acceleration injury, cortical contusion injury, and focal and global cerebral ischemia has repeatedly documented that treatment with magnesium shortly after the induction of injury is effective in limiting the detrimental neural and behavioral consequences of brain trauma (for reviews see: Hoane, 2007; Meloni et al., 2006; Sen and Gulati, 2010). Administration of magnesium prevents the postinjury decline in free magnesium, reduces cortical and hippocampal cell loss, ameliorates cortical alterations in microtubule-associated protein, and enhances cellular bioenergetic status (Enomoto et al., 2005; Heath and Vink, 1999b; Saatman et al., 2001; Turner et al., 2004). Treatment with magnesium can also attenuate the development of brain edema (Feldman et al., 1996), avert apoptotic changes in neurons (Park and Hyun, 2004), and diminish defects in the blood-brain barrier that result from TBI (Esen et al., 2003).

Magnesium also can improve the behavioral consequences of TBI. Heath and Vink (1999a) reported that the administration of magnesium salts after severe TBI resulted not only in dose-related increases in brain intracellular free magnesium, but also led to improvements in motor behavior. Similarly, Hoane et al. (2003) found that magnesium chloride therapy facilitated reduction of sensorimotor deficits in a dose-dependent manner following bilateral damage to the anterior medial cortex.

The effects of magnesium on recovery are not limited to the transient phase of secondary injury, but rather have long-term functional significance. Research has demonstrated that posttraumatic administration of magnesium sulfate diminishes spatial and motor deficits and attenuates anxiety in rats for up to four weeks after the induction of severe diffuse TBI (Vink et al., 2003). Further evidence of the potential long-term effects of magnesium comes from Browne and colleagues, who reported that magnesium given 15 minutes after fluid percussion injury significantly reduced tissue loss in the hippocampus when measured eight months after the induction of brain damage. However, although magnesium did reduce tissue loss, there were no differences observed in cognitive behavior between treated and untreated animals (Browne et al., 2004).

Most studies examining the therapeutic effects of magnesium following TBI in experimental animals have concentrated on recovery of sensory functions, motor functions, or both. Studies conducted since 2000, however, also indicate that magnesium therapy can improve deficits in cognitive function that result from TBI (Enomoto et al., 2005; Hoane, 2007; Hoane et al., 2003). As mentioned in the earlier section on resilience, a significant reduction in ipsilateral hippocampal cell loss was seen when magnesium therapy was administered prior to fluid percussion brain injury; accordingly, the magnesium therapy prevented injury-induced cognitive dysfunction in the Morris water maze (Enomoto et al., 2005). Hoane (2007) similarly reported that rats given magnesium chloride shortly after brain injury displayed fewer deficits in both reference and working memory on the Morris water maze than controls not given magnesium. It should be noted, however, that magnesium did not improve all aspects of cognitive behavior. In fact, daily administration of a high dose of magnesium produced amnesia and impairments in the acquisition of reference memory task on the Morris water maze. These findings indicate that the type of task used must be considered when evaluating the effects of magnesium on recovery of function following TBI.

TBI can affect brain regions and neurotransmitter systems involved in the modulation of mood, making depression and anxiety common occurrences in brain-damaged individuals (Bombardier et al., 2010; Jorge and Starkstein, 2005). It has been hypothesized that magnesium could be useful in alleviating mood disturbances related to TBI. In support of this hypothesis, rats given magnesium sulfate 30 minutes after impact-acceleration injury displayed less anxiety in an open field test 1 and 6 weeks after injury than brain-damaged animals not given magnesium (Fromm et al., 2004).

Taken together, the results of the previous animal studies strongly suggest that magnesium plays a role in the pathophysiological processes following TBI, and that magnesium therapy may be useful in recovery of both neural functioning and behavior. It is important to note, however, that not all studies have confirmed the neuroprotective effects of magnesium (Hoane, 2007; Hoane and Barth, 2002; Meloni et al., 2006); in reviewing studies that investigated the neuroprotective effects of magnesium in animals that had experienced global or focal cerebral ischemia, Meloni et al. (2006) reported that approximately 40 percent of the studies failed to find any positive effect for magnesium. These conflicting findings are important, because they suggest that the types of brain damage; the dose, route, and timing of magnesium administration; the species and strain of animal; and temperature can influence the neuroprotective effects of magnesium (see below).

One obvious factor that could contribute to the discrepancies in the results of studies assessing the neuroprotective effects of magnesium is the dosage used. With few exceptions (Heath and Vink, 1999b; Hoane et al., 2003), researchers have not examined dose-related responses to magnesium. Across studies, doses of magnesium have ranged from 80 mg/kg to more than 2,000 mg/kg, and in some studies animals were given only one dose of magnesium, while in others they were given multiple doses (Meloni et al., 2006). Unfortunately, there are no consistent relationships evident between dosage and the neuroprotective effects of magnesium.

Results of a number of studies suggest that the timing of administration is another important factor in determining whether magnesium can provide neuroprotective effects. Most studies demonstrating such an effect had administered magnesium either immediately before or very shortly (15 to 30 minutes) after the induction of brain injury. It is therefore likely that magnesium levels in the brain were elevated at the time of the injury or shortly thereafter (Meloni et al., 2006). When administration of magnesium was delayed for several hours, neuroprotective effects have been less consistent. For example, although motor behavior improved in response to magnesium treatment provided up to 24 hours after brain damage, earlier treatments provided the most significant benefit (Heath and Vink, 1999a; Hoane and Barth, 2002). Cell death following brain injury was likewise reduced when magnesium was given 15 minutes after injury, but not when it was given either 8 or 24 hours after injury (Hoane and Barth, 2002).

The extent of the damage following TBI may also moderate the neuroprotective effects of magnesium. Following impact-acceleration injury, magnesium treatment improved brain magnesium levels and motor behavior in rats that did not develop subdural hematomas. However, no such improvement was observed in rats that did develop subdural hematomas (Heath and Vink, 2001).

It has been hypothesized that magnesium's neuroprotective effects following the induction of cerebral ischemia are only observed when combined with post-ischemia hypothermia (Campbell et al., 2008; Meloni et al., 2006, 2009; Zhu et al., 2004). Most studies have not considered body temperature following the induction of brain damage. In studies that have monitored body temperature, however, magnesium treatment reduced the death of hippocampal neurons in rats that were mildly hypothermic in the immediate hours after the induction of brain damage, but did not reduce neuronal death in animals that were normothermic (Campbell et al., 2008; Meloni et al., 2006).

CONCLUSIONS AND RECOMMENDATIONS

A number of variables including dose and duration of treatment could modify the neuroprotective effects of magnesium. Findings from both human and animal studies indicate that the most critical issue yet to be addressed is the window of opportunity for magnesium use in the treatment of TBI. Animal studies suggest that the therapeutic window within which neuroprotective effects of magnesium are observed is very brief. As described in preceding paragraphs, most animal studies demonstrating a beneficial effect of magnesium have administered the mineral within 60 minutes following brain damage, which may not be practical or feasible in an uncontrolled environment, such as in combat operations. Results of studies employing longer time intervals between injury and magnesium administration have not been as positive. With respect to clinical trials, results from a small number of patients in the IMAGES trial indicated a beneficial effect of magnesium when it was given within three hours of injury.[3] To further evaluate the importance of rapid treatment with magnesium, the Field Administration of Stroke Therapy—Magnesium (FAST-MAG) phase III clinical trial (Saver et al., 2004) is comparing the effects of magnesium given intravenously by paramedics within 1 to 2 hours of symptom onset on scales of global handicap, neurological deficits, quality of life, and mortality, to placebo three months following injury.[4] Results of this study have yet to be published.

Results of studies employing experimental animals have shown that magnesium can protect against a number of the secondary consequences of traumatic brain injury. Clini-

---

[3] Available online at http://www.fastmag.info/sci_bkg.htm (accessed December 22, 2010).
[4] Available online at http://www.fastmag.info/sci_bkg.htm (accessed December 22, 2010).

cal studies have had more mixed results, however, with several large trials (e.g., IMAGES) failing to observe a beneficial effect of the mineral on recovery from stroke; indeed, a Cochrane review concluded that the evidence does not currently support magnesium therapy in patients with acute brain injury. No large clinical studies have assessed the neuroprotective effects of magnesium on other types of brain injury, including TBI.

At present, there is no clear evidence that magnesium would be useful in the treatment of TBI occurring in military personnel. However, it is recommended that the results of the FAST-MAG trial be monitored to determine if administration of magnesium within a two-hour window after brain damage can alleviate some of the detrimental consequences of TBI.

REFERENCES

Arango, M. F., and D. Bainbridge. 2006. Magnesium for acute traumatic brain injury. *Cochrane Database of Systematic Reviews* (4):CD005400.

Ascherio, A., E. B. Rimm, M. A. Hernan, E. L. Giovannucci, I. Kawachi, M. J. Stampfer, and W. C. Willett. 1998. Intake of potassium, magnesium, calcium, and fiber and risk of stroke among us men. *Circulation* 98(12):1198–1204.

Bareyre, F. M., K. E. Saatman, M. A. Helfaer, G. Sinson, J. D. Weisser, A. L. Brown, and T. K. McIntosh. 1999. Alterations in ionized and total blood magnesium after experimental traumatic brain injury: Relationship to neurobehavioral outcome and neuroprotective efficacy of magnesium chloride. *Journal of Neurochemistry* 73(1):271–280.

Bayir, A., A. Ak, H. Kara, and T. K. Sahin. 2009. Serum and cerebrospinal fluid magnesium levels, Glasgow Coma Scores, and in-hospital mortality in patients with acute stroke. *Biological Trace Element Research* 130(1):7–12.

Begum, R., A. Begum, R. Johanson, M. N. Ali, and S. Akhter. 2001. A low dose ("Dhaka") magnesium sulphate regime for eclampsia. *Acta Obstetricia et Gynecologica Scandinavica* 80(11):998–1002.

Bombardier, C. H., J. R. Fann, N. R. Temkin, P. C. Esselman, J. Barber, and S. S. Dikmen. 2010. Rates of major depressive disorder and clinical outcomes following traumatic brain injury. *Journal of the American Medical Association* 303(19):1938–1945.

Browne, K. D., M. J. Leoni, A. Iwata, X. H. Chen, and D. H. Smith. 2004. Acute treatment with MgSO₄ attenuates long-term hippocampal tissue loss after brain trauma in the rat. *Journal of Neuroscience Research* 77(6):878–883.

Bullock, R., A. Zauner, J. J. Woodward, J. Myseros, S. C. Choi, J. D. Ward, A. Marmarou, and H. F. Young. 1998. Factors affecting excitatory amino acid release following severe human head injury. *Journal of Neurosurgery* 89(4):507–518.

Campbell, K., B. P. Meloni, H. D. Zhu, and N. W. Knuckey. 2008. Magnesium treatment and spontaneous mild hypothermia after transient focal cerebral ischemia in the rat. *Brain Research Bulletin* 77(5):320–322.

Chia, R. Y., R. S. Hughes, and M. K. Morgan. 2002. Magnesium: A useful adjunct in the prevention of cerebral vasospasm following aneurysmal subarachnoid haemorrhage. *Journal of Clinical Neuroscience* 9(3):279–281.

Dhandapani, S. S., A. Gupta, S. Vivekanandhan, B. S. Sharma, and A. K. Mahapatra. 2008. Randomized controlled trial of magnesium sulphate in severe closed traumatic brain injury. *Indian Journal of Neurotrauma* 5(1):27–33.

Dorhout Mees, S. M., W. M. van den Bergh, A. Algra, and G. J. E. Rinkel. 2007. Achieved serum magnesium concentrations and occurrence of delayed cerebral ischaemia and poor outcome in aneurysmal subarachnoid haemorrhage. *Journal of Neurology, Neurosurgery and Psychiatry* 78(7):729–731.

Enomoto, T., T. Osugi, H. Satoh, T. K. McIntosh, and T. Nabeshima. 2005. Pre-injury magnesium treatment prevents traumatic brain injury-induced hippocampal ERK activation, neuronal loss, and cognitive dysfunction in the radial-arm maze test. *Journal of Neurotrauma* 22(7):783–792.

Esen, F., T. Erdem, D. Aktan, R. Kalayci, N. Cakar, M. Kaya, and L. Telci. 2003. Effects of magnesium administration on brain edema and blood-brain barrier breakdown after experimental traumatic brain injury in rats. *Journal of Neurosurgical Anesthesiology* 15(2):119–125.

Faden, A. I., P. Demediuk, S. S. Panter, and R. Vink. 1989. The role of excitatory amino acids and NMDA receptors in traumatic brain injury. *Science* 244(4906):798–800.

Feldman, Z., B. Gurevitch, A. A. Artru, A. Oppenheim, E. Shohami, E. Reichenthal, and Y. Shapira. 1996. Effect of magnesium given 1 hour after head trauma on brain edema and neurological outcome. *Journal of Neurosurgery* 85(1):131–137.

Fleet, J. C., and K. D. Cashman. 2001. Magnesium. In *Present knowledge in nutrition*. 8th ed., edited by R. A. Bowman and R. M. Russell. Washington, DC: International Life Sciences Institute. Pp. 292–301.

Fromm, L., D. L. Heath, R. Vink, and A. J. Nimmo. 2004. Magnesium attenuates post-traumatic depression/ anxiety following diffuse traumatic brain injury in rats. *Journal of the American College of Nutrition* 23(5):529S–533S.

Ghabriel, M. N., A. Thomas, and R. Vink. 2006. Magnesium restores altered aquaporin-4 immunoreactivity following traumatic brain injury to a pre-injury state. *Acta Neurochirurgica—Supplement* 96:402–406.

Gorelick, P. B., and S. Ruland. 2004. IMAGES and FAST-MAG: Magnesium for acute ischaemic stroke. *Lancet Neurology* 3(6):330.

Heath, D. L., and R. Vink. 1998. Blood-free magnesium concentration declines following graded experimental traumatic brain injury. *Scandinavian Journal of Clinical and Laboratory Investigation* 58(2):161–166.

Heath, D. L., and R. Vink. 1999a. Improved motor outcome in response to magnesium therapy received up to 24 hours after traumatic diffuse axonal brain injury in rats. *Journal of Neurosurgery* 90(3):504–509.

Heath, D. L., and R. Vink. 1999b. Optimization of magnesium therapy after severe diffuse axonal brain injury in rats. *Journal of Pharmacology and Experimental Therapeutics* 288(3):1311–1316.

Heath, D. L., and R. Vink. 2001. Subdural hematoma following traumatic brain injury causes a secondary decline in brain free magnesium concentration. *Journal of Neurotrauma* 18(4):465–469.

Hoane, M. R. 2007. Assessment of cognitive function following magnesium therapy in the traumatically injured brain. *Magnesium Research* 20(4):229–236.

Hoane, M. R., and T. M. Barth. 2002. The window of opportunity for administration of magnesium therapy following focal brain injury is 24 h but is task dependent in the rat. *Physiology and Behavior* 76(2):271–280.

Hoane, M. R., S. L. Irish, B. B. Marks, and T. M. Barth. 1998. Preoperative regimens of magnesium facilitate recovery of function and prevent subcortical atrophy following lesions of the rat sensorimotor cortex. *Brain Research Bulletin* 45(1):45–51.

Hoane, M. R., A. A. Knotts, S. L. Akstulewicz, M. Aquilano, and L. W. Means. 2003. The behavioral effects of magnesium therapy on recovery of function following bilateral anterior medial cortex lesions in the rat. *Brain Research Bulletin* 60(1–2):105–114.

IMAGES (Intravenous Magnesium Efficacy in Stroke) Study Investigators. 2004. Magnesium for acute stroke (Intravenous Magnesium Efficacy in Stroke trial): Randomised controlled trial. *Lancet* 363(9407):439–445.

IOM (Institute of Medicine). 1997. *Dietary Reference Intakes for calcium, phosphorus, magnesium, vitamin D, and fluoride*. Washington, DC: National Academy Press.

IOM. 2006. *Mineral requirements for military personnel: Levels needed for cognitive and physical performance during garrison training*. Washington, DC: The National Academies Press.

Iso, H., M. J. Stampfer, J. E. Manson, K. Rexrode, C. H. Hennekens, G. A. Colditz, F. E. Speizer, and W. C. Willett. 1999. Prospective study of calcium, potassium, and magnesium intake and risk of stroke in women. *Stroke* 30(9):1772–1779.

Jorge, R. E., and S. E. Starkstein. 2005. Pathophysiologic aspects of major depression following traumatic brain injury. *Journal of Head Trauma Rehabilitation* 20(6):475–487.

Kerz, T., A. Victor, C. Beyer, I. Trapp, F. Heid, and R. Reisch. 2008. A case control study of statin and magnesium administration in patients after aneurysmal subarachnoid hemorrhage: Incidence of delayed cerebral ischemia and mortality. *Neurological Research* 30(9):893–897.

Kidwell, C. S., K. R. Lees, K. W. Muir, C. Chen, S. M. Davis, D. A. De Silva, C. J. Weir, S. Starkman, J. R. Alger, and J. L. Saver. 2009. Results of the MRI substudy of the Intravenous Magnesium Efficacy in Stroke trial. *Stroke* 40(5):1704–1709.

Lampl, Y., R. Gilad, D. Geva, Y. Eshel, and M. Sadeh. 2001. Intravenous administration of magnesium sulfate in acute stroke: A randomized double-blind study. *Clinical Neuropharmacology* 24(1):11–15.

Larsson, S. C., M. J. Virtanen, M. Mars, S. Mannisto, P. Pietinen, D. Albanes, and J. Virtamo. 2008. Magnesium, calcium, potassium, and sodium intakes and risk of stroke in male smokers. *Archives of Internal Medicine* 168(5):459–465.

McIntosh, T. K., A. I. Faden, I. Yamakami, and R. Vink. 1988. Magnesium deficiency exacerbates and pretreatment improves outcome following traumatic brain injury in rats: 31P magnetic resonance spectroscopy and behavioral studies. *Journal of Neurotrauma* 5(1):17–31.

McIntosh, T. K., R. Vink, I. Yamakami, and A. I. Faden. 1989. Magnesium protects against neurological deficit after brain injury. *Brain Research* 482(2):252–260.

McKee, J. A., R. P. Brewer, G. E. Macy, C. O. Borel, J. D. Reynolds, and D. S. Warner. 2005a. Magnesium neuroprotection is limited in humans with acute brain injury. *Neurocritical Care* 2(3):342–351.

McKee, J. A., R. P. Brewer, G. E. Macy, B. Phillips-Bute, K. A. Campbell, C. O. Borel, J. D. Reynolds, and D. S. Warner. 2005b. Analysis of the brain bioavailability of peripherally administered magnesium sulfate: A study in humans with acute brain injury undergoing prolonged induced hypermagnesemia. *Critical Care Medicine* 33(3):661–666.

Meloni, B. P., H. Zhu, and N. W. Knuckey. 2006. Is magnesium neuroprotective following global and focal cerebral ischaemia? A review of published studies. *Magnesium Research* 19(2):123–137.

Meloni, B. P., K. Campbell, H. D. Zhu, and N. W. Knuckey. 2009. In search of clinical neuroprotection after brain ischemia the case for mild hypothermia (35 degrees C) and magnesium. *Stroke* 40(6):2236–2240.

Natale, J. E., A. M. Guerguerian, J. G. Joseph, R. McCarter, C. Shao, B. Slomine, J. Christensen, M. V. Johnston, and D. H. Shaffner. 2007. Pilot study to determine the hemodynamic safety and feasibility of magnesium sulfate infusion in children with severe traumatic brain injury. *Pediatric Critical Care Medicine* 8(1):1–9.

Park, C. O., and D. K. Hyun. 2004. Apoptotic change in response to magnesium therapy after moderate diffuse axonal injury in rats. *Yonsei Medical Journal* 45(5):908–916.

Saatman, K. E., F. M. Bareyre, M. S. Grady, and T. K. McIntosh. 2001. Acute cytoskeletal alterations and cell death induced by experimental brain injury are attenuated by magnesium treatment and exacerbated by magnesium deficiency. *Journal of Neuropathology and Experimental Neurology* 60(2):183–194.

Saver, J. L., C. Kidwell, M. Eckstein, S. Starkman, and F.-M. P. T. Investigators. 2004. Prehospital neuroprotective therapy for acute stroke—results of the Field Administration of Stroke Therapy-Magnesium (FAST-MAG) pilot trial. *Stroke* 35(5):E106–E108.

Schmid-Elsaesser, R., M. Kunz, S. Zausinger, S. Prueckner, J. Briegel, and H.-J. Steiger. 2006. Intravenous magnesium versus nimodipine in the treatment of patients with aneurysmal subarachnoid hemorrhage: A randomized study. *Neurosurgery* 58(6):1054–1065; discussion 1054–1065.

Sen, A. P., and A. Gulati. 2010. Use of magnesium in traumatic brain injury. *Neurotherapeutics* 7(1):91–99.

Shils, M. E. 1999. Magnesium. In *Modern nutrition in health and disease*. 9th ed., edited by M. E. Shils, J. A. Olson, M. Shike and A. C. Ross. New York: Lippincott Williams & Wilkins. Pp. 169–192.

Song, Y., J. E. Manson, N. R. Cook, C. M. Albert, J. E. Buring, and S. Liu. 2005. Dietary magnesium intake and risk of cardiovascular disease among women. *American Journal of Cardiology* 96(8):1135–1141.

Stippler, M., M. R. Fischer, A. M. Puccio, S. R. Wisniewski, E. B. Carson-Walter, C. E. Dixon, and K. A. Walter. 2007. Serum and cerebrospinal fluid magnesium in severe traumatic brain injury outcome. *Journal of Neurotrauma* 24(8):1347–1354.

Temkin, N. R., G. D. Anderson, H. R. Winn, R. G. Ellenbogen, G. W. Britz, J. Schuster, T. Lucas, D. W. Newell, P. N. Mansfield, J. E. Machamer, J. Barber, and S. S. Dikmen. 2007. Magnesium sulfate for neuroprotection after traumatic brain injury: A randomised controlled trial. *Lancet Neurology* 6(1):29–38.

Turner, R. J., K. W. Dasilva, C. O'Connor, C. van den Heuvel, and R. Vink. 2004. Magnesium gluconate offers no more protection than magnesium sulphate following diffuse traumatic brain injury in rats. *Journal of the American College of Nutrition* 23(5):541S–544S.

Van de Water, J. M. W., W. M. Van den Bergh, R. G. Hoff, A. Algra, and G. J. E. Rinkel. 2007. Hypocalcaemia may reduce the beneficial effect of magnesium treatment in aneurysmal subarachnoid haemorrhage. *Magnesium Research* 20(2):130–135.

van den Bergh, W. M., J. M. W. van de Water, R. G. Hoff, A. Algra, and G. J. E. Rinkel. 2008. Calcium homeostasis during magnesium treatment in aneurysmal subarachnoid hemorrhage. *Neurocritical Care* 8(3):413–417.

Vink, R., and T. K. McIntosh. 1990. Pharmacological and physiological effects of magnesium on experimental traumatic brain injury. *Magnesium Research* 3(3):163–169.

Vink, R., T. K. McIntosh, P. Demediuk, M. W. Weiner, and A. I. Faden. 1988. Decline in intracellular free Mg^{2+} is associated with irreversible tissue injury after brain trauma. *Journal of Biological Chemistry* 263(2):757–761.

Vink, R., C. A. O'Connor, A. J. Nimmo, and D. L. Heath. 2003. Magnesium attenuates persistent functional deficits following diffuse traumatic brain injury in rats. *Neuroscience Letters* 336(1):41–44.

Wong, G. K. C., C. W. K. Lam, M. T. V. Chan, T. Gin, and W. S. Poon. 2009. The effect of hypermagnesemic treatment on cerebrospinal fluid magnesium level in patients with aneurysmal subarachnoid hemorrhage. *Magnesium Research* 22(2):60–65.

Zhu, H. D., B. P. Meloni, S. R. Moore, B. T. Majda, and N. W. Knuckey. 2004. Intravenous administration of magnesium is only neuroprotective following transient global ischemia when present with post-ischemic mild hypothermia. *Brain Research* 1014(1–2):53–60.

13

Eicosapentaenoic Acid (EPA) and Docosahexaenoic Acid (DHA)

Polyunsaturated fatty acids are classified as n-3 (omega-3) or n-6 (omega-6) depending on whether their first double bond is located on the third or sixth carbon from the terminal methyl group (Jones and Kubow, 2006). More than 80 percent of dietary polyunsaturated fatty acids consumed in the United States consist of the 18-carbon, 2 double bond, n-6 (18:2, n-6) linoleic acid, with an average intake of about 17 g/day (IOM, 2005). The major dietary n-3 fatty acid is alpha-linolenic acid (ALA) (18:3, n-3), which is derived from certain nuts and vegetable oils (Kris-Etherton et al., 2000). Although the long-chain n-3 fatty acids eicosapentaenoic acid (EPA) (20:5, n-3) and docosahexaenoic acid (DHA) (22:6, n-3) can be synthesized from linolenic acid, the efficiency (yield) of the enzymatic reactions involved is rather low (Jones and Kubow, 2006).

Epidemiological studies have indicated that Inuit populations in Greenland whose diets contain a high level of fish (and concomitant high levels of EPA and DHA) have low incidences of cardiovascular disease and rheumatoid arthritis, conditions with a significant inflammatory etiology (Dyerberg, 1993). Several mechanisms affected by n-3 fatty acids may account for these findings. Polyunsaturated fatty acids serve as the precursor molecules for eicosanoids. The primary precursor is arachidonic acid (20:4, n-6), which is enzymatically transformed into inflammatory prostaglandins or leukotrienes that contain two and four double bonds, respectively. Prostaglandins and leukotrienes synthesized from n-3 fatty acids contain three and five double bonds, respectively, and are less biologically active (Jones and Kubow, 2006). Dietary fish oil supplementation reduces synthesis of inflammatory cytokines such as interleukin-1 (IL-1) and tumor necrosis factor (TNF) (Endres et al., 1989). Supplementation with n-3 fatty acids likewise reduces reactive oxygen species (ROS) production by leukocytes (Massaro et al., 2008). EPA and DHA are also the precursors for resolvins, which bring about a programmed resolution of the inflammatory process (Schwab et al., 2007), and DHA serves as the precursor for synthesis of protectins that have anti-inflammatory and neuroprotective activities (Serhan, 2006).

EPA AND DHA AND THE BRAIN

Long-chain polyunsaturated fatty acids are important structural components in cell membrane phospholipid bilayers, with EPA and DHA concentrated in synaptic membranes in the brain and in the retina (Dyall and Michael-Titus, 2008). Variations in the ratio of n-3:n-6 composition may affect membrane fluidity, thickness, or other characteristics, as well as influence how proteins embedded in the membrane move and function (Lauritzen et al., 2001). There is evidence that n-3 fatty acids protect normal mitochondrial function and reduce excitotoxicity (reviewed in Dyall and Michael-Titus, 2008). Human studies (years 1990 and later) addressing the influence of EPA/DHA on resilience or treatment of central nervous system (CNS) injuries or disorders, such as stroke, epilepsy, and subarachnoid hemorrhage, are presented in Table 13-1. Likewise, Table 13-1 also lists animal studies on the effects of EPA/DHA on TBI.

There are various models that explain the transportation of fatty acids through the blood-brain barrier, most of them involving complexes with albumin and circulating lipoproteins. Other models propose that there are no specific transporters that participate in this process (Hamilton and Brunaldi, 2007).

USES AND SAFETY

There are insufficient data to correlate reduced concentrations of n-3 fatty acids with functional impairments; therefore, no Estimated Average Requirements (EARs) have been established. An Adequate Intake (AI) for alpha-linolenic acid, based on the average daily intake by apparently healthy people that is therefore assumed to be adequate, has been set at 1.6 g/day for adult men and 1.1 g/day for adult women (IOM, 2005). Any intake of EPA and DHA, which normally accounts for about 10 percent of total n-3 fatty acids in the diet, is considered to contribute to the AI for ALA. The most effective way to increase body stores of EPA and DHA is through increased dietary intake of oil from cold-water fish species and from krill.

Intake of up to 1 g/day of n-3 fatty acids from dietary fish intake is generally regarded as having very low risk, but higher intakes can increase the risk of gastrointestinal upset as well as increases in blood glucose and concentrations of low-density lipoprotein (LDL) cholesterol (Kris-Etherton et al., 2002). Increased intake of n-3 fatty acids will decrease the synthesis of the eicosanoid thromboxane A_2, which promotes platelet aggregation (Kramer et al., 1996). Excessive intake can therefore increase the risk of bleeding, although this was not generally observed in a number of randomized clinical trials of fish-oil supplementation (Huang et al., 2007; Javierre et al., 2006). Environmental contaminants such as mercury and polychlorinated biphenyls can accumulate in certain species of fish, presenting another potential risk. The risk from mercury toxicity can be diminished, however, by avoiding some fish species (e.g., swordfish, mackerel), and ingestion of other contaminants can be diminished by removing the skin and fat from fish before cooking. Alternatively, purified EPA and DHA can be taken in capsule form.

Although increased dietary n-3 fatty acid intake reduces cellular production of ROS, the increased desaturation (double bonds) of these fatty acids increases susceptibility to lipid peroxidation, which may have detrimental effects on specific cellular processes, such as T cell–mediated immune function (Wu and Meydani, 1998). This can be ameliorated, however, by adequate supplementation with the antioxidant vitamin E (Wu and Meydani, 1998).

TABLE 13-1 Relevant Data Identified for n-3 Fatty Acids (DHA, EPA, ALA)

Reference	Type of Injury/Insult	Type of Study and Subjects	Treatment	Findings/Results
Tier 1: Clinical trials				
Garbagnati et al., 2009	Ischemic stroke	Randomized, double-blind, placebo-controlled trial n^a=72 stroke patients	Postinjury, n-3 polyunsaturated fatty acids (PUFA, 500 mg), antioxidants, PUFA and antioxidants, or placebo for 12 months	Neurological and function status was not significantly affected by any supplements. Although PUFA was associated with lower mortality rate, the trend was not statistically significant. No adverse effects were observed.
Poppitt et al., 2009	Ischemic stroke	Randomized, placebo-controlled trial n=102 stroke patients	3 g/day of fish oil capsules containing approx 1.2 g total n-3 fatty acid (0.7 DHA, 0.3 EPA) or placebo for 12 weeks	Fish oil had no effect on triglyceride level, though there was a nonsignificant 7% increase in the fish oil-treated group and a nonsignificant 3% decrease in the placebo group. Fish oil also had no significant effect on total cholesterol level, high-density lipoprotein cholesterol, low-density lipoprotein cholesterol (LDL-C), LDL particle size, different sized LDL-C, high sensitivity C-reactive protein, erythrocyte sedimentation, ferritin, or fibrinogen. Analysis of the 28-item General Health Questionnaire showed that fish oil–treated group had a mean 1.41 point decrease in total score (95% CI[b]: –2.76 to –0.06; p=0.04) and a mean 1.24 point decrease in social dysfunction (95% CI: –2.33 to –0.14; p=0.03). There was no change in scores for somatic symptoms, anxiety and insomnia, or depression. Adverse effects related to treatment were not assessed.

TABLE 13-1 Continued

Reference	Type of Injury/Insult	Type of Study and Subjects	Treatment	Findings/Results
Bromfield et al., 2008	Intractable focal or generalized epilepsy	Randomized, double-blind trial for 12 weeks, then open-label for 4 weeks n=21	PUFA supplement (EPA + DHA) at 2.2 mg/day in 3:2 ratio or placebo	During the double-blind phase, the number of subjects experiencing a > 50% reduction in seizure frequency was not significantly higher than baseline. Median seizure frequency during this study phase also showed no significant difference between the two groups. PUFA treatment also had no effect on quality of life, as measured by Quality of Life in Epilepsy survey. During the open-label phase, 79% of patients experienced decreased seizure frequency, with 33% of these patients experiencing a > 50% reduction. Analysis of serum drug concentration showed a 16% decrease in lamotrigine levels ($p < 0.05$); there were no changes in other drugs. Although not significant, nausea and/or diarrhea was reported more frequently in the treatment group (p=0.18).
DeGiorgio et al., 2008	Refractory epilepsy	Randomized, double-blind, cross-over clinical trial n=11	9,600 mg of fish oil/day (2,800 mg of n-3 fatty acids) or same quantity of placebo	An average 11% increase in seizure frequency from baseline was observed in patients taking fish oil, and an average 14% increase was observed in those taking placebo, but these increases were not significant (p=0.051). There was no significant change of seizure severity from baseline in either group. Fish oil treatment also had no effect on total cholesterol level, LDL level, high-density lipoprotein level, mean arterial pressure, or heart rate variability. However, fish oil treatment was inversely correlated with heart rate variability (SDNN[c]) in the highest risk patients ($r_s{}^d=-0.65$, p=0.03); there was no correlation between placebo and heart rate variability (SDNN).

continued

TABLE 13-1 Continued

Reference	Type of Injury/Insult	Type of Study and Subjects	Treatment	Findings/Results
Tanaka et al., 2008	Stroke	Prospective, randomized, open-label, blinded endpoint trial n=18,645	EPA (1,800 mg/day) supplementing statin or statin alone for approximately 5 years	During the study period, subjects with no history of stroke who were taking EPA had significantly greater reduction in total cholesterol level (17.6% vs. 17.0%; p < 0.0001) and triglyceride level (7.3% vs. 2.6%; p < 0.0001) than subjects in the same subgroup who were not taking EPA. EPA subjects with history of stroke had greater reduction of triglyceride level (p < 0.001) than subjects not taking EPA. EPA supplementation had no significant effect in preventing stroke in subjects without a history of stroke, but it significantly reduced total stroke incident in subjects who had a history of stroke (HR[c]=0.80, 95% CI: 0.64–0.997; p=0.047). No adverse effects were mentioned.
Yoneda et al., 2008	Subarachnoid hemorrhage (SAH)	Prospective, non-randomized trial n=101 SAH patients	Oral administration of EPA (1,800 mg) daily for 10 days (day 4–14); control group did not receive EPA	EPA supplementation significantly reduced the incidence of symptomatic vasospasm in the treatment group compared to the control group (14% vs. 36%, p=0.019). The EPA group also had a lower level of low-density areas attributable to vasospasm than the controls (4% vs. 29%, p=0.001). More patients from the EPA group had a good outcome at 1 month after onset of SAH (85% vs. 64% in control group, p=0.022). The control group had more deaths than the EPA group (11% vs. 0%, p=0.020). No adverse effects were observed.
Puri et al., 2007	Chronic refractory epilepsy	Pilot, randomized, double-blind, placebo-controlled trial n=7 patients average age: 50.7±13.6 years	EPA (1 g) + DHA (0.7 g) or placebo daily for 12 weeks	Treatment with n-3 fatty acids had no significant effect on the percentage change of phosphodiesters, γ-nucleotide triphosphate, or broadband component. No adverse effects were mentioned.

TABLE 13-1 Continued

Reference	Type of Injury/Insult	Type of Study and Subjects	Treatment	Findings/Results
Yuen et al., 2005	Epilepsy	Randomized, placebo-controlled, double-blind trial for 12 weeks, followed by open-label trial for another 12 weeks when all patients received PUFA n=57	1 g of EPA + 0.7 g of DHA or matching placebo daily	Greater proportion of patients on PUFA than on placebo had a > 50% seizure reduction in the first 6 weeks (17% vs. 0%, 95% CI: 1.5–3.6%; p < 0.05), but there was no difference between weeks 6 and 12. During the open-label period (weeks 13–24), total seizure and complex partial seizure in previously placebo-treated patients was reduced in weeks 13–18 compared to the first 6 weeks of the trial (p=0.051). There was no significant difference in rescue medication doses between the two groups during the blind period. But the PUFA group had greater decrease during weeks 19–24, with 1.2 from previous range of 1.9–2.3. There was no significant difference in serum antiepileptic drug concentration. Sleepiness, fatigue and breathlessness, diarrhea, recurrence of depression and paranoia, and status epilepticus were reported among only a small number of subjects on supplements (n=5, one subject reporting per adverse effect).

continued

TABLE 13-1   Continued

Reference	Type of Injury/Insult	Type of Study and Subjects	Treatment	Findings/Results
GISSI-Prevenzione Investigators, 1999	Myocardial infarction (MI), stroke, and death from cardiovascular causes (primary outcome events)	Randomized, placebo-controlled, multi-center, open-label trial (Gruppo Italiano per lo Studio della Sopravvivenza nell'Infarto miocardico) n=11,324 patients aged 49–70 years with recent (≤ 3 months) MI	2×2 factorial design: vitamin E (300 mg synthetic α-tocopherol) or placebo and n-3 PUFA (850–882 mg EPA and DHA as ethyl esters in average ratio of EPA/DHA 1:2)	At 6 months, patients taking PUFA had decreased triglyceride concentration compared to controls (p < 0.05). Two-way analysis of PUFA treatment (vs. no PUFA) for the entire study period showed that PUFA-treatment patients were at lower risk for combined endpoints of death, non-fatal MI, and non-fatal stroke (RR/=0.90, 95% CI: 0.82–0.99; p=0.048). Four-way analysis of all four treatment groups confirmed that PUFA group was at lower risk for combined endpoints of death, non-fatal MI, and non-fatal stroke (RR=0.85, 95% CI: 0.74–0.98; p=0.023) and combined endpoints of cardiovascular disease (CVD) death, non-fatal MI, and non-fatal stroke (RR=0.80, 95% CI: 0.68–0.95; p=0.008). PUFA patients also had reduced risk of individual mortality events: CVD death (RR=0.70, 95% CI: 0.56–0.87; p=0.042), coronary death (RR=0.65, 95% CI: 0.51–0.84; p=0.0226), and sudden death (RR=0.55, 95% CI: 0.40–0.76; p=0.01). Analyzing the combined effects of PUFA and vitamin E showed that treatment reduced the risk for combined endpoints of death, non-fatal MI, and non-fatal stroke (RR=0.86, 95% CI: 0.74–0.99) and for CVD death, non-fatal MI, and non-fatal stroke (RR=0.88, 95% CI: 0.75–1.03). Total mortality also was reduced in PUFA + vitamin E group (RR=0.80, 95% CI: 0.67–0.95) compared to controls. The risk of combined death, non-fatal MI, and non-fatal stroke in PUFA + vitamin E patients was similar to patients taking PUFA alone. Gastrointestinal disturbances and nausea were reported as the most frequent side effects among 4.9% and 1.4% of n-3 PUFA recipients, respectively.

TABLE 13-1 Continued

Reference	Type of Injury/Insult	Type of Study and Subjects	Treatment	Findings/Results
Tier 2: Observational studies				
Mozaffarian et al., 2005	Ischemic stroke	Prospective cohort study n=4,775 > 65 years old, with no history of cerebrovascular disease at baseline follow-up at approximately 12 years	Fish consumption (tuna, other baked or broiled fish, and fried fish or fish sandwich. Note: intake of tuna and other baked or broiled fish is positively correlated with DHA+EPA levels, but fried fish and fish sandwich are not)	Tuna/other baked or broiled fish: compared to subjects with consumption of < 1 time/month, HR (adjusted for CVD risk factors) for those with intake of 1–3 times/month was 0.86 (95% CI: 0.65–1.13), 1–4 times/week was 0.74 (95% CI: 0.57–0.97), and ≥ 5 times/week was 0.72 (95% CI: 0.53–0.98); this trend was significant (p for trend=0.02). Further analysis of the trend showed that the significance existed for period between baseline and 6 years (p=0.03), but not years 6 to 12. Risk of ischemic stroke was reduced in tuna/other fish consumers: HR=0.85 for 1–3 times/month (95% CI: 0.63–1.15), HR=0.72 for 1–4 times/week (95% CI: 0.54–0.96), and HR=0.68 for ≥ 5 times/week (95% CI: 0.48–0.95; p for trend=0.009). Again, the trend was significant from baseline to 6 years (p=0.02), but not from years 6 to 12. Intake frequency had no significant impact on hemorrhagic stroke. Fried fish/fish sandwich: compared to those who ate < 1 time/month, total stroke risk was increased in those who consumed 1–3 times/month (HR=1.15, 95% CI: 0.95–1.39) and ≥ 1 time/week (HR=1.30, 95% CI: 1.04–1.61; p for trend=0.02). Analysis of follow-up period breakdown was not significant. Increased risk of ischemic stroke also was observed in these two groups consuming fried fish/fish sandwiches (1–3 times/month: HR=1.17, 95% CI: 0.96–1.43; ≥ 1 time/week: HR=1.36, 95% CI: 1.08–1.72; p for trend=0.008). This trend was significant during years 6 to 12 (p=0.03). Intake frequency had no significant impact on hemorrhagic stroke. Apart from the increased risk of stroke associated with fried fish/fish sandwich consumption, no other adverse effects were mentioned.

continued

TABLE 13-1 Continued

Reference	Type of Injury/Insult	Type of Study and Subjects	Treatment	Findings/Results
Caicoya, 2002	Stroke	Population-based, case-control study n=913	Fish consumption	Using intake of > 1 g/day as reference, stroke risk in subjects eating 1–22.5 g of fish per day was 70% lower (adjusted OR^g=0.30, 95% CI: 0.12–0.78). Adjusted OR was 0.44 in those with intake of 23–45 g/day (95% CI: 0.18–1.41), 0.59 in those with intake of 46–90 g/day (95% CI: 0.24–1.47), and 0.76 in those with intake of 91–250 g/day (95% CI: 0.27–2.1). Risk of stroke increased with consumption of n-3 fatty acid. Compared to those consuming < 115 mg/day, adjusted OR for 116–319 mg/day was 1.14 (95% CI: 0.60–1.88), for 320–659 mg/day was 1.37 (95% CI: 0.91–2.20), and for > 659 mg/day was 1.76 (95% CI: 0.96–3.26); the trend was significant (χ^2 for trend=2.7, p=0.01). Compared to those with fish intake of < 11.2 g/day, adjusted OR for cerebral infarction in those consuming 11.3–28.7 g/day was 1.05 (95% CI: 0.64–1.65), intake of 28.8–46.5g/day had OR=0.90 (95% CI: 0.55–1.48), and intake of > 46.5 g/day had OR=1.98 (95% CI: 1.08–3.45); the trend was not significant. OR of small, deep cerebral infarction in subjects consuming > 46.5 g/day was 3.21 (95% CI: 1.11–9.20); however, OR for superficial cerebral infarction and intraparenchymatous hemorrhage were not significant. Cerebral infarction in those consuming > 659 mg/day of n-3 fatty acid had adjusted OR=1.89 (95% CI: 0.95–3.75). Besides finding that increased fish consumption was associated with increased risk of stroke and cerebral infarction, no other significant adverse effects were mentioned.

TABLE 13-1 Continued

Reference	Type of Injury/Insult	Type of Study and Subjects	Treatment	Findings/Results
He et al., 2002	Stroke	Prospective cohort study (Health Professional Follow-up Study) n=43,671 men	Fish consumption	Men who consumed fish > 1 time/month had significantly lower risk of ischemic stroke than those who consumed fish < 1 time/month (p < 0.05). Specifically, cumulative consumption of 1–3 times/month had a 43% reduction in risk (RR=0.57, 95% CI: 0.35–0.95), once/week had a 44% reduction (RR=0.56, 95% CI: 0.37–0.84), 2–4 times/week had 45% reduction (RR=0.36–0.85), and ≥ 5 times/week had a 46% reduction (RR=0.54, 95% CI: 0.31–0.94); however, test for trend was not significant.
				Compared to men whose cumulative intake of n-3 PUFA was < 0.05 g/day, those with higher intake had lower risk of ischemic stroke. Intake of 0.05–0.2 g/day was associated with 44% risk reduction (RR=0.56, 95% CI: 0.35–0.88), 0.2–0.4 g/day was associated with 36% reduction (RR=0.63, 95% CI: 0.40–0.98), and 0.4–0.6 g/day was associated with 46% reduction (RR=0.54, 95% CI: 0.32–0.91). Intake of > 0.06 g/day did not significantly reduce risk of ischemic stroke. And test for trend was also not significant.
				Fish consumption and n-3 PUFA intake had no effect on hemorrhagic stroke. And effects of fish consumption on ischemic stroke were not modified by use of fish oil, vitamin E, aspirin, or linolenic acid.
Schlanger et al., 2002	Epilepsy secondary to other CNS diseases	n=5 observation period: 6 months	5 g/day of a spread containing 65% n-3 PUFAs	After 6 months, seizures of grand mal stopped completely in 3 patients, reduced to once a month in 1 patient, and reduced to 3 times/week in another patient. 1 patient experienced seizure of petit mal. In this patient, frequency of petit mal was reduced to once/week from 5 times/week.
				None of the patients experienced adverse effects.

continued

TABLE 13-1 Continued

Reference	Type of Injury/Insult	Type of Study and Subjects	Treatment	Findings/Results
Iso et al., 2001	Stroke	Prospective cohort study (Nurses Health Study) n=79,839 women with no history of stroke, cancer, CVD, diabetes, or high cholesterol level 14-year observation period	Fish and seafood consumption	Increase of fish intake was inversely associated with risk (adjusted for age and smoking) of total stroke (p for trend=0.005), ischemic stroke (p=0.04), thrombotic infarction (p=0.02), and lacunar infarction (p=0.008). After further adjusting for CVD risk factors, intake of fruits and vegetables, saturated and *trans* fat, linoleic acid, animal protein, and calcium, inverse association was still significant for thrombotic infarction (p=0.03) and lacunar infarction (p=0.007). For thrombotic infarction, compared to fish intake of < 1 time/month, multivariate RR for intake of 1–3 times/month was 0.77 (95% CI: 0.46–1.30) and for > 2 times/week was 0.52 (95% CI: 0.27–0.99). For lacunar infarction, multivariate RR for fish intake of 1–3 times/month was 0.63 (95% CI: 0.32–1.24) and for > 2 times/week was 0.28 (95% CI: 0.12–0.67). Increase in PUFA intake was inversely associated with risk of total stroke (p for trend=0.01), lacunar infarction (p=0.01), hemorrhagic stroke (p=0.03), and SAH (p=0.03). After further adjustment for CVD risk factors and dietary pattern, the inverse association remained significant only for lacunar infarction (p=0.004). Compared to PUFA intake in the lowest quintile (median intake of 0.077 g/day), multivariate RR for lacunar infarction was 0.89 (95% CI: 0.55–1.43) in the 2nd quintile and 0.37 (95% CI: 0.19–0.73) in the 5th quintile. When n-3 fatty acid intake exceeded 3 g/day (or, approximately the consumption of fish 3 times or more per day), bleeding time was prolonged.

TABLE 13-1 Continued

Reference	Type of Injury/Insult	Type of Study and Subjects	Treatment	Findings/Results
Tier 3: Animal studies				
Mills et al., 2010; Bailes and Mills, 2010	Traumatic axonal injury, impact acceleration injury	Adult, male Sprague-Dawley rats	Postinjury, oral supplementation of n-3 fatty acids (10 or 40 mg/kg/day) or no treatment	Immunohistochemical analysis showed that injured rats without n-3 fatty acids supplement had significantly increased amyloid precursor protein-labeled axons than sham-injured rats ($p < 0.05$) and rats receiving n-3 fatty supplements ($p < 0.05$); there was no significant difference between supplemented rats and sham-injured rats.
				Further immunohistochemical analysis showed that sham-injured rats and rats receiving n-3 supplementation had significantly fewer caspase-3 positive axons than injured, unsupplemented rats ($p < 0.05$).
Wu et al., 2007	TBI, mild fluid percussion injury (FPI)	Sprague-Dawley rats	Preinjury, diet supplemented with n-3 fatty acids (1.4% DHA and 13.5% EPA) or regular diet for 4 weeks	Injury significantly reduced Sir2α expression ($p < 0.05$ vs. sham-injured rats), but n-3 fatty acid supplementation significantly restored it ($p < 0.05$). Level of oxidized protein was increased after injury ($p < 0.01$ vs. sham), but was reduced by n-3 fatty acid supplementation ($p < 0.01$). Sir2α expression was negatively correlated with oxidized protein level ($r'=-0.67$, $p < 0.05$).
				AMPK and p-AMPK levels were significantly reduced by injury ($p < 0.05$ vs. sham), but were increased to the same level as sham-injured rats by n-3 fatty acid supplementation. In sham-injured and n-3 fatty acid treated rats, Sir2α was correlated with AMPK ($r=0.82$, $p < 0.05$) and p-AMPK ($r=0.96$, $p < 0.05$). The correlations were not significant in injured rats.
				Ubiquitous mitochondrial creatine kinase was significantly reduced in injured rats ($p < 0.05$ vs. sham), but was restored in n-3 fatty acid treated rats.

continued

TABLE 13-1   Continued

Reference	Type of Injury/Insult	Type of Study and Subjects	Treatment	Findings/Results
Wu et al., 2004	TBI, mild fluid percussion injury model	Male, Sprague-Dawley rats	Preinjury, diet supplemented with fish oil (12.4% DHA and 13.5 EPA) or regular diet for 4 weeks before injury and for 1 week after injury	Learning ability in rats was assessed with Morris water maze. Rats fed with fish oil supplemented diet performed significantly better than rats fed with regular diet (p < 0.05) and were similar to sham-injured rats. Swimming speed was similar across all groups.

Levels of BDNF, CREB, and synapsin I were significantly reduced by injury (p < 0.05 vs. sham), but were restored to normal levels with n-3 fatty acid supplementation.

Compared to sham-injured rats, injured rats on regular diet had higher level of oxidized protein (p < 0.01). But injured rats fed with n-3 fatty acid supplemented diet had significantly lower level of oxidized protein compared to injured rats on regular diet and sham-injured rats on both diets (p < 0.01). |

[a] n: sample size.

[b] CI: confidence interval.

[c] SDNN: standard deviation of all normal R-R intervals for 1 hour, where R-R is the time between two r-waves on the ECG.

[d] rs: Spearman's correlation.

[e] HR: hazard ratio.

[f] RR: relative risk.

[g] OR: odds ratio.

[h] χ2: Chi-square.

[i] r: correlation coefficient.

EVIDENCE SUGGESTING INCREASED RESILIENCE

Human Studies

There have been no human studies examining the role of EPA/DHA in providing resilience to traumatic brain injury (TBI). However, several randomized clinical trials have examined the effect of EPA/DHA on other neurological diseases, such as epilepsy and stroke, with mixed results. In a clinical trial including 942 Japanese hypercholesterolemic patients with stroke, use of EPA (1,800 mg/day for approximately five years) led to a significant reduction of stroke recurrence (Tanaka et al., 2008). Use of n-3 fatty acids also was associated with a lower risk of mortality in stroke patients in a small trial (n = 72) (Garbagnati et al., 2009). In another trial including 102 ischemic stroke patients, however, fish oil supplementation (1,200 mg/day) for 12 weeks produced no significant differences from placebo in any lipids, inflammatory, hemostatic, or composite mood parameters (Poppitt et al., 2009). In a small trial including 51 epilepsy patients, seizure frequency was reduced over the first six weeks of supplementation with n-3 fatty acids (1,700 mg/day), but the protective effect was not sustained thereafter (Yeun et al., 2005). Additional studies (from 1990) addressing the influence of EPA/DHA on other CNS injuries or disorders in humans, such as stroke, epilepsy, subarachnoid hemorrhage, and Alzheimer's disease are presented in Table 13-1. The occurrence or absence of adverse effects in humans is included if reported by the authors.

Animal Studies

A series of animal studies (Wu et al., 2004, 2007) showed that preinjury intake of an n-3 fatty acid–enriched diet (8 percent of total energy) could counteract some of the damaging effects of TBI by, for example, normalizing levels of molecular systems associated with energy homeostasis (e.g., Sir2α), ameliorating protein oxidation, and improving learning ability (Table 13-1). These results suggest potential neuroprotective effects of n-3 fatty acids on TBI.

EVIDENCE INDICATING EFFECT ON TREATMENT

Human Studies

There have been no clinical trials conducted to determine the efficacy of n-3 fatty acid infusion for treatment of TBI. Nevertheless, n-3 fatty acid infusion into healthy human subjects affects several inflammatory pathways in a way that could be beneficial for TBI patients: platelet aggregation and thromboxane B_2 synthesis were reduced within 60 minutes of infusion (Elmadfa et al., 1993). In a different study, the ratio of n-3 to n-6 fatty acids in monocyte membranes likewise increased, monocyte synthesis of interleukin-1 and TNF decreased, and monocyte adhesion/transendothelial migration decreased within 48 hours after initiation of infusion (Mayer et al., 2003).

Animal Studies

In a 2010 study using an impact acceleration head injury model, 40 adult male Sprague-Dawley rats were assigned to four groups (n = 10 per group), of which two groups received dietary supplementation of n-3 fatty acids (EPA:DHA = 2:1) at a dosage of 10 or 40 mg/kg/day, starting on postinjury day one (Mills et al., 2010). The authors found that, compared to injured rats on the control diet, n-3 fatty acids significantly reduced the number of beta-amyloid precursor protein-positive (injured) axons at 30 days postinjury, achieving levels similar to those in uninjured animals.

CONCLUSIONS AND RECOMMENDATIONS

The n-3 fatty acid status of the active-duty military population is unknown. A survey by Lieberman et al. (2010) sought to determine the current usage of dietary supplements in U.S. Army soldiers on active duty. Fish oil was grouped in an "other" category that included supplements such as melatonin, caffeine, coenzyme Q10, and lycopene. The authors reported that 11 percent of military personnel in combat-arms positions and 23 percent of those in Special Forces were taking "other" supplements. Data on the EPA and DHA concentrations measured in frozen serum (some archived for up to several years) from military personnel suggest that the levels are lower than in the civilian population (Lewis et al., 2011). There were a number of methodological differences, however, in the comparison civilian studies, such as measurement of fresh (not frozen) serum samples, expression of DHA as a percentage of fatty acids in serum phospholipids (rather than total fatty acids), or measurement of DHA levels in red blood cell membranes (rather than serum). Differences in DHA concentrations between military and civilian populations might thus be attributable to methodological issues. In order to definitively determine if such differences exist, it will be necessary to conduct a prospective study in which samples from both populations are collected, stored, processed, and assayed in a uniform manner. By better determining the n-3 fatty acid status of military personnel, these data will also provide a basis for recommending increases in intake of n-3 fatty acid should future research findings indicate a role in resilience to TBI.

It is well documented that fish-oil supplementation will decrease inflammation. The influences of n-3 fatty acids on prostaglandin, leukotriene, cytokine, and ROS were described earlier in this chapter, and extensive reviews are available (Calder, 2006; Massaro et al., 2008). When taken orally, the effects of n-3 fatty acids are not evident for days to weeks because of their slow incorporation into cellular membranes. Initiation of oral administration after TBI therefore may not be of immediate benefit (although when evaluated 30 days after injury, the 2010 animal study by Mills and colleagues showed reductions in neuronal toxicity). On the other hand, evidence from human subjects indicates that intravenous administration of n-3 fatty acids can have more immediate effects. This is especially relevant to military operational settings, where the feasibility of a feeding tube or oral administration is greatly reduced immediately following injury. Overall, continuous administration—whether enteral, parenteral, or intravenous—is considered to be most effective in the early phase of severe TBI.

RECOMMENDATION 13-1. DoD should conduct animal studies that examine the effectiveness of preinjury and postinjury oral administration of current commercial preparations of purified n-3 fatty acids on TBI outcomes.

RECOMMENDATION 13-2. Based on the evidence that fish oil decreases inflammation within hours of continuous administration, human clinical trials that investigate fish oil or purified n-3 fatty acids as a treatment of TBI are recommended. For acute cases of TBI, it should be noted that there are intravenous fish oil formulations available in Europe, but these are not approved by the Food and Drug Administration. Continuous enteral feeding with a feeding formula containing fish oil should provide equivalent effects for this purpose in the early phase of severe TBI when enteral access becomes available.

REFERENCES

Bailes, J. E., and J. D. Mills. 2010. Docosahexaenoic acid reduces traumatic axonal injury in a rodent head injury model. *Journal of Neurotrauma* 27(9):1617–1624.

Bromfield, E., B. Dworetzky, S. Hurwitz, Z. Eluri, L. Lane, S. Replansky, and D. Mostofsky. 2008. A randomized trial of polyunsaturated fatty acids for refractory epilepsy. *Epilepsy and Behavior* 12(1):187–190.

Caicoya, M. 2002. Fish consumption and stroke: A community case-control study in Asturias, Spain. *Neuroepidemiology* 21(3):107–114.

Calder, P. C. 2006. N-3 polyunsaturated fatty acids, inflammation, and inflammatory diseases. *American Journal of Clinical Nutrition* 83(6 Suppl.):1505S–1519S.

DeGiorgio, C. M., P. Miller, S. Meymandi, and J. A. Gornbein. 2008. N-3 fatty acids (fish oil) for epilepsy, cardiac risk factors, and risk of sudep: Clues from a pilot, double-blind, exploratory study. *Epilepsy and Behavior* 13(4):681–684.

Dyall, S. C., and A. T. Michael-Titus. 2008. Neurological benefits of omega-3 fatty acids. *Neuromolecular Medicine* 10(4):219–235.

Dyerberg, J. 1993. Epidemiology of n-3 fatty acids and disease. In *Fatty acids and vascular disease*, edited by R. De Caterina, S. Endres, S. D. Kristensen and E. B. Schmidt. London: Springer-Verlag.

Elmadfa, I., S. Stroh, K. Brandt, and E. Schlotzer. 1993. Influence of a single parenteral application of a 10% fish oil emulsion on plasma fatty acid pattern and the function of thrombocytes in young adult men. *Annals of Nutrition and Metabolism* 37(1):8–13.

Endres, S., R. Ghorbani, V. E. Kelley, K. Georgilis, G. Lonnemann, J. W. M. van der Meer, J. G. Cannon, T. S. Rogers, M. S. Klempner, P. C. Weber, E. J. Schaefer, S. M. Wolff, and C. A. Dinarello. 1989. The effect of dietary supplementation with n-3 polyunsaturated fatty acids on the synthesis of interleukin-1 and tumor necrosis factor by mononuclear cells. *The New England Journal of Medicine* 320(5):265–271.

Garbagnati, F., G. Cairella, A. De Martino, M. Multari, U. Scognamiglio, V. Venturiero, and S. Paolucci. 2009. Is antioxidant and n-3 supplementation able to improve functional status in poststroke patients? Results from the Nutristroke Trial. *Cerebrovascular Diseases* 27(4):375–383.

GISSI (Gruppo Italiano per lo Studio della Sopravvivenza nell'Infarto miocardico)-Prevenzione Investigators. 1999. Dietary supplementation with n-3 polyunsaturated fatty acids and vitamin E after myocardial infarction: Results of the GISSI-Prevenzione Trial. *Lancet* 354(9177):447–455.

Hamilton, J., and K. Brunaldi. 2007. A model for fatty acid transport into the brain. *Journal of Molecular Neuroscience* 33(1):12–17.

He, K., E. B. Rimm, A. Merchant, B. A. Rosner, M. J. Stampfer, W. C. Willett, and A. Ascherio. 2002. Fish consumption and risk of stroke in men. *The Journal of the American Medical Association* 288(24):3130–3136.

Huang, W. L., V. R. King, O. E. Curran, S. C. Dyall, R. E. Ward, N. Lal, J. V. Priestley, and A. T. Michael-Titus. 2007. A combination of intravenous and dietary docosahexaenoic acid significantly improves outcome after spinal cord injury. *Brain* 130(Pt 11):3004–3019.

IOM (Institute of Medicine). 2005. *Dietary Reference Intakes for energy, carbohydrate, fiber, fat, fatty acids, cholesterol, protein, and amino acids (macronutrients).* Washington, DC: The National Academies Press.

Iso, H., K. M. Rexrode, M. J. Stampfer, J. E. Manson, G. A. Colditz, F. E. Speizer, C. H. Hennekens, and W. C. Willett. 2001. Intake of fish and omega-3 fatty acids and risk of stroke in women. *Journal of the American Medical Association* 285(3):304–312.

Javierre, C., J. Vidal, R. Segura, M. A. Lizarraga, J. Medina, and J. L. Ventura. 2006. The effect of supplementation with n-3 fatty acids on the physical performance in subjects with spinal cord injury. *Journal of Physiology and Biochemistry* 62(4):271–279.

Jones, P. J. H., and S. Kubow. 2006. Lipids, sterols, and their metabolites. In *Modern nutrition in health and disease.* 10th ed., edited by M. E. Shils, M. Shike, A. C. Ross, B. Caballero and R. J. Cousins. Baltimore, MD: Lippincott Williams & Wilkins. Pp. 92–122.

Kramer, H. J., J. Stevens, F. Grimminger, and W. Seeger. 1996. Fish oil fatty acids and human platelets: Dose dependent decrease in dienoic and increase in trienoic thromboxane generation. *Biochemical Pharmacology* 52(8):1211–1217.

Kris-Etherton, P. M., D. S. Taylor, S. Yu-Poth, P. Huth, K. Moriarty, V. Fishell, R. L. Hargrove, G. Zhao, and T. D. Etherton. 2000. Polyunsaturated fatty acids in the food chain in the United States. *American Journal of Clinical Nutrition* 71(1 Suppl.):179S–188S.

Kris-Etherton, P. M., W. S. Harris, L. J. Appel, and AHA (American Heart Association) Nutrition Committee. 2002. Fish consumption, fish oil, omega-3 fatty acids, and cardiovascular disease. *Circulation* 106(21):2747–2757.

Lauritzen, L., H. S. Hansen, M. H. Jorgensen, and K. F. Michaelsen. 2001. The essentiality of long chain n-3 fatty acids in relation to development and function of the brain and retina. *Progress in Lipid Research* 40(1–2):1–94.

Lewis, M. D., J. R. Hibbeln, J. E. Johnson, Y. H. Lin, D. Y. Hyun, and J. D. Loewke. 2011. Suicide deaths of active duty U.S. military and omega-3 fatty acid status: A case control comparison. *The Journal of Clinical Psychiatry* 72 (forthcoming).

Lieberman, H. R., T. B. Stavinoha, S. M. McGraw, A. White, L. S. Hadden, and B. P. Marriott. 2010. Use of dietary supplements among active-duty U.S. Army soldiers. *American Journal of Clinical Nutrition* 92(4):985–995.

Massaro, M., E. Scoditti, M. A. Carluccio, and R. De Caterina. 2008. Basic mechanisms behind the effects of n-3 fatty acids on cardiovascular disease. *Prostaglandins Leukotrienes and Essential Fatty Acids* 79(3–5):109–115.

Mayer, K., S. Meyer, M. Reinholz-Muhly, U. Maus, M. Merfels, J. Lohmeyer, F. Grimminger, and W. Seeger. 2003. Short-time infusion of fish oil-based lipid emulsions, approved for perenteral nutrition, reduces monocyte proinflammatory cytokine generation and adhesive interaction with endothelium in humans. *Journal of Immunology* 171(9):4837–4843.

Mills, J. D., J. E. Bailes, C. L. Sedney, H. Hutchins, and B. Sears. 2010. Omega-3 fatty acid supplementation and reduction of traumatic axonal injury in a rodent head injury model. *Journal of Neurosurgery* 114(1):77–84.

Mozaffarian, D., W. T. Longstreth Jr, R. N. Lemaitre, T. A. Manolio, L. H. Kuller, G. L. Burke, and D. S. Siscovick. 2005. Fish consumption and stroke risk in elderly individuals: The cardiovascular health study. *Archives of Internal Medicine* 165(2):200–206.

Poppitt, S. D., C. A. Howe, F. E. Lithander, K. M. Silvers, R. B. Lin, J. Croft, Y. Ratnasabapathy, R. A. Gibson, and C. S. Anderson. 2009. Effects of moderate-dose omega-3 fish oil on cardiovascular risk factors and mood after ischemic stroke: A randomized, controlled trial. *Stroke* 40(11):3485–3492.

Puri, B. K., M. J. Koepp, J. Holmes, G. Hamilton, and A. W. C. Yuen. 2007. A 31-phosphorus neurospectroscopy study of omega-3 long-chain polyunsaturated fatty acid intervention with eicosapentaenoic acid and docosa-hexaenoic acid in patients with chronic refractory epilepsy. *Prostaglandins Leukotrienes and Essential Fatty Acids* 77(2):105–107.

Schlanger, S., M. Shinitzky, and D. Yam. 2002. Diet enriched with omega-3 fatty acids alleviates convulsion symptoms in epilepsy patients. *Epilepsia* 43(1):103–104.

Schwab, J. M., N. Chiang, M. Arita, and C. N. Serhan. 2007. Resolvin E1 and protectin D1 activate inflammation-resolution programmes. *Nature* 447(7146):869–874.

Serhan, C. N. 2006. Resolution phase of inflammation: Novel endogenous anti-inflammatory and proresolving lipid mediators and pathways. *Annual Review of Immunology* 25:101–137.

Tanaka, K., Y. Ishikawa, M. Yokoyama, H. Origasa, M. Matsuzaki, Y. Saito, Y. Matsuzawa, J. Sasaki, S. Oikawa, H. Hishida, H. Itakura, T. Kita, A. Kitabatake, N. Nakaya, T. Sakata, K. Shimada, and K. Shirato. 2008. Reduction in the recurrence of stroke by eicosapentaenoic acid for hypercholesterolemic patients: Subanalysis of the JELIS trial. *Stroke* 39(7):2052–2058.

Wu, A., Z. Ying, and F. Gomez-Pinilla. 2004. Dietary omega-3 fatty acids normalize BDNF levels, reduce oxidative damage, and counteract learning disability after traumatic brain injury in rats. *Journal of Neurotrauma* 21(10):1457–1467.

Wu, A. G., Z. Ying, and F. Gomez-Pinilla. 2007. Omega-3 fatty acids supplementation restores mechanisms that maintain brain homeostasis in traumatic brain injury. *Journal of Neurotrauma* 24(10):1587–1595.

Wu, D., and S. N. Meydani. 1998. N-3 polyunsaturated fatty acids and immune function. *Proceedings of the Nutrition Society* 57(4):503–509.

Yeun, A. W., J. W. Sander, D. Fluegel, P. N. Patsalos, G.S. Bell, T. Johnson, and M.J. Koepp. 2005. Omega-3 fatty acid supplementation in patients with chronic epilepsy: A randomized trial. *Epilepsy & Behavior* 7(2):253–258.

Yoneda, H., S. Shirao, T. Kurokawa, H. Fujisawa, S. Kato, and M. Suzuki. 2008. Does eicosapentaenoic acid (EPA) inhibit cerebral vasospasm in patients after aneurysmal subarachnoid hemorrhage? *Acta Neurologica Scandinavica* 118(1):54–59.

Yuen, A. W. C., J. W. Sander, D. Fluegel, P. N. Patsalos, G. S. Bell, T. Johnson, and M. J. Koepp. 2005. Omega-3 fatty acid supplementation in patients with chronic epilepsy: A randomized trial. *Epilepsy and Behavior* 7(2):253–258.

14

Polyphenols

Polyphenols are a diverse group of naturally occurring compounds widely distributed in many plant-based foods and plant-derived beverages. More than 8,000 have been identified in various plant species, and commonly consumed phytonutrient-rich foods include cocoa, tea, soy products, apples, onions, and *Ginkgo biloba*. Polyphenols arise from the common intermediate phenylalanine, or a precursor, shikimic acid. The main classes of polyphenols, based on their structure, are phenolic acids, flavonoids, stilbenes, and lignans. In food, these compounds are usually found complexed to sugar groups that must be removed by intestinal or colonic microfloral enzymatic hydrolysis. This process makes the identification of all the metabolites and evaluation of biological activity difficult, but the increase in antioxidant capacity of the plasma after consumption of polyphenol-rich foods provides evidence of absorption through the gut barrier (Pandey and Rizvi, 2009) (see Doré in Appendix C). There is interest in this group of compounds because of human and animal studies suggesting that long-term consumption is associated with protection against many chronic diseases such as cancer, cardiovascular diseases, and neurodegenerative diseases. It is important to note, however, that although studies on plasma levels and dietary intakes can be used to initiate hypotheses about nutrient status and health outcomes, their findings often vary, making it difficult to reach conclusions. It is obvious that these bioactive compounds are a heterogeneous group, with different structures and pharmacological properties.

Although few studies have been conducted to test their effects in traumatic brain injury (TBI), their mechanism of action in protecting against cardiovascular and neurodegenerative diseases suggests that they warrant attention as neuroprotectants against this disease. Flavonoids, for example, are able to interact with neuronal signaling pathways critical in controlling neuronal survival (see Doré in Appendix C). The committee selected flavonoids, specifically the flavonoid curcumin, and a stilbene, resveratrol, for review because their health effects have been studied most extensively. A list of human studies evaluating the effectiveness of these compounds in providing resilience or treating TBI or related diseases or conditions (i.e., subarachnoid hemorrhage, intracranial aneurysm, stroke, anoxic or hypoxic ischemia, epilepsy) in the acute phase is presented in Tables 14-1 (flavonoids) and 14-2 (resveratrol), which also include supporting evidence from animal models of TBI. All studies included in these tables are from 1990 and after. The occurrence or absence of adverse effects in humans is included if reported by the authors.

FLAVONOIDS

Flavonoids are the group of polyphenols most studied. Their structure consists of two aromatic rings bound together by three carbons that form an oxygenated heterocycle. More than 4,000 flavonoids have been identified and categorized into seven subclasses, based on their structure: flavonols (e.g., quercetin), flavones (e.g., apigenin), flavanones (e.g., hesperetin), flavan-3-ols (e.g., epicatechin), anthocyanins (e.g., cyanidin), polymers (e.g., proanthocyanidins), and isoflavones (e.g., genistein). In addition to their antioxidant capacity, flavonoids can also alleviate neuroinflammation and regulate mitochondrial function and neuronal cell signaling cascades (Ramassamy, 2006; Spencer, 2008; Vafeiadou et al., 2007). Because of these properties and their ability to pass through the blood-brain barrier (BBB) (Dreiseitel et al., 2009; Youdim et al., 2004), flavonoids have been suggested as potential neuroprotective agents. Below is an overview of selected human trials that summarizes the evidence on flavonoid use for the prevention of cardiovascular diseases, a group of diseases that share some common pathways (e.g., oxidative stress and inflammation) with TBI (see Table 14-1 for both human and animal studies from 1990 and later). The results from animal studies on flavonoids and TBI are also presented. The committee highlights curcumin as one flavonoid for which there is substantial evidence of neuroprotectant effects in animal models of TBI.

In light of the work of Miller and colleagues (2005), any trials undertaken should ensure that dose levels of flavonoids do not approach levels that might cause adverse events, such as higher risk of mortality.

Evidence Indicating Effects on Resilience

Human Studies

Hollman and colleagues reviewed six prospective observational studies (n = 111,067) addressing the effects of dietary intake of flavonol on stroke risk (Hollman et al., 2010). In this review, the pooled RR of stroke, for the highest versus the lowest intake of flavonol, was 0.80. In a sample of 9,208 Finnish men and women, apple consumption was significantly associated with a reduced risk of developing thrombotic stroke during a 28-year follow-up period (Knekt et al., 2000). However, the authors failed to find any significant association between quercetin and stroke (Knekt et al., 2000). Consumption of tea, as well as catechin, was not associated with significantly lower risks of stroke in the Zutphen Elderly study (806 men aged 65–84 years at baseline) in the Netherlands (Arts et al., 2001), or the College Alumni Health Study in Japan (17,228 participants with a mean age of 59.5 years at baseline) (Sesso et al., 2003b). The Women's Health study, a large, randomized, clinical control trial that looked at vitamin E and cardiovascular disease, examined the association of food intakes of flavonols and flavones and primary food sources of flavonoids with cardiovascular disease (Sesso et al., 2003a). The study found no clear association with stroke. The authors observed nonsignificant inverse associations of the consumption of broccoli, apples, and tea with important vascular events. It is, however, noteworthy that estimation of total flavonoid intake in this study was based on an obsolete food composition table, which included only two flavonoid subclasses (flavonols and flavones). The potential neuroprotective effects of

TABLE 14-1 Relevant Data Identified for Flavonoids

Reference	Type of Injury/ Insult	Type of Study and Subjects	Treatment	Findings/Results
Tier 1: Clinical trials				
Cao et al., 2008	Acute cerebral infarction	Meta-analysis of 9 randomized and quasi-randomized controlled clinical trials n^d=723 male and female patients	Dengzhanhua (Erigeron breviscapus) alone or as supplement to another treatment vs. placebo or no treatment	None of the outcome measures of this meta-analysis (death from any cause at the end of follow-up period, death or dependence at the end of follow-up period, quality of life, and adverse events) were included in any of the selected trials. However, post hoc analysis showed that, compared to controls, patients taking dengzhanhua were more likely to have at least 45% improvement in neurologic condition (RR^b=1.53, 95% CI^c: 1.36–1.72). Study heterogeneity was 0%.
Chan et al., 2008	Brachial flow-mediated dilatation	Randomized, double-blind, placebo-controlled n=102	Postinjury, isoflavone supplement (80 mg/day) or placebo for 12 weeks	Compared with controls, isoflavone-treated patients had greater flow-mediated dilatation (FMD; 1.2% vs. –0.1%, p=0.035) and lower prevalence of impaired FMD (58% vs. 79%, p=0.023) at 12 weeks. Adjusted for baseline differences in FMD, isoflavone treatment was found to be associated with lower prevalence of FMD impairment (OR^d=0.32, 95% CI: 0.13–0.80; p=0.014). Treatment effect on brachial FMD was inversely related to baseline FMD (r^e=–0.514, p < 0.001). Isoflavone treatment had greater effect on current or past smokers than non-smokers (p=0.045) and on non-diabetics than diabetics (p=0.030). Moreover, isoflavone treatment for 12 weeks lowered high sensitivity-C-reactive protein level (treatment effect =–1.7%, 95% CI: –3.3 to –0.1%; p=0.033). There was no significant effect on nitroglycerin-mediated dilatation, blood pressure, heart rate, serum levels of fasting glucose and insulin, hemoglobin A1c, or oxidative stress. No significant adverse effects from the isoflavone treatment were mentioned.

continued

TABLE 14-1   Continued

Reference	Type of Injury/ Insult	Type of Study and Subjects	Treatment	Findings/Results
Le Bars et al., 2000	Dementia (uncomplicated Alzheimer's disease or multi-infarct dementia)	Double-blind, placebo-controlled, fixed dose, parallel-group, multicenter study	*Ginkgo biloba* extract (EGb), 120 mg dose (40 mg t.i.d.), 26-week treatment	Compared to baseline, the placebo group had a significant 1.3 point increase on Alzheimer's Disease Assessment Scale Cognitive Subscale (ADAS-Cog, p=0.01), while EGb group had a 0.7 point decrease at 26 weeks; the difference of 2 points between the two groups was significant (p=0.007).
		n=224		Compared to baseline value of the Geriatric Evaluation by Relative's Rating Instrument, the placebo group had a worsening of 0.06 points, while the EGb group had an improvement of 0.06 points (p=0.02). The placebo group's mean rating on the Clinical Global Impression of Change worsened compared to baseline (p=0.008), while the EGb group experienced no change; the difference between groups was not significant.
				Over the course of the study, 87 patients reported 149 adverse events, of which 69 were mild, 60 were moderate, and 20 were severe. Of the 20 severe adverse events, 13 were reported by patients in the EGb group, 7 by patients in the placebo group. Adverse events were distributed equally between the two groups, except those related to gastrointestinal system, which occurred more frequently in EGb group.

Tier 2: Observational studies

Hollman et al., 2010	Stroke	Meta-analysis of 7 prospective cohort studies with data from individuals free of CVD or stroke at baseline (data from 6 cohorts) n_{pooled}=111,067	Flavonol intake	Compared to subjects with the lowest amount of flavonoid consumption, those with the highest consumption had a significantly reduced risk of fatal or non-fatal stroke (pooled RR=0.80, 95% CI: 0.65–0.98, p=0.05). However, there was significant heterogeneity among the studies (54%, p=0.05) and publication bias (p=0.01). No adverse effects were mentioned.

TABLE 14-1 Continued

Reference	Type of Injury/ Insult	Type of Study and Subjects	Treatment	Findings/Results
Mursu et al., 2008	Cardiovascular disease (CVD), especially strokes	Prospective, population-based trial (Kuopio Ischaemic Heart Disease Risk Factor Study) n=1,950 Finnish men aged 42–60 years, free of prior coronary heart disease or stroke average follow-up period=15.2 years	Flavonoids and flavonoid subclasses from non-controlled diet	Intake of flavonols, a subclass of flavonoids, was inversely associated with risk of ischemic stroke (p for trend=0.027). The risk of ischemic stroke in men taking the highest amount of flavonols was 48% lower than in men taking the lowest amount (RR=0.52, 95% CI: 0.30–0.90). However, total flavonoids intake and intake of other subclasses had no significant effect on risk of ischemic stroke. Although there was a nonsignificant inverse association between flavones and risk of CVD mortality, total flavonoid intake and intake of other subclasses had no effect on CVD mortality. No adverse effects of flavonoid intake were mentioned.
Kokubo et al., 2007	Cerebral and myocardial infarctions (MI)	Japan Public Health Center-Based Study Cohort n=40,462 participants, aged 40–59 years, without prior CVD or cancer at baseline average follow-up period=12.5 years	Soy and isoflavone intake	Soy intake had no significant association with cerebral infarction, MI, or ischemic CVD mortality in men. But in women, risk of cerebral infarction was inversely associated with intake of soy (multivariable HR[f]=0.64, 95% CI: 0.43–0.95, p=0.037) and beans (HR=0.62, 95% CI: 0.39–0.97, p=0.018). Risk of MI was inversely associated with intake of soy (HR=0.45, 95% CI: 0.23–0.88, p=0.024). Risk for cerebral infarction and MI combined was reduced with increased intake of soy (HR=0.64, p=0.008) and beans (HR=0.65, p=0.022). High level of soy intake also reduced ischemic CVD mortality in women (multivariable HR=0.31, 95% CI: 0.13–0.74). Isoflavone intake was only associated with risk of CI in men (HR=1.16, 95% CI: 0.84–1.61, p=0.046). In women, isoflavone intake reduced risk of cerebral infarction (multivariable HR=0.35, 95% CI: 0.21–0.59, p=0.015), MI (multivariable HR=0.37, 95% CI: 0.14–0.98, p=0.006), and combined cerebral infarction and MI (multivariable HR=0.39, 95% CI: 0.25–0.60, p < 0.001). Isoflavone also reduced risk of ischemic CVD mortality (HR=0.56, 95% CI: 0.21–1.44, p=0.01). Risk of ischemic CVD was significantly reduced in post-menopausal women taking isoflavone (multivariable HR=0.25, 95% CI: 0.14–0.45, p < 0.001) but not in pre-menopausal women. No adverse effects were mentioned.

continued

TABLE 14-1   Continued

Reference	Type of Injury/ Insult	Type of Study and Subjects	Treatment	Findings/Results
Sesso et al., 2003a	CVD and important vascular events (MI, stroke, and cardiovascular death)	Randomized, double-blind, placebo-controlled trial (Women's Health Study) n=38,445 female U.S. health professionals free of CVD and cancer, aged 45–89 years	Flavonols and flavones (quercetin, kaempferol, myricetin, apigenin, luteolin) and primary food sources of flavonoids (tea, broccoli, apples, onions, tofu)	Total and individual flavonoid intake had no significant effect on CVD, major vascular events, MI, or stroke. There also was no inverse association between flavonoid intake and CVD death. No effect was seen after adjusting for confounders. Analysis of select food intake showed beneficial effect of broccoli on CVD (age-adjusted RR=0.58, 95% CI: 0.38–0.89, p=0.027), apples on CVD (age-adjusted RR=0.58, 95% CI: 0.41–0.81, p=0.015), and apples on important vascular events (age-adjusted RR=0.49, 95% CI: 0.32–0.76, p=0.015). However, these effects were not significant after further adjusting for CVD risk factors and dietary pattern. No adverse effects of flavonoid intake were mentioned.
Sesso et al., 2003b	CVD, coronary heart disease, and stroke	Prospective study (College Alumni Health Study) n=17,228 (95.6% male; mean age of 59.5 years), free of prior CVD and cancer at baseline average follow-up period=15 years	Tea consumption— specifically catechin intake	Consumption of tea had no significant association with risk of CVD, coronary heart disease, stroke, or CVD death. Stratifying subjects by age, gender, and hypertension and diabetes statuses also showed no effect for tea consumption. Analysis of original group of subjects (male Harvard alumni) showed that men who drank tea throughout the follow-up period had a 36% reduction in stroke risk compared to those who never drank tea (age-adjusted RR=0.64, p < 0.05). No adverse effects were mentioned.

TABLE 14-1   Continued

Reference	Type of Injury/ Insult	Type of Study and Subjects	Treatment	Findings/Results
Polidori et al., 2002	Acute ischemic stroke	Case-control study n=104 (28 stroke patients and 76 controls), age 76.9 ± 8.7 years	Measured level of 6 carotenoids (lutein, zeaxanthin, beta-cryptoxanthin, lycopene, alpha- and beta-carotene) and compared to healthy, normolipidemic control group	Upon admission, the stroke patients had significantly lower plasma levels of lutein (p < 0.04), lycopene (p < 0.001), α-carotene (p < 0.001), and β-carotene (p < 0.004) and significantly higher levels of malondialdehyde (MDA, p < 0.001) than controls. During follow-up, all stroke patients had a decrease in plasma carotenoid levels in the first 24 hours; the levels return to normal in the following days, except in patients who experienced a decline in functional independence between 2 weeks prior to stroke and admission or 1 week after stroke. These patients had lower levels of lutein (p < 0.01) and higher levels of MDA (p < 0.05) than controls. There was an inverse relationship between MDA levels and Canadian Neurological Score (CNS) score on day 1 of follow up (r=−0.37, p < 0.05) and a positive correlation between lutein levels and CNS score on day 7 (r=0.51, p < 0.03). No significant adverse effects were mentioned.
Arts et al., 2001	Ischemic heart disease and stroke	Prospective cohort study (Zutphen Elderly Study) n=806 men aged 65–84 years	Examine tea consumption— specifically catechin intake and the risk of cardiovascular disease	There was significant inverse relationship between catechin intake and risk of ischemic heart disease mortality (RR=0.49, 95% CI: 0.27–0.88, p=0.17; RR adjusted for age, MI and angina pectoris at baseline, CVD risk factors, and dietary patterns). The inverse relationship between catechin intake and MI incidence was only significant in the age-adjusted model (RR=0.54, 95% CI: 0.32–0.93, p=0.026). Catechin had no effect on stroke mortality or incidence. Catechin intake was highly correlated to tea consumption (r=0.98) and flavonol intake (r=0.85), but tea intake was not significantly related to risk of ischemic heart disease mortality. And effects of catechin and flavonol from sources other than tea were not significant. No adverse effects were mentioned.

continued

TABLE 14-1   Continued

Reference	Type of Injury/ Insult	Type of Study and Subjects	Treatment	Findings/Results
Knekt et al., 2000	Cerebrovascular disease (CVA)	Cohort study n=9,208 men and women, aged 15 years or older and initially free of CVA	Studying relation between quercetin intake and subsequent incidence of CVA	Quercetin intake had no significant effect on CVA in men or women. However, apple consumption was inversely associated with risk of thrombosis or embolisms in women (RR=0.61, 95% CI: 0.33–1.12, p for trend=0.02). Consumption of onion was associated with risk of acute strokes (RR=1.37, 95% CI: 0.91–2.08, p=0.01) and thrombosis or embolisms (RR=1.44, 95% CI: 0.90–2.31, p=0.008). High quercetin intake increased the risk of thrombotic stroke in both men and women who had diabetes (men: RR=18.5, 95 CI: 2.77–123.5; women: RR=2.79, 95% CI: 1.18–2.36; both: $p < 0.05$).
Keli et al., 1996	Stroke	Cohort study (Zutphen Study) n=552 men, aged 50–69 years follow-up period=15 years	Examining flavonoid intake	Flavonoid intake was greater in men who had not had a stroke than in those who had (23.8 mg/day vs. 20.7 mg/day, $p < 0.01$). The risk of stroke was reduced in men who had the highest intake of flavonoids (≥ 28.6 mg/day) compared to men with the lowest intake (< 18.3 mg/day, RR=0.27, 95% CI: 0.11–0.70, p=0.004). Flavonoid intake was correlated with tea consumption (r=0.94, $p < 0.001$), which is inversely associated with stroke incidence (RR=0.31, 95% CI: 0.31–0.84, p=0.02). Flavonoid intake was also correlated with solid fruit consumption (R=0.31, $p < 0.001$), which has a nonsignificant inverse association on stroke incidence. No adverse effects were mentioned.

TABLE 14-1 Continued

Reference	Type of Injury/ Insult	Type of Study and Subjects	Treatment	Findings/Results
Tier 3: Animal studies				
Laird et al., 2010	TBI (cerebral edema), moderate controlled cortical impact	Male CD-1 mice	Curcumin 15 minutes pre- and 30 minutes or 1 hour postinjury, 75, 150 or 300 mg/kg or DMSO placebo (dimethyl sulfoxide)	Edema in the ipsilateral cortex was reduced with pretreatment of 75 mg/kg ($p < 0.05$ compared to placebo-treated mice and sham-injured mice) and 150 mg/kg ($p < 0.001$ against placebo-treated mice) of curcumin. Treatment with 150 mg/kg and 300 mg/kg of curcumin 30 minutes after injury was also effective in reducing edema (both $p < 0.05$ vs. placebo). However, curcumin did not reduce lesion size.
				In postinjury tests of neurological functions, mice pretreated with curcumin had greater amount of locomotor activity ($p < 0.05$ vs. placebo; similar to sham mice) and spent more time exploring new objects ($p < 0.05$ vs. placebo; similar to sham mice).
				Pre-treatment with 150 mg/kg of curcumin reduced the induction of AQP4 ($p < 0.05$ vs. placebo; not significantly different from sham mice). Posttreatment with 300 mg/kg also reduced AQP4 expression ($p < 0.05$ vs. placebo and sham). Pretreatment with 150 mg/kg of curcumin reduced expression of interleukin-1β to the level of sham-injured mice at 6 hours ($p < 0.05$ vs. placebo) and 12 hours ($p < 0.001$ vs. placebo). Pretreatment with 150 mg/kg of curcumin also reduced the expression of GFAP (Glial fibrillary acid protein) after injury to the level of sham-injured mice ($p < 0.05$ vs. placebo).
Sharma et al., 2009	TBI, mild fluid percussion injury	Male Sprague-Dawley rats Age: approximately 2 months	Preinjury, diet supplemented with 500 ppm curcumin or regular diet for 4 weeks	pAMPK/AMPK ratio, ubiquitous mitochondrial creatine kinase level, and UCP2 level were significantly reduced by injury ($p < 0.05$ vs. sham), but were restored by curcumin supplementation ($p < 0.05$ vs. injured, regular diet rats).
				Further, injury also deceased the level of COX-II in rats ($p < 0.05$ vs. sham). But curcumin supplementation restored the COX-II level to 96% of sham-injured rats ($p < 0.01$ vs. injured, regular diet rats). Sir2 level decreased to 71% after injury ($p < 0.01$ vs. sham), but curcumin restored Sir2 level to 105% ($p < 0.01$ vs. injured, regular diet rats).

continued

TABLE 14-1 Continued

Reference	Type of Injury/ Insult	Type of Study and Subjects	Treatment	Findings/Results
Di Giorgio et al., 2008	TBI, moderate lateral fluid percussion TBI	Adult, male Sprague-Dawley rats	Pre- and postinjury, curcumin (3, 30, 300 mg/kg), α-tocopherol (100 mg/kg), DMSO (1 ml/ kg), or saline (1 ml/kg), 30 minutes prior to injury, then 30 and 90 minutes after injury	Compared to rats treated with saline, rats that received curcumin (at all 3 dosages), DMSO, and α-tocopherol had significantly less neuron degeneration ($p < 0.05$). But there was no significant difference between the 3 treatment groups.
Wu et al., 2006	TBI, mild fluid percussion injury model	Male, Sprague-Dawley rats	Preinjury, regular diet, regular diet with curcumin (500ppm), high-fat diet, or high-fat diet with curcumin (500ppm), for 4 weeks	Rats on diets without curcumin had significantly higher level of oxidized proteins compared to sham-injured rats ($p < 0.01$), but rats on diets with curcumin had lower oxidized protein level than sham-injured rats ($p < 0.01$). Curcumin had no effect on sham-injured rats.
				Injury lowered BDNF level, CREB, synapsin I and phosphorylated-synapsin I expression in the hippocampus ($p < 0.05$ vs. sham-injured rats on regular diet), but curcumin supplementation restored them to normal level (~100% of sham-injured rats on regular diet). While the 2 diets had no effect on BDNF level in sham-injured rats, curcumin supplementation increased it ($p < 0.05$ vs. sham-injured rats on regular diet).
				Injured rats on diets without curcumin had worse performance in Morris water maze than sham-injured rats ($p < 0.05$), with injured rats on high-fat diet having the lowest performance ($p < 0.05$); but the addition of curcumin to diets reversed the effect of TBI on the rats' performance. Curcumin also increased the swim speed of injured rats on high-fat diet. Performance of sham-injured rats in Morris water maze was not affected by high-fat diet or curcumin.

[a] n: sample size.
[b] RR: relative risk.
[c] CI: confidence interval.
[d] OR: odds ratio.
[e] r: correlation coefficient.
[f] HR: hazard ratio.

several other important flavonoids, such as flavan-3-ols, isoflavone, and anthocyanins, could therefore not be evaluated.

Despite these disappointing results, other human studies have found better cerebrovascular disease outcomes from the consumption of flavonoids. In a large Japanese cohort (n=40,462), greater intake of soy and isoflavone was significantly associated with lower risk of cerebral infarctions in women (adjusted RRs ranged from 0.35 to 0.64, comparing two extreme intake categories), though not in men (adjusted RR ranged from 0.95 to 1.21, comparing two extreme intake categories) (Kokubo et al., 2007). Another large prospective population-based study found an inverse association between high intakes of flavonoid subclasses and stroke, suggesting that high intakes of certain flavonoids could be neuroprotective (Mursu et al., 2008). This was supported by an earlier, smaller study that also tested the association between flavonoids and incidence of stroke (Keli et al., 1996). In a 2009 review, Macready and colleagues summarized 15 human dietary intervention studies that examined associations between administration of flavonoid pure supplements or a flavonoid-rich herbal extract (e.g., *Ginkgo biloba*) and cognitive function. The results are encouraging: nine studies reported that flavonoid supplementation provided greater neuroprotection than placebo. However, due to the great variations in exposure and outcome assessments across studies, results based on this review should be interpreted with caution.

Evidence Indicating Effects on Treatment

Human Studies

The committee found no clinical trials that tested the potential benefits of flavonoids in TBI, but did find evidence for other diseases or conditions included in the review of the literature (subarachnoid hemorrhage, intracranial aneurysm, stroke, anoxic or hypoxic ischemia, epilepsy). Included here are the results from two clinical trials and two meta-analyses that may be relevant to the hypothesis that flavonoids are beneficial for TBI. In a randomized, double-blind, placebo-controlled trial including 102 individuals with acute ischemic stroke, there was significant inverse association between isoflavone supplementation and impairment of brachial flow-mediated dilatation and serum C-reactive protein concentrations (Chan et al., 2008). A double-blind trial conducted among 309 dementia patients also found that after 26 weeks of treatment with *Ginkgo biloba* extract, participants had significantly better cognitive performance, as assessed by the Alzheimer's Disease Assessment Scale-Cognitive subscale (ADAS-cog), than controls (Le Bars et al., 2000). In contrast, a meta-analysis failed to show significant protective effects of puerarin, an isoflavone found mainly in *Pueraria*, on acute ischemic stroke (only one trial was included) (Tan et al., 2008). Another meta-analysis including nine studies found that treatment with dengzhanhua, an herb widely used in China, produced "marked neurological improvement" in acute cerebral infarction patients, but the overall quality of the included studies was low (i.e., there was a "high risk of bias") (Cao et al., 2008). Thus, no firm conclusion on the use of flavonoids could be reached.

CURCUMIN

Curcumin is a flavonoid derived from the spice turmeric, which has been used as a therapeutic agent in China and India (Sun et al., 2008). Many studies have demonstrated its antioxidant and anti-inflammatory properties, but more recent studies have also pointed to a potential ability to bind amyloid and prevent fibril and oligomer formation.

Curcumin and the Brain

Although neurodegenerative diseases are not included in this review, it is noteworthy that curcumin is being studied for potential benefits for Parkinson's disease and Alzheimer's disease (AD). Curcumin was shown to protect against oxidative damage and synaptophysin loss, and to lower the level of oxidized proteins and cytokines in animal models of AD. Neuroprotective effects against Parkinson's disease were hypothesized to result from a protection of the BBB (Sun et al., 2008). The mechanism of action of curcumin is not fully elucidated, but the array of molecular targets found for curcumin (e.g., transcription factors, growth factors, antioxidant enzymes, cell-surviving kinases and signaling molecules) suggests the multifaceted mode of action of this flavonoid. Recently, several animal studies have investigated the potential effects of curcumin on TBI and on diseases with mechanistic similarities to TBI. The committee did not identify any human studies on this topic.

Uses and Safety

In a review that examined published papers included in the database MEDLINE that addressed the safety of curcumin, the investigators found no safety concerns reported in six human trials. One human trial with 25 subjects used up to 8,000 mg/day of curcumin for three months, and the other five human trials used 1,125–2,500 mg/day of curcumin (Chainani-Wu, 2003). It is, however, worth noting that curcumin may slow down blood clotting, especially when administered with anticoagulant drugs or dietary supplements having a similar effect.[1]

Humans and rodents metabolize curcumin differently (i.e., curcumin hydrolyzes in the gastrointestinal tract in humans but not in rodents), so investigators should ensure that they use a form of curcumin that is physiologically stable and absorbable by humans.

Evidence Indicating Effect on Resilience

Human Studies

There have been no human trials or observational studies conducted to study curcumin's potential to impart resilience against TBI. Likewise, there are no human studies to assess the effect of curcumin on subarachnoid or intracranial hemorrhage, intracranial aneurysm, ischemia, stroke, or epilepsy.

Animal Studies

A small number of studies employing animal epilepsy models (e.g., Sharma et al., 2010), using a pentylenetetrazol-induced oxidative stress model, and Gupta et al. (2009) using a kainic acid–induced model, have consistently shown that curcumin is anticonvulsant. This finding may have relevance in TBI, because epilepsy is an effect seen in both its acute and long-term phases.

Studies also have assessed the neuroprotective effects of curcumin, using moderate or mild fluid percussion as a model of TBI. In an animal study of TBI using male CD-1 mice (8–10 weeks old; n = 8–12 per group), pretreatment with intraperitoneal injection of curcumin (75 or 150 mg/kg) resulted in significantly lower brain water content and neuroinflammation as well as better neurological function, as assessed by the open field activity test

---

[1] Available online: http://www.nlm.nih.gov/medlineplus/druginfo/natural/662.html (accessed March 1, 2011).

and a two-trial novel object recognition task, than controls treated by the vehicle [dimethyl sulfoxide (DMSO)] only (Laird et al., 2010). In another animal study, however, giving adult male Sprague-Dawley rats DMSO alone conferred neuroprotective effects against neuron death due to TBI that were similar to the curcumin treatment group. In other words, there was no difference between the two treatment groups (Di Giorgio et al., 2008). Oral administration of curcumin prior to injury also has been shown to improve neurobehavioral and cognitive performance, promote membrane homeostasis, regulate energy homeostasis, reduce infarct area, and reduce lipid peroxidation in other animal studies of TBI or ischemic stroke (Sharma et al., 2009; Shukla et al., 2008; Wu et al., 2006).

Evidence Indicating Effect on Treatment

Human Studies

There have been no studies conducted with TBI patients. Likewise, there have been no human studies conducted to assess the effect of curcumin on subarachnoid or intracranial hemorrhage, intracranial aneurysm, ischemia, stroke, or epilepsy.

Animal Studies

Various animal studies conducted to test outcomes that are mechanistically similar to the pathology of TBI have shown that curcumin holds promise to lessen the effects of TBI. For example, curcumin given after injury in models of cerebral ischemia and reperfusion resulted in decreases in oxidative stress as measured by levels of malondialdehyde, cytochrome c, and cleaved caspase 3 and mitochondrial Bcl-2 expression (Zhao et al., 2010). In addition to lowering indicators of stress using similar models (Wang et al., 2005), studies have shown improved behavioral outcomes (Yang et al., 2009), attenuated neurological deficits and reactive oxygen species (Dohare et al., 2008; Jiang et al., 2007), and reduction in infarct and edema volume (Jiang et al., 2007; Thiyagarajan and Sharma, 2004).

The animal study by Laird and colleagues (2010) also included experiments with animals treated with curcumin intraperitoneally after the injury. As with preinjury administration, curcumin was found to be neuroprotective against deteriorative events caused by TBI, such as lipid peroxidation, inflammation, and cognitive impairment. Similar findings were reported in an earlier study by Shukla and colleagues (2008), where curcumin was given both pre- and postinjury. The authors of this study could make no conclusions about whether the effects of curcumin were due to its administration before the injury, or after (Shukla et al., 2008).

RESVERATROL

Resveratrol (3,5,4′-trihydroxy-trans-stilbene) belongs to a class of polyphenolic compounds called stilbenes. Resveratrol and other stilbenes are produced by some types of plants in response to stress and injury (for example, when under attack by bacteria or fungi), presumably to aid in recovery. Resveratrol was first isolated from the roots of white hellebore in 1940, but it began to attract more interest in 1992, when its potential protective effects on the cardiovascular system were hypothesized. Resveratrol is now the subject of numerous animal and human studies on its anti-inflammatory and anticarcinogenic effects as well as its potential to confer protection from heart disease, aging, and the effects of brain damage after a stroke (Baur and Sinclair, 2006).

Resveratrol and the Brain

Resveratrol has been shown to exert anti-inflammatory and anti-aging effects in vitro and in animal models. Resveratrol inhibits the activity of several inflammatory enzymes in vitro, including cyclooxygenase and lipoxygenase, resulting in a suppressive effect upon inflammatory and oxidative stress (Ghanim et al., 2010). Resveratrol also may inhibit pro-inflammatory transcription factors, such as NFκB or AP-1. Other mechanisms by which resveratrol may improve brain injury effects are restoration of cerebral blood flow, repair of neural loss, and scavenging of free radicals.

Recent evidence suggests that SIRT1[2] inhibitors may be neuroprotective; however, resveratrol does not appear to act directly as a SIRT1 inhibitor (Tang, 2010), because it does not activate SIRT1 during the acute phase of neuronal cell demise. Resveratrol may indirectly increase SIRT1 activity in recovering or spared cells via elevation by 5′ AMP-activated protein kinase (AMPK) of NAD^+ levels, which then translates into an overall beneficial outcome (activation of AMPK, another enzyme with a key role in cellular energy homeostasis, may be neuroprotective). Table 14-2 lists studies (from 1990 and after) evaluating the effectiveness of resveratrol in providing resilience or treating TBI or related diseases or conditions (i.e., subarachnoid hemorrhage, intracranial aneurysm, stroke, anoxic or hypoxic ischemia, epilepsy) in the acute phases.

Uses and Safety

An expanding body of preclinical evidence suggests resveratrol may be beneficial in treating a variety of human diseases. For this reason, resveratrol is being sold as a dietary supplement, despite the absence of definitive information about resveratrol's effects in humans, and while research into the potential health benefits of resveratrol is continuing. As with other food components, it appears that the health benefits of resveratrol are dose-dependent. Low doses of resveratrol have been found to lead to beneficial health outcomes, while high doses of resveratrol can be detrimental to health (Mukherjee et al., 2010). High doses of resveratrol may, however, be required for treatment of pathological conditions, such as destruction of cancer cells (Mukherjee et al., 2010).

A 2011 review describes the available clinical data on safety and potential mechanisms of action following multiple dosing with resveratrol (Patel et al., 2011). The review acknowledged that a complete picture of the safety of resveratrol could not be asserted, because out of 16 clinical trials, only 5 included information on adverse effects, and only 1 of these studies included a placebo control group. Still, the authors found resveratrol to be safe and reasonably well tolerated at doses of up to 5 g/day. The review found some mild to moderate side effects, such as gastrointestinal disturbances, if used at doses higher than 1 g/day.

Evidence Indicating Effect on Resilience

Human Studies

There have been no human trials or observational studies conducted to study resveratrol's potential to impart resilience against TBI. Likewise, there are no human studies to assess the effect of resveratrol on subarachnoid or intracranial hemorrhage, intracranial aneurysm, ischemia, stroke, or epilepsy.

---

[2]The NAD-dependent deacetylase sirtuin-1 (SIRT1) is an enzyme that deacetylates proteins contributing to cellular regulation, including reaction to stressors.

TABLE 14-2 Relevant Data Identified for Resveratrol

Reference	Type of Injury/Insult	Type of Study and Subjects	Treatment	Findings/Results
Tier 1: Clinical trials				
None found				
Tier 2: Observational studies				
None found				
Tier 3: Animal studies				
Sönmez et al., 2007	Percussion TBI model for immature rats	Randomized, placebo-controlled study 7-day-old Wistar albino rat pups	Postinjury, a single dose of intraperitoneal resveratrol (100 mg/kg), saline, or no treatment	Locomotor activity in injured rats treated with saline was 38% lower than control rats and 36.2% lower than resveratrol-treated rats ($p < 0.01$). Performances on discrimination index, used to assess posttraumatic memory, were higher in both control rats (0.65 ± 0.06, $p < 0.01$) and resveratrol-treated rats (0.43 ± 0.06, $p < 0.05$) compared to saline-treated rats (0.17 ± 0.07).
				Treatment with resveratrol increased the density of neurons in all ipsilateral and contralateral hippocampal regions in comparison to the injured, saline-treated animals ($p < 0.001$). There was a significant neuronal loss despite the treatment, however, in the ipsilateral hipoccampal CA1 ($p < 0.001$), CA2 ($p < 0.01$), CA3 ($p < 0.05$), and DG ($p < 0.001$) regions when compared to control rats.
Ates et al., 2007	TBI model by weight drop technique	Randomized, placebo-controlled study adult albino male Wistar rats	Postinjury, a single dose of intraperitoneal resveratrol (100 mg/kg), saline, or no treatment	Saline-treated injured rats had increased levels of MDA ($p < 0.05$), nitric oxide (NO, $p < 0.05$), and xanthine oxidase (XO, $p < 0.05$) and decreased levels of gluthatione (GSH, $p < 0.05$) compared to control rats. But injured rats treated with resveratrol showed reduced levels of MDA ($p < 0.05$), NO ($p < 0.05$), and XO ($p < 0.05$) and increased levels of GSH ($p < 0.05$).
				The resveratrol group also showed significantly lower cerebral edema 24 hours after injury ($p < 0.05$) and smaller lesion area 14 days after injury ($p < 0.05$) compared to untreated group.

continued

TABLE 14-2   Continued

Reference	Type of Injury/Insult	Type of Study and Subjects	Treatment	Findings/Results
Singleton et al., 2010	Control cortical impact	Randomized, placebo-controlled study adult male Sprague-Dawley rats	Postinjury, 10 or 100 mg/kg of resveratrol or vehicle administered intraperitoneally at 5 minutes, 1 day, and 2 days after injury	Injured rats treated with 100 mg/kg of resveratrol and sham-injured rats treated with vehicle showed significantly better motor performance on beam-balance (p < 0.01), beam walk score (p < 0.01), and beam walk (p < 0.01 tests compared to injured, vehicle-treated rats). Rats treated with 10 mg/kg of resveratrol were not significantly different from vehicle-treated rats. Cognitive performance on Morris water maze was significantly better in sham rats (p < 0.001) and in rats treated with 100 mg/kg of resveratrol (p < 0.05) than vehicle-treated rats. Rats treated with 100 mg/kg of resveratrol had a mean contusion volume that was 10.6 mm³ smaller than injured, vehicle-treated rats (p < 0.028). Rats treated with 100 mg/kg resveratrol had more cells in the CA1 region (difference: 334.9, p < 0.001) and the CA3 region (difference: 102.5, p=0.001) of the hippocampus than injured, vehicle-treated rats. Thus, resveratrol (100 mg/kg) was significantly associated with hippocampal preservation (p=0.033).

Animal Studies

Numerous studies using rat models of ischemia reperfusion have demonstrated the ability of resveratrol, administered either intravenously or orally, to improve ischemia outcomes. The outcomes evaluated include cerebral blood flow, infarct volume, indicators of oxidative stress and inflammation, apoptotic cell death, and mitochondrial function. Studies have looked at the effects of intake of resveratrol as early as 21 days before the injury (Sinha et al., 2002), but even oral intake 3 days before the injury showed positive effects. For example, in an ischemia model in rats, infarct volume decreased when resveratrol was given orally once daily for three days before the injury, but there was no decrease when it was given one hour prior to injury (Inoue et al., 2003). Likewise, when administered intraperitoneally immediately after occlusion and at the time of reperfusion, oxyresveratrol (an analogue of resveratrol) at 10 and 20 mg/kg reduced the infarct volume and, in the range of 10–30 mg/kg, improved neurological outcomes. It also reduced apoptotic cell death and damage to the mitochondria. Similar results in infarct volume reduction were reported by Gao and colleagues (2006) when resveratrol was given seven days before the injury at 50 mg/kg, and by Li and colleagues (2010) when rats were injected with 30 mg/kg of resveratrol intraperitoneally for 6 days before the injury. Li and colleagues (2010) also showed a reduction in neurological deficit scores when evaluated with a neuromotor test two hours after reperfusion. When the release of neurotransmitters was measured, rats that received resveratrol showed lower levels of glutamine and aspartate and higher levels of gamma-aminobutyric acid, glycine, and taurine than control ischemic rats. The excitotoxicity index, measured as excitation versus inhibition (i.e., glutamate × glycine/gamma-aminobutyric acid), was also lower in resveratrol-treated animals than in the injured controls. Resveratrol's effects on resilience were also observed in younger animals. When administered before injury, resveratrol showed dose-dependent protection (but not at ≤ 0.002 mg/kg) against caspase-3 activation and also decreased the number of necrotic cells and reduced tissue loss in a neonatal model of ischemia (West et al., 2007).

Resveratrol also was beneficial in increasing the latency of pentylenetetrazol-induced epilepsy, as well as decreasing convulsions at doses ranging from 20 to 80 mg/kg. This enhanced protection also was observed when resveratrol was administered in combination with other known anticonvulsants (Gupta et al., 2002).

Evidence Indicating Effect on Treatment

Human Studies

There have been no studies conducted with TBI patients. Likewise, there have been no human studies conducted to assess the effect of resveratrol on subarachnoid or intracranial hemorrhage, intracranial aneurysm, ischemia, stroke, or epilepsy.

Animal Studies

One of the earliest investigations of the effect of resveratrol in brain injury used a model of ischemic injury in Mongolian gerbils that were given resveratrol immediately after injury and again 24 hours after injury (Wang et al., 2002). The decrease in neuronal cell death and decreased activation of astrocytes and glial cells led the authors to propose this polyphenol as a protective agent against ischemic injury. This study also demonstrated that resveratrol can cross the BBB, and has often been subsequently mentioned as a pivotal investigation. Given these positive findings, many studies have investigated the benefits of resveratrol, typically using ischemia reperfusion models in rodents. Improved measures of oxidative stress, brain damage, and blood flow indicate that the use of resveratrol is beneficial to ischemia outcomes. For example, resveratrol was found to reduce infarct volume when administered before or after injury at very low intravenous doses (10^{-9} and 10^{-10} mg/kg) (Huang et al., 2001). A single dose of resveratrol significantly increased the level of nitric oxide and decreased the hydroxyl radical level (Kwok et al., 2006) in a cerebral ischemia model in rats. Subsequent research in humans not suffering from brain damage demonstrated that oral administration resulted in dose-dependent increases in cerebral blood flow (Kennedy et al., 2010). In an effort to more precisely determine the time window of resveratrol's efficacy after ischemia, and considering that patients will not have access to care immediately after injury, a 2010 study of mice given resveratrol three hours after ischemia showed it to be effective in suppressing indicators of inflammation, microglial activation, and reactive oxidation species (Shin et al., 2010). Yousuf and colleagues (2009) conducted a very thorough study measuring functional and histopathological indicators after a rat model of ischemia. All indicators, including mitochondrial function, energy metabolism, oxidation, apoptosis, cell death, neurological behavior, reduced DNA fragmentation, and brain damage, suggested that resveratrol was beneficial in preserving anatomy and function of the brain after injury.

Animal models of TBI also have demonstrated the benefits of resveratrol. In a fluid percussion model of TBI for rat pups, those rats treated with 100 mg/kg resveratrol immediately after trauma showed that posttraumatic memory decline (evaluated using the novel object recognition test) was restored to 66 percent of the uninjured control (Sönmez et al., 2007). In the same experiment, locomotor activity was normalized in the rats treated with resveratrol. In a weight-drop animal model of TBI, immediate treatment with a single dose of 100 mg/kg of resveratrol reduced lesion volume and brought the levels of oxidative stress indicators (malondialdehyde, nitric oxide, xanthine oxidase, and glutathione) back to preinjury levels (Ates et al., 2007). Reinforcing these positive results are the results found by Singleton and colleagues (2010) in a trial with a TBI rat model, a controlled cortical impact model. In this case, resveratrol was given intraperitoneally at 10 or 100 mg/kg three times after injury (i.e., 5 minutes, 1 day, and 2 days after injury). Motor control and coordination of the animals were tested on days 1–5 after injury, and a cognitive test (the Morris water maze) was given on days 14–20 after the injury. The 100 mg/kg dose demonstrated benefits in all measures. Contusion volume was less and hippocampal preservation increased. Cognitive test results and motor skills were improved in animals treated with the highest level of resveratrol. Animals given the 10 mg/kg dose did not see the same behavior improvements when compared to the injured controls.

CONCLUSIONS AND RECOMMENDATIONS

Given the oxidative and inflammatory processes associated with TBI, the committee supports efforts to provide a high-quality diet that supplies a mix of polyphenols. This would concur with the *Dietary Guidelines for Americans, 2010*, which recommends consuming a greater amount and variety of fruits and vegetables.[3]

The evidence presented of potential benefits of polyphenols on TBI suggests several conclusions. This review suggests that polyphenols fall into a category of compounds that exert their effects via not only their antioxidant properties, but also through modulation of enzymes important for the progression of the disease. This characteristic distinguishes this class of compounds from other antioxidants and gives them an advantage in protecting against a disease process as complex as TBI. Because there are many biological activities attributed to the flavonoids, some of which could be either beneficial or detrimental depending on specific circumstances, further studies in both the laboratory and with patient populations are warranted.

Curcumin has not been tested in humans who have experienced a TBI event. However, in animal models of TBI, curcumin administration has consistently resulted in positive outcomes such as improved neurological function and neurobehavioral performance, as well as reduced neuroinflammation and lipid oxidation. Although resveratrol has not been tested in a human TBI trial, the positive findings from studies using animal models of ischemia and TBI described above likewise support the notion that resveratrol may also be beneficial for resilience or treatment of TBI in humans.

Although caution must be exerted because the mechanisms of action of curcumin and resveratrol have not been completely elucidated, there have been no adverse effects reported from the studies reviewed. The committee concluded there is enough evidence to concur that further research needs to be conducted to confirm the results seen so far in small-animal studies and duplicate them in humans.

RECOMMENDATION 14-1. Based on positive outcomes with curcumin and resveratrol in small-animal models of TBI, DoD should consider conducting human trials. In addition, other flavonoids (e.g., isoflavones, flavanols, epicatechin, theanine) should be evaluated in animal models of TBI.

---

[3] Available online: http://www.cnpp.usda.gov/DGAs2010-PolicyDocument.htm (accessed March 1, 2011).

REFERENCES

Arts, I. C., P. C. Hollman, E. J. Feskens, H. B. Bueno de Mesquita, and D. Kromhout. 2001. Catechin intake might explain the inverse relation between tea consumption and ischemic heart disease: The Zutphen Elderly Study. *American Journal of Clinical Nutrition* 74(2):227–232.

Ates, O., S. Cayli, E. Altinoz, I. Gurses, N. Yucel, M. Sener, A. Kocak, and S. Yologlu. 2007. Neuroprotection by resveratrol against traumatic brain injury in rats. *Molecular and Cellular Biochemistry* 294(1–2):137–144.

Baur, J. A., and D. A. Sinclair. 2006. Therapeutic potential of resveratrol: The in vivo evidence. *Nature Reviews Drug Discovery* 5(6):493–506.

Cao, W., W. Liu, T. Wu, D. Zhong, and G. Liu. 2008. Dengzhanhua preparations for acute cerebral infarction. *Cochrane Database of Systematic Reviews* (4):CD005568.

Chainani-Wu, N. 2003. Safety and anti-inflammatory activity of curcumin: A component of tumeric (curcuma longa). *Journal of Alternative and Complementary Medicine* 9(1):161–168.

Chan, Y.-H., K.-K. Lau, K.-H. Yiu, S.-W. Li, H.-T. Chan, D. Y.-T. Fong, S. Tam, C.-P. Lau, and H.-F. Tse. 2008. Reduction of c-reactive protein with isoflavone supplement reverses endothelial dysfunction in patients with ischaemic stroke. *European Heart Journal* 29(22):2800–2807.

Di Giorgio, A. M., Y. Hou, X. Zhao, B. Zhang, B. G. Lyeth, and M. J. Russell. 2008. Dimethyl sulfoxide provides neuroprotection in a traumatic brain injury model. *Restorative Neurology & Neuroscience* 26(6):501–507.

Dohare, P., P. Garg, V. Jain, C. Nath, and M. Ray. 2008. Dose dependence and therapeutic window for the neuroprotective effects of curcumin in thromboembolic model of rat. *Behavioural Brain Research* 193(2):289–297.

Dreiseitel, A., B. Oosterhuis, K. V. Vukman, P. Schreier, A. Oehme, S. Locher, G. Hajak, and P. G. Sand. 2009. Berry anthocyanins and anthocyanidins exhibit distinct affinities for the efflux transporters BCRP and MDR1. *British Journal of Pharmacology* 158(8):1942–1950.

Gao, D., X. Zhang, X. Jiang, Y. Peng, W. Huang, G. Cheng, and L. Song. 2006. Resveratrol reduces the elevated level of MMP-9 induced by cerebral ischemia-reperfusion in mice. *Life Sciences* 78(22):2564–2570.

Ghanim, H., C. L. Sia, S. Abuaysheh, K. Korzeniewski, P. Patnaik, A. Marumganti, A. Chaudhuri, and P. Dandona. 2010. An antiinflammatory and reactive oxygen species suppressive effects of an extract of polygonum cuspidatum containing resveratrol. *Journal of Clinical Endocrinology Metabolism* 95(9):E1–8.

Gupta, Y. K., G. Chaudhary, and A. K. Srivastava. 2002. Protective effect of resveratrol against pentylenetetrazole-induced seizures and its modulation by an adenosinergic system. *Pharmacology* 65(3):170–174.

Gupta, Y. K., S. Briyal, and M. Sharma. 2009. Protective effect of curcumin against kainic acid induced seizures and oxidative stress in rats. *Indian Journal of Physiology & Pharmacology* 53(1):39–46.

Hollman, P. C. H., A. Geelen, and D. Kromhout. 2010. Dietary flavonol intake may lower stroke risk in men and women. *Journal of Nutrition* 140(3):600–604.

Huang, S. S., M. C. Tsai, C. L. Chih, L. M. Hung, and S. K. Tsai. 2001. Resveratrol reduction of infarct size in long-evans rats subjected to focal cerebral ischemia. *Life Sciences* 69(9):1057–1065.

Inoue, H., X. F. Jiang, T. Katayama, S. Osada, K. Umesono, and S. Namura. 2003. Brain protection by resveratrol and fenofibrate against stroke requires peroxisome proliferator-activated receptor alpha in mice. *Neuroscience Letters* 352(3):203–206.

Jiang, J., W. Wang, Y. J. Sun, M. Hu, F. Li, and D. Y. Zhu. 2007. Neuroprotective effect of curcumin on focal cerebral ischemic rats by preventing blood-brain barrier damage. *European Journal of Pharmacology* 561(1–3):54–62.

Keli, S. O., M. G. L. Hertog, E. J. M. Feskens, and D. Kromhout. 1996. Dietary flavonoids, antioxidant vitamins, and incidence of stroke—the Zutphen Study. *Archives of Internal Medicine* 156(6):637–642.

Kennedy, D. O., E. L. Wightman, J. L. Reay, G. Lietz, E. J. Okello, A. Wilde, and C. F. Haskell. 2010. Effects of resveratrol on cerebral blood flow variables and cognitive performance in humans: A double-blind, placebo-controlled, crossover investigation. *American Journal of Clinical Nutrition* 91(6):1590–1597.

Knekt, P., S. Isotupa, H. Rissanen, M. Heliovaara, R. Jarvinen, S. Hakkinen, A. Aromaa, and A. Reunanen. 2000. Quercetin intake and the incidence of cerebrovascular disease. *European Journal of Clinical Nutrition* 54(5):415–417.

Kokubo, Y., H. Iso, J. Ishihara, K. Okada, M. Inoue, S. Tsugane, and J. S. Group. 2007. Association of dietary intake of soy, beans, and isoflavones with risk of cerebral and myocardial infarctions in Japanese populations: The Japan Public Health Center-Based (JPHC) Study Cohort I. *Circulation* 116(22):2553–2562.

Kwok, T. L., R. Y. Y. Chiou, G. C. Li, H. C. Ming, T. T. Wan, T. H. Hsiang, and L. Y. Yi. 2006. Neuroprotective effects of resveratrol on cerebral ischemia-induced neuron loss mediated by free radical scavenging and cerebral blood flow elevation. *Journal of Agricultural and Food Chemistry* 54(8):3126–3131.

Laird, M. D., S. Sukumari-Ramesh, A. E. Swift, S. E. Meiler, J. R. Vender, and K. M. Dhandapani. 2010. Curcumin attenuates cerebral edema following traumatic brain injury in mice: A possible role for aquaporin-4? *Journal of Neurochemistry* 113(3):637–648.

Le Bars, P. L., M. Kieser, and K. Z. Itil. 2000. A 26-week analysis of a double-blind, placebo-controlled trial of the ginkgo biloba extract EGB 761 in dementia. *Dementia & Geriatric Cognitive Disorders* 11(4):230–237.

Li, C., Z. Yan, J. Yang, H. Chen, H. Li, Y. Jiang, and Z. Zhang. 2010. Neuroprotective effects of resveratrol on ischemic injury mediated by modulating the release of neurotransmitter and neuromodulator in rats. *Neurochemistry International* 56(3):495–500.

Macready, A. L., O. B. Kennedy, J. A. Ellis, C. M. Williams, J. P. E. Spencer, and L. T. Butler. 2009. Flavonoids and cognitive function: A review of human randomized controlled trial studies and recommendations for future studies. *Genes and Nutrition* 4(4):227–242.

Miller, E. R., 3rd, R. Pastor-Barriuso, D. Dalal, R. A. Riemersma, L. J. Appel, and E. Guallar. 2005. Meta-analysis: High-dosage vitamin E supplementation may increase all-cause mortality. *Annals of Internal Medicine* 142(1):37–46.

Mukherjee, S., J. I. Dudley, and D. K. Das. 2010. Dose-dependency of resveratrol in providing health benefits. *Dose Response* 8(4):478–500.

Mursu, J., S. Voutilainen, T. Nurmi, T.-P. Tuomainen, S. Kurl, and J. T. Salonen. 2008. Flavonoid intake and the risk of ischaemic stroke and CVD mortality in middle-aged Finnish men: The Kuopio Ischaemic Heart Disease Risk Factor Study. *British Journal of Nutrition* 100(4):890–895.

Pandey, K. B., and S. I. Rizvi. 2009. Plant polyphenols as dietary antioxidants in human health and disease. *Oxidative Medicine and Cellular Longevity* 2(5):270–278.

Patel, K. R., E. Scott, V. A. Brown, A. J. Gescher, W. P. Steward, and K. Brown. 2011. Clinical trials of resveratrol. *Annals of the New York Academy of Sciences* 1215(1):161–169.

Polidori, M. C., A. Cherubini, W. Stahl, U. Senin, H. Sies, and P. Mecocci. 2002. Plasma carotenoid and malondialdehyde levels in ischemic stroke patients: Relationship to early outcome. *Free Radical Research* 36(3):265–268.

Ramassamy, C. 2006. Emerging role of polyphenolic compounds in the treatment of neurodegenerative diseases: A review of their intracellular targets. *European Journal of Pharmacology* 545(1):51–64.

Sesso, H. D., J. M. Gaziano, S. Liu, and J. E. Buring. 2003a. Flavonoid intake and the risk of cardiovascular disease in women. *American Journal of Clinical Nutrition* 77(6):1400–1408.

Sesso, H. D., R. S. Paffenbarger, Jr., Y. Oguma, and I. M. Lee. 2003b. Lack of association between tea and cardiovascular disease in college alumni. *International Journal of Epidemiology* 32(4):527–533.

Sharma, S., Y. Zhuang, Z. Ying, A. Wu, and F. Gomez-Pinilla. 2009. Dietary curcumin supplementation counteracts reduction in levels of molecules involved in energy homeostasis after brain trauma. *Neuroscience* 161(4):1037–1044.

Sharma, V., B. Nehru, A. Munshi, and A. Jyothy. 2010. Antioxidant potential of curcumin against oxidative insult induced by pentylenetetrazol in epileptic rats. *Methods & Findings in Experimental & Clinical Pharmacology* 32(4):227–232.

Shin, J. A., H. Lee, Y. K. Lim, Y. Koh, J. H. Choi, and E. M. Park. 2010. Therapeutic effects of resveratrol during acute periods following experimental ischemic stroke. *Journal of Neuroimmunology* 227(1–2):93–100.

Shukla, P. K., V. K. Khanna, M. M. Ali, M. Y. Khan, and R. C. Srimal. 2008. Anti-ischemic effect of curcumin in rat brain. *Neurochemical Research* 33(6):1036–1043.

Singleton, R. H., H. Q. Yan, W. Fellows-Mayle, and C. E. Dixon. 2010. Resveratrol attenuates behavioral impairments and reduces cortical and hippocampal loss in a rat controlled cortical impact model of traumatic brain injury. *Journal of Neurotrauma* 27(6):1091–1099.

Sinha, K., G. Chaudhary, and Y. K. Gupta. 2002. Protective effect of resveratrol against oxidative stress in middle cerebral artery occlusion model of stroke in rats. *Life Science* 71(6):655–665.

Sönmez, U., A. Sönmez, G. Erbil, I. Tekmen, and B. Baykara. 2007. Neuroprotective effects of resveratrol against traumatic brain injury in immature rats. *Neuroscience Letters* 420(2):133–137.

Spencer, J. P. E. 2008. Flavonoids: Modulators of brain function? *British Journal of Nutrition* 99(E Suppl. 1):ES60–77.

Sun, A. Y., Q. Wang, A. Simonyi, and G. Y. Sun. 2008. Botanical phenolics and brain health. *NeuroMolecular Medicine* 10(4):259–274.

Tan, Y., M. Liu, and B. Wu. 2008. Puerarin for acute ischaemic stroke. *Cochrane Database of Systematic Reviews*(1):CD004955.

Tang, B. L. 2010. Resveratrol is neuroprotective because it is not a direct activator of Sirt1-A hypothesis. *Brain Research Bulletin* 81(4–5):359–361.

Thiyagarajan, M., and S. S. Sharma. 2004. Neuroprotective effect of curcumin in middle cerebral artery occlusion induced focal cerebral ischemia in rats. *Life Sciences* 74(8):969–985.

Vafeiadou, K., D. Vauzour, and J. P. E. Spencer. 2007. Neuroinflammation and its modulation by flavonoids. *Endocrine Metabolic & Immune Disorders-Drug Targets* 7(3):211–224.

Wang, Q., J. Xu, G. E. Rottinghaus, A. Simonyi, D. Lubahn, G. Y. Sun, and A. Y. Sun. 2002. Resveratrol protects against global cerebral ischemic injury in gerbils. *Brain Research* 958(2):439–447.

Wang, Q., A. Y. Sun, A. Simonyi, M. D. Jensen, P. B. Shelat, G. E. Rottinghaus, R. S. MacDonald, D. K. Miller, D. E. Lubahn, G. A. Weisman, and G. Y. Sun. 2005. Neuroprotective mechanisms of curcumin against cerebral ischemia-induced neuronal apoptosis and behavioral deficits. *Journal of Neuroscience Research* 82(1):138–148.

West, T., M. Atzeva, and D. M. Holtzman. 2007. Pomegranate polyphenols and resveratrol protect the neonatal brain against hypoxic-ischemic injury. *Developmental Neuroscience* 29(4–5):363–372.

Wu, A., Z. Ying, and F. Gomez-Pinilla. 2006. Dietary curcumin counteracts the outcome of traumatic brain injury on oxidative stress, synaptic plasticity, and cognition. *Experimental Neurology* 197(2):309–317.

Yang, C., X. Zhang, H. Fan, and Y. Liu. 2009. Curcumin upregulates transcription factor Nrf2, HO-1 expression and protects rat brains against focal ischemia. *Brain Research* 1282:133–141.

Youdim, K. A., B. Shukitt-Hale, and J. A. Joseph. 2004. Flavonoids and the brain: Interactions at the blood-brain barrier and their physiological effects on the central nervous system. *Free Radical Biology and Medicine* 37(11):1683–1693.

Yousuf, S., F. Atif, M. Ahmad, N. Hoda, T. Ishrat, B. Khan, and F. Islam. 2009. Resveratrol exerts its neuroprotective effect by modulating mitochondrial dysfunctions and associated cell death during cerebral ischemia. *Brain Research* 1250(C):242–253.

Zhao, J., S. Yu, W. Zheng, G. Feng, G. Luo, L. Wang, and Y. Zhao. 2010. Curcumin improves outcomes and attenuates focal cerebral ischemic injury via antiapoptotic mechanisms in rats. *Neurochemical Research* 35(3):374–379.

15

Vitamin D

The requirement for the essential nutrient vitamin D can be met by a combination of de novo synthesis and intake, either from dietary sources or supplements. The form of vitamin D derived from plant sources is D_2, while D_3 is the form derived from the intake of animal-based foods. Vitamin D_3 also can be synthesized from cholesterol by exposure of the skin to ultraviolet light. Both of these forms of vitamin D act as prohormones. Modified first by the liver enzyme 25-hydroxylase, vitamin D is then transported to the kidney microsomes where it is converted to the active hormonal form known as 1,25-dihydroxyvitamin D, or calcitriol.

The function of the hormonal form of vitamin D is mediated by the nuclear receptor vitamin D receptor (VDR), which acts as a DNA-binding protein to regulate the transcription of vitamin D–responsive genes. This mechanism of action is responsible for enhanced intestinal calcium absorption, kidney calcium reabsorption, and bone resorption of calcium. In this way, vitamin D regulates serum calcium and phosphate levels as well as bone metabolism. Although vitamin D's role in calcium balance is most prominent in the literature, it is clear that vitamin D also plays a key role in the molecular processes that control cellular proliferation, differentiation, and survival (Fleet, 2007). Consequently, in addition to the development of rickets and osteopenia, vitamin D deficiency has been linked to a variety of illnesses including hypertension and heart disease, obesity, diabetes, rheumatoid arthritis, and an increased risk of cancer (Holick, 2007; Martini and Wood, 2008; Wood, 2008).

VITAMIN D AND THE BRAIN

Although the role of vitamin D in calcium absorption, serum calcium balance, and bone metabolism has long been recognized, its essential role in the brain and central nervous system (CNS) has only recently been appreciated. It is now known that the human brain expresses the enzyme 1 alpha-hydroxylase, responsible for the hydroxylation of 25-hydroxyvitamin D to its active, hormonal form, 1,25-dihydroxyvitamin D; as well as the nuclear receptor for vitamin D, VDR.

TABLE 15-1 Relevant Data Identified for Vitamin D

Reference	Type of Injury/Insult	Type of Study and Subjects	Treatment	Findings/Results
Tier 1: Clinical trials				
None found				
Tier 2: Observational studies				
Buell et al., 2010	Stroke	Prospective cohort study (Nutrition and Memory in Elders)		25(OH)D insufficiency (10–20 ng/mL) was associated with twice the risk of stroke (OR[b]=2.29, 95% CI[c]: 1.09–4.83, p=0.03). But the association with stroke was not significant after stratifying for presence or absence of dementia.
		n[a]=318 patients ≥ 60 years old		Compared to patients taking sufficient levels (> 20 ng/mL) of 25(OH)D, deficient (< 10 ng/mL) patients had higher geometric mean white matter hypersensitivity (WMH) volume (p=0.004), higher WMH grade (p=0.02), and higher prevalence of large vessel infarcts (p < 0.01).
Tier 3: Animal studies				
None found				

[a] n: sample size.
[b] OR: relative risk.
[c] CI: confidence interval.

Although the roles of vitamin D in the CNS are not well understood, it appears that its function is largely mediated by VDR. This member of the steroid-thyroid nuclear receptor family is widely expressed in both the human and rodent cortex, spinal cord, amygdala, hypothalamus, cerebellum, mesopontine area, and diencephalon. VDR is particularly high in the hippocampus, a region of the brain associated not only with learning and memory, but also with emotion (Eyles et al., 2005). When the hormonal form of vitamin D associates with VDR in the nucleus, this complex can combine with the retinoic acid receptor RXR to produce heterodimers. Together, these two nutrients (vitamin D in the form of $1,25(OH)_2\text{-}D_3$ and vitamin A in the form of 9-cis-retinoic acid) and their respective nuclear receptors (VDR and RXR) bind to specific sequences of DNA known as vitamin D response elements (VDREs). Binding of this complex to VDREs in the 5′-flanking region of vitamin D–responsive genes results in the regulation of gene transcription in the CNS, where it is now believed to participate in cell proliferation and neuronal differentiation and neuronal function (Levenson and Figueirôa, 2008).

Table 15-1 includes limited supporting evidence (1990 and later) from human studies on vitamin D supplementation for CNS injuries. Any adverse effects in humans are also listed.

USES AND SAFETY

The current Recommended Dietary Allowance (RDA) for vitamin D is 600 International Units (IU) per day for both male and female adults up to the age of 70 (IOM, 2010). At age 70, the RDA increases to 800 IU. There are a number of considerations to take into account when applying these recommendations to military populations and others at risk for traumatic brain injury (TBI). First, the current RDAs for vitamin D were developed under conditions of minimal sun exposure (IOM, 2010), and therefore do not factor in the vitamin D synthesized in the skin through exposure to sunlight. More importantly, the Institute of Medicine (IOM) set the current RDA for vitamin D at a level found to be sufficient to maintain bone health and normal calcium metabolism in healthy people, the only outcome found to be associated with vitamin D status. It is not known whether the dietary vitamin D requirement for optimal brain function under normal or injured conditions should be different.

Median estimates of vitamin D intake from foods are below the Estimated Average Requirements (EARs) of 400 IU recently established by the IOM. However, vitamin D also is synthesized in the skin, and therefore vitamin D status is not accurately reflected exclusively by dietary intake. Using National Health and Nutrition Examination Survey (NHANES) data from 2000 to 2006, levels of 25-hydroxyvitamin D in serum, a depiction of total vitamin D exposure, were above 50 nmol/mL, the level identified as meeting the needs of most of the population. The IOM concluded that the population of North America, with the possible exception of the aging population and those with dark skin, is meeting its needs for vitamin D.

NHANES (2005–2006) data show that 37 percent of the U.S. population reported using vitamin D supplements. This is likely to be predominantly in the form of multivitamin supplements or as an adjunct to calcium supplementation. The current Tolerable Upper Intake Level (UL) for adults is 4,000 IU. Excess dietary intake of vitamin D has been shown to cause vitamin D intoxication, which leads to hypercalcemia and, eventually, soft tissue calcification and resultant renal and cardiovascular damage.

EVIDENCE INDICATING EFFECT ON RESILIENCE

Human Studies

There have been no clinical trials to address the possibility that vitamin D supplementation may promote resilience to subsequent TBI. However, human data (in elderly populations) does indicate that failure to maintain adequate vitamin D nutriture is associated with diminished neurocognitive health. For example, plasma 25-hydroxy vitamin D concentrations of less than 20 ng/mL in individuals 65–99 years of age were associated with increased prevalence of dementia, and concentrations below 10 ng/mL were associated with increased cranial indicators (detected via magnetic resonance imaging [MRI]) of cerebrovascular disease such as white matter hyperintensity volume and large vessel infarcts (Buell et al., 2010).

Animal Studies

Maintaining adequate vitamin D nutrition prior to injury may be critical for post-TBI treatment with progesterone, the only agent that has thus far shown therapeutic benefit in randomized, placebo-controlled clinical trials. This possibility is based on a 2009 study conducted in aged rats (Cekic et al., 2009): vitamin D–replete animals showed a 50 percent reduction in spontaneous locomotor activity following contusion to the medial frontal cortex, but progesterone treatment fully restored activity. Rats deficient in vitamin D exhibited a similar reduction in locomotor activity following contusion, but treatment with either progesterone alone or vitamin D alone had no restorative effect. Although treatment with progesterone plus vitamin D did completely restore locomotor activity, the possible efficacy of vitamin D as an adjunct to progesterone therapy is supported by in vitro data showing that pretreatment of cultured rat cortical neurons with either progesterone or vitamin D protected the cells from glutamate-induced excitotoxicity. Pretreatment with progesterone in combination with some lower doses of vitamin D was more protective than progesterone alone (Atif et al., 2009).

This requirement for vitamin D is important in light of two very encouraging human studies involving progesterone. In the first, Wright and colleagues (2007) conducted a phase II clinical trial with TBI patients. The treated patient group achieved a significantly lower mortality rate at 30 days and improved scores on disability rating scales at 30 days and 1 year postinjury, compared to the placebo-treated patients; there were no serious adverse events observed. In the second study, Xiao and coworkers (2008) performed a human trial involving patients with severe TBI. These patients had significantly improved functional independence and Glasgow Outcome Scale scores at three and six months postinjury, and lower mortality at six months, compared to placebo-treated controls. Progesterone administration to patients with severe TBI is currently in phase III clinical trials.

Progesterone is best known as a steroid hormone involved in the regulation of reproductive function (Cannon, 1998), and in immunosuppression during pregnancy to guard against immunological rejection of the fetus (Arck et al., 2007). Progesterone is, however, also produced in the cerebral cortex, hypothalamus, and other areas of the brains of both men and women, primarily by astrocytes (Micevych and Sinchak, 2008); receptors for progesterone are also located in the brain, many in regions associated with cognitive function (Wagner, 2008). There is growing evidence that neuroprogesterone produced in the brain can influence neurons by modulating membrane-bound receptors (including gamma-aminobutyric acid type A [$GABA_A$] and glutamate receptors) and subsequently influencing neuronal excitotoxicity and apoptosis (reviewed in Leskiewicz et al., 2006). Progesterone may also promote myelin repair (Chesik and De Keyser, 2010; Labombarda et al., 2009). Potential neuroprotective mechanisms have been reviewed in the context of TBI by Stein (2008).

Although no published work has directly tested the hypothesis that vitamin D supplementation improves resilience to TBI in otherwise vitamin D–adequate animals, an examination of data collected using other models of brain injury suggests the need for more work in this area. For example, eight days of treatment with 1,25 dihydroxyvitamin-D_3 reduced tissue damage in the rat brain subjected to the middle cerebral artery occlusion model of stroke (Wang et al., 2000). Interestingly, four days of vitamin D treatment were ineffective, suggesting a dose-response curve that needs to be examined.

EVIDENCE INDICATING EFFECT ON TREATMENT

Human Studies

There have been no clinical trials to assess the efficacy of vitamin D as a treatment for TBI or for other related diseases or conditions included in the review of the literature (subarachnoid hemorrhage, intracranial aneurysm, stroke, anoxic or hypoxic ischemia, epilepsy).

Animal Studies

No published studies have used vitamin D supplementation to treat TBI. In vitro work, however, has shown that vitamin D has direct neuroprotective and antiapoptotic functions, and protects cultured cortical neurons against excitotoxic damage (Kajta et al., 2009). The same report further showed that administration of a single dose of 1,25 dihydroxyvitamin D_3 (2 µg/kg) 30 minutes after hypoxia-ischemia in seven-day-old rats effectively reduced brain damage in these animals (Kajta et al., 2009). Although clearly very different from the accepted models of TBI, these data do suggest that future studies to examine the possible effectiveness of vitamin D in TBI models are warranted.

CONCLUSIONS AND RECOMMENDATIONS

An examination of the literature on the possible role of vitamin D in improving resilience to TBI and in the treatment of TBI has identified a number of unanswered questions that reveal gaps in our current knowledge. It is not known whether chronic vitamin D supplementation alone improves resilience. There also is no clear evidence yet to show the extent to which vitamin D supplementation is effective in treating TBI, the therapeutic window for treatment after TBI, or the optimal dose. Although it appears that adequate vitamin D status is necessary to the action of effective treatments such as progesterone, it is not currently known if vitamin D supplementation that exceeds recommended doses would improve progesterone efficacy or enhance other treatments. It is, however, recommended that military personnel ensure adequate intakes to meet the RDA for vitamin D. Because the current vitamin D status of military personnel is not definitive, the committee recommends in Chapter 5 that dietary assessments be conducted across military settings. A retrospective assessment of pre- and postinjury nutrition status is likewise recommended in Chapter 5. This should include investigating serum vitamin D levels in patients during the acute phase of TBI, with a range of severity from mild/concussion to severe injuries, to explore whether preinjury vitamin D levels are associated with different outcomes.

Progesterone was not included for independent evaluation in this report because, although it is incorporated in some dietary supplements, there was no evidence that these preparations will have positive effects on TBI. Although progesterone can be taken orally in a micronized form that enhances solubility in aqueous solutions and absorption in the gastrointestinal tract (Fitzpatrick and Good, 1999), it appears that its positive effects in TBI are achieved only via intravenous administration and at therapeutic doses (Wright et al., 2005, 2007; Xiao et al., 2008). Although some phytoprogestins have been identified by their ability to bind progesterone receptors on the breast carcinoma cell line T47D (Zava et al., 1998), none of the herbal extracts that bound the receptors were agonists. They were either neutral or were progestin antagonists (examples include red clover, licorice, and nutmeg). Altogether, there is no evidence that oral administration of progesterone or phytoprogestins will provide a benefit as treatment for TBI.

> **RECOMMENDATION 15-1.** The committee recommends more animal studies be conducted to determine if vitamin D enhances the beneficial actions of progesterone in the treatment of TBI. If this synergistic effect is confirmed in animals, then studies in humans should be conducted to evaluate the extent to which vitamin D supplementation might improve the efficacy of progesterone treatment.

> **RECOMMENDATION 15-2.** Based on animal studies showing a requirement of vitamin D for the efficacy of progesterone therapy, future animal studies are recommended to test the efficacy of using vitamin D supplements to improve resilience to TBI. Should the data from animal studies support use of this steroid hormone, human trials should be implemented to test the efficacy of vitamin D in populations at high risk for TBI.

REFERENCES

Arck, P., P. J. Hansen, B. M. Jericevic, M.-P. Piccinni, and J. Szekeres-Bartho. 2007. Progesterone during pregnancy: Endocrine-immune cross talk in mammalian species and the role of stress. *Journal of Reproductive Immunology* 58(3):268–279.

Atif, F., I. Sayeed, T. Ishrat, and D. G. Stein. 2009. Progesterone with vitamin D affords better neuroprotection against excitotoxicity in cultured cortical neurons than progesterone alone. *Molecular Medicine* 15(9–10):328–336.

Buell, J. S., B. Dawson-Hughes, T. M. Scott, D. E. Weiner, G. E. Dallal, W. Q. Qui, P. Bergethon, I. H. Rosenberg, M. F. Folstein, S. Patz, R. A. Bhadelia, and K. L. Tucker. 2010. 25-Hydroxyvitamin D, dementia, and cerebrovascular pathology in elders receiving home services. *Neurology* 74(1):18–26.

Cannon, J. G. 1998. Adaptive interactions between cytokines and the hypothalamic-pituitary-gonadal axis. *Annals of the New York Academy of Sciences* 856:234–242.

Cekic, M., S. M. Cutler, J. W. vanLandingham, and D. G. Stein. 2009. Vitamin D deficiency reduces the benefits of progesterone treatment after brain injury in aged rats. *Neurobiology of Aging.* Published electronically May 29, 2009. doi:10.1016/jneurobiolaging.2009.04.017.

Chesik, D., and J. De Keyser. 2010. Progesterone and dexamethasone differentially regulate the IGF system in glial cells. *Neuroscience Letters* 468(3):178–182.

Eyles, D. W., S. Smith, R. Kinobe, M. Hewison, and J. J. McGrath. 2005. Distribution of the vitamin D receptor and 1α-hydroxylase in human brain. *Journal of Chemical Neuroanatomy* 29(1):21–30.

Fitzpatrick, L. A., and A. Good. 1999. Micronized progesterone: Clinical indications and comparison with current treatments. *Fertility and Sterility* 72(3):389–397.

Fleet, J. C. 2007. What have genomic and proteomic approaches told us about vitamin D and cancer? *Nutrition Reviews* 65(8):S127–S130.

Holick, M. F. 2007. Vitamin D deficiency. *The New England Journal of Medicine* 357(3):266–281.

IOM (Institute of Medicine). 2010. *Dietary Reference Intakes for calcium and vitamin D.* Washington, DC: The National Academies Press.

Kajta, M., D. Makarewicz, E. Zieminska, D. Jantas, H. Domin, W. Lason, A. Kutner, and J. W. Lazarewicz. 2009. Neuroprotection by co-treatment and post-treating with calcitriol following the ischemic and excitotoxic insult in vivo and in vitro. *Neurochemistry International* 55(5):265–274.

Labombarda, F., S. L. Gonzalez, A. Lima, P. Roig, R. Guennoun, M. Schumacher, and A. F. de Nicola. 2009. Effects of progesterone on oligodendrocyte progenitors, oligodendrocyte transcription factors, and myelin proteins following spinal cord injury. *Glia* 57(8):884–897.

Leskiewicz, M., B. Budziszewska, A. Basta-Kaim, A. Zajac, M. Kacinski, and W. Lason. 2006. Effects of neurosteroids on neuronal survival: Molecular basis and clinical perspectives. *Acta Neurobiologiae Experimentalis* 66(4):359–367.

Levenson, C. W., and S. M. Figueirôa. 2008. Gestational vitamin D deficiency: Long-term effects on the brain. *Nutrition Reviews* 66(12):726–729.

Martini, L. A., and R. J. Wood. 2008. Vitamin D and blood pressure connection: Update on epidemiologic, clinical, and mechanistic evidence. *Nutrition Reviews* 66(5):291–297.

Micevych, P., and K. Sinchak. 2008. Minireview: Synthesis and function of hypothalamic neuroprogesterone in reproduction. *Endocrinology* 149(6):2739–2742.

Stein, D. G. 2008. Progesterone exerts neuroprotective effects after brain injury. *Brain Research Reviews* 57(2):386–397.

Wagner, C. K. 2008. Minireview: Progesterone receptors and neural development: A gap between bench and bedside? *Endocrinology* 149(6):2743–2749.

Wang, Y., Y. H. Chiang, T. P. Su, T. Hayashi, M. Morales, B. J. Hoffer, and S. Z. Lin. 2000. Vitamin D-3 attenuates cortical infarction induced by middle cerebral arterial ligation in rats. *Neuropharmacology* 39(5):873–880.

Wood, R. J. 2008. Vitamin D and adipogenesis: New molecular insights. *Nutrition Reviews* 66(1):40–46.

Wright, D. W., J. C. Ritchie, R. E. Mullins, A. L. Kellermann, and D. D. Denson. 2005. Steady-state serum concentrations of progesterone following continuous intravenous infusion in patients with acute moderate to severe traumatic brain injury. *Journal of Clinical Pharmacology* 45(6):640–648.

Wright, D. W., A. L. Kellermann, V. S. Hertzberg, P. L. Clark, M. Frankel, F. C. Goldstein, J. P. Salomone, L. L. Dent, O. A. Harris, D. S. Ander, D. W. Lowery, M. M. Patel, D. D. Denson, A. B. Gordon, M. M. Wald, S. Gupta, S. W. Hoffman, and D. G. Stein. 2007. ProTECT: A randomized clinical trial of progesterone for acute traumatic brain injury. *Annals of Emergency Medicine* 49(4):391–402.

Xiao, G., J. Wei, W. Yan, W. Wang, and Z. Lu. 2008. Improved outcomes from the administration of progesterone for patients with acute severe traumatic brain injury: A randomized controlled trial. *Critical Care* 12(2):R61.

Zava, D. T., C. M. Dollbaum, and M. Blen. 1998. Estrogen and progestin bioactivity of foods, herbs and spices. *Proceedings of the Society for Experimental Biology and Medicine* 217(3):369–378.

16

Zinc

The trace element zinc is essential to at least 80 different enzymes in the human central nervous system (CNS), including DNA (deoxyribonucleic acid) and RNA (ribonucleic acid) polymerases, metalloproteinases, and many dehydrogenases in intermediary metabolism, such as lactate dehydrogenase and pyruvate carboxylase (Tapiero and Tew, 2003). Zinc also is a structural component of a family of DNA-binding transcription factors known as zinc-finger proteins that are essential for gene expression (Klug and Schwabe, 1995; O'Halloran, 1993). Nuclear receptors, such as those that mediate the transcriptional roles of thyroid hormones, glucocorticoids, retinoic acid, vitamin D, and estrogen, are all zinc-finger proteins (Freedman and Luisi, 1993), and function as key players in the CNS.

ZINC AND THE BRAIN

In addition to the zinc that is bound to enzymes, transcription factors, and other proteins, about 10 percent of CNS zinc is in the free form and is associated with presynaptic vesicles of glutamatergic neurons. Although neurons containing free zinc are found in many regions of the brain, including the cortex, amygdala, and olfactory bulb, the neurons of the hippocampus have the highest concentrations of free zinc. The zinc in these vesicles is released into the synaptic cleft, where it modulates the activity of a variety of postsynaptic receptors including N-methyl-D-aspartate (NMDA) receptors, gamma-aminobutyric acid (GABA) receptors, and voltage-gated calcium channels (Matias et al., 2006; Stoll et al., 2007). Regulation of NMDA receptor subunit expression also has been shown to be regulated by zinc (Levenson, 2006).

In addition to the important neuromodulatory roles of free zinc, it has been repeatedly shown that excessive release of zinc from synaptic boutons can result in postsynaptic neuronal death. Neurons in brain regions with high concentrations of free zinc, such as the hippocampus, are thus particularly vulnerable to zinc-mediated damage and death. Additionally, after CNS injury, large quantities of free zinc can be released, not only from presynaptic vesicles but also from metalloproteins and from mitochondrial zinc pools, result-

233

ing in neuronal damage and death in a variety of brain regions (Frederickson et al., 2004; Sensi and Jeng, 2004).

Traumatic brain injury (TBI) induces a variety of damaging oxidative processes, and a number of studies show a role for zinc deficiency in the induction of reactive oxygen species (ROS). Zinc deficiency may therefore exacerbate the oxidative damage associated with TBI. This hypothesis is supported by work in cultured rat neurons (differentiated PC12 cells) showing that deficiencies in extracellular zinc resulted in an increase in neuronal oxidation via the activation of the NMDA receptor. This in turn led to calcium influx and to the calcium-mediated activation of protein kinase C/NADPH (nicotinamide adenine dinucleotide phosphate) oxidase as well as nitric oxide synthase (Aimo et al., 2010). Other work has implicated zinc deficiency in mitochondrial accumulation and release of ROS (Corniola et al., 2008). This mechanism is dependent on the tumor suppressor protein p53. Nuclear targets of p53 in zinc deficiency include genes that arrest the cell cycle and induce apoptotic mechanisms leading to cell death (Corniola et al., 2008). Finally, in response to TBI, antioxidant mechanisms are increased in the brain. For example, increases in several isoforms (I, II, and III) of the zinc- and copper-binding protein metallothionein have been reported after brain injury (Penkowa et al., 2001; Yeiser et al., 1999). Zinc deficiency blunts this response. Because the metal-binding metallothioneins have been shown to play an antioxidant role, these data suggest that zinc deficiency may impair antioxidant mechanisms that are needed to protect neurons and other cell types in the brain after TBI.

A relevant selection of human and animal studies (from the year 1990) examining the effectiveness of zinc supplementation on providing resilience or treating TBI in the acute and subacute phases of injury is presented in Table 16-1. This table also includes some supporting evidence from human studies on zinc supplementation for other CNS injuries, such as stroke and seizure. The occurrence or absence of adverse effects in humans is included if reported by the authors.

USES AND SAFETY

Dietary requirements for zinc are determined not only by the roles of zinc in the brain, but also by the necessity of adequate zinc for immune function, tissue repair and replacement, nutrient digestion, and energy metabolism in all organ systems. There is, however, no single widely accepted or routinely available biomarker for zinc status (IOM, 2006). Marginal zinc deficiency is particularly difficult to identify and is thus likely to go unrecognized. The Committee on Mineral Requirements for Cognitive and Physical Performance of Military Personnel (IOM, 2006) reported that high-intensity exercise can increase urinary zinc excretion by 20–40 percent. This, combined with severe environmental conditions that promote sweating, means that many active-duty military personnel have high zinc losses. These losses must be replaced by dietary intake.

The current Recommended Dietary Allowance (RDA) for zinc in the general population is 9 mg/day for females between the ages of 14 and 18, 8 mg/day for females 19 years and older, and 11 mg/day for males 14 years and older. In the general population, data from the National Health and Nutrition Examination Survey (2002) suggest that 11 percent of males and 17 percent of females have regular intakes below the recommended amounts. Owing to the increased requirements resulting from physical activity and potential increased excretion (via sweat and urine, as well as increased muscle turnover), the Military Daily Recommended Intake (MDRI) for zinc is 12 mg/day for females and 15 mg/day for males (IOM, 2006). Revisions to the MDRIs, based on current DRIs, are imminent.

Because of zinc's important role in the modulation of immunity, zinc supplements have

TABLE 16-1 Relevant Data Identified for Zinc

Reference	Type of Injury/Insult	Type of Study and Subjects	Treatment	Findings/Results
Tier 1: Clinical trials				
Aquilani et al., 2009	Subacute stroke patients with low Zn^{2+} intake (< 6.6 mg/day)	Randomized, prospective, placebo-controlled, double-blind trial n^a=26	Postinjury, Zn^{2+} supplementation at 10 mg/day or placebo	Compared to baseline values, all patients had significantly greater daily carbohydrate (p=0.03) and zinc intake (p < 0.001) and lower National Institute of Health Stroke Scale (NIHSS) scores (p < 0.001) at 30 days. Compared to patients assigned to placebo, patients assigned to zinc supplementation had greater body weight (p=0.002), daily energy intake (p=0.02), protein intake (p=0.04), lipid intake (p=0.01), and zinc level (p < 0.001) at 30 days. Zinc-treated patients also had higher level of serum albumin (p=0.001) and greater improvement in NIHSS score (p=0.04) than controls. And zinc intake was inversely correlated to NIHSS score (r^b=-0.46, p < 0.02). No adverse effects of zinc were mentioned.
Young et al., 1996	Severe TBI	Randomized, prospective, double-blind, placebo-controlled trial n=68 TBI patients	Postinjury, elemental zinc at standard level of 2.5 mg or supplementation at 12 mg for 15 days, then tablets of 22 mg elemental zinc or placebo for 3 months	Although there was no difference between the standard (2.5 mg) group and the supplemented (12 mg) group on serum zinc level, the supplemented group had significantly higher levels of zinc in urine at days 2 (p=0.0001) and 10 (p=0.01). But the significance disappeared at week 3. Supplemented group also had higher mean serum pre-albumin level (p=0.003) and mean retinol-binding protein levels (p=0.01) at 3 weeks. After adjusting for baseline value, supplemented group had higher mean Glasgow Coma Scale (GCS) score at day 28 (p=0.03) and mean motor GCS score at days 15 (p=0.005) and 21 (p=0.02), although there was no statistically significant difference in the raw GCS scores. No adverse effects were mentioned.
Tier 2: Observational studies				
None found				

continued

TABLE 16-1   Continued

Reference	Type of Injury/Insult	Type of Study and Subjects	Treatment	Findings/Results
Tier 3: Animal studies				
Hellmich et al., 2008	TBI	Adult, male Sprague-Dawley rats	Calcium ethylenediaminetetraacetic acid (EDTA)	Compared to saline-treated rats, rats pretreated with CaEDTA had significantly fewer Flouro-Jade (FJ, showing injured cells) stained cells in CA1 ($p < 0.05$) and rats treated with CaEDTA after TBI had reduced FJ-stained cells in CA3 ($p < 0.02$).
				Although both pre- and postinjury administration of CaEDTA increased the expression of antiapoptotic gene Bcl-2, only pretreatment was significant when compared to saline-treated rats ($p < 0.05$). And only postinjury treatment with CaEDTA increased the expression of Bax ($p < 0.05$ vs. saline-treated and pretreated rats) and caspase 3 genes ($p < 0.05$ vs. saline-treated rats only).
				CaEDTA treatment had no significant effect on spatial memory. And injured rats with and without CaEDTA treatment and treated, sham-injured rats all had significantly worse performance on the Morris water maze test ($p < 0.05$) compared to untreated, sham-injured rats.
Hellmich et al., 2007	TBI, fluid percussion injury (FPI)	Adult, male Sprague-Dawley rats	Lamotrigine or nicardipine	At 4 hours post-TBI, injured rats had significant increase in number of neurons with Flouro-Jade (FJ, showing injured cells) and Newport Green (NG, showing zinc positive cells) staining in CA1, CA3, and dentate gyrus regions of the hippocampus ($p < 0.05$). At 24 hours after injury, increased number of FJ- and NG-positive cells was seen in the CA1 and CA2 regions ($p < 0.05$), with stained cells seen in rats with severe injury. In the dentate gyrus, increase in stained cells was seen only in moderately injured rats ($p < 0.05$).
				Both lamotrigine and nicardipine led to a decrease on FJ- and NG-stained neurons in CA1 ($p < 0.05$), and lamotrigine led to decrease of stained cells in CA3 ($p < 0.05$).
				There was no significant difference in the expression of Bcl-2, caspase 3 and caspase 9, and Hsp 70 between the two staining methods. However, within-rat variability was smaller for FJ staining than NG.

TABLE 16-1   Continued

Reference	Type of Injury/Insult	Type of Study and Subjects	Treatment	Findings/Results
Hellmich et al., 2004	TBI, FPI	Male Sprague-Dawley rats	Preinjury, calcium EDTA (100mM) 30 minutes before injury or no treatment	Treatment with EDTA was significantly associated with increased expression of neuroprotective genes and antioxidant enzymes.
				EDTA also significantly increased expression of cell cycle regulatory genes and reduced apoptotic cell death after TBI up to 85%. Results were consistent with microarray studies describing changes in the expression of genes in several signaling and cellular pathways after TBI.
Yeiser et al., 2002	TBI, unilateral cortical stab wounds	Adult, male Sprague-Dawley rats	Postinjury, zinc diets (standard: 30 mg/kg; moderately deficient: 5 mg/kg; and supplemental: 180 mg/kg)	Compared to rats fed with standard amount of zinc (controls), serum zinc level was significantly lower in zinc-deficient rats ($p \leq 0.05$) and was not significantly different in zinc-supplemented rats. There was no significant between-group difference regarding zinc levels in the brain.
				Compared to controls, deficient rats had greater number of cells stained with terminal deoxynucleotidyl transferase dUTP nick end labeling ($p \leq 0.05$).

continued

TABLE 16-1 Continued

Reference	Type of Injury/Insult	Type of Study and Subjects	Treatment	Findings/Results
Penkowa et al., 2001	TBI	Adult, male Sprague-Dawley rats	Preinjury, normal diet (43.3 mg Zn/kg, 6.5 mg Cu/kg), zinc-deficient diet (1.9 mg Zn/kg), copper-deficient diet (0.8 mg Cu/kg), or zinc pair-fed diet (43.3 mg Zn/kg)	Compared to uninjured controls, zinc-deficient rats had lower food consumption, lower level of brain zinc, and decreased weight gain ($p < 0.05$ for all three). Zinc-deficient rats had decreased weight gain compared to pair-fed rats, too ($p < 0.05$).
				Injured, zinc-deficient rats had greater number of round hypertrophic microphages at the periphery of the lesion and in the parenchyma than injured, normally fed rats ($p < 0.05$) and uninjured controls ($p < 0.001$). Both injured and uninjured zinc-deficient rats had decreased astrogliosis around the lesion and long thin processes than corresponding normally fed rats ($p < 0.05$ for both).
				Injured zinc-deficient rats had more apoptotic cells (neurons, astrocytes, and microglia/microphages) than uninjured controls ($p < 0.001$) and injured normally fed rats ($p < 0.05$). Expression of metallothionein (MT) isoforms I and II in injured, zinc-deficient rats was greater compared to uninjured controls ($p < 0.001$), but lower compared to injured, normally fed rats ($p < 0.05$). Expression of MT-III was higher in injured, zinc-deficient rats compared to both controls ($p < 0.001$) and injured, normally fed rats ($p < 0.05$).
				Analysis of oxidative stress markers showed that injured, zinc-deficient rats had increased levels of MDA (malondialdehyde), NITT (protein tyrosine nitration), and NF-κB (nuclear factor kappa B) compared to both uninjured controls ($p < 0.001$ for all three markers) and injured, normally fed rats ($p < 0.05$ for all three).

TABLE 16-1 Continued

Reference	Type of Injury/Insult	Type of Study and Subjects	Treatment	Findings/Results
Suh et al., 2000	Moderate and severe TBI, induced by weight drop model	Male Sprague-Dawley rat	Postinjury, calcium EDTA (for ion zinc chelation), zinc-EDTA (prevents zinc chelation), or saline	Vesicular zinc was loss from boutons in impacted area within 6 hours of injury. In rats that underwent severe trauma, neurons stained with N-(6-methoxy-8-quinolyl)-para-toluenesulfonamide (TSQ) can be seen 1 hour after TBI, especially in the hilar and infragranular regions in dentate gyrus. TSQ-labeled neurons can be seen in the cortex and thalamic regions after 24 hours. The main difference between severe and moderate trauma was there was more florescent neurons in the dentate granule layer and subgranular hilar regions. Results from TSQ florescence were confirmed by eosin staining showing neuron degeneration. Administration of calcium EDTA reduced the number of eosinophilic neurons in the dentate gyrus, hilus, and CA1 regions (p < 0.05 vs. saline for all three). The number of eisonophilic neurons was not affected by zinc-EDTA.

[a] n: sample size.
[b] r: correlation coefficient.

been used in a variety of settings to improve immune function and reduce inflammation (see Prasad, 2009; Scrimgeour and Condlin, 2009 for recent reviews). A 2008 meta-analysis of the four available randomized trials of zinc supplementation and clinical outcomes in critically ill patients showed only small, statistically insignificant improvements in mortality and length of stay in intensive care (Heyland et al., 2008). However, zinc supplementation appears to be associated with improvements in markers of immune function in a variety of other noncritically ill patients. For example, a 2010 report showed that 18 months of daily zinc supplementation (12 mg for women and 15 mg for men) significantly reduced the likelihood of immunological failure, rate of diarrhea, and mortality in HIV-infected adults (Baum et al., 2010). The use of zinc to treat cold and flu symptoms also has become very popular, albeit with conflicting scientific evidence on efficacy. Although some studies have reported no improvements in cold symptoms (Eby and Halcomb, 2006), a meta-analysis of double-blind, randomized, controlled trials suggested that zinc gluconate may be effective in reducing the symptoms and duration of the common cold in healthy people when administered within 24 hours of onset of symptoms (Singh and Das, 2011). To produce these effects, however, the daily dose varied between 30 mg zinc in syrup preparation and 80–190 mg zinc in lozenge form (Singh and Das, 2011).

This raises the issue of zinc overload. Currently, the Tolerable Upper Intake Level (UL) for zinc is set at 40 mg/day; the minimum effective dose discussed for treatment of colds would significantly exceed this amount. A number of recent reports have shown that prolonged excessive zinc overload from misuse of dental preparations results in potentially fatal copper deficiency, characterized by pancytopenia and myelopolyneuropathy (Afrin, 2010; Hedera et al., 2009). These data suggest that recommendations to supplement zinc for any reason, including for the treatment of TBI, should include cautionary advice not to chronically exceed the UL for zinc intake.

EVIDENCE INDICATING EFFECT ON RESILIENCE

Human Studies

As with other nutrients or food components, the committee found no human studies that have examined the potential benefits of zinc in TBI or in other related diseases or conditions included in the review of the literature (subarachnoid hemorrhage, intracranial aneurysm, stroke, anoxic or hypoxic ischemia, epilepsy).

Animal Studies

Given the evidence, both clinical and experimental, showing a possible role for the use of zinc as a treatment in TBI, a 2010 study (Cope et al., unpublished) sought to test the hypothesis that zinc supplementation prior to injury could increase resilience and improve outcomes of brain injury. The effect of diet was assessed using the controlled cortical injury model of TBI in adult rats. This model of severe injury induced anhedonia, a depression-like symptom, in the rat, as measured by the two-bottle saccharin preference test. Although this symptom was observed in injured animals that were fed a diet with adequate zinc (30 ppm), four weeks of zinc supplementation (180 ppm) prior to the injury prevented the appearance of anhedonia following TBI.

Animals also were monitored for the appearance of anxiety-like behaviors. Four weeks of a diet with marginal zinc deficiency (5 ppm) resulted in anxiety, as measured by the elevated plus maze, even in the absence of brain injury. The development of anxiety has been previously reported in zinc-deficient rats (Takeda et al., 2008; Tassabehji et al., 2008) and reviewed in 2010 (Cope and Levenson). The earlier reports used diets that were more severely limited in zinc (< 3 ppm), used weanling animals that are highly susceptible to zinc deficiency, or both. The most recent work is the first report to show that even diets marginally deficient in zinc may result in anxiety. Cortical injury produced additional evidence of anxiety; however, animals fed the zinc-supplemented diet prior to injury appeared to have greater resilience to the effects of injury on anxiety. Not only did supplementation partially prevent anxiety-like behaviors, supplemented animals also showed prevention of significant increases in adrenal weight measured two weeks after TBI (Cope et al., unpublished).

Because loss of cognitive function can be one of the most debilitating deficits associated with TBI, the 2010 study also examined whether zinc supplementation could prevent losses in spatial learning and memory. While controlled cortical impact resulted in significant performance deficits on the Morris water maze test in animals fed a diet adequate in zinc, rats that were fed the zinc-supplemented diet (180 ppm) prior to TBI showed no differences from sham-operated control rats at any point during the 10-day cognitive trial, suggesting that zinc supplementation may improve cognitive resilience in the event of brain injury (Cope et al., unpublished). Future work will be needed to determine the possible uses of zinc supplementation to improve resilience across the range of traumatic brain injuries, including mild TBI.

EVIDENCE INDICATING EFFECT ON TREATMENT

Human Studies

Traumatic brain injury results in significantly depressed serum zinc levels as well as increased urinary zinc excretion. A 1986 report showed that urinary zinc excretion was proportional to the severity of the brain injury (McClain et al., 1986). The most severely injured patients in this study had mean urinary zinc levels that were 14 times normal values, suggesting rapid zinc depletion. Additionally, patients with severe head injuries develop hypoalbuminemia (most likely secondary to increased interleukin-1-mediated transendothelial movement of albumin), as well as evidence of inflammation, including increases in acute-phase proteins (e.g., C-reactive protein, ceruloplasmin), and elevated white blood cell counts (McClain et al., 1988; Young et al., 1988). The impact of these factors on zinc availability and zinc metabolism is potentially significant. Because albumin is the major serum transport protein for zinc, hypoalbuminemia would potentially impair both zinc transport and availability. Induction of cytokines such as interleukin-1 may further compromise zinc availability and reduce zinc stores that are already significantly depleted by increased urinary excretion.

Given the apparent role of TBI in compromising zinc status, Young et al. (1996) sought to test the effectiveness of using zinc supplementation after TBI to reduce zinc losses, maintain protein balance, and improve neurological outcomes. Within 72 hours of injury, 68 patients with severe closed head injuries were randomly assigned to either an adequate zinc (2.5 mg/day) or supplemental zinc (12 mg/day) treatment group. These zinc levels were administered intravenously as zinc sulfate in conjunction with total parenteral nutrition. Supplements were administered in a double-blind fashion for the initial 15 days and followed by 22 mg intravenous zinc (as zinc gluconate) or placebo for the remainder of the study. Zinc supplementation resulted in increased levels of serum pre-albumin and retinol-binding protein, suggesting improved protein synthesis and a role for supplemental zinc in maintaining visceral protein in TBI patients. Two weeks after injury, patients in the zinc-supplemented group had better Glasgow Coma Scale scores than control patients given adequate zinc. These improvements were maintained at 21 and 28 days. Interestingly, the differences between the groups were seen despite the fact that neither serum zinc concentrations nor zinc levels in cerebral spinal fluid were changed by zinc supplementation, suggesting that the zinc is taken up into tissues after administration, and illustrating the fact that serum zinc levels are not a good indicator of zinc status. One month after TBI, mortality in the control group receiving adequate zinc was 26 percent, compared to 12 percent in the group receiving supplemental zinc. Caution should be exercised, however, when interpreting the mortality data, because a larger number of patients in the control group (13 vs. 6 in the zinc-supplemented group) required craniotomies for hematoma evacuation during the course of the study.

The efficacy of treatment with zinc also has been tested after ischemic injury. A small (26 patients assigned to receive either zinc supplementation or placebo) human study sought to explore the effectiveness of replacing zinc in stroke patients who had dietary zinc intakes that were lower than two-thirds of the RDA. In these patients, zinc replacement (10 mg/day) improved outcomes measured by the National Institutes of Health Stroke Scale 30 days after stroke (Aquilani et al., 2009). Although this work does not address the effect of zinc supplementation using levels that are higher than the RDA as a treatment for neuronal injury, it does suggest that, at the very least, maintaining adequate zinc levels after injury is important for recovery.

Finally, as many as 40 percent of patients hospitalized with TBI develop major depression, making it the most common long-term complication of TBI (Jorge and Starkstein, 2005). Although there are no data on the use of supplemental zinc to improve antidepressant drug treatment in patients with TBI-associated depression and although this report does not further review long-term health disorders associated with TBI, the use of zinc to improve mood may be effective among this patient population.

Animal Studies

Zinc Deficiency

Because military personnel may be at risk for developing zinc deficiency, and TBI further increases zinc losses, it is important to understand the possible effects of zinc deficiency on the cellular and molecular mechanisms associated with TBI. Animal models not only permit the study of these mechanisms in a controlled fashion, but also have provided useful information about the role of zinc in TBI. For example, an examination of DNA damage after infliction of a unilateral cortical stab wound in adult rats found that zinc deficiency (induced with a moderately deficient diet that did not result in anorexia) led to a significant increase in terminal deoxynucleotidyl transferase-mediated biotinylated dUTP nick-end labeling (TUNEL)-positive cells at the site of injury compared to animals with adequate zinc. TUNEL staining, a marker of DNA fragmentation and cell death, in combination with nuclear morphology and cell-specific markers, revealed that moderate zinc deficiency caused both apoptosis and necrosis of macrophages and ameboid microglia involved in the clearance of debris following TBI (Yeiser et al., 2002). More severely zinc-deficient diets that induced anorexia resulted in increased neuronal death and significant increases in gliosis at the site of injury (Penkowa et al., 2001). These data combine to suggest that zinc deficiency not only increases the severity of damage after TBI, but also may prevent debris clearance and inhibit repair at the site of the injury.

Zinc Toxicity

Animal models also have been used to show that TBI can result in the accumulation of free zinc that leads to neuronal death (Hellmich et al., 2004; Yeiser et al., 1999). In addition to affecting the site of injury, TBI produced either by fluid percussion injury (Hellmich et al., 2004) or mechanical cortical trauma (Suh et al., 2000) resulted in neuronal death in the dentate gyrus, hilus, and CA1 regions of the hippocampus. Not only does the neuronal death appear to be associated with presynaptic zinc release (Hellmich et al., 2007), but also the cell death was largely prevented by treatment with the zinc chelator calcium disodium ethylenediamine tetraacetate (Hellmich et al., 2004, 2008), suggesting that zinc in high concentrations after TBI is neurotoxic. Despite histological evidence of neuronal survival, however, chelation of zinc after TBI did not improve the spatial memory deficits associated with brain injury (Hellmich et al., 2008).

This understanding of the possible role of free zinc in neuronal death raises the question of whether clinicians should be treating brain-injured patients with supplemental zinc, particularly in acute periods after severe injury when the blood-brain barrier that regulates brain zinc uptake has been disrupted. An animal model of TBI showed that four weeks of dietary zinc supplementation (180 ppm) after TBI did not significantly increase cell death (as measured by TUNEL labeling) in any cell type examined, including microglia, macrophages, neurons, or oligodendrocytes at the site of injury or any other region of the CNS (Yeiser et al., 2002). These data suggest that concerns about the potential neurotoxicity of enteral zinc supplementation in TBI patients are unwarranted. Reports that intraperitoneal injections of zinc significantly increased the infarct size and impaired motor behavior after focal ischemia in subject rats suggest, however, that caution is warranted when using zinc parenterally in moderately to severely injured patients (Levenson, 2005; Shabanzadeh et al., 2004).

CONCLUSIONS AND RECOMMENDATIONS

Although the available evidence suggests that zinc may be an effective treatment for TBI, there are many unanswered questions that prevent its optimal use in the clinical setting. Future research will be needed to determine the best practices for zinc administration after TBI and to populations at risk of TBI. The safety of zinc supplementation, especially in patients with moderate to severe TBI, also must be evaluated.

In the acute care situation, the available clinical evidence suggests that after TBI, zinc deficiency should be prevented to maintain visceral protein and optimize the potential for neurological recovery. The only acute dose of supplemental zinc that has been tested in a clinical setting is 12 mg/day administered intravenously for the first 15 days after injury. After day 15, an oral dose of 22 mg/day was used. With the UL set at 40 mg/day, these doses are not likely to have adverse effects. However, the impact of parenteral administration of zinc has not been independently investigated, nor has it been compared to enteral feeding in a TBI model. Doses of up to 30 mg/day have been provided to critically ill patients without obvious adverse clinical impacts.

Although there have been no studies to determine the possible efficacy of zinc supplementation in TBI patients who are being treated for depression and depression-related disorders, the available clinical evidence suggests that this approach may be warranted.

RECOMMENDATION 16-1. Based on a report showing efficacy in humans, the committee recommends that animal studies be conducted to determine the best practices for zinc administration after concussion/mild, moderate, and severe TBI, such as determining the therapeutic window for zinc administration, the length of treatment time for greatest efficacy, and the optimal level of zinc to improve outcomes. These trials should also evaluate the safety of zinc, based on concerns about toxicity and overload. Results from these studies should be used to design human clinical trials using zinc as a treatment for TBI.

RECOMMENDATION 16-2. Future work is needed in both humans and animal models to determine the extent to which chronic preinjury zinc supplementation can improve resilience in the event of a TBI.

REFERENCES

Afrin, L. B. 2010. Fatal copper deficiency from excessive use of zinc-based denture adhesive. *American Journal of the Medical Sciences* 340(2):164–168.

Aimo, L., G. N. Cherr, and P. I. Oteiza. 2010. Low extracellular zinc increases neuronal oxidant production through NADPH oxidase and nitric oxide synthase activation. *Free Radical Biology and Medicine* 48(12):1577–1587.

Aquilani, R., P. Baiardi, M. Scocchi, P. Iadarola, M. Verri, P. Sessarego, F. Boschi, E. Pasini, O. Pastoris, and S. Viglio. 2009. Normalization of zinc intake enhances neurological retrieval of patients suffering from ischemic strokes. *Nutritional Neuroscience* 12(5):219–225.

Baum, M. K., S. H. Lai, S. Sales, J. B. Page, and A. Campa. 2010. Randomized, controlled clinical trial of zinc supplementation to prevent immunological failure in HIV-infected adults. *Clinical Infectious Diseases* 50(12):1653–1660.

Cope, E. C., and C. W. Levenson. 2010. Role of zinc in the development and treatment of mood disorders. *Current Opinion in Clinical Nutrition and Metabolic Care* 13(6):685–689.

Cope, E. C., J. W. VanLandingham, A. G. Scrimgeour, and C. W. Levenson. (unpublished). *Zinc supplementation improves behavioral resilience to traumatic brain injury in the rat.*

Corniola, R. S., N. M. Tassabehji, J. Hare, G. Sharma, and C. W. Levenson. 2008. Zinc deficiency impairs neuronal precursor cell proliferation and induces apoptosis via p53-mediated mechanisms. *Brain Research* 1237:52–61.

Eby, G. A., and W. W. Halcomb. 2006. Ineffectiveness of zinc gluconate nasal spray and zinc orotate lozenges in common-cold treatment: A double-blind, placebo-controlled clinical trial. *Alternative Therapies in Health and Medicine* 12(1):34–38.

Frederickson, C. J., W. Maret, and M. P. Cuajungco. 2004. Zinc and excitotoxic brain injury: A new model. *Neuroscientist* 10(1):18–25.

Freedman, L. P., and B. F. Luisi. 1993. On the mechanism of DNA-binding by nuclear hormone receptors—A structural and functional perspective. *Journal of Cellular Biochemistry* 51(2):140–150.

Hedera, P., A. Peltier, J. K. Fink, S. Wilcock, Z. London, and G. J. Brewer. 2009. Myelopolyneuropathy and pancytopenia due to copper deficiency and high zinc levels of unknown origin II. The denture cream is a primary source of excessive zinc. *Neurotoxicology* 30(6):996–999.

Hellmich, H. L., C. J. Frederickson, D. S. DeWitt, R. Saban, M. O. Parsley, R. Stephenson, M. Velasco, T. Uchida, M. Shimamura, and D. S. Prough. 2004. Protective effects of zinc chelation in traumatic brain injury correlate with upregulation of neuroprotective genes in rat brain. *Neuroscience Letters* 355(3):221–225.

Hellmich, H. L., K. A. Eidson, B. A. Capra, J. M. Garcia, D. R. Boone, B. E. Hawkins, T. Uchida, D. S. Dewitt, and D. S. Prough. 2007. Injured fluoro-jade-positive hippocampal neurons contain high levels of zinc after traumatic brain injury. *Brain Research* 1127(1):119–126.

Hellmich, H. L., K. Eidson, J. Cowart, J. Crookshanks, D. K. Boone, S. Shah, T. Uchida, D. S. DeWitt, and D. S. Prough. 2008. Chelation of neurotoxic zinc levels does not improve neurobehavioral outcome after traumatic brain injury. *Neuroscience Letters* 440(2):155–159.

Heyland, D. K., N. Jones, N. Z. Cvijanovich, and H. Wong. 2008. Zinc supplementation in critically ill patients: A key pharmaconutrient? *Journal of Parenteral and Enteral Nutrition* 32(5):509–519.

IOM (Institute of Medicine). 2006. *Mineral requirements for military personnel: Levels needed for cognitive and physical performance during garrison training.* Washington, DC: The National Academies Press.

Jorge, R. E., and S. E. Starkstein. 2005. Pathophysiologic aspects of major depression following traumatic brain injury. *Journal of Head Trauma Rehabilitation* 20(6):475–487.

Klug, A., and J. W. R. Schwabe. 1995. Protein motifs .5. Zinc fingers. *The Federation of American Societies for Experimental Biology Journal* 9(8):597–604.

Levenson, C. W. 2005. Zinc supplementation: Neuroprotective or neurotoxic? *Nutrition Reviews* 63(4):122–125.

Levenson, C. W. 2006. Regulation of the NMDA receptor: Implications for neuropsychological development. *Nutrition Reviews* 64(9):428–432.

Matias, C. M., N. C. Matos, M. Arif, J. C. Dionisio, and M. E. Quinta-Ferreira. 2006. Effect of the zinc chelator N,N,N',N'-tetrakis (2-pyridylmethyl)ethylenediamine (TPEN) on hippocampal mossy fiber calcium signals and on synaptic transmission. *Biological Research* 39(3):521–530.

McClain, C. J., D. L. Twyman, L. G. Ott, R. P. Rapp, P. A. Tibbs, J. A. Norton, E. J. Kasarskis, R. J. Dempsey, and B. Young. 1986. Serum and urine zinc response in head-injured patients. *Journal of Neurosurgery* 64(2):224–230.

McClain, C. J., B. Hennig, L. G. Ott, S. Goldblum, and A. B. Young. 1988. Mechanisms and implications of hypoalbuminemia in head-injured patients. *Journal of Neurosurgery* 69(3):386–392.

O'Halloran, T. V. 1993. Transition-metals in control of gene-expression. *Science* 261(5122):715–725.

Penkowa, M., M. Giralt, P. S. Thomsen, J. Carrasco, and J. Hidalgo. 2001. Zinc or copper deficiency-induced impaired inflammatory response to brain trauma may be caused by the concomitant metallothionein changes. *Journal of Neurotrauma* 18(4):447–463.

Prasad, A. S. 2009. Zinc: Role in immunity, oxidative stress and chronic inflammation. *Current Opinion in Clinical Nutrition and Metabolic Care* 12(6):646–652.

Scrimgeour, A. G., and M. L. Condlin. 2009. Zinc and micronutrient combinations to combat gastrointestinal inflammation. *Current Opinion in Clinical Nutrition and Metabolic Care* 12(6):653–660.

Sensi, S. L., and J. M. Jeng. 2004. Rethinking the excitotoxic ionic milieu: The emerging role of Zn^{2+} in ischemic neuronal injury. *Current Molecular Medicine* 4(2):87–111.

Shabanzadeh, A. P., A. Shuaib, T. Yang, A. Salam, and C. X. Wang. 2004. Effect of zinc in ischemic brain injury in an embolic model of stroke in rats. *Neuroscience Letters* 356(1):69–71.

Singh, M., and Das, R. R. 2011. Zinc for the common cold. *Cochrane Database of Systematic Reviews* 2:CD001364.

Stoll, L., J. Hall, N. Van Buren, A. Hall, L. Knight, A. Morgan, S. Zuger, H. Van Deusen, and L. Gentile. 2007. Differential regulation of ionotropic glutamate receptors. *Biophysical Journal* 92(4):1343–1349.

Suh, S. W., J. W. Chen, M. Motamedi, B. Bell, K. Listiak, N. F. Pons, G. Danscher, and C. J. Frederickson. 2000. Evidence that synaptically-released zinc contributes to neuronal injury after traumatic brain injury. *Brain Research* 852(2):268–273.

Takeda, A., H. Itoh, K. Yamada, H. Tamano, and N. Oku. 2008. Enhancement of hippocampal mossy fiber activity in zinc deficiency and its influence on behavior. *Biometals* 21(5):545–552.

Tapiero, H., and K. D. Tew. 2003. Trace elements in human physiology and pathology: Zinc and metallothioneins. *Biomedicine and Pharmacotherapy* 57(9):399–411.

Tassabehji, N. M., R. S. Corniola, A. Alshingiti, and C. W. Levenson. 2008. Zinc deficiency induces depression-like symptoms in adult rats. *Physiology and Behavior* 95(3):365–369.

Yeiser, E. C., A. A. Lerant, R. M. Casto, and C. W. Levenson. 1999. Free zinc increases at the site of injury after cortical stab wounds in mature but not immature rat brain. *Neuroscience Letters* 277(2):75–78.

Yeiser, E. C., J. W. Vanlandingham, and C. W. Levenson. 2002. Moderate zinc deficiency increases cell death after brain injury in the rat. *Nutritional Neuroscience* 5(5):345–352.

Young, A. B., L. G. Ott, D. Beard, R. J. Dempsey, P. A. Tibbs, and C. J. McClain. 1988. The acute-phase response of the brain-injured patient. *Journal of Neurosurgery* 69(3):375–380.

Young, B., L. Ott, E. Kasarskis, R. Rapp, K. Moles, R. J. Dempsey, P. A. Tibbs, R. Kryscio, and C. McClain. 1996. Zinc supplementation is associated with improved neurologic recovery rate and visceral protein levels of patients with severe closed head injury. *Journal of Neurotrauma* 13(1):25–34.

Part III

Recommendations

17

Summary of Recommendations

Traumatic brain injury (TBI) is the beginning of an ongoing process that affects multiple organs and systems and may cause or accelerate other diseases and disorders that can reduce life quality and expectancy. As the physiological mechanisms associated with TBI, such as oxidation and inflammation, are elucidated, it becomes clear that nutrition may play a role in ameliorating primary and secondary (i.e., acute, or within minutes; and subacute, or within 24 hours) as well as long-term effects of TBI. The ability of any intervention to improve the outcomes of TBI will largely depend on its ability to inhibit disease progression either by solo action, or by acting synergistically with other interventions or endogenous recovery factors. Specific approaches need to be targeted to the pathophysiology of the disease, and will differ depending on the mechanisms involved in the disease progression. Broadly speaking, different processes—such as hypoxia, excitotoxicity, or proteinopathies—will respond to different interventions. Some interventions also may be most beneficial when administered over an extended period of time, while others may provide optimal benefit with one-time administration. The timing of administration is also critical, as there may be a time window of efficacy for some nutrients; that is, some interventions might be beneficial within minutes, while others will be effective later. For these reasons, it is important to identify promising interventions of two different kinds: those that will target primary and secondary effects early after injury, and those that will target long-term effects of TBI.

In addition to the evidence indicating that nutrition can affect the disease pathophysiology, there is increasing information indicating that nutrition affects brain function and that nutritional strategies may improve resilience or support treatment of brain disorders. With this in mind, an IOM expert committee reviewed the evidence supporting the potential role for nutrition in the acute and subacute phases of TBI. Based on the evidence reviewed, the committee concluded that nutritional interventions could be important both to augment mechanisms that defend against the effects of TBI, and to serve as an integral component of multidisciplinary postinjury treatment to lessen the primary and secondary effects of TBI. With the exception of a recommendation to follow a specific energy- and protein-feeding regimen early after injury for patients with severe TBI, the committee concluded there is a need to either refine study protocols or confirm the effectiveness of nutritional approaches in lessening the health outcomes of TBI. Because of the paucity of data about the efficacy of most of the nutrition approaches reviewed, the committee thought it premature to direct DoD to adopt any of them at this time. For some approaches for which enough preclinical and, in some cases, clinical data exist the committee sees the potential benefits and reached consensus about research needed in some promising areas. The research recommended will serve to confirm published results and to refine the protocols (i.e., optimal route of administration, timing, and dose). There is even less data being generated about the effectiveness of nutritional interventions in combination, either with one another or with other forms of treatment. Investigating the synergistic or antagonistic effects of nutrients is an important area of research for the future. However, there are more pressing areas to investigate that are highlighted below.

It is important to note that, as requested in the statement of task, this report has reviewed nutritional interventions only for primary (i.e., acute) and secondary (i.e., subacute) effects. The effects of TBI are conceptually categorized as primary, secondary, and long-term effects, based on the amount of time elapsed since the injury; but in reality, the boundaries of these definitions are ambiguous. For example, the impact of some of the early pathogenic events related to cell death may linger in the more chronically injured brain, into the time when there is upregulation of growth factors linked to plasticity and ongoing angiogenesis. Moreover, events such as angiogenesis, typically associated with wound healing, are initiated within the more acutely injured brain. Because of these challenges, this report includes, in addition to acute effects, some studies that also evaluate outcomes that are seemingly long-term but that might be initiated in the acute phase of the disease. This report does not address other outcomes such as neurodegenerative (e.g., Alzheimer's disease, Parkinson's disease), neuroendocrine, psychiatric, and other nonneurological disorders that appear later in life and for which a causal relationship with the original injury has not been clearly established.

The report is limited in that it did not evaluate the role of nutritional therapies in the rehabilitation phase and did not address the long-term effects of TBI, despite evidence indicating that nutritional therapies may be beneficial. Based on the literature searches the committee concluded that conducting a review of the nutrition approaches to improve long-term effects of TBI, which was part of the initial task and later excluded because of financial constraints, would also be important. Specifically, it would be important to review the alterations in metabolism associated with TBI, together with the nutritional interventions that could enhance or impair recovery from those long-term health disorders in the areas of motor dysfunction and cognitive, neuropsychiatric, and neurodegenerative states, should be reviewed (see also workshop papers by Metzger, Gomez-Pinilla, and Sands in Appendix C).

RECOMMENDATIONS

The committee concluded that there is already sufficient evidence to indicate that nutrition should be added to the toolbox of interventions for TBI treatment and recovery. A summary of the committee's recommendations follows. Only one recommendation calls for updating evidence-based guidelines for severe TBI, to provide patients with energy and protein (Box 17-1). The remaining recommendations identify additional research needs in study methodologies (Box 17-2), nutritional assessments (Box 17-3), and specific recommendations for research on nutritional interventions that have been prioritized into the most promising (Box 17-4) and other research (Box 17-5). Finally, the committee includes a general recommendation to develop evidence-based clinical nutritional guidelines, and to continue to update them as more evidence becomes available (Box 17-6).

BOX 17-1
Standardize the Provision of Energy and Protein to Patients with Severe TBI

RECOMMENDATION 6-1. The committee recommends that evidence-based guidelines include the provision of early (within 24 hours after injury) nutrition (more than 50 percent of total energy expenditure and 1–1.5 g/kg protein) for the first two weeks after injury. This intervention is critical to limit the intensity of the inflammatory response due to TBI, and to improve outcome.

BOX 17-2
Continue Improving Animal Models and Identifying Biomarkers

RECOMMENDATION 3-1. The committee recommends that the Department of Defense (DoD), in cooperation with others, refine existing animal models to investigate the potential benefits of nutrition throughout the spectrum of TBI injuries, that is, concussion/mild, moderate, severe, and penetrating, as well as repetitive and blast injuries. Development of animal models is particularly urgent for concussion/mild TBI and brain injuries due to blast as well as for repetitive injuries. These models also will aid in understanding the pathobiology of TBI, which is particularly needed for concussion/mild TBI, blast, and repetitive injuries.

RECOMMENDATION 3-2. The committee recommends that DoD, in cooperation with others, continue to develop better clinical biomarkers of TBI (i.e., concussion/mild, moderate, severe, penetrating, repetitive, and blast injuries) for the purposes of diagnosis, treatment, and outcome assessment. In addition, the committee recommends the identification of biomarkers specifically related to proposed mechanisms of action for individual nutritional interventions.

BOX 17-3
Assessing Nutrition Status

RECOMMENDATION 5-1. DoD should conduct dietary intake assessments in different military settings (e.g., when eating in military dining facilities or when subsisting on a predominantly ration-based diet) both predeployment and during deployment to determine the nutritional status of soldiers as a basis for recommending increases in intake of specific nutrients that may provide resilience to TBI.

RECOMMENDATION 5-2. Routine dietary intake assessments of TBI patients in medical treatment facilities should be undertaken as soon after hospitalization as possible to estimate preinjury nutrition status as well as to provide optimal nutritional intake throughout the various stages of treatment.

RECOMMENDATION 5-3. In individuals with TBI, DoD should estimate preinjury and postinjury dietary intake or status for those nutrients, dietary supplements, and diets that might show a relationship to TBI outcome. For example, based on the current evidence, the committee recommends collecting those estimates for creatine, n-3 fatty acids, choline, and vitamin D. The data could be used to investigate potential relationships between preinjury nutritional intake or status and recovery progress. Such data also would show possible synergistic effects between nutrients and dietary supplements.

Energy and Protein to Patients with Severe TBI

The committee made one urgent recommendation to standardize the feeding regimen for TBI patients early after a severe injury. This important recommendation focuses on including specific energy and protein provisions for patients with severe TBI in the current evidence-

BOX 17-4
Most Promising Research Recommendations on Nutritional Interventions

RECOMMENDATION 6-2. DoD should conduct human trials to determine appropriate levels of blood glucose following TBI to minimize morbidity and mortality. These should be clinical trials of early feeding using intense insulin therapy to maintain blood glucose concentrations at less than 150–160 mg/dL versus current usual care of acute TBI in intensive care unit (ICU) settings for the first two weeks.

RECOMMENDATION 6-3. DoD should conduct clinical trials of the benefits of insulin therapy for care of acute TBI in inpatient settings with total parenteral nutrition (TPN) alone (or plus enteral feeding) versus enteral feeding alone. The goals for blood glucose in the TPN group should be lower (e.g., less than 120 mg/dL) than in the enteral group (e.g., less than 150–160 mg/dL). Variables to measure include clinical outcomes and incidence of hypoglycemia.

RECOMMENDATION 6-4. DoD should conduct studies to determine the optimal goals for nutrition (e.g., when to begin meeting total energy expenditure for optimal lean tissue maintenance or repletion) after the first two weeks following severe injury.

RECOMMENDATION 8-1. DoD should continue to monitor the literature on the effects of nutrients, dietary supplements, and diets on TBI, particularly those reviewed in this report but also others that may emerge as potentially effective in the future. For example, although the evidence was not sufficiently compelling to recommend that research be conducted on branched-chain amino acides, DoD should monitor the scientific literature for relevant research.

RECOMMENDATION 9-1. DoD should monitor the results of the Citicoline Brain Injury Treatment (COBRIT) trial, a human experimental trial examining the effect of CDP-choline and genomic factors on cognition and functional measures in severe, moderate, and complicated mild TBI. If the results of that trial are positive, DoD should conduct animal studies to define the optimal clinical dose and duration of treatment for choline (CDP-choline) following TBI, as well as to explore choline's potential to promote resilience to TBI when used as a preinjury supplement.

RECOMMENDATION 10-1. Based on the evidence supporting the effects of creatine on brain function and behavior after brain injury in children and adolescents, DoD should initiate studies in adults to assess the value of creatine for treating TBI patients.

RECOMMENDATION 13-1. DoD should conduct animal studies that examine the effectiveness of preinjury and postinjury oral administration of current commercial preparations of purified n-3 fatty acids on TBI outcomes.

RECOMMENDATION 13-2. Based on the evidence that fish oil decreases inflammation within hours of continuous administration, human clinical trials that investigate fish oil or purified n-3 fatty acids as a treatment for TBI are recommended. For acute cases of TBI, it should be noted that there are intravenous fish oil formulations available in Europe, but these are not approved by the Food and Drug Administration (FDA). Continuous enteral feeding with a feeding formula containing fish oil should provide equivalent effects for this purpose in the early phase of severe TBI when enteral access becomes available.

RECOMMENDATION 16-1. Based on a report showing efficacy in humans, the committee recommends that animal studies be conducted to determine the best practices for zinc administration after concussion/mild, moderate, and severe TBI, such as determining the therapeutic window for zinc administration, the length of treatment time for greatest efficacy, and the optimal level of zinc to improve outcomes. These t also rials should evaluate the safety of zinc, based on concerns about toxicity and overload. Results from these studies should be used to design human clinical trials using zinc as a treatment for TBI.

BOX 17-5
Other Research Recommendations

RECOMMENDATION 7-1. Based on the literature from animal and human trials concerning stroke and epilepsy, DoD should consider a clinical trial with TBI patients using an array of antioxidants in combination (e.g., vitamins E and C, selenium, beta-carotene).

RECOMMENDATION 11-1. DoD should conduct animal studies to examine the specific effects of ketogenic diets, other modified diets (e.g., structured lipids, low-glycemic-index carbohydrates, fructose), or precursors of ketone bodies that affect energetics and have potential value against TBI. These animal studies should specifically consider dose, time, and clinical correlates with injury as variables. Results from these studies should be used to design human studies with these various diets to determine if they improve outcome against severe TBI. These studies should include time as a variable to determine whether there is an optimal initiation point and length of use.

RECOMMENDATION 11-2. If these studies show benefits, then DoD should further investigate whether the potential beneficial effect of such ketogenic or modified diets or precursors to ketone bodies applies to concussion/mild and moderate TBI. Before conducting these studies, DoD should consider the feasibility (i.e., how to ensure compliance with a modified diet) of using diets that affect the metabolic energy available, such as ketogenic diets, for the treatment of TBI.

RECOMMENDATION 14-1. Based on positive outcomes in small-animal models of TBI with curcumin and resveratrol, DoD should consider conducting human trials. In addition, other flavonoids (e.g., isoflavones, flavanols, epicatechin, theanine) should be evaluated in animal models of TBI.

RECOMMENDATION 15-1. The committee recommends more animal studies be conducted to determine if vitamin D enhances the beneficial actions of progesterone in the treatment of TBI. If this synergistic effect is confirmed in animals, then studies in humans should be conducted to evaluate the extent to which vitamin D supplementation might improve the efficacy of progesterone treatment.

RECOMMENDATION 15-2. Based on animal studies showing a requirement of vitamin D for the efficacy of progesterone therapy, future animal studies are recommended to test the efficacy of using vitamin D supplements to improve resilience to TBI. Should the data from animal studies support use of this steroid hormone, human trials should be implemented to test the efficacy of vitamin D in populations at high risk for TBI.

RECOMMENDATION 16-2. Future work is needed in both humans and animal models to determine the extent to which chronic preinjury zinc supplementation can improve resilience in the event of a TBI.

BOX 17-6
Future Update of Evidence-Based Guidelines

RECOMMENDATION 2-1. Evidence-based nutrition guidelines specific for severe TBI should be updated. These guidelines should address unique nutritional concerns of severe TBI when different from generic critical illness nutrition guidelines (e.g., meeting energy needs and benefits of specific nutrients, food components, or diets). In addition, current guidelines to manage mild and moderate TBI should include recommendations for nutritional interventions. The guidelines should be developed in a collaborative manner with the various key stakeholders (e.g., American Dietetic Association, Department of Veterans Affairs, DoD).

based guidelines. Such nutritional intervention should be implemented immediately, and will achieve significant positive outcomes by reducing the inflammatory response, which is likely to be at its height during the first two weeks after injury.

Research Needs

The rest of the recommendations concern research questions about the potential benefits and adverse effects of nutritional interventions for TBI. The committee made research recommendations for animal studies as well as for both observational and randomized controlled trials in humans. Despite the expressed need for more research in the TBI patient population, the committee recognizes that clinical TBI is extremely complex and that the understanding of the differences in pathophysiology between mild and severe injuries is continuously evolving. Furthermore, the translation of experimental models to clinical care is limited by a number of factors, such as differences between animal species and variations in the mechanisms of injury producing the various types of TBIs. In addition, patients with TBI often suffer from polytrauma, which adds another level of complexity to an already multifaceted injury. Given the diverse nature of the injury, randomized clinical trials in a population with TBI are difficult to carry out, and long-term prospective studies among high-risk populations are costly, from both a financial and human resources perspective. Still, the committee emphasizes the need to follow best practices when designing such studies. Instead of providing specifics about the design of the research studies that might be challenging to meet, the committee offers the following list of considerations for future investigators in this discipline:

- A note of caution is offered on extrapolating findings from animal models to humans; although there are good animal models for severe injuries, there is a need for better animal models for other types of TBI, especially concussion/mild TBI and blast TBI (see recommendation 3-1).
- There are limitations, such as poor sensitivity and specificity, on the use of biomarkers as indicators of injury and recovery. Better predictability might be attained by using several biomarkers in conjunction with clinical data (see recommendation 3-2).
- Unless specified in the recommendations, research should be conducted on the full spectrum of TBI, from mild/concussion to severe injuries.
- Although not specifically mentioned in the research recommendations, adverse effects from any studies should be recorded, taking into consideration that TBI patients may experience more frequent adverse effects than a healthy population exposed to the same intervention. The reader is also referred to the 2008 Institute of Medicine (IOM) report *Use of Dietary Supplements by Military Personnel*, in which a framework to review the safety of dietary supplements in military settings was developed.
- In general, and based on results from previous studies, the committee advises that gender and age differences be considered in the study design.
- The committee emphasizes that commercial food components and nutrient supplements vary in their purity, and this variation will likely have an effect in the results of a study. Therefore, investigators should pay particular attention to the quality (i.e., purity) of these compounds.
- The chemistry (and source) of each compound of interest affects its bioavailability, metabolism, and ability to reach the target area, which in turn influence the effectiveness of a nutritional intervention.

- Before any definitive conclusions can be made about efficacy, the route and timing of administration and dosage are key considerations that investigators need to optimize in study designs.
- Investigators should consider synergistic and antagonistic effects with nutrients, dietary supplements, food components, or other substances in the diets of military personnel.

Although not related to nutrition specifically, the committee thought it important to mention the significance of appropriate methodologies. There are still substantial deficiencies in the biomarkers and animal models currently used. On that point, the committee made two general recommendations: first, to continue to develop better animal models, and second, to identify biomarkers of both injury and improved brain function.

There also is a need to assess the nutritional status of military personnel to determine whether there are nutrients that need to be added to the diets of military personnel to maintain optimal readiness and mission performance goals. The committee found there are not enough nutritional assessments of military personal conducted in various settings, specifically during deployments.

In addition to providing protein and energy after severe injury, there are other nutritional interventions that are promising but for which many questions persist about exact protocols (e.g., dosage, time, and route of administration), and more research is critically needed in order to provide optimal treatment to military members with TBI. For example, based on recent reports that mortality and morbidity of TBI patients are affected by early feeding, the committee strongly supports elucidation of the best practices during the early postinjury period. Fundamental questions remain, however, about the appropriate serum levels of glucose and insulin to be achieved within the first 24 hours after severe TBI. More information is also needed on the best nutrition goals for the two weeks following that period. In addition to these urgent questions about protein and energy needs shortly after injury, research gaps also were identified in other promising areas. Based on the existing evidence from animal and human research studies, the nutritional interventions selected for review by the committee were energy and protein provision, antioxidants (e.g., vitamins E and C), polyphenols (e.g., flavonoids, resveratrol, and curcumin), branched-chain amino acids, choline, creatine, ketogenic and similar modified diets, magnesium, n-3 fatty acids, vitamin D, and zinc. Chapter 4 describes how these nutrition interventions were selected. For some of the selected nutrients, such as resveratrol, studies have demonstrated benefits of the nutrient in animal models of TBI or brain injury. However, there are as yet no clinical trials that confirm similar beneficial effects in humans. For other nutrients, such as creatine, there are human trials with promising results that could be extended to military personnel. In other cases, such as magnesium, choline, and n-3 fatty acids, human trials are under way, and the military should review those studies as the results are made public.

The committee recognizes the need for the Department of Defense (DoD) to prioritize the research recommendations. Although there will undoubtedly be other criteria that will be used to guide such ranking, the committee offers here its reflections on the prioritization of research based on its opinions about the likelihood of positive results for lessening the effects of TBI. Research on interventions for which human trials to explore efficacy in improving the outcomes of TBI already exist or are ongoing have been presented as "most promising research" (Box 17-4). Research on interventions for which animal studies in TBI or human studies in associated conditions have shown improvements in outcomes is presented as "other research" (Box 17-5). Although the research recommendations are directed to DoD as the sponsor of this study, the committee recognizes that this research agenda would entail a tremendous effort. Because the problem of TBI is not unique to military personnel but is also a concern for the civilian population, the research questions would likely be of interest to other organizations. DoD is encouraged to conduct research internally, to support extramural research, or to collaborate with others in order to obtain answers in the most effective manner.

Ultimately, any potential interventions must be applied to clinical care situations to benefit TBI patients. The committee found that, except for guidance on energy intake, the majority of clinical guidelines for critical care and TBI patients do not include specific recommendations for adequate nutrition either early after injury or in the long term. In addition, discussions with critical care and rehabilitation clinicians indicate there is diversity in clinical practices, and that the small number of current nutrition guidelines is followed by few practitioners. This picture is even more worrisome when considering the lack of specific, evidence-based guidelines for the use of dietary supplements or food components for TBI, and the frequent use of dietary supplements by military personnel discussed in the 2008 IOM report *Use of Dietary Supplements by Military Personnel* (IOM, 2008). The committee therefore also reflected on the application of the research recommended in this report to improve the clinical guidelines. The findings of the research gaps outlined above would present an opportunity to update the existing clinical guidelines with evidence-based nutritional interventions. To that effect, a table (see Appendix B) was developed with questions for which the evidence does not currently exist, but that will benefit clinicians as they create evidence-based guidelines in the future. These questions are outlined in the PICO (Population/Participant, Intervention, Comparator, Outcomes) format, which is used to present questions for the purpose of creating evidence-based guidelines. Topics include designation of biomarkers, optimal feeding regimens (e.g., sources of energy, percentage of energy needs to be met, route of administration), and novel nutrition therapies. The committee hopes that in addition to creating a research agenda to answer questions about TBI, these recommendations will serve to update clinical guidelines.

Appendixes

A

Agenda

Workshop on Nutrition and Neuroprotection in Military Personnel
June 23–24, 2010
VENABLE
575 Seventh St., NW, Washington, DC 20004

Wednesday, June 23, 2010: Day 1

1:30 pm   Welcome, Introductions, and Purpose of Open Session
           John Erdman, Committee Chair

SESSION 1: BACKGROUND AND OVERVIEW

Objective: To understand possible differences in pathophysiology and metabolic response between acute injury and injury from repeated low-severity events due to blast overpressure.

1:40   **Moderator: Cathy Levenson, Committee on Nutrition, Trauma, and the Brain**

1:45   Central nervous system (CNS)-related neurotrauma in the military
           environment
           Col. Michael Jaffee, M.D., USAF
           Director, Defense and Veterans Brain Injury Center

2:15   Pathophysiology and mechanisms of neurotrauma: Blast and civilian
           Mårten Risling, M.D., Ph.D.
           Associate Professor, Department of Neuroscience
           Karolinska Institutet, Sweden

2:45   Recurrent sports-related traumatic brain injury (TBI) and tauopathy
            Robert Stern, Ph.D.
            Associate Professor of Neurology
            Co-Director, Center for the Study of Traumatic Encephalopathy
            Co-Director, Alzheimer's Disease Clinical & Research Program
            Boston University School of Medicine

3:15   Panel Discussion

4:15   Public Comments

4:45   Adjourn

Thursday, June 24, 2010: Day 2

8:30 am   Welcome
            John Erdman, Committee Chair

SESSION 2: CLINICAL TREATMENT AND REHABILITATION

Objectives:
  • To gain understanding of the acute phase of injury in the civilian world (What
    treatments are available in early phases and rehabilitation; long-term strategies?)
  • To gain understanding of the acute phase of injury in the military (What treatments
    are available in early phases and rehabilitation; long-term strategies?)

8:35   **Moderator: Ross Zafonte, Committee on Nutrition, Trauma, and the Brain**

8:40   Clinical management in the field
            Col. Geoffrey Ling, M.D., Ph.D.
            Medical Corps, U.S. Army
            Program Manager, Defense Sciences Office
            DARPA

9:10   Stateside acute care and rehabilitation
            Maj. Megumi Vogt, M.D.
            Medical Corps, U.S. Air Force
            Deputy Director, TBI Clinical Standards of Care
            Defense Center of Excellence for Psychological Health and Traumatic
            Brain Injury

SESSION 3: NUTRITIONAL CONSIDERATIONS IN CLINICAL TREATMENT

Objective: To gain understanding of existing clinical guidance and standards of practice
on nutritional interventions for concussion and other CNS-related neurotrauma treatment
and recovery.

9:40   **Moderator: Wayne Askew, Committee on Nutrition, Trauma, and the Brain**

9:45   The perspective of an R.D. working with civilian TBI
            Natalia Bailey, M.S., R.D., C.D.
            Neurological Trauma/Surgery ICU Nutrition Support Dietitian
            Harborview Medical Center
            University of Washington Level I Trauma Center

| 10:05 | The perspective of a neurosurgeon
Jamshid Ghajar, M.D., Ph.D., FACS
President, Brain Trauma Foundation
Clinical Professor of Neurological Surgery
Weill Cornell Medical College, Cornell University |
|---|---|

10:05   The perspective of a neurosurgeon
Jamshid Ghajar, M.D., Ph.D., FACS
President, Brain Trauma Foundation
Clinical Professor of Neurological Surgery
Weill Cornell Medical College, Cornell University

10:25   The perspective of an R.D. working in the military environment
Maj. Kelli Metzger, R.D.
Medical Specialist Corps, U.S. Army
Chief, Nutrition Marketing and Integration Services
Walter Reed Army Medical Center

10:55   Break

11:10   Panel Discussion

12:10 pm   Lunch

SESSION 4: ROLE OF NUTRITION IN RESILIENCE AND RECOVERY

Objective: To gather information about the state of research on the role of diets, food products, and/or nutritional interventions in the enhancement or impairment of recovery from CNS-related neurotrauma.

1:10   **Moderator: John Erdman, Committee on Nutrition, Trauma, and the Brain**

1:20   The ability of nutrients to promote brain plasticity and cognitive health
Fernando Gómez-Pinilla, Ph.D.
Professor, Depts. of Neurosurgery and Physiological Science
University of California, Los Angeles

1:50   Resolvins and Protectins: Specialized proresolving mediators in inflammation, and organ protection from essential fatty acids
Charles Serhan, Ph.D.
Director, Center for Experimental Therapeutics and Reperfusion Injury
The Simon Gelman Professor of Anesthesia
Brigham and Women's Hospital and Harvard Medical School

2:20   Mechanisms of nutritional neuroprotection: Flavanols
Sylvain Doré, Ph.D.
Associate Professor of Anesthesiology and Critical Care Medicine, and
Pharmacology and Molecular Sciences
Johns Hopkins University School of Medicine

2:50   Overview of therapeutics for TBI
Edward Hall, Ph.D.
Director, Spinal Cord & Brain Injury Research Center
Professor of Anatomy & Neurobiology, Neurosurgery, Neurology, and
Physical Medicine & Rehabilitation, Chandler Medical Center
University of Kentucky

3:20   Panel Discussion

4:20   Public Comments

Meeting 2 of the Committee on Nutrition, Trauma, and the Brain

September 23, 2010
The Keck Center of the National Academies
500 Fifth Street, NW, Washington, DC 20001
Room 205

OPEN SESSION AGENDA

10:00 am   Welcome
            John Erdman
            Chair, Committee on Nutrition, Trauma, and the Brain

10:05 am   The need for glucose control in critically ill patients: Risks and benefits
            Stanley Nasraway, M.D.
            Tufts University School of Medicine & Tufts Medical Center

11:05 am   Targeting mitochondrial dysfunction following TBI using creatine and fasting
            Patrick Sullivan, Ph.D.
            The University of Kentucky Chandler College of Medicine

12:05 pm   Nutritional Support of TBI at the VA
            Stephanie Sands, R.D.
            James A. Haley Veterans Hospital

B

Evidence-Based Guidelines for Traumatic Brain Injury

TABLE B-1   Content of Evidence-Based Guidelines (EBG) for Acute Traumatic Brain Injury (TBI) in Intensive Care Unit (ICU) Setting (e.g., Critical Illness)

Guideline/ Step of Care Process with Nutrition Implications	Brain Trauma Foundation (BTF) *Guidelines for the Management of Severe Traumatic Brain Injury*[a]	American Society for Parenteral and Enteral Nutrition Critically Ill Patient[b]
Nutrition-related assessment information		A1. Traditional nutrition assessment tools (albumin, pre-albumin, and anthropometry) are not validated in critical care. Before initiation of feedings, assessment should include evaluation of weight loss and previous nutrient intake prior to admission, level of disease severity, comorbid conditions, and function of the gastrointestinal (GI) tract. (Grade: E)
		C1. The target goal of enteral nutrition (EN) (defined by energy requirements) should be determined and clearly identified at the time of initiation of nutrition support therapy. (Grade: C) Energy requirements may be calculated by predictive equations or measured by indirect calorimetry. Predictive equations should be used with caution, because they provide a less accurate measure of energy requirements than indirect calorimetry in the individual patient. In the obese patient, the predictive equations are even more problematic without availability of indirect calorimetry. (Grade: E)

American Dietetic Association—Critical Illness[c]	American Association of Neuroscience Nurses—Nursing Management of Adults with Severe TBI[d]

CI: Indirect calorimetry to determine RMR
Indirect calorimetry is the standard for determination of resting metabolic rate (RMR) in critically ill patients because RMR based on measurement is more accurate than estimation using predictive equations.

Rating: Strong
Imperative

CI: RMR Predictive equations for nonobese patients
If predictive equations are needed in nonobese, critically ill patients, consider using one of the following, as they have the best prediction accuracy of equations studied (listed in order of accuracy): Penn State, 2003a (79%), Swinamer (55%), and Ireton-Jones, 1992 (52%). In some individuals, errors between predicted and actual energy needs will result in under- or over-feeding.

Rating: Fair
Conditional

CI: Inappropriate RMR predictive equations for this population
The Harris-Benedict (with or without activity and stress factors), the Ireton-Jones, 1997, and the Fick equations should not be considered for use in RMR determination in critically ill patients, because these equations do not have adequate prediction accuracy. In addition, the Mifflin-St. Jeor equation should not be considered for use in critically ill patients, as it was developed for healthy people and has not been well researched in the critically ill population.

Rating: Strong
Imperative

CI: RMR predictive equations for obese patients
If predictive equations are needed for critically ill, mechanically ventilated individuals who are obese, consider using Ireton-Jones, 1992 or Penn State, 1998, because they have the best prediction accuracy of equations studied. In some individuals, errors between predicted and actual energy needs will result in under- or over-feeding.

Rating: Fair
Conditional

CI: Rest periods and RMR
Allow a rest of 30 minutes prior to RMR measurement in critically ill patients.

Rating: Consensus
Imperative

CI: Rest period and accuracy of RMR
If the critically ill patient has undergone a nursing activity or medical procedure (e.g., suctioning, wound care, central venous access or ventilator setting change), then employ a 30-minute rest after procedures to achieve a resting state during RMR measurement. Measuring RMR before the 30-minute period may be inaccurate because patient instability or ventilator gas re-equilibration.

Rating: Consensus
Conditional

continued

TABLE B-1   Continued

Guideline/ Step of Care Process with Nutrition Implications	Brain Trauma Foundation (BTF) *Guidelines for the Management of Severe Traumatic Brain Injury[a]*	American Society for Parenteral and Enteral Nutrition Critically Ill Patient[b]

American Dietetic Association—Critical Illness[c]	American Association of Neuroscience Nurses—Nursing Management of Adults with Severe TBI[d]

CI: Impact of environmental factors on RMR
Ensure that the room is comfortably quiet, and the light is not providing heat or discomfort for the patient. Noise and light may cause erroneous measures of RMR if the critically ill patient's state of rest is disturbed.

Rating: Consensus
Imperative

CI: Impact of room temperature on RMR
Recommend a room temperature 20 to 25 degrees Celsius (68 to 77 degrees Fahrenheit). When the room's temperature is too cold, RMR is overestimated in critically ill patients by shivering or non-shivering thermogenesis, as the body adapts.

Rating: Weak
Imperative

CI: Environmental factors and RMR
Ensure that each critically ill patient is in a physically comfortable posture before proceeding with the test, because discomfort will result in erroneously high RMR measures. Make sure that repeated measures are taken in the same position to ensure comparability of data.

Rating: Insufficient Evidence
Imperative

CI: Steady state measurement of RMR
For ventilated patients, if a steady state is achieved, then a single measure is adequate to describe RMR. To achieve a steady state, discard the first five minutes of measurement. Then achieve a five-minute period with CV = 5% for oxygen consumption and carbon dioxide production. An alternate protocol can be 25 minutes in duration if a CV of 10% is achieved. If proper attention is given to achieving resting conditions, 80% or more of RMR measures in ventilator patients will be in steady state. Sedation improves the likelihood of obtaining steady state measures.

Rating: Strong
Imperative

CI: Non-steady state measurement conditions
There are published data that were not in steady state, but were still reasonably close to steady state measures. When steady state is not achieved, interpret the results carefully. If the non-steady state conditions are chronic (e.g., patient posturing), then higher measures may reflect actual energy expenditure. If non-steady state conditions are episodic (e.g., ventilator change, nursing intervention, anxiety, coughing, sneezing, movement), RMR measures should be taken at a separate time.

Rating: Consensus
Conditional

continued

TABLE B-1 Continued

Guideline/ Step of Care Process with Nutrition Implications	Brain Trauma Foundation (BTF) *Guidelines for the Management of Severe Traumatic Brain Injury[a]*	American Society for Parenteral and Enteral Nutrition Critically Ill Patient[b]
Specific nutrition interventions	Level II. Patients should be fed to attain full caloric replacement by day 7 postinjury Data show that starved traumatic brain injury (TBI) patients lose sufficient nitrogen to reduce weight by 15% per week; 100 to 140% replacement of Resting Metabolism Expenditure with 15 to 20% nitrogen calories reduces nitrogen loss. Data in non-TBI injured patients show that a 30% weight loss increased mortality rate. The data support feeding at least by the end of the first week. It has not been established that any method of feeding is better than another or that early feeding prior to 7 days improves outcome. Based on the level of nitrogen wasting documented in TBI patients and the nitrogen sparing effect of feeding, it is a Level II recommendation that full nutritional replacement be instituted by day 7 postinjury.	A2. Nutrition support therapy in the form of enteral nutrition (EN) should be initiated in the critically ill patient who is unable to maintain volitional intake. (Grade: C) A3. EN is the preferred route of feeding over parenteral nutrition (PN) for the critically ill patient who requires nutrition support therapy. (Grade: B) A4. Enteral feeding should be started early within the first 24–48 hours following admission. (Grade: C) The feedings should be advanced toward goal over the next 48–72 hours. (Grade: E) A5. In the setting of hemodynamic compromise (patients requiring significant hemodynamic support including high dose catecholamine agents, alone or in combination with large volume fluid or blood product resuscitation to maintain cellular perfusion), EN should be withheld until the patient is fully resuscitated and/or stable. (Grade: E) A6. In the ICU patient population, neither the presence nor absence of bowel sounds nor evidence of passage of flatus and stool is required for the initiation of enteral feeding. (Grade: B) A7. Either gastric or small bowel feeding is acceptable in the ICU setting. Critically ill patients should be fed via an enteral access tube placed in the small bowel if at high risk for aspiration or after showing intolerance to gastric feeding. (Grade: C) Withholding of enteral feeding for repeated high gastric residual volumes alone may be sufficient reason to switch to small bowel feeding (the definition for high gastric residual volume is likely to vary from one hospital to the next, as determined by individual institutional protocol). (Grade: E)

American Dietetic Association—Critical Illness[c]

American Association of Neuroscience Nurses—Nursing Management of Adults with Severe TBI[d]

CI: Respiratory quotient

If Respiratory Quotient (RQ) is below 0.7 or above 1.0, then repeated measures are necessary under more optimal conditions. An RQ under 0.70 suggests hypoventilation (inadequate removal of metabolic carbon dioxide from the blood to the lung) or prolonged fasting. An RQ above 1.0, in the absence of overfeeding, suggests hyperventilation (removal of carbon dioxide from the blood to the lung in excess of the amount produced by metabolism) or inaccurate gas collection.

Rating: Strong
Conditional

CI: Enteral vs. parenteral nutrition

If the critically ill ICU patient is hemodynamically stable with a functional GI tract, then EN is recommended over PN. Patients who received EN experienced less septic morbidity and fewer infectious complications than patients who received PN. In the critically ill patient, EN is associated with significant cost savings when compared to PN. There is insufficient evidence to draw conclusions about the impact of EN or PN on length of stay (LOS) and mortality.

Rating: Strong
Conditional

CI: Timing of enteral nutrition

If the critically ill patient is adequately fluid resuscitated, then EN should be started within 24 to 48 hours following injury or admission to the ICU. Early EN is associated with a reduction in infectious complications and may reduce LOS. The impact of timing of EN on mortality has not been adequately evaluated.

Rating: Strong
Conditional

CI: Immune-enhancing enteral nutrition

Immune-enhancing EN is not recommended for routine use in critically ill patients in the ICU. Immune-enhancing EN is not associated with reduced infectious complications, LOS, reduced cost of medical care, days on mechanical ventilation or mortality in moderately to less severely ill ICU patients. Their use may be associated with increased mortality in severely ill ICU patients, although adequately powered trials evaluating this have not been conducted. For the trauma patient, it is not recommended to routinely use immune-enhancing EN, because its use is not associated with reduced mortality, reduced LOS, reduced infectious complications or fewer days on mechanical ventilation.

Rating: Fair
Imperative

Administering intensive insulin therapy may reduce intercranial pressure (ICP) (Level 3)

Isolated patients with severe TBI treated with intensive insulin therapy had lower mean and maximal ICPs than subjects in a randomized control group who were treated with insulin only when their glucose levels exceeded 220 mg/dl. The intensive insulin therapy group did not experience more hypoglycemic episodes and required less vasopressors to achieve the same cerebral perfusion pressure as the control group.

Initiating adequate nutrition within 72 hours of injury may improve outcomes (Level 3)

A study of the effect of malnutrition on rehabilitation length of stay found that patients with malnutrition had lengths of stay that were 28 days longer than patients with adequate nutrition. Two systematic reviews found a trend toward improved mortality and less disability with early feeding in patients with severe TBI. The BTF *Guidelines for the Management of Severe TBI* recommend patients be fed so that full caloric requirements are met by postinjury day 7 (Bratton et al., 2007).

continued

TABLE B-1   Continued

Guideline/ Step of Care Process with Nutrition Implications	Brain Trauma Foundation (BTF) *Guidelines for the Management of Severe Traumatic Brain Injury*[a]	American Society for Parenteral and Enteral Nutrition Critically Ill Patient[b]
		(See guideline D4 for recommendations on gastric residual volumes, identifying high-risk patients, and reducing chances for aspiration.)
		B1. If early EN is not feasible or available the first 7 days following admission to the ICU, no nutrition support therapy (i.e., standard therapy) should be provided. (Grade: C)
		In the patient who was previously healthy prior to critical illness with no evidence of protein calorie malnutrition, use of PN should be reserved and initiated only after the first 7 days of hospitalization (when EN is not available). (Grade: E)
		B2. If there is evidence of protein-calorie malnutrition on admission and EN is not feasible, it is appropriate to initiate PN as soon as possible following admission and adequate resuscitation. (Grade: C)
		B3. If a patient is expected to undergo major upper GI surgery and EN is not feasible, PN should be provided under very specific conditions: If the patient is malnourished, PN should be initiated 5–7 days preoperatively and continued into the postoperative period. (Grade: B)
		PN should not be initiated in the immediate postoperative period but should be delayed for 5–7 days (should EN continue not to be feasible). (Grade: B)
		PN therapy provided for a duration of < 5–7 days would be expected to have no outcome effect and may result in increased risk to the patient. Thus, PN should be initiated only if the duration of therapy is anticipated to be ≥ 7 days. (Grade: B)
		C2. Efforts to provide > 50–65% of goal calories should be made in order to achieve the clinical benefit of EN over the first week of hospitalization. (Grade: C)
		C3. If unable to meet energy requirements (100% of target goal calories) after 7–10 days by the enteral route alone, consider initiating supplemental PN. (Grade: E) Initiating supplemental PN prior to this 10-day period in the patient already receiving EN does not improve outcome and may be detrimental to the patient. (Grade: C)

American Dietetic Association—Critical Illness[c]	American Association of Neuroscience Nurses—Nursing Management of Adults with Severe TBI[d]
CI: Feeding tube placement EN administered into the stomach is acceptable for most critically ill patients. Consider placing feeding tube in the small bowel when patient is in supine position or under heavy sedation. If your institution's policy is to measure gastric residual volume (GRV), then consider small bowel tube feeding placement in patients who have more than 250 ml GRV or formula reflux in two consecutive measures. Small bowel tube placement is associated with reduced GRV. Adequately powered studies have not been conducted to evaluate the impact of GRV on aspiration pneumonia. There may be specific disease states or conditions that may warrant small bowel tube placement (e.g., fistulas, pancreatitis, gastroparesis); however, they were not evaluated at this phase of the analysis. **Rating: Fair Conditional**	**Providing continuous intragastric feeding may improve tolerance (Level 3)** Continuous feeding was better tolerated and achieved 75% of nutritional goals faster than bolus feeding in patients admitted to a neurosurgical ICU (20% of whom had sustained a severe TBI). Feeding via percutaneous endoscopic gastrostomy in patients with moderate-to-severe TBI was well tolerated without complication in 97% of patients. **Prokinetic agents have shown no effect on feeding tolerance (Level 2)** A prospective randomized double-blind study of patients with severe TBI that compared metoclopramide with normal saline found no difference in feeding intolerance or complication rates between the groups. Prokinetic agents demonstrated no improvement in feeding tolerance in patients in barbiturate-induced comas for refractory intracranial hypertension. The amount of time it took to achieve nutritional goals was not reduced with the use of prokinetic agents in a neurosurgical ICU in which 20% of patients had severe TBI. **Administering intensive insulin therapy for serum glucose greater than 110 mg/dl improves outcomes (Level 2)** Glucose levels exceeding 170 mg/dl during the first 5 days post-severe TBI correlate with prolonged hospital length of stay and increased mortality. Administering intensive insulin therapy for elevated serum glucose can improve outcomes. A glucose level higher than 200 mg/dl that goes untreated during the first 24 hours post-severe TBI has been associated with worse outcomes and is related to increased ICP and impaired pupillary reaction.

continued

TABLE B-1 Continued

Guideline/ Step of Care Process with Nutrition Implications	Brain Trauma Foundation (BTF) *Guidelines for the Management of* *Severe Traumatic Brain Injury*[a]	American Society for Parenteral and Enteral Nutrition Critically Ill Patient[b]
		C4. Ongoing assessment of adequacy of protein provision should be performed. The use of additional modular protein supplements is a common practice, as standard enteral formulations tend to have a high nonprotein calorie:nitrogen ratio. In patients with body mass index (BMI) < 30, protein requirements should be in the range of 1.2–2.0 g/kg actual body weight per day, and may likely be even higher in burn or multi-trauma patients. (Grade: E)
		C5. In the critically ill obese patient, permissive underfeeding or hypocaloric feeding with EN is recommended. For all classes of obesity where BMI is > 30, the goal of the EN regimen should not exceed 60–70% of target energy requirements or 11–14 kcal/kg actual body weight per day (or 22–25 kcal/kg ideal body weight per day). Protein should be provided in a range ≥ 2.0 g/kg ideal body weight per day for Class I and II patients (BMI 30–40), ≥ 2.5 g/kg ideal body weight per day for Class III (BMI ≥ 40). Determining energy requirements is discussed in guideline C1. (Grade: D)
		D1. In the ICU setting, evidence of bowel motility (resolution of clinical ileus) is not required in order to initiate EN in the ICU. (Grade: E)
		D3. Use of enteral feeding protocols increases the overall percentage of goal calories provided and should be implemented. (Grade: C)
		E1. Immune-modulating enteral formulations (supplemented with agents such as arginine, glutamine, nucleic acid, n-3 fatty acids, and antioxidants) should be used for the appropriate patient population (major elective surgery, trauma, burns, head and neck cancer, and critically ill patients on mechanical ventilation), with caution in patients with severe sepsis. (For surgical ICU patients, Grade: A) (For medical ICU patients, Grade: B) ICU patients not meeting criteria for immune-modulating formulations should receive standard enteral formulations. (Grade: B)
		E2. Patients with Acute respiratory distress syndrome (ARDS) and severe acute lung injury (ALI) should be placed on an enteral formulation characterized by an anti-inflammatory lipid profile (i.e., n-3 fish oils, borage oil) and antioxidants. (Grade: A)
		E3. To receive optimal therapeutic benefit from the immune-modulating formulations, at least 50–65% of goal energy requirements should be delivered. (Grade: C)

American Dietetic Association—Critical Illness[c]	American Association of Neuroscience Nurses—Nursing Management of Adults with Severe TBI[d]

continued

TABLE B-1 Continued

Guideline/ Step of Care Process with Nutrition Implications	Brain Trauma Foundation (BTF) *Guidelines for the Management of Severe Traumatic Brain Injury*[a]	American Society for Parenteral and Enteral Nutrition Critically Ill Patient[b]
		E4. If there is evidence of diarrhea, soluble-fiber-containing or small peptide formulations may be utilized. (Grade: E)
		F1. Administration of probiotic agents has been shown to improve outcome (most consistently by decreasing infection) in specific critically ill patient populations involving transplantation, major abdominal surgery, and severe trauma. (Grade: C)
		No recommendation can currently be made for use of probiotics in the general ICU population because of a lack of consistent outcome effect. It appears that each species may have different effects and variable impact on patient outcome, making it difficult to make broad categorical recommendations. Similarly, no recommendation can currently be made for use of probiotics in patients with severe acute necrotizing pancreatitis, based on the disparity of evidence in the literature and the heterogeneity of the bacterial strains utilized.
Monitoring and evaluations of nutrition-related indicators		D2. Patients should be monitored for tolerance of EN (determined by patient complaints of pain and/or distention, physical exam, passage of flatus and stool, abdominal radiographs). (Grade: E)
		Inappropriate cessation of EN should be avoided. (Grade: E) Holding EN for gastric residual volumes < 500 mL in the absence of other signs of intolerance should be avoided. (Grade: B)
		The time period that a patient is made nil per os (NPO; no food or drink thourhg the mouth) prior to, during, and immediately following the time of diagnostic tests or procedures should be minimized to prevent inadequate delivery of nutrients and prolonged periods of ileus. Ileus may be propagated by NPO status. (Grade: C)
		D4. Patients placed on EN should be assessed for risk of aspiration. (Grade: E) Steps to reduce risk of aspiration should be employed. (Grade: E) The following measures have been shown to reduce risk of aspiration: In all intubated ICU patients receiving EN, the head of the bed should be elevated 30–45 degrees. (Grade: C) For high-risk patients or those shown to be intolerant to gastric feeding, delivery of EN should be switched to continuous infusion. (Grade: D)

American Dietetic Association—Critical Illness[c]	American Association of Neuroscience Nurses—Nursing Management of Adults with Severe TBI[d]

CI: Blue dye use and critically ill patients
Blue dye should not be added to EN for detection of aspiration. The
risk of using blue dye outweighs any perceived benefit. The presence of
blue dye in tracheal secretions is not a sensitive indicator for aspiration.

Rating: Strong
Imperative

CI: Monitoring patient position
Evaluating patient position should be part of an EN monitoring plan.
To decrease the incidence of aspiration pneumonia and reflux of gastric
contents into the esophagus and pharynx, critically ill patients should
be placed in a 45-degree head of bed elevation, if not contraindicated.

Rating: Strong
Imperative

continued

TABLE B-1   Continued

Guideline/ Step of Care Process with Nutrition Implications	Brain Trauma Foundation (BTF) *Guidelines for the Management of Severe Traumatic Brain Injury*[a]	American Society for Parenteral and Enteral Nutrition Critically Ill Patient[b]
		Agents to promote motility such as prokinetic drugs (metoclopramide and erythromycin) or narcotic antagonists (naloxone and alvimopan) should be initiated where clinically feasible. (Grade: C) Diverting the level of feeding by post-pyloric tube placement should be considered. (Grade: C) Use of chlorhexidine mouthwash twice a day should be considered to reduce risk of ventilator-associated pneumonia. (Grade: C)
		D5. Blue food coloring and glucose oxidase strips, as surrogate markers for aspiration, should not be used in the critical care setting. (Grade: E)
		D6. Development of diarrhea associated with enteral tube feedings warrants further evaluation for etiology. (Grade: E)
		F2. A combination of antioxidant vitamins and trace minerals (specifically including selenium) should be provided to all critically ill patients receiving specialized nutrition therapy. (Grade: B)
		F3. The addition of enteral glutamine to an EN regimen (not already containing supplemental glutamine) should be considered in burn, trauma, and mixed ICU patients. (Grade: B)
		F4. Soluble fiber may be beneficial for the fully resuscitated, hemodynamically stable critically ill patient receiving EN who develops diarrhea. Insoluble fiber should be avoided in all critically ill patients. Both soluble and insoluble fiber should be avoided in patients at high risk for bowel ischemia or severe dysmotility. (Grade: C)

American Dietetic Association—Critical Illness[c]	American Association of Neuroscience Nurses—Nursing Management of Adults with Severe TBI[d]

CI: Monitoring gastric residual volume

Evaluating GRV in critically ill patients is an optional part of a monitoring plan to assess tolerance of EN. Enteral nutrition should be held when a GRV greater than or equal to 250 ml is documented on two or more consecutive occasions. Holding EN when GRV is less than 250 ml is associated with delivery of less EN. Gastric residual volume may not be a useful tool to assess the risk of aspiration pneumonia. Adequately powered studies have not been conducted to evaluate the impact of GRV on aspiration pneumonia.

Rating: Consensus
Imperative

CI: Monitoring and promotility agents

If the patient exhibits a history of gastroparesis or repeated high GRVs, then consider the use of a promotility agent in critically ill ICU patients, if there are no contraindications. The use of a promotility agent (e.g., metoclopramide) has been associated with increased GI transit, improved feeding tolerance, improved EN delivery, and possibly reduced risk of aspiration.

Rating: Strong
Conditional

CI: Monitoring delivery of energy

Monitoring plan of critically ill patients must include a determination of daily actual EN intake. Enteral nutrition should be initiated within 48 hours of injury or admission and average intake actually delivered within the first week should be **at least** 60–70% of total estimated energy requirements as determined in the assessment. Provision of EN within this time frame and at this level may be associated with a decreased LOS, days on the mechanical ventilation, and infectious complications.

Rating: Fair
Imperative

Glucose Monitoring Recommendation was removed and is under revision (Sep 2009)

CI: Thermic effect of continuous feeding on RMR

If a critically ill patient is continuously receiving any energy source (e.g., intravenous fluids, EN or PN), the rate and concentration should remain unchanged during the 24-hour period before and during RMR measure. After 24-hour equilibration, the impact of the thermal effect of food (TEF) on RMR is constant and indirect calorimetry measurements can proceed.

Rating: Fair
Conditional

CI: Thermic effect of intermittent feeding on RMR

If a critically ill patient receives intermittent EN above 400 kcal per feeding, then hold feedings for a minimum of five hours before measuring RMR. When a five-hour fast is not clinically feasible or when a small feeding (< 400 kcal) is given, a four-hour fast is allowed. Measuring RMR during the time of the TEF will produce inaccurately high values.

Rating: Weak
Conditional

continued

TABLE B-1   Continued

Guideline/ Step of Care Process with Nutrition Implications	Brain Trauma Foundation (BTF) *Guidelines for the Management of Severe Traumatic Brain Injury[a]*	American Society for Parenteral and Enteral Nutrition Critically Ill Patient[b]
		G1. If EN is not available or feasible, the need for PN therapy should be evaluated (see guidelines B1, B2, B3, C3). (Grade: C) If the patient is deemed to be a candidate for PN, steps to maximize efficacy (regarding dose, content, monitoring, and choice of supplemental additives) should be used. (Grade: C)
		G2. In all ICU patients receiving PN, mild permissive underfeeding should be considered at least initially. Once energy requirements are determined, 80% of these requirements should serve as the ultimate goal or dose of parenteral feeding. (Grade: C) Eventually, as the patient stabilizes, PN may be increased to meet energy requirements. (Grade: E) For obese patients (BMI ≥ 30), the dose of PN with regard to protein and caloric provision should follow the same recommendations given for EN in guideline C5. (Grade: D)
		G3. In the first week of hospitalization in the ICU, when PN is required and EN is not feasible, patients should be given a parenteral formulation without soy-based lipids. (Grade: D)
		G4. A protocol should be in place to promote moderately strict control of serum glucose when providing nutrition support therapy. (Grade: B) A range of 110–150 mg/dL may be most appropriate. (Grade: E)
		G5. When PN is used in the critical care setting, consideration should be given to supplementation with parenteral glutamine. (Grade: C)
		G6. In patients stabilized on PN, periodically repeated efforts should be made to initiate EN. As tolerance improves and the volume of EN calories delivered increases, the amount of PN calories supplied should be reduced. PN should not be terminated until ≥ 60% of target energy requirements are being delivered by the enteral route. (Grade: E)
		H1. Specialty high-lipid low-carbohydrate formulations designed to manipulate the respiratory quotient and reduce CO_2 production are not recommended for routine use in ICU patients with acute respiratory failure. (Grade: E) (This is not to be confused with guideline E2 for ARDS/ALI).
		H2. Fluid-restricted calorically dense formulations should be considered for patients with acute respiratory failure. (Grade: E)
		H3. Serum phosphate levels should be monitored closely and replaced appropriately when needed. (Grade: E)

American Dietetic Association—Critical Illness[c]	American Association of Neuroscience Nurses—Nursing Management of Adults with Severe TBI[d]

continued

TABLE B-1 Continued

Guideline/ Step of Care Process with Nutrition Implications	Brain Trauma Foundation (BTF) *Guidelines for the Management of Severe Traumatic Brain Injury*[a]	American Society for Parenteral and Enteral Nutrition Critically Ill Patient[b]
		(NOT including renal pancreatitis and end of life)

[a] Bratton et al., 2007.
[b] McClave et al., 2009.
[c] ADA, 2006.
[d] Mcilvoy and Meyer, 2008.

TABLE B-2 Summary Table for Nutrition Content of Existing EBGs for Non-ICU Acute TBI

Guideline/Care Process	**Guidelines for the Field Management of Combat-Related Head Trauma**[a] Mild TBI-Acute Nondeployed Care; Mild TBI Sub-Acute Interdisciplinary team (referrals to PT, OT, Speech & Language pathology, pharmacy, audiology/vestibular and optometry)	**VA Management of Concussion/Mild Traumatic Brain Injury**[b] (Adults, nonacute, not management of moderate or severe TBI)
Nutrition-related assessment information	Neurobehavioral Symptom Inventory (includes nausea, change in appetite, taste or smell) Patient Health Questionnaire (includes changes in appetite) Sub-Acute Cognitions (normalize nutrition) BMI > 30 (Refer for Sleep Study)	Nausea, vomiting Change in appetite Change in taste or smell
Specific nutrition interventions	Novel therapy (nutritional supplements)	Limit caffeine and alcohol. Minimize caffeine and avoid herbal diet supplements such as "energy" products as some contain agents that cross-react with psychiatric mediation and lead to a hypertensive crisis. Novel therapy (hyperbaric oxygen, nutritional supplements) modalities in the management of concussion/mTBI are being explored in the field as potential treatment approaches. It is the recommendation of the Working Group that interventions that lack sufficient empirical support should occur only under the auspices of an IRB-reviewed protocol.
Monitoring and evaluations of nutrition-related indicators		

[a] Knuth, 2005.
[b] Department of Veterans Affairs and Department of Defense (VA/DoD), 2009.

American Dietetic Association—Critical Illness[c]

American Association of Neuroscience Nurses—Nursing Management of Adults with Severe TBI[d]

TABLE B-3   Questions to Guide Future Research Searches to Support Future Evidence-Based Guidelines for Nutrition in TBI Patients[a,b,c]

Population	Intervention (Assessment factor of interest)	Comparator (Alternative assessment factor)	Outcome
Assessment questions			
Acute TBI patients	Selected biomarkers or constellation of biomarkers (e.g., Ca^{2+}, ROS, protein carbonyls, lipid peroxidase, S-100B, neuron specific enolase, glial fibrillary acidic protein, myelin basic protein, phosphorylated neurofilament H, ubiquitin C-Terminal hydrolase, a-II spectrin, microtubule-binding protein Tau, F2-isoprostane, and 4-hydroxynonenol)	Other biomarkers and neuroimaging studies	Sensitive and specific predictor of the level of brain damage and oxidative stress (vs. other types of injuries or conditions) Or Sensitive and specific predictor of mitochondrial function post injury
TBI patients	Remeasurement of energy needs at specific intervals	Monitoring weight and nutrition intake	Maintaining optimal body composition
Acute TBI patients being considered for progesterone treatment for TBI	Serum 25-hydroxyvitamin D	Vitamin D intake	Vitamin D adequacy
Treatment/intervention questions			
Acute TBI in ICU setting	Parenteral nutrition	Enteral nutrition	Tight glucose control Range of control with decreased risk of hypoglycemia and accounting for risks of hypoglycemia (limits to be defined)
Acute TBI in ICU setting	Adjustment of nutrition and medication to maintain "tight" glucose control (e.g., 80–110 mg/dl)	Adjustment of nutrition and medication to maintain "moderate" glucose control (less than 150 mg/dl)	Recovery parameters to severe TBI (e.g., intracranial pressure, increase the level of consciousness, duration of ICU stay or duration of intubation)
Acute TBI in ICU setting in first 24 hours to 7 days	Permissive underfeeding (50–80% of estimated energy needs using specified method to estimate energy needs)	Higher percentage of estimated energy needs (e.g., greater than 80%)	Recovery parameters (See above)

TABLE B-3 Continued

Population	Intervention (Assessment factor of interest)	Comparator (Alternative assessment factor)	Outcome
Acute TBI with severe reduction in mitochondrial function as shown by selected biomarker levels *(NOTE: Only practical if assessment methods are able to identify patients with reduction in mitochondrial function—see related assessment question)*	Alternative energy sources (e.g., ketones from a ketogenic diet)	Traditional sources of energy (carbohydrate, protein, fat)	Minimize depressed mitochondrial functioning using biomarkers from assessment (e.g., lactate production would indicate use of ketones)
Acute severe TBI injury	IV n-3 fatty acid as additional or sole source of fat (dose TBD)	Normal IV fat emulsion (fatty acid dose TBD)	Recovery factors for severe TBI or research parameters of resolvins, protectins, tumor necrosis factor, fatty acid profile
Mild TBI injury or repeated mild TBI injury	Postoperative supplemental n-3 fatty acid (dose TBD)	Normal or nonsupplemented diet n-3 fatty acid (dose TBD)	Resolvins, protectins, tumor necrosis factor
Mild TBI injury or repeated mild TBI injury (by time period, 14–30 days or 45–50 days for repeated injuries)	Eucaloric ketogenic diet (dose TBD)	Normal diet (TBD)	Reduce impact on mitochondrial function deficit with corresponding improvement in clinical symptoms *(Note: Ideally have assessment methods to measure level of mitochondrial function versus relying on clinical symptoms)*
Postacute phase severe TBI	Eucaloric ketogenic diet (dose TBD)	Normal diet (TBD)	Reduce impact on mitochondrial function deficit with corresponding improvement in clinical symptoms *(Note: Ideally have assessment methods to measure level of mitochondrial function versus relying on clinical symptoms)*
Postacute phase of either mild or severe TBI	Choline supplementation (dose above Daily Recommended Intake)	Normal dietary choline content (dose TBD)	Cognitive functioning indicator e.g., National Institute of Child Health and Human Development combined TBI outcome statistic as well as identify potential negative side effects
Postacute phase severe TBI (by gender)	Creatine supplementation (dose TBD)	Nonsupplemented diet (Baseline dose TBD)	Signs and symptoms of TBI, e.g., reduction in headaches, fatigue, and depression and improved cognitive function as well as identifying potential negative side effects

continued

TABLE B-3   Continued

Population	Intervention (Assessment factor of interest)	Comparator (Alternative assessment factor)	Outcome
Postacute phase severe TBI	Preinjury creatine supplementation	Preinjury nonsupplemented diet	Signs and symptoms of TBI, e.g., reduction in headaches, fatigue, and depression and improved cognitive function as well as identifying potential negative side effects
Acute moderate to severe TBI	Zinc administration above DRI level (timing—e.g., hours postinjury, dose and duration—TBD)	Zinc at optimal levels (DRI)	Enhanced memory, reduction in depression, and anxiety symptoms as well as identifying potential negative side effects
Chronic TBI patient	Various counseling theories and strategies (e.g., memory books, motivational interviewing, problem-solving, self-monitoring)	Comparator counseling theories and strategies	Optimal dietary intake matching nutrient needs
Severe TBI with multiple trauma injuries, postacute phase	Branched-chain amino acids as % of total amino acid intake (IV or diet with varying amounts of leucine, isoleucine, and valine—doses TBD, duration < 1 week)	Normal amino acid formula or nonsupplemented diet (baseline dose TBD)	Disability Rating Scale Score, memory or cognitive functioning
TBI, chronic	Novel nutrition therapies sold as dietary supplements (e.g., combinations of resveratrol, curcumin, polyphenols, creatine and CDP-choline)	Nonsupplemented diet (baseline doses TBD)	Improved cognitive function (indicator TBD) as well as identifying potential negative side effects
Monitoring/evaluating questions			
TBI patients (by mild, moderate, severe over specified time and event intervals)	Reassessment of energy needs (RMR)	Original RMR	Significant differences between original RMR and reassessed RMR
TBI patients	Brain-specific biomarkers for improvement in brain function	Other assessment biomarkers	Improved brain function

[a]To aid those preparing future clinical practice guidelines for severe TBI, the questions have been formatted in the Population/Participant, Intervention, Comparator, Outcome (PICO) format. The questions are organized by the step in the care process to which the questions apply, i.e., assessment procedures, types of interventions to be selected, and the types of monitoring and evaluating parameters to be used.

[b]Strauss, S. E., W. S. Richardson, P. Glasziou, and R. B. Haynes. 2005. *Evidence-based medicine: How to practice and teach EBM.* Edinburgh: Churchill Livingstone.

[c]Guyatt, G., R. Drummond, M. O. Meade, and D. J. Cook, eds. 2008. *Users' guides to the medical literature: Amanual for evidence-based clinical practice, 2nd Edition.* Chicago: American Medical Association.

REFERENCES

ADA (American Dietetic Association). 2006. *Critical illness evidence-based nutrition practice guideline.* American Dietetic Association. http://www.adaevidencelibrary.com/topic.cfm?cat=2799 (accessed October 26, 2010).

Bratton, S. L., R. M. Chestnut, J. Ghajar, F. F. McConnell Hammond, O. A. Harris, R. Hartl, G. T. Manley, A. Nemecek, D. W. Newell, G. Rosenthal, J. Schouten, L. Shutter, S. D. Timmons, J. S. Ullman, W. Videtta, J. E. Wilberger, and D. W. Wright. 2007. Guidelines for the management of severe traumatic brain injury. XII. Nutrition. *Journal of Neurotrauma* 24 (Suppl. 1):S77–S82.

Knuth, T., P. B. Letarte, G. Ling, L. E. Moores, P. Rhee, D. Tauber, and A. Trask. 2005. *Guidelines for the field management of combat-related head trauma.* New York: Brain Trauma Foundation.

McClave, S. A., R. G. Martindale, V. W. Vanek, M. McCarthy, P. Roberts, B. Taylor, J. B. Ochoa, L. Napolitano, and G. Cresci. 2009. Guidelines for the provision and assessment of nutrition support therapy in the adult critically ill patient: Society of Critical Care Medicine (SCCM) and American Society for Parenteral and Enteral Nutrition (A.S.P.E.N.). *Journal of Parenteral and Enteral Nutrition* 33(3):277–316.

Mcilvoy, L., and K. Meyer. 2008. *Nursing management of adults with severe traumatic brain injury.* Glenview, IL: American Association of Neuroscience Nurses.

VA/DoD (Department of Veterans Affairs and Department of Defense). 2009. VA/DoD *clinical practice guideline for management of concussion/mild traumatic brain injury.* http://www.healthquality.va.gov/mtbi/concussion_mtbi_full_1_0.pdf (accessed January 19, 2011).

C

Workshop Speakers' Papers

Overview of Traumatic Brain Injury Within the Department of Defense

Kimberly S. Meyer[1] and Michael S. Jaffee[2]

INTRODUCTION

Traumatic brain injury (TBI) has been declared by the media as the signature injury of the current conflicts in Iraq and Afghanistan. The Department of Defense (DoD) defines TBI as a traumatic blow or jolt to the head resulting in an alteration or loss of consciousness (DoD, 2007).

TBI surveillance efforts within DoD began in 2000 and, through the fourth quarter of 2010, 202,281 service members have been diagnosed with TBI.[3] The majority of these injuries (77 percent) are classified as mild TBI (mTBI) or concussion. The severity of injury for the remainder of cases is as follows: moderate (16.8 percent), severe (1 percent), and penetrating (1.7 percent). A small proportion (3.5 percent) is of undetermined severity, likely because of coding incongruencies. Since 2000, the frequency of diagnosis has increased each year (Table C-1), which is likely a result of the aggressive pursuit of increased screening efforts instituted by DoD in 2006.

SCREENING

Screening of TBI occurs at various time points following combat activities. During the acute stages, screening takes place in theater. Early efforts regarding TBI screening required

---

[1] Defense & Veterans Brain Injury Center.
[2] San Antonio Uniformed Services Health Education Consortium.
[3] Available online: http://www.dvbic.org/TBI-Numbers.aspx (accessed March 25, 2011).

TABLE C-1 The Number of DoD Service Members
(All Armed Forces) Diagnosed with TBI, 2000–2010[a]

Year	Number of Service Members
2000	10,963
2001	11,830
2002	12,470
2003	12,898
2004	13,312
2005	12,192
2006	16,946
2007	23,160
2008	28,555
2009	29,252
2010[b]	30,703
Total	202,281

[a]Available online: http://www.dvbic.org/TBI-Numbers.aspx (accessed March 25, 2011).
[b]As of quarter 4 of 2010, as of February 17, 2011.

evaluation when an individual presented to medical care with symptoms concerning for TBI. An in-theater assessment of TBI care sponsored by the Joint Chiefs of Staff, however, found that individuals at risk for TBI failed to seek medical evaluation; consequently, mandatory event-based screening protocols were implemented in July 2010. These protocols include obligatory medical evaluations for all individuals within 50 meters of a blast, those who were located in a building or vehicle damaged by a blast, and those with certain other indications like blunt trauma to the head.

The Military Acute Concussion Evaluation (MACE) is the tool used in acute TBI screening (Figure C-1). The MACE tool was instituted in 2006 and assesses the following four domains: history of the traumatic event, including presence or absence of changes in consciousness; current symptoms; neurological exam; and, if indicated, a brief cognitive appraisal. The MACE tool is based on the Standardized Assessment of Concussion used for sports-related injuries where scores of 25 or less are indicative of cognitive impairment (McCrea et al., 2000). A validation study of MACE use in an austere environment is currently under way. Preliminary evidence suggests cognitive scores slightly less than 25 in a deployed setting may be normal because simple orientation may be affected by lack of differentiation during daily routines. Further validation testing is ongoing to optimize the use of this cognitive evaluation in theater.

Initially, the only documentation required when utilizing MACE was the numeric score associated with the cognitive assessment, which led to incomplete capture of the TBI exposure and an immediate written record in a member's medical history. Subsequently, documentation requirements were modified and the following were added: *c*ognitive score, *n*eurological assessment, and current *s*ymptoms (CNS). Using this additional documentation facilitates the identification of a temporal relationship between the traumatic event and symptom onset in addition to changes in symptom profiles over time. Although MACE is not a definitive diagnostic tool for TBI, positive screens trigger a detailed clinical exam to confirm the diagnosis or determine the differential diagnosis for ongoing symptoms.

Service members evacuated to Landstuhl Regional Medical Center (LRMC) for any injury or illness undergo additional screening using the MACE tool. From May 2006 to October 2008, approximately 18,000 patients (approximately 12,200 inpatients and 5,800

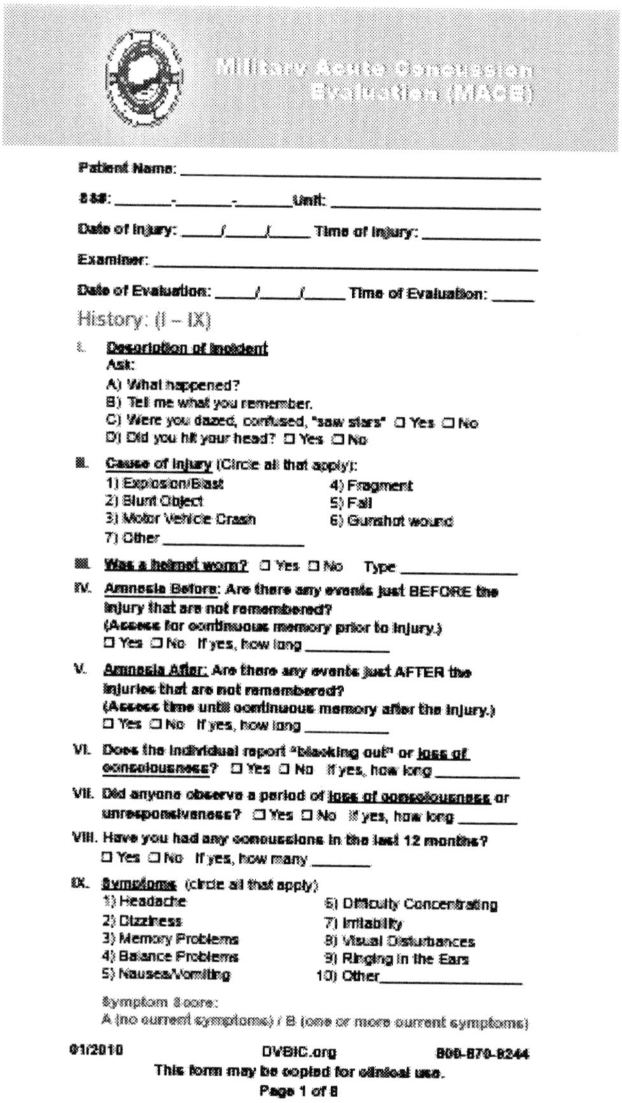
Military Acute Concussion
Evaluation (MACE)

Patient Name: ____________________

SS#: ____-____-____ Unit: ____________

Date of Injury: ___/___/___ Time of Injury: ________

Examiner: ____________________

Date of Evaluation: ___/___/___ Time of Evaluation: ____

History: (I – IX)

I. Description of Incident
Ask:
A) What happened?
B) Tell me what you remember.
C) Were you dazed, confused, "saw stars" ☐ Yes ☐ No
D) Did you hit your head? ☐ Yes ☐ No

II. Cause of Injury (Circle all that apply):
1) Explosion/Blast
2) Blunt Object
3) Motor Vehicle Crash
4) Fragment
5) Fall
6) Gunshot wound
7) Other ________

III. Was a helmet worn? ☐ Yes ☐ No Type ________

IV. Amnesia Before: Are there any events just BEFORE the injury that are not remembered?
(Assess for continuous memory prior to injury.)
☐ Yes ☐ No If yes, how long ______

V. Amnesia After: Are there any events just AFTER the injuries that are not remembered?
(Assess time until continuous memory after the injury.)
☐ Yes ☐ No If yes, how long ______

VI. Does the individual report "blacking out" or loss of consciousness? ☐ Yes ☐ No If yes, how long ______

VII. Did anyone observe a period of loss of consciousness or unresponsiveness? ☐ Yes ☐ No If yes, how long ______

VIII. Have you had any concussions in the last 12 months?
☐ Yes ☐ No If yes, how many ____

IX. Symptoms (circle all that apply)
1) Headache
2) Dizziness
3) Memory Problems
4) Balance Problems
5) Nausea/Vomiting
6) Difficulty Concentrating
7) Irritability
8) Visual Disturbances
9) Ringing in the Ears
10) Other ________

Symptom Score:
A (no current symptoms) / B (one or more current symptoms)

01/2010 DVBIC.org 800-870-9244
This form may be copied for clinical use.
Page 1 of 8

FIGURE C-1 An example of a MACE form.
SOURCE: Available online: http://www.dvbic.org/Providers/TBI-Screening.aspx (accessed April 5, 2011).

outpatients) completed the initial MACE screening at LRMC. Sixteen percent of outpatients screened positively as being at risk for TBI. Additional screening revealed that 78 percent of the positive screens described symptoms associated with TBI. Thirty-one percent of inpatients screened positively as being at risk for TBI. Of those inpatients screening positive, 66 percent reported associated symptoms (Dempsey et al., 2009). Those with significant findings are triaged to a stateside military medical facility with appropriate resources to further evaluate and treat TBI. Increased funding has led to allocation of resources at most military installations, thereby allowing those with mTBI to be treated at their home base. The U.S. Army has credentialed its hospitals based on resources available (Figure C-2). Similarly, the U.S. Navy and U.S. Air Force have declared certain facilities as TBI centers. Those deter-

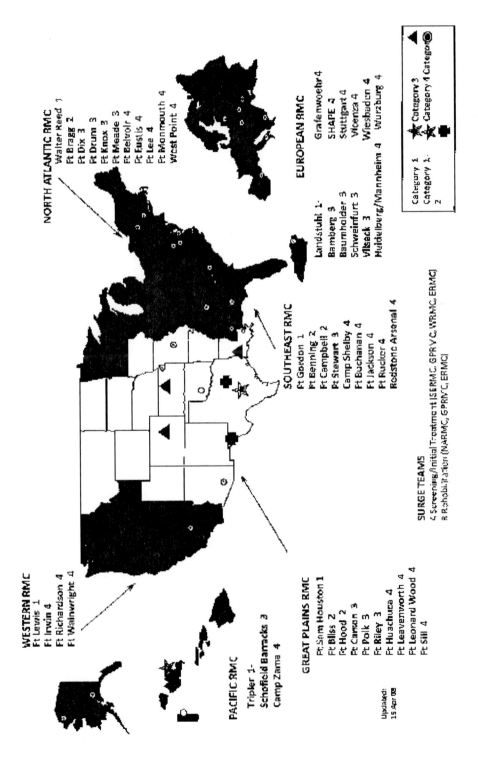

FIGURE C-2 U.S. Army TBI medical assets.

mined to need specialized services (i.e., severe and penetrating TBI patients), however, are directed to Walter Reed Army Medical Center (WRAMC) or National Naval Medical Center (NNMC) for additional acute and subacute care.

Active-duty service members undergo a final screening during mandatory Post-Deployment Health Assessment (PDHA, DD-Form 2796). This assessment is not limited to TBI and covers symptoms associated with a variety of other medical and psychological conditions. The TBI component consists of the following four questions, which are based on the Brief Traumatic Brain Injury Screen (Schwab et al., 2006):

1. During this deployment, did you experience any of the following events?
   - Blast or explosion
   - Vehicular accident
   - Fragment wound or bullet wound above the shoulders
   - Fall
   - Other event causing injury to the head
2. Did any of the following happen to you, or were you told happened to you, IMMEDIATELY after any of the event(s)?
   - Lost consciousness or got "knocked out"
   - Felt dazed, confused, or "saw stars"
   - Didn't remember the event
   - Had a concussion
   - Had a head injury
3. Did any of the following problems begin or get worse after the event(s)?
   - Memory problems or lapses
   - Balance problems or dizziness
   - Ringing in the ears
   - Sensitivity to bright light
   - Irritability
   - Headaches
   - Sleep problems
4. In the past week, have you had any of the symptoms you indicated?
   - Memory problems or lapses
   - Balance problems or dizziness
   - Ringing in the ears
   - Sensitivity to bright light
   - Irritability
   - Headaches
   - Sleep problems

One study of a returning U.S. Army Combat Brigade Team revealed that 22.8 percent of soldiers who reported injury during assessment with PDHA sustained a clinician-confirmed TBI (Terrio et al., 2009). The majority were mTBIs (i.e., concussions). Although 33.4 percent of this sample reported multiple symptoms immediately following the injury, symptom reporting decreased to 7.5 percent in the postdeployment period. These results suggest that most individuals recover within weeks to months of concussion injury, which is consistent with findings among the civilian population.

Further screening occurs for those entering the Veterans Health Administration (VHA) for care. Affirmative responses on all questions are required to be a positive screen. This serves to identify those still in need of medical care for TBI-related symptoms but does not enhance current TBI surveillance methods.

NEUROCOGNITIVE ASSESSMENT TESTING

In accordance with the congresional National Defense Authorization Act of 2007, predeployment neurocognitive testing was implemented in 2008. To date, 723,981 service members have completed this testing, which currently uses the Automated Neurocognitive Assessment Metrics (ANAM). This is a brief computerized battery that is designed to detect speed and accuracy of attention, memory, and thinking ability. By completing the ANAM within 12 months of deployment, each service member establishes an individual preinjury baseline; thus, if a TBI is sustained in theater, the ANAM can be repeated to allow for pre- and postinjury comparison and to better inform return-to-duty determinations. Pending inclusion in the electronic medical record, test results are stored in a central repository. Health-care providers can obtain these results from the helpdesk by emailing pertinent demographic information to anam.baselines@amedd.army.mil. To date, there have been 5,820 requests for baseline scores with 1,826 from Afghanistan, 202 from Iraq, and 3,792 from the Continental United States.

TREATMENT

Clinical practice guidelines have been developed to guide the evaluation and management of TBI in both the acute and chronic settings. These guidelines incorporate available evidence and expert consensus. Acute care begins on the battlefield with theater-based guidelines, which incorporate the tactical requirements of the combat setting. Previous guidelines were only useful if the service member sought a medical evaluation. Recent revisions, supported by the Joint Chiefs of Staff, require all service members involved in a traumatic event to undergo screening and a mandatory 24-hour rest period. Those with serious neurologic injury are evacuated to facilities with imaging capabilities. Those with symptoms of concussion, such as headache or dizziness, are managed aggressively with local medical assets. Once symptoms resolve, exertional testing is performed prior to return to duty to ensure that symptoms do not return with physiologic stress. Those with persistent symptoms undergo combat stress evaluations and more detailed medical examinations. Because of concerns that multiple concussions may result in slower recovery or, in more severe cases, chronic traumatic encephalopathy (Guskiewicz et al., 2003; McKee et al., 2009), service members sustaining three or more concussions in a 12-month period are required to undergo a complete neurological and psychological evaluation. The result of this exam may lead to one of the three following dispositions: stateside evacuation, restricted duty, or return to full duty.

Subacute and chronic TBI care is guided by the Department of Veterans Affairs (VA) and DoD *Evidence-Based Clinical Practice Guideline for the Management of Concussion/ Mild Traumatic Brain Injury* (2009). This document was developed under the auspices of the VHA and DoD with the intent of providing evidence-based recommendations to patients and their providers, reduce practice variability, and provide structure for measurement of patient outcomes. The guidelines include three algorithms: initial presentation, symptom management, and follow-up of persistent symptoms. More detailed guidance is included for the use of pharmacotherapy and management of common physical symptoms associated with concussion.

TELEMEDICINE

Various telemedicine modalities are currently used in the care of TBI patients within the Military Health System (MHS). For example, *TBI.consult* is an electronic consult service available to deployed providers, and it is staffed by neurologists, neurosurgeons, and nurse practitioners with expertise in TBI. A confidential history and physical record are transmitted to the consult team via email. The team considers local resources and within two to three hours of consult receipt an initial response is provided. The team makes individualized recommendations based on the patient's medical condition. Resources such as the theater clinical practice guidelines (Brain Trauma Foundation, 2005) and MACE are provided when needed as well as in-theater contacts for specialty care. In some cases, collaboration occurs with other specialty services (i.e., ear, nose, and throat services for hearing loss associated with TBI), with TBI staff in theater, or with LRMC staff to facilitate necessary evacuations. Stateside TBI care in more remote locations is supported by the virtual TBI (vTBI) clinic. The vTBI clinic currently provides symptom management and neuropsychological screening via videoconferencing. Plans are in process to increase capabilities to include mass screening and some components of neurorehabilitation.

The Defense Centers of Excellence for Psychological Health and Traumatic Brain Injury (DCoE) has established a 24/7 Outreach Center. Service members can contact the center via email, live online chat, or telephone for immediate assistance. After immediate concerns are addressed by trained operators, callers are connected with appropriate TBI resources, most often through the Defense and Veterans Brain Injury Center (DVBIC).

CARE COORDINATION

In the acute care phase, service members sustaining severe or penetrating TBI are assigned a federal recovery coordinator to facilitate coordination of care across the health-care continuum. Those with mTBI may also require coordination of services during their recovery. This is accomplished by the DVBIC Care Coordination Program. Once identified with TBI, service members are contacted by a regional care coordinator (RCC), who conducts assessments and identifies patient needs. The RCC works with the individual's case managers to identify ongoing needs and local TBI resources for up to two years. Data from this program indicate that physical symptom reporting decreases with time while psychological symptom reporting increases. Further work is needed to determine the cause and implications of these findings.

EDUCATION

TBI-related educational efforts within DoD are aimed at two main consumers: providers and patients/families. Three websites have been developed to assist patients and their families with their understanding of TBI.

- www.traumaticbraininjuryatoz.org
  Sponsored by the U.S. Air Force Center of Excellence for Medical Multimedia, this award-winning site provides an overview of TBI by severity, expected courses of recovery, and personal stories of service members with TBI. In addition, there are

downloadable components to the congressionally mandated DoD/VA TBI Family Caregiver Curriculum.
- www.afterdeployment.org (mTBI)
  Developed by the DCoE's National Center for Telehealth and Technology, this website provides an overview of mTBI. Self-assessments are available for many common symptoms or conditions associated with mTBI. A resource library is also included.
- www.brainline.org
  A service of WETA[4] public communications with funding by DVBIC, this website provides information about TBI for patients, families, and providers. Various research topics, TBI experts, and other headlines are presented.

The National Defense Authorization Act of 2007 established a 15-member panel to develop a curriculum to train family caregivers of service members and veterans with TBI. Panel members were appointed by the DoD and the Department of Health and Human Services on March 6, 2008. The members of the panel include professionals from DoD and the VA specializing in TBI, family caregivers, and experts in the development of curricula. The curricula were approved for distribution in April 2010. The curricula are presently being disseminated by recovery coordinators at WRAMC and NNMC to family members of patients with significant TBI. They are also available to the public for download at www.dvbic.org, in addition to other currently approved patient and provider materials.

Many modalities are used to ensure that DoD providers have an adequate understanding of TBI. Since 2007, DVBIC has hosted the annual TBI military training conference. The 2010 event registered more than 850 participants from all branches of service for the two-day conference. Experts from across the country contributed to education through case studies, panel discussions, and podium presentations. The DCoE and DVBIC host regularly scheduled webinars to further facilitate provider education. TBI education is also provided at deployment platforms. The U.S. Army Proponency Office for Rehabilitation and Reintegration convened a panel of subject-matter experts—both military and civilian—to develop a series of TBI materials ranging from a public service announcement (101) to treatment paradigms.

- TBI 101: Introduction and Awareness—Army
- TBI 101: Introduction and Awareness—Joint
- TBI 201: TBI Overview for Healthcare Personnel
- TBI 401: Primary Care Assessment and Management for Concussion

This program is available for use at deployment platforms and, most recently, has been included on the MHS Learning Portal (MHS Learn), accompanied by appropriate continuing medical education credits. Thirteen other TBI-related lessons are also available on MHS Learn.

RESEARCH

In 2009, more than $40 million were allocated for TBI and psychological health research through the Congressionally Directed Medical Research Program (CDMRP). Funding priorities included cellular regeneration and interconnection strategies for the central

---

[4] WETA is the flagship, not-for-profit public broadcasting station serving Washington, DC; Virginia; and Maryland.

nervous system, evidence-based prevention and rehabilitation strategies, three-dimensional models of blast injury, and advanced diagnostic modalities (e.g., neuroimaging, biomarkers). Figure C-3 depicts an overview of current CDMRP-funded studies.

Key collaborations with academia and industry are likely to provide high-yield information in the upcoming years. A partnership between DVBIC and the Armed Forces Institute of Pathology established a state-of-the-art research lab. This alliance also introduced an organizational structure for the development of a "brain bank" allowing for detailed neuropathological examinations. In addition, the lab has a small animal imaging facility featuring a 7 Tesla horizontal bore imager used in various preclinical research protocols. In conjunction with Massachusetts Institute of Technology and the Institute of Soldier Nanotechnology, DoD scientists have developed the most comprehensive computerized simulation model of the interactions between blast and brain. It is anticipated that this initial effort will lead to further work on the utilization of nanotechnology to protect and improve survivability of wounded service members.

Findings from the U.S. Army Medical Research and Materiel Command Blast Symposium reveal pathological differences in blast and blunt trauma seen on diffusion tensor imaging. Data presented at the symposium from functional Magnetic Resonance Imaging (fMRI) showed statistically significant differences between breacher instructors and students. During their training to be breachers, students are exposed to 50 to 70 blasts of weapons-grade explosives. Finally, animal models suggest axonal, neuronal, and glial damage following blast injury as well as physiologic, histologic, and behavioral differences between blunt and blast injury. Proceedings from this symposium are scheduled to be published in an upcoming special issue of the journal *Neuroimage*. Other studies still in progress include helmet sensor studies, a 15-year longitudinal study of TBI, and the Head to Head Study of computerized neurocognitive tools. All of these studies will greatly enhance the understanding of TBI and its consequences.

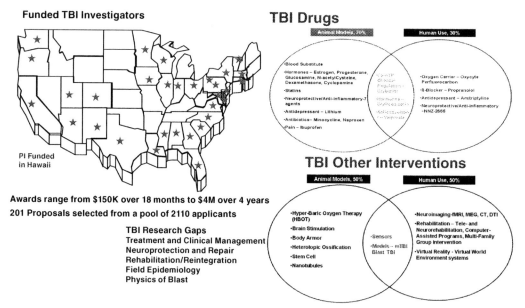

FIGURE C-3   CDMRP-funded studies and their locations.
SOURCE: Jaffee, 2010.

TABLE C-2 Key Combat-Related TBI Scholarly Papers, 2003–2009

Category	Reference	Title
Screening	Ivins et al., 2009	Performance on the Automated Neuropsychological Assessment Metrics in a nonclinical sample of soldiers screened for mTBI after return returning from Iraq and Afghanistan: A descriptive analysis
	Terrio et al., 2009	Traumatic brain injury screening: Preliminary findings in a U.S. Army Brigade Combat Team
	Ivins et al., 2003	Traumatic brain injury in U.S. Army paratroopers: Prevalence and character
Clinical Findings	Bell et al., 2009	Military traumatic brain and spinal column injury: A 5-year study of the impact blast and other military grade weaponry on the central nervous system
	Brahm et al., 2009	Visual impairment and dysfunction in combat-injured service members with traumatic brain injury
	Hoge et al., 2008	Mild traumatic brain injury in U.S. soldiers returning from Iraq
Blast Neurotrauma	Ling et al., 2009	Explosive blast neurotrauma
	Moore et al., 2009	Computational biology—Modeling of primary blast effects on the central nervous system
	Dewitt et al., 2009	Blast-induced brain injury and posttraumatic hypotension and hypoxemia
TBI & Post-Traumatic Stress Disorder	Stein and McAllister, 2009	Exploring the convergence of posttraumatic stress disorder and mild traumatic brain injury
	Nelson et al., 2009	Relationship between processing speed and executive functioning performance among OEF/OIF veterans: Implications for post deployment rehabilitation
	Kennedy et al., 2007	Posttraumatic stress disorder and posttraumatic stress disorder-like symptoms and mild traumatic brain injury
Imaging	Moore et al., 2009	Diffusion tensor imaging and mTBI—A case-control study of blast (+) in returning service members following OIF and OEF
	Huang et al., 2009	Integrated imaging approach with MEG and DTI to detect mild traumatic brain injury in military and civilian patients
Outcomes	Bjork and Grant, 2009	Does traumatic brain injury increase risk for substance abuse?
	Han et al., 2009	Clinical, cognitive, and genetic predictors of change in job status following traumatic brain injury in a military population
	Gottshall et al., 2003	Objective vestibular tests as outcome measures in head injury patients
	Drake et al., 2000	Factors predicting return to work following mild traumatic brain injury: A discriminant analysis

continued

TABLE C-2   Continued

Category	Reference	Title
Rehabilitation	Lew et al., 2009	The potential utility of driving simulators in the cognitive rehabilitation of combat-returnees with traumatic brain injury
	Vanderploeg et al., 2008	Rehabilitation of traumatic brain injury in active-duty military personnel and veterans: Defense and Veterans Brain Injury Center randomized controlled trial of two rehabilitation approaches
	Trudel et al., 2007	Community-integrated brain injury rehabilitation: Treatment models and challenges for civilian, military, and veteran populations
	Walker et al., 2007	Motor impairment after severe traumatic brain injury: A longitudinal multicenter study
Miscellaneous	Cote et al., 2007	A mixed integer programming model to locate traumatic brain injury treatment units in the Department of Veterans Affairs: A case study
	Warden, 2006	Military TBI during the Iraq and Afghanistan wars
	Ivins et al., 2006	Hospital admissions associated with traumatic brain injury in the U.S. Army during peacetime: 1990s trends

Clinicians continue to contribute to the understanding of combat-related TBI. Table C-2 summarizes recent observations of providers involved in the day-to-day care of those with TBI. These efforts identify some of the consequences associated with TBI and lead to additional scientific inquiry.

SUMMARY

Much work remains to be done in order to fully understand TBI and its long-term consequences. Efforts within DoD to rapidly transform bench science and observed best practice to clinical practice continue. This is most readily evident by the annual revisions of educational materials, clinical practice guidelines, and screening techniques.

REFERENCES

Brain Trauma Foundation. 2005. *Guidelines for field management of combat-related head trauma.* New York, NY: Brain Trauma Foundation.

Dempsey, K. E., W. C. Dorlac, K. Martin, R. Fang, C. Fox, B. Bennett, K. Williams, and S. Flaherty. 2009. Landstuhl Regional Medical Center: Traumatic brain injury screening program. *Journal of Trauma Nursing* 16(1):6–12.

DoD (Department of Defense). 2007. *Traumatic brain injury: Definition and reporting.* Memorandum. HA Policy 07-030. Dated October 1, 2007. Available online at http://mhs.osd.mil/content/docs/pdfs/policies/2007/07-030.pdf (accessed March 25, 2011).

Guskiewicz, K. M., M. McCrea, S. W. Marshall, R. C. Cantu, C. Randolph, W. Barr, J. A. Onate, and J. P. Kelly. 2003. Cumulative effects associated with recurrent concussion in collegiate football players: The NCAA Concussion Study. *The Journal of the American Medical Association* 290(19):2549–2555.

Jaffee, M. S. 2010. *Overview of Combat Related Traumatic Brain Injury and DoD TBI Initiatives.* Presented at Institute of Medicine's Workshop on Nutrition and Neuroprotection in Military Personnel, Washington, DC, June 23, 2010.

McKee, A. C. M., R. C. M. Cantu, C. J. A. Nowinski, E. T. M. Hedley-Whyte, B. E. P. Gavett, A. E. M. Budson, V. E. M. Santini, H.-S. M. Lee, C. A. Kubilus, and R. A. P. Stern. 2009. Chronic traumatic encephalopathy in athletes: Progressive tauopathy after repetitive head injury. *Journal of Neuropathology & Experimental Neurology* 68(7):709–735.

Schwab, K. A., G. Baker, B. Ivins, M. Sluss-Tiller, W. Lux, and D. Warden. 2006. The brief traumatic brain injury screen (BTBIS): Investigating the validity of a self-report instrument for detecting traumatic brain injury (TBI) in troops returning from deployment in Afghanistan and Iraq. *Neurology* 66(5)(Suppl. 2):A235.

Terrio, H., L. A. Brenner, B. J. Ivins, J. M. Cho, K. Helmick, K. Schwab, K. Scally, R. Bretthauer, and D. Warden. 2009. Traumatic brain injury screening: Preliminary findings in a U.S. Army brigade combat team. *Journal of Head Trauma Rehabilitation* 24(1):14–23.

VA/DoD (Department of Veterans Affairs and Department of Defense). 2009. *VA/DoD clinical practice guideline for management of concussion/mild traumatic brain injury.* http://www.healthquality.va.gov/mtbi/concussion_mtbi_full_1_0.pdf (accessed January 19, 2011).

Pathophysiology and Mechanisms of Neurotrauma: Blast and Civilian

Mårten Risling[5]

Traumatic brain injury (TBI) is not only a leading cause of death and disability in young active people, but also a significant health problem in elderly people. It is a fundamental type of trauma in both civilian life and at the battlefield. However, the spectrum of the injuries seems to be different in these two areas, and has also changed over time. For example, the signature TBI in recent military conflicts has evidently changed from penetrating TBI to blast-induced TBI. Below we will first describe a basic classification of TBI. All types of TBI may occur in both the civilian and military setting. However, there are some important considerations for TBI on the battlefield, mostly relating to the extreme energy transfer.

CLASSIFICATION

The term TBI includes a number of different injuries, ranging from mild to severe lesions. Several mechanisms contribute to the induction of the injury. The World Health Organization (WHO) publishes an International Classification of Diseases (ICD), where trauma and head injury are included in the chapter "Injury and poisoning." The latest edition, ICD-10, lists the injuries as:

SO6 Intracranial injury
  SO6.0 Concussion
  • Commotio cerebri
  SO6.1 Traumatic cerebral edema
  SO6.2 Diffuse brain injury
  Cerebral:
  • contusion NOS
  • laceration NOS
  • traumatic compression of brain NOS
  SO6.3 Focal brain injury
  Focal:
  • cerebral:
    ○ contusion
    ○ aceration
  • traumatic intracerebral haemorrhage

[5] Department of Neuroscience, Karolinska Institutet, Sweden

SO6.4 Epidural hemorrhage
SO6.5 Traumatic subdural hemorrhage (SDH)
SO6.6 Traumatic subarachnoid hemorrhage (SAH)
SO6.7 Intracranial injury with prolonged coma
SO6.8 Other intracranial injuries
SO6.9 Intracranial injury, unspecified

Adoption of ICD-10 seems to be slow in the United States. Since 1999, the ICD-10 (without clinical extensions) was adopted for reporting mortality, but ICD-9-CM is apparently still often used for morbidity, unlike the situation in many European countries. The causes of the injuries have been systematically listed in the International Classification of External Causes of Injury (ICECI). It contains seven modules for the mechanism of injury (objects/substances producing injury, place of occurrence, activity when injured, the role of human intent, use of alcohol, use of psycho-active drugs) and five additional modules referring to special topics (violence, transport, place, sports, occupational injury). The ICECI contains a module V7—TYPE OF CONFLICT, which includes war.

This type of classification is requisite for meaningful statistics and epidemiology. According to data from the U.S. Centers for Disease Control and Prevention (CDC), the annual incidence for TBI in the United States is approximately 1.5 million. Among these, around 50,000 die and a larger number (around 85,000 people) survive with long-term disabilities. Because many of the victims are young at the time of the injury, the accumulated number of people with disabilities caused by TBI is assumed to be more than 5 million. Sport activities, firearms, and road traffic accidents represent common causes of TBI in young people, whereas fall injury is a common cause in the elderly.

MILD TBI

A TBI is often classified as mild (concussion or commotion) if loss of consciousness or confusion is shorter than 30 minutes. Magnetic resonance imaging (MRI) and computerized axial tomography (CAT) scans are usually normal but the patient may have headache and cognitive problems (memory problems, mood disturbance, attention deficits), and the effect on the patient can be devastating. The majority of blast-induced TBI fall into this category, although the pathophysiology is largely unknown. Cerebral concussion is often associated with other types of brain injury.

MODERATE AND SEVERE TBI

These injuries can be divided into closed head injuries and penetrating injuries. The penetrating TBI will always induce a focal injury and often diffuse secondary injuries. Closed head injuries may be both diffuse and focal (Reilly and Bullock, 2005).

DIFFUSE TBI

The most common diffuse injury is the diffuse axonal injury (DAI). With increasing sensitivity in imaging techniques, the proportion of DAIs will probably increase in statistics. DAI is defined as the presence of diffuse damage to axons in the cerebral subcortical parasagittal white matter, corpus callosum, brain stem, and cerebellum (Reilly and Bullock, 2005). Another type of diffuse injury is diffuse vascular injury (DVI) (Reilly and Bullock, 2005). DAI is often, but not always, also associated with vascular injury. Different parts of the brain move at different speeds because of their relative density. This can lead to shearing injury and DAI (Anderson and McLean, 2005). Beta-amyloid precursor protein (APP) is a membrane-spanning glycoprotein originating from a gene on chromosome 21. APP, which is transported by fast axoplasmic transport, has been proven to be an excellent marker for axonal injury in histology (Sherriff et al., 1994). Modern imaging techniques, such as MRI with diffusion tensor imaging (DTI), have provided improved possibilities to detect DAI.

FOCAL TBI

Vascular injury can result in intracerebral hemorrhage, subdural hemorrhage, epidural hemorrhage, or subarachnoid hemorrhage. Extradural hematomas (EDH) are the result of bleeding that occurs between the calvarium and the dura mater, most frequently in the temporo-parietal region near the middle meningeal arteries. There are two main types of traumatic acute subdural hematoma (ASDH). In traumatic ASDH related to contusions and lacerations, the hematoma is located adjacent to damaged brain. The second type of ASDH is the result of rupture of the bridging veins (Reilly and Bullock, 2005).

Cerebral contusions are focal injuries. Bleeding from damaged blood vessels is usually the most obvious feature upon macroscopic or microscopic examination. Contrecoup contusions occur opposite the impact site. Fracture contusions occur beneath the site of a fracture. Gliding contusions occur in the parasagittal regions and are often associated with DAI. In a simple contusion the pia–glial membrane is intact. Disruption of this membrane with tearing of the underlying tissue constitutes a laceration. Contusions and lacerations form a continuum of tissue injury.

Lacerations of the brain may be defined as primary disruptions of the brain tissue at the moment of injury. In direct lacerations the tissue disruption is caused by a penetrating injury from various types of missiles or an open depressed fracture of the skull with penetration of the brain by fragments of bone and foreign bodies.

SCREENING AND EXAMINATION AFTER TBI

In the acute phase physical examination, CAT scans and biomarkers are used to differentiate from more severe injuries. The Glasgow Coma Scale (GCS) is a 15-point scale for estimating the acute effect of TBI. The test measures the motor response, verbal response, and eye-opening response. The score is determined by adding the values of these three parameters. Mild TBI should have a score between 13 and 15 (Servadei et al., 2001). Lower scores indicate a more severe injury, that is, a moderate or severe TBI. This test is useful for screening in the emergency room, and repeated tests can be useful for monitoring. However, GCS seems to be less reliable for penetrating injuries and maybe also blast injuries with late onset of symptoms. Therefore, there is an interest for additional tools for screening after TBI, especially in the military setting.

Biomarkers such as the calcium-binding protein S100B can be used as a screening tool. S100B can be detected in serum samples after TBI (Berger et al., 2002; Elting et al., 2000; Pelinka et al., 2003). It has a short half-life in serum, and it has been suggested that repeated samples can be used to monitor the progress of a TBI and make predictions on the outcome. Some guidelines for mild TBI in children advocate the use of S100B instead of CAT scans in order to reduce the exposure to radiation. Several research programs focus on the development of more sensitive and more CNS-specific biomarkers, such as various axonal markers.

Imaging techniques such as CAT scans and MRIs have increased the precision and sensitivity for exact diagnosis after TBI. The resolution and protocols are improving. For example, DTI can be used to visualize fiber tracts in the brain and enhance the diagnosis of diffuse TBI. Additional techniques such as PET (positron emission tomography) scanning may, for example, add knowledge on metabolic parameters after the injury but are not employed as a screening tool.

In the neurointensive-care unit (NICU) additional techniques can be used to monitor the TBI patients (Matz and Pitts, 1997). Microdialysis is a technique to monitor the chemistry of the extracellular space in the brain (Alessandri et al., 2000). The microdialysis probe consists of a semi-permeable catheter that is constantly perfused with a physiological solution. The perfusate can give information on the metabolic state in the injured brain. Digital electroencephalography (EEG) can provide information on the occurrence of post-TBI seizures or to monitor sedative treatment after the injury. Microdialysis studies in the NICU have revealed that the level of glucose in the brain is difficult to predict from analysis of peripheral blood or samples from fat tissue (Rostami and Bellander, 2011). However, microdialysis is a difficult technique and probably very dependent on the position of the catheter. It is more useful for the monitoring of patients in the NICU than for prediction of secondary events in the injury.

SECONDARY INJURIES

Secondary traumatic brain damage occurs as a complication of the different types of TBI and includes ischemic and hypoxic damage, swelling, raised intracranial pressure, and infection (Figure C-4). Neurochemical alterations, such as excitatory stress, may mediate important components of brain physiology associated with TBI, and such alterations may be responsive to pharmacologic therapy (Miller et al., 1990; Palmer et al., 1993). The secondary TBI is potentially reversible with adequate treatment. A part of the treatment is to reduce the metabolic load by controlled sedation. It should be mentioned that there is some evidence that neurons reduce their metabolic load after injuries in the central nervous system by active removal of excitatory synapses.

Thus, the secondary injuries are extremely important because they represent the components of the injury that could be treated or prevented if the mechanism and threshold have been identified. Becaquse TBI from high-energy incidents may be induced by more than one mechanism (e.g., primary blast + acceleration movements), we can assume to find more than one threshold for these secondary assaults.

The blood-brain barrier (BBB) can be assumed to have a key function in the aftermath

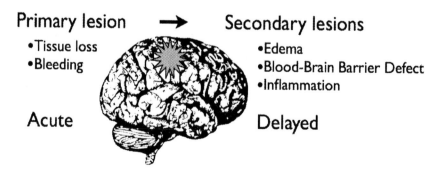

FIGURE C-4   A schematic representation of the relation between primary and secondary traumatic brain damage after TBI. The interval between the primary acute lesion and the secondary lesions can vary from hours to days.

of TBI. The BBB is the result of a complex interaction of astrocyte endfeet and the endothelium of the capillaries in the central nervous system. On the molecular level, the BBB is a complicated interaction of specialized contact proteins at junctions between the cells and active transporters for essential compounds, like the Glut-1 glucose transporter (Stark et al., 2000). The BBB can be rapidly distorted after TBI, resulting in extracellular edema and infiltration with inflammatory cells. The threshold for BBB defects after TBI has not been established, but could possibly be different after different types of injury. The BBB function following TBI is usually restored within four weeks, although more permanent BBB defects have been observed after lesions in the spinal cord (Risling et al., 1989).

Axonal damage in both DAI and focal injuries interferes with axoplasmic transport. Severe traumatic injury results in primary axonal disruption, termed primary axotomy, which can initiate a series of poorly understood events culminating in secondary axonal degeneration or secondary axotomy (Maxwell et al., 1997). Thus, adequate treatment could probably limit the axonal damage.

Edema is an important and variable secondary response to TBI, the causes and consequences of which are only partly understood. Effective treatment is lacking. Impairment of the BBB leads to accumulation of fluid in the extracellular space. The localized edema around contusions and penetrating TBI is mostly vasogenic. Cytotoxic edema occurs in association with hypoxic-ischemic damage where there is a disturbance of ionic gradients leading to an accumulation of intracellular fluid. Energy crisis and mitochondria malfunction can be important components of the cytotoxic edema (Castejon and Castejon, 2000; Castejon and de Castejon, 2004; Clausen et al., 2001; Klatzo, 1987). Severe blast-induced TBI is often complicated by acute edema. The mechanisms for this edema formation have still to be identified. Decompressive craniotomy is often needed (Ling et al., 2009).

COMPLICATIONS WITH LATE ONSET

Epilepsy occurs in many TBI patients. Recent studies indicate an association between TBI and the subsequent development of Alzheimer's disease (Emmerling et al., 2000; Uryu et al., 2002). Genetic background, such as changes in the APO-E gene can increase the risk for trauma-related Alzheimer dementia, and it has been suggested that the APOE-epsilon4 genotype may result in an earlier onset of the disease, rather than increased incidence (Hartman et al., 2002).

RISK ASSESSMENT

Several measures have been developed in an attempt to quantify the tolerance of the head to impact in terms of the magnitude of both the resulting acceleration of the head and the duration of the impact. The Head Injury Criterion (HIC) is the most widely used. Such values have a definite role for improved car crash safety and body armor. However, although HIC can provide an assessment of the risk for fractures of head it does not seem to give a reliable description of the risk for diffuse injuries, such as DAI (Margulies and Thibault, 1992).

BLAST-INDUCED BRAIN INJURIES—THE GRAND CHALLENGE IN TBI RESEARCH

The U.S. government has initiated the largest coordinated research programs ever in neurotrauma to get insight on mechanisms and to provide better treatment for blast-induced traumatic brain injuries (Risling, 2010). TBI has been identified as a major health problem in military personnel returning from service. The injuries range from severe multitrauma to a number of mild TBIs that still has to be settled (Jaffee and Meyer, 2009; Ling et al., 2009).

The enormous energy transfer in blast TBI creates a number of specific problems:

- Propagation of blast waves is very complex. It could involve both direct propagation through the skull and indirect propagation via blood vessels (Cernak and Noble-Haeusslein, 2010). If the latter mechanism is important, we could expect effects from vascular disturbance. Several lines of evidence seem to point in that direction.
- It is not known whether blast TBI is a specific type of injury that will require specific and new types of treatment, or if, for example, the mild TBI from blast exposure is more like a classical type of concussion injury (Hoge et al., 2009).
- A reliable borderline between mild blast-induced TBI and posttraumatic stress syndrome (PTSD) has yet to be identified. Many of the symptoms are similar, and many patients might suffer from both TBI and PTSD (Jaffee and Meyer, 2009).
- There is some debate about whether blast-induced TBI is an entirely new problem. The shellshock syndrome (Anderson, 2008) that was seen after the enormous artillery battles during World War I had similarities to blast-induced TBI and post blast-induced TBI symptoms, but for many years it has been regarded as PTSD rather than physical injuries. The new situation with improvised explosive devices (IEDs) is that the explosive often detonates at short distances, and improved body armor and helmets protect much better against penetration from fragments.
- Although the epidemiology of blast-induced TBI has been established in terms of approximate numbers of people injured, it is very difficult to assess the injury mechanisms in individual cases. The actual situation during exposure to an IED is usually very complicated because of complex propagation and reflection of the primary supersonic blast wave, effects from acceleration and rotation (Moss et al., 2009), effects from impact of fragments, effects from heating, and effects from emitted gases and electromagnetic waves (Figure C-5). Well-designed experimental models as well as data from acceleration probes and pressure sensors that have been mounted into helmets and body armor are required to increase the knowledge of the critical mechanisms.

EXAMPLE OF ONGOING EXPERIMENTAL RESEARCH

As indicated earlier, it may be assumed that several mechanisms contribute to the injury. This study was an attempt to characterize the presumed components of blast-induced TBI (Risling et al., 2011). Our experimental models included a blast tube in which an anesthetized rat can be exposed to controlled detonations of explosives that result in a pressure wave with a magnitude between 130 and 260 kPa. In this model, the animal is fixed with a metal net to avoid head acceleration forces. The second model is a controlled penetration of a 2-mm thick needle. In the third model, the animal is subjected to a high-speed sagittal rotation angular acceleration.

Immunohistochemical labeling for amyloid precursor protein revealed signs of DAI in the penetration and rotation models. Signs of punctuate inflammation were observed after focal and rotation injury. Exposure in the blast tube did not induce DAI or detectable cell death but did not functional changes. Affymetrix gene arrays showed changes in the expression in a large number of gene families including cell death, inflammation, and neurotransmitters in the hippocampus after both acceleration and penetration injuries. Exposure to the

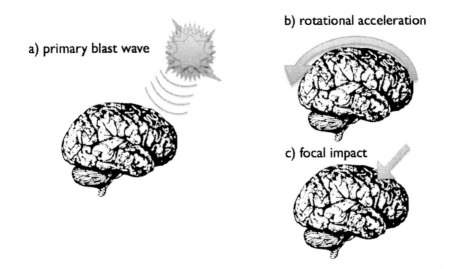

a) primary blast wave

b) rotational acceleration

c) focal impact

FIGURE C-5 Primary blast wave, rotational acceleration, and focal impact can be assumed to represent key components in the injury mechanism of blast TBI.

primary blast wave induced limited shifts in gene expression in the hippocampus. The most interesting findings were a downregulation of genes involved in neurogenesis and synaptic transmission. These experiments indicate that rotational acceleration may be a critical factor for DAI and other acute changes after blast-TBI. The further exploration of the mechanisms of blast-induced TBI will have to include a search for long-term effects.

The microarray data indicated that the metabolic load and mitochondrial function were very different in the three models (Risling et al., 2011). For example, 47 different mitochondrial genes showed a changed expression in the cortex surrounding the penetrating TBI, whereas no mitochondrial gene showed any sign of significant expression changes in the primary blast model. A number of genes for the metabolic cytochrome p450 (CYP) enzymes also showed significant changes in the cortex subjected to penetrating TBI. It may be assumed that such expression changes could have implications for drug and hormone metabolism. The relatively modest changes in the employed primary blast model could be related to the simple pulse form and short duration of the primary peak that is achieved by a detonation at short distance (1 meter) in this type of blast tube (Clemedson and Criborn, 1955). This may be relevant for some types of IED at short distance but in a protected vehicle, could be very different (Courtney and Courtney, 2011). Preliminary data from experiments employing a rigid body protection for the torso and a higher load of explosive, indicate a rapid induction of GFAP and s-fos, indicators of TBI pathology, but without any signs of DAI. Thus, these data indicate that blast-induced TBI may be the result of a number of simultaneous mechanisms with different thresholds.

REFERENCES

Alessandri, B., M. Reinert, H. F. Young, and R. Bullock. 2000. Low extracellular (ECF) glucose affects the neurochemical profile in severe head-injured patients. *Acta Neurochirurgica. Supplement* 76:425–430.

Anderson, R. J. 2008. Shell shock: An old injury with new weapons. *Molecular Interventions* 8(5):204–218.

Anderson, R., and J. McLean. 2005. Biomechanics of closed head injury. In *Head injury. pathophysiology and management*, edited by P. L. Reilly and R. Bullock. London: Hodder Arnold. Pp. 26–40.

Berger, R. P., M. C. Pierce, S. R. Wisniewski, P. D. Adelson, and P. M. Kochanek. 2002. Serum s100b concentrations are increased after closed head injury in children: A preliminary study. *Journal of Neurotrauma* 19(11):1405–1409.

Castejon, O. J., and H. V. de Castejon. 2000. Oligodendroglial cell behaviour in traumatic oedematous human cerebral cortex: A light and electron microscopic study. *Brain Injury* 14(4):303–317.

Castejon, O. J., and H. V. de Castejon. 2004. Structural patterns of injured mitochondria in human oedematous cerebral cortex. *Brain Injury* 18(11):1107–1126.

Cernak, I., and L. J. Noble-Haeusslein. 2010. Traumatic brain injury: An overview of pathobiology with emphasis on military populations. *Journal of Cerebral Blood Flow and Metabolism* 30(2):255–266.

Clausen, T., A. Zauner, J. E. Levasseur, A. C. Rice, and R. Bullock. 2001. Induced mitochondrial failure in the feline brain: Implications for understanding acute post-traumatic metabolic events. *Brain Research* 908(1):35–48.

Clemedson, C. J., and C. O. Criborn. 1955. A detonation chamber for physiological blast research. *The Journal of Aviation Medicine* 26(5):373–381.

Courtney, M. W., and A. C. Courtney. 2011. Working toward exposure thresholds for blast-induced traumatic brain injury: Thoracic and acceleration mechanisms. *Neuroimage* 54(Suppl. 1):S55–S61.

Elting, J. W., A. E. de Jager, A. W. Teelken, M. J. Schaaf, N. M. Maurits, J. van der Naalt, C. T. Sibinga, G. A. Sulter, and J. De Keyser. 2000. Comparison of serum s-100 protein levels following stroke and traumatic brain injury. *Journal of the Neurological Sciences* 181(1–2):104–110.

Emmerling, M. R., M. C. Morganti-Kossmann, T. Kossmann, P. F. Stahel, M. D. Watson, L. M. Evans, P. D. Mehta, K. Spiegel, Y. M. Kuo, A. E. Roher, and C. A. Raby. 2000. Traumatic brain injury elevates the alzheimer's amyloid peptide a beta 42 in human CSF. A possible role for nerve cell injury. *Annals of the New York Academy of Sciences* 903:118–122.

Hartman, R. E., H. Laurer, L. Longhi, K. R. Bales, S. M. Paul, T. K. McIntosh, and D. M. Holtzman. 2002. Apolipoprotein E4 influences amyloid deposition but not cell loss after traumatic brain injury in a mouse model of Alzheimer's disease. *Journal of Neuroscience* 22(23):10083–10087.

Hoge, C. W., H. M. Goldberg, and C. A. Castro. 2009. Care of war veterans with mild traumatic brain injury—flawed perspectives. *The New England Journal of Medicine* 360(16):1588–1591.

Jaffee, M. S., and K. S. Meyer. 2009. A brief overview of traumatic brain injury (TBI) and post-traumatic stress disorder (PTSD) within the Department of Defense. *Clinical Neuropsychologist* 23(8):1291–1298.

Klatzo, I. 1987. Pathophysiological aspects of brain edema. *Acta Neuropathologica* 72(3):236–239.

Ling, G., F. Bandak, R. Armonda, G. Grant, and J. Ecklund. 2009. Explosive blast neurotrauma. *Journal of Neurotrauma* 26(6):815–825.

Margulies, S. S., and L. E. Thibault. 1992. A proposed tolerance criterion for diffuse axonal injury in man. *Journal of Biomechanics* 25(8):917–923.

Matz, P. G., and L. Pitts. 1997. Monitoring in traumatic brain injury. *Clinical Neurosurgery* 44:267–294.

Maxwell, W. L., J. T. Povlishock, and D. L. Graham. 1997. A mechanistic analysis of nondisruptive axonal injury: A review. *Journal of Neurotrauma* 14(7):419–440.

Miller, L. P., B. G. Lyeth, L. W. Jenkins, L. Oleniak, D. Panchision, R. J. Hamm, L. L. Phillips, C. E. Dixon, G. L. Clifton, and R. L. Hayes. 1990. Excitatory amino acid receptor subtype binding following traumatic brain injury. *Brain Research* 526(1):103–107.

Moss, W. C., M. J. King, and E. G. Blackman. 2009. Skull flexure from blast waves: A mechanism for brain injury with implications for helmet design. *Physical Review Letters* 103(10):108702.

Palmer, A. M., D. W. Marion, M. L. Botscheller, P. E. Swedlow, S. D. Styren, and S. T. DeKosky. 1993. Traumatic brain injury-induced excitotoxicity assessed in a controlled cortical impact model. *Journal of Neurochemistry* 61(6):2015–2024.

Pelinka, L. E., E. Toegel, W. Mauritz, and H. Redl. 2003. Serum s100b: A marker of brain damage in traumatic brain injury with and without multiple trauma. *Shock* 19(3):195–200.

Reilly, P. L., and R. Bullock. 2005. *Head injury. Pathophysiology & management.* 2nd ed.: Hodder Arnold.

Risling, M. 2010. Blast induced brain injuries—a grand challenge in TBI research. *Frontiers in Neurotrauma* 1(1):1–2.

Risling, M., H. Linda, S. Cullheim, and P. Franson. 1989. A persistent defect in the blood-brain barrier after ventral funiculus lesion in adult cats: Implications for CNS regeneration? *Brain Research* 494(1):13–21.

Risling, M., S. Plantman, M. Angeria, E. Rostami, B. M. Bellander, M. Kirkegaard, U. Arborelius, and J. Davidsson. 2011. Mechanisms of blast induced brain injuries, experimental studies in rats. *Neuroimage* 54(Suppl. 1):S89–S97.

Rostami, E., and B.-M. Bellander. 2011. Monitoring of glucose in brain, adipose tissue and peripheral blood in patients with traumatic brain injury, a microdialysis study. *Journal of Diabetes Science and Technology* 5(3):596–604.

Servadei, F., G. Teasdale, and G. Merry. 2001. Defining acute mild head injury in adults: A proposal based on prognostic factors, diagnosis, and management. *Journal of Neurotrauma* 18(7):657–664.

Sherriff, F. E., L. R. Bridges, and S. Sivaloganathan. 1994. Early detection of axonal injury after human head trauma using immunocytochemistry for beta-amyloid precursor protein. *Acta Neuropathologica* 87(1):55–62.

Stark, B., T. Carlstedt, S. Cullheim, and M. Risling. 2000. Developmental and lesion-induced changes in the distribution of the glucose transporter Glut-1 in the central and peripheral nervous system. *Experimental Brain Research* 131(1):74–84.

Uryu, K., H. Laurer, T. McIntosh, D. Pratico, D. Martinez, S. Leight, V. M. Lee, and J. Q. Trojanowski. 2002. Repetitive mild brain trauma accelerates Abeta deposition, lipid peroxidation, and cognitive impairment in a transgenic mouse model of Alzheimer amyloidosis. *Journal of Neuroscience* 22(2):446–454.

Recurrent Sports-Related Traumatic Brain Injury and Tauopathy

Robert A. Stern,[6] Brandon E. Gavett,[7] Christine Baugh,[8] Christopher J. Nowinski,[9]
Robert C. Cantu,[10] and Ann C. McKee[11]

Dementia pugilistica and related terms (e.g., punch drunk, slug nutty) have evolved over the previous century (Millspaugh, 1937; Parker, 1934). The origin of these terms can be traced to boxers that were perceived by the lay public to have developed serious cognitive and movement abnormalities as a result of being repeatedly punched in the head in their sport (Critchley, 1957). The first neuropathological examination of a "punch drunk" boxer was conducted by Harrison Martland in 1928 (Martland, 1928). One half-century later, a more comprehensive neuropathological study of the brains of boxers was carried out by Corsellis and colleagues, who examined 15 deceased retired boxers and found a characteristic pattern of brain injury that was distinct from other known causes of neurodegeneration (Corsellis et al., 1973).

As research into the link between the long-term effects of repeated head injury grew, it became clear that this condition was not restricted to boxers, but rather, could result from other causes of head injury. Similar neuropathological findings were found in individuals with a common history of head trauma of various causes, including soccer (Geddes et al., 1999), head-banging behavior (Geddes et al., 1999), and domestic abuse (Roberts et al., 1990b). As such, the term chronic traumatic encephalopathy (CTE) became the most commonly used term to describe what had previously been referred to as dementia pugilistica (Miller, 1966). Chronic traumatic encephalopathy is a progressive neurodegenerative disease, similar to Alzheimer's disease, but with unique features (McKee et al., 2009). It is believed to be caused by repeated trauma to the brain, including mild concussions and subconcussive blows. Its symptoms occur years or decades following head trauma and continue to worsen; these symptoms are distinct from the acute or post-acute (e.g., postconcussion syndrome) effects of a head injury. The early symptoms of CTE are believed to include memory and cognitive difficulties, depression, impulse control problems, and behavior changes. Later on,

---

[6] Alzheimer's Disease Clinical and Research Program, Boston University School of Medicine.

[7] Alzheimer's Disease Clinical and Research Program, Boston University School of Medicine.

[8] Center for the Study of Traumatic Encephalopathy, Boston University School of Medicine.

[9] Center for the Study of Traumatic Encephalopathy, Boston University School of Medicine.

[10] Center for the Study of Traumatic Encephalopathy, Boston University School of Medicine.

[11] Departments of Neurology and Pathology, Boston University School of Medicine.

movement abnormalities (including Parkinsonism) become more common, and, in many cases, full-blown dementia occurs. CTE is the only preventable cause of dementia.

Recently, our group combined a review of the existing CTE neuropathology literature with a neurological and clinical case series of three athletes (McKee et al., 2009). At the time of the McKee et al. publication, there were 52 cases of neuropathologically verified CTE in the world's literature (including the three cases in that case series). Since that time, our group has examined more than 35 cases of CTE (well over half of the known cases) and helped to refine its neuropathological characterization.

The microscopic pathology of CTE includes neurofibrillary degeneration in the form of extensive tau-immunoreactive neurofibrillary tangles, glial tangles, and neuropil neurites throughout the brain in a widespread distribution. Within the cerebral cortex, the frontal and temporal lobes are commonly affected, with very dense neuropathology in the medial temporal lobe structures—the amygdala, hippocampus, and entorhinal cortex. Tau-immunoreactive inclusions are also found in the subcortical white matter, thalamus, hypothalamus, mammillary bodies, and brainstem (Corsellis et al., 1973; McKee et al., 2009).

CTE may be similar to Alzheimer's disease (AD), both in terms of clinical presentation and neuropathological changes. Both are progressive, incurable, neurodegenerative diseases, and both are currently only diagnosed through postmortem examination of brain tissue. However, there are a number of important distinctions between CTE and AD. Age of onset in AD is usually later than in CTE; while sporadic AD most often occurs after age 65, the onset of CTE has been found to range from ages 20 to 50. Neuropathologically, AD is associated with an abundance of both tau-immunoreactive inclusions and significant deposition of neuritic beta-amyloid plaques (Braak and Braak, 1991). In contrast, fewer than half of the neuropathologically documented cases of CTE showed evidence of amyloid deposition, and when amyloid is present, the plaques tend to be very modest and diffuse, as opposed to neuritic (Clinton et al., 1991; Roberts et al., 1990a).

Athletic participation is ubiquitous amongst people of all ages, especially children. The link between sports-related head injuries and CTE is alarming considering that an estimated 1.6 to 3.8 million people suffer sports-related concussions each year (Langlois et al., 2006). This highlights the importance of expanding the study of CTE beyond boxing. Within the past decade, CTE has been documented in a number of professional athletes who were not boxers. The first five of these cases included four professional football players and one professional wrestler. Mike Webster was a retired National Football League (NFL) center who died at age 50 because of a myocardial infarction; in addition to suffering from depression and cognitive problems, he was also unemployed and homeless at the time of his death in 2002. Terry Long was a retired NFL guard who committed suicide in 2005 at the age of 45. Andre Waters was a retired NFL safety who committed suicide in 2007 at the age of 44. Justin Strzelczyk, a retired NFL offensive lineman, was 36 years old at death; his life had begun to slip into a "downward spiral" of depression and behavioral changes. His death in 2004 was caused by erratic behavior leading to a high-speed police chase that ended when he drove his truck into a tractor trailer. Chris Benoit was a 40-year-old professional wrestler when he committed suicide in 2007 after murdering his wife and child (Cajigal, 2007; Omalu et al., 2005, 2006, 2010a, 2010b).

Following the report of these five cases, the Boston University (BU) Center for the Study of Traumatic Encephalopathy (CSTE) was established to further investigate the relationship between head trauma and later neurodegenerative disease. The CSTE (McKee et al., 2009) first reported on John Grimsley, a retired NFL linebacker who died at the age of 45 after a 10-year career with the Houston Oilers and Miami Dolphins. There was no evidence that he used performance-enhancing drugs in his lifetime, and he reportedly suffered at least eight concussions during his NFL career. He died of a gunshot wound to his chest while cleaning his gun, and his death was ruled an accident. For the five years prior to his death, he reportedly experienced worsening memory and cognitive functioning, as well as an increasingly "short fuse." Neuropathologically, Mr. Grimsley's brain was characteristic of CTE and was noteworthy for the dense tau-immunoreactive inclusions in the medial temporal lobes. Tom McHale was a retired offensive lineman who spent 10 years in the NFL with the Tampa Bay Buccaneers. He was a graduate of Cornell University, former restaurateur, husband, and father of three boys. It was reported that, during his playing career, he suffered two to three concussions, but as lineman, he suffered routine subconcussive blows. He died from a drug overdose after a multi-year battle with drug addiction. Of note, Mr. McHale's drug abuse problems began late in his life, after retiring from the NFL. Neuropathologically, Mr. McHale's brain was consistent with CTE and contained numerous areas of dense tau-immunoreactivity in the cerebral cortex. The first member of the Professional Football Hall of Fame and the first participant in the NFL's "88 Plan" to pass away and undergo neuropathological examination for CTE was Lou Creekmur. Mr. Creekmur died at the age of 82. He played 10 seasons as an offensive lineman for the Detroit Lions and was an eight-time Pro Bowler. He was famous for suffering at least 13 broken noses while playing without a facemask. He died from complications of dementia while in a nursing home after a 30-year decline that included cognitive and behavioral issues, memory loss, problems with attention and organization, and angry and aggressive outbursts. His wife referred to him as "punchy" for the last 30 years of his life. Neuropathological findings revealed extensive tau-immunoreactive inclusions throughout the cortex and medial temporal lobes consistent with CTE. Remarkably, there was no neuropathological evidence of AD in this 82-year-old.

In addition to finding evidence of CTE in professional athletes, recent evidence suggests that CTE can occur following shorter athletic careers. Mike Borich played football in college, but did not play football professionally. He died at age 42 after exhibiting a pattern of erratic behavior throughout much of his adult life. His college-playing career included stints with Snow College and Western Illinois University in the 1980s. He was known to have approximately 10 concussions during his college football career with no subsequent concussions or head injuries after college. He worked as a Division I college football coach, and was named Offensive Coordinator of the Year in 2001 while coaching at Brigham Young University. He also coached for the NFL's Chicago Bears in 1999–2000. He left coaching in 2003 while struggling with overwhelming drug and alcohol addictions, and ultimately died from a drug overdose in February 2009 at the age of 42. Neuropathological examination of Mr. Borich's brain revealed less pathology overall than many previous cases of confirmed CTE, but was consistent with CTE nonetheless. Of particular salience was the patchy, superficial distribution of tau protein throughout Mr. Borich's frontal cortex and medial temporal lobes.

Although evidence of CTE has become increasingly common in retired football players, it has been found in other sports as well. The first professional ice hockey player to be examined for CTE was Reggie Fleming, who died at the age of 73 in 2009. Fleming was a defensemen and forward for six National Hockey League (NHL) teams from 1959 to 1971. His 13 seasons and 749 NHL games were part of a storied professional career that lasted more than 20 years. He is remembered today for his hard-nosed play and combative style that led to 108 NHL goals, 1,468 penalty minutes, and a Stanley Cup with the 1961 Chicago Blackhawks. He reportedly exhibited symptoms of CTE for decades; he was diagnosed with "manic depression" in his early 40s because of frequent extreme behavioral outbursts. He was described as "out of control" because of significant problems controlling his eating, drinking, gambling, and temper. He reportedly suffered from significant attention, concentration, memory, and executive impairment that progressed to frank dementia in his final two years of life. Neuropathologically, examination of Mr. Fleming's brain was also consistent with CTE, as evidenced by the extensive tau-immunoreactive inclusions distributed throughout the neocortex and medial temporal lobes, particularly at the depths of sulci.

Although much of the proceeding discussion has emphasized the ubiquity of tau protein abnormalities in the pathogenesis of CTE, more recent evidence also suggests the involvement of a second abnormal protein in CTE: Tar-DNA Binding Protein-43 (TDP-43). This abnormal protein has been found in 85 percent of CTE-positive cases (King et al., 2010; McKee et al., 2010). It is also associated with other neurodegenerative diseases like frontotemporal lobar degeneration, and, in some cases, may be associated with motor neuron disease that mimics amyotrophic lateral sclerosis (King et al., 2010; McKee et al., 2010; Tatom et al., 2009).

The prevalence of CTE is currently unknown, but appears to be more common than was previously thought. All 13 of the 13 football players examined by the BU CSTE have had CTE. However, the athletes examined are not representative of the general population or even the population of retired athletes, thus calling into question the denominator used to estimate CTE prevalence. However, assuming that neuropathological findings observed in the next 87 football players to come to autopsy are negative, this would nonetheless suggest a prevalence rate of 13 percent in this population. Clearly, there is a need for longitudinal research with a large, representative sample to more precisely estimate prevalence and identify potential risk and protective factors of CTE.

Such a longitudinal study has recently been implemented through the CSTE's Brain Donation Registry. Recruitment for this registry began approximately 12 months ago and currently, approximately 300 active or retired athletes have agreed to participate in annual telephone interviews and to donate their brains at death. The goal of the CSTE is to recruit a total of 750 athletes altogether. The annual evaluations consist of telephone interviews regarding cognitive and behavioral symptoms, athletic, concussion, and medical history, and include a brief cognitive assessment. The CSTE is also beginning a new registry for combat veterans, another population at risk for brain trauma due to blast injuries caused by improvised explosive devices.

Many combat veterans exposed to blast injuries, like athletes who may suffer incidental blows to the head, experience repetitive *subconcussive* trauma. In other words, trauma caused by forces that are not substantial enough to cause symptoms of concussion. It is believed that concussions are just the tip of the iceberg when it comes to repetitive head trauma; the chronic neurodegeneration seen in CTE also may be influenced by a large number of subconcussive blows to the head that in and of themselves are not acutely problematic. It is believed that the long-term progressive tauopathy of CTE is caused by repetitive blows to the head, including mild, non-symptomatic, subconcussive trauma. However, this hypothesis has yet to be tested empirically.

In addition to the contribution of subconcussive blows to the pathogenesis of CTE, there are many other research questions that have yet to be answered. How common is CTE in athletes at all levels? Is CTE found in combat veterans? What are the risk factors of CTE? Is risk influenced by genetics? How does the type of trauma (loss of consciousness, severity of concussion, subconcussive blows) influence CTE? Can the impact of blast injuries (single, repetitive) lead to CTE? Can the frequency and time interval between successive head traumas affect CTE? For athletes, how can the positions and sports played (i.e., "load" of trauma) influence CTE? Does the age of the individual at time of injury(ies) and the duration of exposure affect CTE? How can we detect and diagnose CTE prior to death? What treatments and prevention strategies will be effective? Is CTE triggered by repetitive blast injury in a similar fashion to repetitive (sub)concussive trauma? What roles do diffuse axonal injury and microhemorrhages play in CTE's pathogenesis?

Returning to the discussion of blast injuries in a military combat setting, the long-term consequences of repetitive blast injuries are currently unknown. In athletes, the clinical symptoms of CTE begin years or decades following trauma. If the physical mechanics of athletic trauma and blast injuries are both capable of initiating the same metabolic cascade that may initiate CTE pathogenesis (Giza and Hovda, 2001), it is possible that, in several decades, we may see a growing epidemic of progressive dementia in veterans. One confounding factor that must be better understood is the fact that the symptoms of CTE and of posttraumatic stress disorder can manifest similarly. A second confound pertains to the fact that many members of the military also may have had previous and/or concurrent contact sport involvement.

Given that the risk factors for CTE are currently not well characterized, how can the risk of CTE be reduced, especially in young people? Under ideal circumstances, the best method to reduce CTE risk is to avoid head trauma. However, short of banning sports and preventing all accidents, head trauma cannot be completely avoided. Proper management of head trauma then becomes paramount. In sports, the following strategies are often recommended to reduce the overall trauma load suffered by an athlete: limit repetition (e.g., "return to play" guidelines); make changes to helmet technology to better absorb the force of the impact; identify the players who may be at increased risk (e.g., based on position, stature, style of play, etc.); and change rules to reduce head injuries without affecting the overall "feel" of the sport.

CTE research is in its infancy. However, a number of important changes have already been made, including changes to rules, increased public awareness, and increased research participation. It is hoped that these efforts can contribute to the prevention of this fully preventable neurodegenerative disease.

REFERENCES

Braak, H., and E. Braak. 1991. Neuropathological stageing of Alzheimer-related changes. *Acta Neuropathologica* 82(4):239–259.

Cajigal, S. 2007. Brain damage may have contributed to former wrestler's violent demise. *Neurology Today* 7(18):15–16.

Clinton, J., M. W. Ambler, and G. W. Roberts. 1991. Post-traumatic Alzheimer's disease: Preponderance of a single plaque type. *Neuropathology and Applied Neurobiology* 17(1):69–74.

Corsellis, J. A. N., C. J. Bruton, and D. Freeman Browne. 1973. The aftermath of boxing. *Psychological Medicine* 3(3):270–303.

Critchley, M. 1957. Medical aspects of boxing, particularly from a neurological standpoint. *British Medical Journal* 1(5015):357–362.

Geddes, J. F., G. H. Vowles, J. A. R. Nicoll, and T. Révész. 1999. Neuronal cytoskeletal changes are an early consequence of repetitive head injury. *Acta Neuropathologica* 98(2):171–178.

Giza, C. C., and D. A. Hovda. 2001. The neurometabolic cascade of concussion. *Journal of Athletic Training* 36(3):228–235.

King, A., F. Sweeney, I. Bodi, C. Troakes, S. Maekawa, and S. Al-Sarraj. 2010. Abnormal TDP-43 expression is identified in the neocortex in cases of dementia pugilistica, but is mainly confined to the limbic system when identified in high and moderate stages of Alzheimer's disease. *Neuropathology* 30(4):408–419.

Langlois, J. A., W. Rutland-Brown, and M. M. Wald. 2006. The epidemiology and impact of traumatic brain injury: A brief overview. *Journal of Head Trauma Rehabilitation* 21(5):375–378.

Martland, H. 1928. Punch drunk. *Journal of the American Medical Association* 91(15):1103–1107.

McKee, A. C., R. C. Cantu, C. J. Nowinski, E. T. Hedley-Whyte, B. E. Gavett, A. E. Budson, V. E. Santini, H. S. Lee, C. A. Kubilus, and R. A. Stern. 2009. Chronic traumatic encephalopathy in athletes: Progressive tauopathy after repetitive head injury. *Journal of Neuropathology and Experimental Neurology* 68(7):709–735.

McKee, A. C., B. E. Gavett, R. A. Stern, C. J. Nowinski, R. C. Cantu, N. W. Kowall, D. P. Perl, E. T. Hedley-Whyte, B. Price, C. Sullivan, P. Morin, H. S. Lee, C. A. Kubilus, D. H. Daneshvar, M. Wulff, and A. E. Budson. 2010. TDP-43 proteinopathy and motor neuron disease in chronic traumatic encephalopathy. *Journal of Neuropathology and Experimental Neurology* 69(9):918–929.

Miller, H. 1966. Mental after-effects of head injury. *Proceedings of the Royal Society of Medicine* 59(3):257–261.

Millspaugh, J. 1937. Dementia pugilistica. *United States Naval Medical Bulletin* 35(3):297–303.

Omalu, B. I., S. T. DeKosky, R. L. Minster, M. I. Kamboh, R. L. Hamilton, and C. H. Wecht. 2005. Chronic traumatic encephalopathy in a National Football League player. *Neurosurgery* 57(1):128–133.

Omalu, B. I., S. T. DeKosky, R. L. Hamilton, R. L. Minster, M. I. Kamboh, A. M. Shakir, and C. H. Wecht. 2006. Chronic traumatic encephalopathy in a National Football League player: Part II. *Neurosurgery* 59(5):1086–1092.

Omalu, B. I., J. Bailes, J. L. Hammers, and R. P. Fitzsimmons. 2010a. Chronic traumatic encephalopathy, suicides and parasuicides in professional American athletes: The role of the forensic pathologist. *American Journal of Forensic Medicine and Pathology* 31(2):130–132.

Omalu, B. I., R. L. Hamilton, M. I. Kamboh, S. T. DeKosky, and J. Bailes. 2010b. Chronic traumatic encephalopathy (CTE) in a National Football League player: Case report and emerging medicolegal practice questions. *Journal of Forensic Nursing* 6(1):40–46.

Parker, H. 1934. Traumatic encephalopathy ('punch drunk') of professional pugilists. *Journal of Neurology and Psychopathology* 15(57):20–28.

Roberts, G. W., D. Allsop, and C. Bruton. 1990a. The occult aftermath of boxing. *Journal of Neurology, Neurosurgery, & Psychiatry* 53(5):373–378.

Roberts, G. W., H. L. Whitwell, P. R. Acland, and C. J. Bruton. 1990b. Dementia in a punch-drunk wife. *Lancet* 335(8694):918–919.

Tatom, J. B., D. B. Wang, R. D. Dayton, O. Skalli, M. L. Hutton, D. W. Dickson, and R. L. Klein. 2009. Mimicking aspects of frontotemporal lobar degeneration and Lou Gehrig's disease in rats via TDP-43 overexpression. *Molecular Therapy* 17(4):607–613.

Standardized Clinical Management of Traumatic Brain Injury by the U.S. Military

Geoffrey S. F. Ling[12]

INTRODUCTION

Traumatic brain injury (TBI) is a common disorder associated with military service. For Operation Iraqi Freedom (OIF) and Operation Enduring Freedom (Afghanistan) (OEF), TBI has been referred to as the "signature injury of the war" (Warden, 2006).

The exact incidence and prevalence of this disease among OIF and OEF troops is uncertain. There are estimates that as many as 19.5–40.0 percent of those deployed are affected. For civilians, the TBI rates also are uncertain with estimates suggesting that as many as 8 million head injuries occur each year in the United States alone. The reasons for the uncertainty are that many patients receive care by non-medical professionals, do not seek medical attention at all, or are improperly diagnosed. This is particularly true for mild TBI (mTBI), where signs and symptoms may be subtle. For moderate to severe TBI, where diagnosis is more certain, among U.S. civilians there are an estimated 1.7 million new cases per year.

Recently, the U.S. military, in response to this rising TBI problem, has instituted a system-wide standardized approach to diagnosis and clinical management of TBI. Critical elements of this approach are criteria for TBI screening; return to duty; neuroimaging; and, especially important, clinical practice guidelines for prehospital, in-hospital, and chronic treatment. As this is a collaborative effort between the Department of Defense (DoD) and

[12] Department of Neurology, Uniformed Services University of the Health Sciences, Bethesda, MD.

the Veterans Administration (VA), it is national in scope. This may be the first such large system-wide effort to apply clinical practice guidelines (CPGs) for TBI patients. Importantly, this has been endorsed and mandated at the highest level of command, which ensures its adoption and execution by medical care providers.

SEVERITY OF TRAUMATIC BRAIN INJURY

There are three major TBI categories: mild, moderate, and severe. These are differentiated by the patient's presenting Glasgow Coma Scale (GCS). A traumatic injury to the brain leading to a GCS of 13–15 is defined as mild. If the GCS is 9–12, it is moderate TBI, and if 8 or less, then it is severe.

Mild TBI is further clarified by the Mild Traumatic Brain Injury Section of the American Congress of Rehabilitation Medicine (1993) as the loss of consciousness, loss of memory preceding or following injury (amnesia), alteration in mental status at time of injury, and/or focal neurological deficit. The American Academy of Neurology's (AAN's) Quality Standards Subcommittee (1997) reports that mTBI and concussion is often associated with brief (< 5 min) loss of consciousness or situational awareness where the person suffers a performance decrement within his/her required environmental context.

In clinical practice, mTBI and concussion are used interchangeably. However, they are distinct. Concussion is altered function following injury. Mild TBI is a pathological state of brain resulting from injury.

Concussion has three grades of severity (ANN, 1997). The grades are differentiated by duration of altered mental status and any loss of conscious. Although not part of the original AAN criteria, amnesia is an independent diagnostic indicator of TBI severity, with the loss of memory preceding (retrograde) or following (posttraumatic or anterograde) injury. Grade 1 concussion is defined as injury leading to altered mental status lasting less than 15 minutes without loss of consciousness. Grade 2 concussion is altered mental status lasting more than 15 minutes without loss of consciousness. Grade 3 concussion is any loss of consciousness.

Moderate TBI is usually associated with prolonged loss of consciousness and/or neurological deficit (Geocadin, 2004). These patients require advanced medical care including neurosurgical and neurointensive care. Later, as they recover, they may develop postconcussion syndrome (Jarell et al., 2003).

Severe TBI is when injury causes the patient to be significantly neurologically compromised such as obtundation or coma. Typically, this is associated with significant neurological injury, often with structural brain or skull lesions revealed by neuroimaging, e.g., head computerized tomography (CT) scan revealing skull fracture, intracranial hemorrhage, and early diffuse cerebral edema. Severe TBI patients require advanced medical care even in the pre-hospital setting. After initial resuscitation and stabilization in the field, severe TBI patients should be quickly evacuated directly to the nearest combat support hospital (CSH) with neurosurgical capability. These patients need airway protection, mechanical ventilation, neurosurgical evaluation, neurocritical care, intracranial pressure (ICP) monitoring, and highly skilled nursing in a trauma or neurointensive care unit. For these patients, recovery will be prolonged and often incomplete with many not surviving to 1 year (Ashwal et al., 1994; BTF, 2007; Bullock et al., 2006).

Mild TBI

Diagnosis and therapy begins at the site of injury, whether the battlefield or the playing field. It is now required that all troops at risk of TBI be evaluated as soon as possible after exposure. During combat operations, at risk is defined as being within a certain distance of an explosive blast. That distance is different depending on circumstances, such as being mounted or dismounted when exposed. Evaluation is done using the military's standardized MACE[13] or military acute concussion evaluation. This is a paper-based tool developed by the Defense and Veterans Brain Injury Center (DVBIC). It begins with obtaining relevant patient information including history, especially exposure details, e.g., blast versus impact, etc. Embedded within the MACE is the standardized assessment of concussion (SAC). The SAC is a neuropsychological clinical test of orientation, concentration, memory, processing, etc. It is based on a similar test used by the National Football League. At present, there are six versions of the SAC so as to minimize the effect of learning the test.

Without a history of altered mental status, if the SAC is normal and the patient does not have any symptoms, he/she does not have TBI and is returned to duty. However, some patients may have symptoms, such as dizziness, for which other non-TBI etiologies are considered such as dehydration. This and other mild symptoms are treated conservatively with simple therapies such as rehydration or sleep hygiene. The patient may need to be referred to an advanced medical care provider such as the battalion surgeon, who is typically a physician.

With a history of change in mental status after injury and abnormal SAC (score < 25) then the patient has suffered mTBI with impairment and is referred to an advanced medical care provider. A more detailed history and neurological exam is performed. If there are any neurological deficits, the patient is evacuated to the nearest CT for neuroimaging. If CT is normal, patients are returned to their unit to be managed. These patients are automatically taken off of combat operation duty ("take a knee") for a prescribed period of time, on the order of a few days. During this time, patients are treated symptomatically based on the VA/DoD *Clinical Practice Guidelines for Management of Concussion/mTBI* (2009). These guidelines have both pharmacological and nonpharmacological (such as sleep, physical therapy, etc.) treatment recommendations. Patients are given crossword puzzles, Sudoku and similar cognitive games. Finally, there are daily education sessions to teach each patient about his/her disease, including possible symptoms (headache, dizziness, insomnia, etc.) and expectations of recovery. An important aspect of this care is that each patient is purposely kept with his/her unit. By doing so, the service member has an important support group and is able to maintain a sense of normality and purpose (Bell et al., 2009).

If the SAC remains abnormal or symptoms persist beyond seven days, patients are referred to an in-theater restoration center, which is clinically staffed with a neurologist and/or occupational therapist and is located near a CSH so that more advanced medical care can be rendered. The neurologist is able to perform more detailed neurological and medical assessments, treat with a wider selection of medications, and test with more sophisticated methods. The occupational therapist can provide a more focused nonpharmacologic treatment plan. Typically, patients stay up to 14 days. If they still have not recovered, then they are evacuated out of theater (Linquist et al., 2010).

This approach has been very successful. Most service members are able to stay with their unit throughout treatment. The majority of those that have been referred to the restoration centers have been able to return to their units. The recovery rate exceeds 90 percent (Bell et al., 2009).

If a service member incurs three concussions over the course of his/her deployment, he/she is removed from further combat operations. The service members call this the "three strikes and you are out" rule (Hancock, 2008).

---

[13] Available online: www.pdhealth.mil/downloads/MACE.pdf (access March 30, 2011).

Moderate to Severe TBI

It is especially important for medical care for moderate to severe TBI to begin at the site of injury. In 2000, the Brain Trauma Foundation published the first edition of *Guidelines for the Prehospital Management of Severe TBI*, which is now in its second edition. Recognizing the need for similar CPGs for the battlefield, the Brain Trauma Foundation and the U.S. military developed the *Guidelines for the Field Management of Combat-Related Head Trauma*. These CPGs are specific treatment recommendations and goals to be used by medics, corpsmen, and other prehospital medical care providers for use on the battlefield. The emphasis is on maintaining optimal physiology to support the injured brain and prevent exacerbation of injury while under the constraints of military operations (Badjatia et al., 2008; Knuth et al., 2005).

Key guidelines are preventing hypoxia, maintaining perfusion (systolic blood pressure > 90 mmH), and avoiding potentially deleterious interventions (prophylactic hyperventilation). This is accomplished by placing an artificial airway if the patient's GCS $\leq$ 8, supporting breathing and oxygenation if oxygen saturation < 90 percent, and maintaining systolic blood pressure > 90 mmHg. Unless a patient is actively herniating, hyperventilation and mannitol are to be avoided. They are not effective for prophylaxis. Mannitol also should not be used when maintenance of intravascular volume can be assured. Other guidelines are analgesic and sedation use, which are important to optimize patient safety, particularly during evacuation. Of note, no particular resuscitation fluid is endorsed because none have sufficient evidence to show clear superiority. However, hypertonic fluids are preferred because they may have benefit in maintaining serum osmolality, which could be beneficial for intracranial pressure (ICP) management (Knuth et al., 2005).

The GPG salso include triage and evacuation. As early as reasonably possible, a GCS for each patient should be determined as well as evaluation of pupillary function. Patients with GCS < 13 should be evacuated as early as possible to a CSH with a neurosurgeon.

Military in-hospital care of moderate to severe TBI treatment has benefited from advances previously developed for civilian TBI. The same civilian-developed CPGs are used in OEF and OIF CSHs. These in-hospital CPGs are directed at optimizing the general physiology; avoiding exacerbation of injury; careful clinical monitoring; and preventing conditions that could worsen outcome, such as deep vein thrombosis (DVT). The key guidelines are placing an artificial airway if the GCS $\leq$ 8, placing an ICP monitor for GCS $\leq$ 8, developing criteria to obtain neuroimaging, maintaining ICP < 25 mmHg, systolic blood pressure > 90 mmHg, pO_2 > 60 mmHg or O_2 saturation > 90 percent, normothermia, and hematocrit $\geq$ 28. Cerebral perfusion pressure (CPP) is kept between 50 to 70 mmHg if fluids or vasoactive agents are needed to achieve this range. If assistive therapy is not required to keep CPP above 50, then it is permitted to be at any level above that. To optimize cerebral venous drainage, the patient's head is to be keep midline and the head of the bed at 30°. Antiepileptic medications are given for only the first seven days to minimize the occurrence of early posttraumatic seizures. To prevent DVT, anticoagulation begins as soon as hemorrhages are stable. The approach is using sequential compression devices (SCDs) and anticoagulation with low molecular weight heparin (LMWH) or low dose unfractionated heparin (LDUH), with or without mechanical compression devices such as graduated compression stockings and SCDs. If intracerebral hemorrhage is present, then it is recommended that only SCDs are used until the risk of further bleeding decreases, at which time anticoagulation may be started. Also important is early institution of nutritional support and gastrointestinal prophylaxis to prevent stress ulcers (BTF, 2007; Geerts et al., 2008).

In the event of cerebral herniation, mannitol and hyperventilation can be considered.

Again, mannitol can be used so long as the patient's intravascular volume can be maintained. Hyperventilation should be to pCO_2 34–36 mmHg. Neither should be used as prophylaxis against herniation. Because many combat wounded suffer from hemorrhagic shock and/ or dehydration, hypertonic saline solutions are often considered, including 3 percent saline infusion or 23 percent saline bolus. Hemicraniectomy is also a therapeutic option frequently used, especially with long evacuation times from theater back to the United States during which managing ICP can be challenging (Ling et al., 2009).

Nutrition is now recognized to be an important component of proper TBI care. The patient should be fed as soon as practical. In moderate to severe TBI, patients usually need nasogastric or orogastric tubes. This is preferred over using parenteral nutrition as enteric feeding more easily allows meeting metabolic needs. Another benefit is that by minimizing free water, enteral feeds can help maintain the intravascular osmolar gradient used in treating intracranial hypertension. Because most TBI patients have some cerebral edema, hyperosmotic feeds are typically used. Because the injured brain is hypermetabolic, TBI patients typically require 140 percent of their basal metabolic caloric needs (BTF, 2007).

A concern is the risk of cerebral vasospasm. Armonda et al. (2006) reported that close to 50 percent of a series of patients with blast-related severe TBI developed cerebral vasospasm that led to symptomatic neurological deterioration. This is diagnosed with neurological examination, transcranial Doppler, and cerebral angiogram. It is often responsible for delayed or late neurological deterioration. Treatment with intra-arterial nicardipine at the site of spasm is effective in reversing this and restoring neurological function (Armonda et al., 2006).

Close neurological monitoring is essential for optimal outcome. While in the acute period, all TBI patients need to be examined neurologically on a regular basis—at least every hour for the first 24 hours and then less often as clinically indicated. Patients with intracranial lesions require continuous ICP and CPP measurements. Typically, the most critical period is during the 48 to 96 hours following injury when cerebral edema is greatest. Thereafter, edema gradually resolves and the patient should improve clinically.

CONCLUSION

Sadly, TBI is a common consequence of armed conflict. Clinical estimates of prevalence are high. In light of this, the military has enacted a comprehensive system-wide program to identify, treat, and rehabilitate TBI wounded service members. It uses evidence-based CPGs. Even though there is not yet a specific "brain rescue" or neuroprotective drug, evidenced-based CPG for treatment and return to duty provide a rational approach to proper management of the TBI patient. It must be emphasized that this is merely a beginning. To be truly effective, the CPGs must be regularly updated. More research and quality assurance follow-up are essential. The system in place is imperfect so there is ample opportunity for improvement. The ultimate goal is that every TBI service member will receive the highest level of medical care—no matter where they are.

DISCLAIMER

The opinions expressed herein belong solely to the author. They do not nor should they be interpreted as representative of or endorsed by the Uniformed Services University of the Health Sciences, Defense Advanced Research Projects Agency, U.S. Army, or Department of Defense.

REFERENCES

AAN (American Academy of Neurology). 1997. Practice parameter: The management of concussion in sports (summary statement). *Neurology* 48(3):581–585.

American Congress of Rehabilitation Medicine. 1993. Definition of mild traumatic brain injury. *Journal of Head Trauma Rehabilitation* 8(3):86–87.

Armonda, R. A., R. S. Bell, A. H. Vo, G. Ling, T. J. DeGraba, B. Crandall, J. Ecklund, and W. W. Campbell. 2006. Wartime traumatic cerebral vasospasm: Recent review of combat casualties. *Neurosurgery* 59(6):1215–1225.

Ashwal, S., R. Cranford, J. L. Bernat, G. Celesia, D. Coulter, H. Eisenberg, E. Myer, F. Plum, M. Walker, C. Watts, and T. Rogstad. 1994. Medical aspects of the persistent vegetative state (first of two parts). *The New England Journal of Medicine* 330(21):1499–1508.

Badjatia, N., N. Carney, T. J. Crocco, M. E. Fallat, H. M. A. Hennes, A. S. Jagoda, S. Jernigan, P. B. Letarte, E. B. Lerner, T. M. Moriarty, P. T. Pons, S. Sasser, T. Scalea, C. L. Schelein, and D. W. Wright. 2008. Guidelines for prehospital management of traumatic brain injury, 2nd ed. *Prehospital Emergency Care* 12(Suppl. 1).

Bell, J., K. Nasky, and W. Skipton. 2009. Personal communication from Afghanistan.

Bullock, M. R., R. Chestnut, J. Ghajar, D. Gordon, R. Hartl, D. W. Newell, F. Servadia, B. C. Waters, and J. E. Wilberger. 2006. Guidelines for the surgical management of traumatic brain injury. *Neurosurgery* 58(3):S2-1–S2-62.

BTF (Brain Trauma Foundation). 2007. Guidelines for the management of severe traumatic brain injury, 3rd ed. *Journal of Neurotrauma* 24(Suppl. 1):S1–S106.

Geerts, W. H., D. Bergqvist, G. F. Pineo, J. A. Heit, C. M. Samama, M. R. Lassen, C. W. Colwell, and P. American College of Chest. 2008. Prevention of venous thromboembolism: American College of Chest Physicians evidence-based clinical practice guidelines (8th ed.). *Chest* 133(6 Suppl.):381S–453S.

Geocadin, R. 2004. Traumatic brain injury. In *Handbook of neurocritical care*, edited by A. Bharwaj, M. A. Mirski and J. A. Ulatowski. Totowa, NJ: Humana Press.

Hancock, J. 2008. Personal communication from Afghanistan.

Jarell, A., J. M. Ecklund, and G. Ling. 2003. Traumatic brain injury. In *Combat medicine*, edited by G. Tsokos and J. Atkinson. Totowa, NJ: Humana Press.

Knuth, T., P. B. LeTarte, G. S. F. Ling, L. E. Moores, P. Rhee, D. Tauber, and A. Trask. 2005. *Guidelines for the field management of combat-related head trauma*. New York: Brain Trauma Foundation.

Ling, G., F. Bandak, R. Armonda, G. Grant, and J. Ecklund. 2009. Explosive blast neurotrauma. *Journal of Neurotrauma* 26(6):815–825.

Linquist, J., K. Radcliff, and M. Wagner. 2010. Personal communication from Afghanistan.

VA/DoD. 2009. The clinical practice guidelines for management of concussion/mild traumatic brain injury. *Journal of Rehabilitation Research and Development* 46(6):CP1–68.

Warden, D. 2006. Military TBI during the Iraq and Afghan wars. *The Journal of Head Trauma Rehabilitation* 21(5):398–402.

The Perspective of an R.D. Working with Civilian Traumatic Brain Injury

Natalia Bailey[14]

INTRODUCTION

Traumatic brain injury (TBI) causes a very serious assault to the body, not only because of the primary or secondary injuries, but also because of the effects it has on all of the body's systems. Brain injury results in a significant increase in metabolism and catabolism that, if left unchecked, can lead to malnutrition. It has been shown that adequate nutrition support can attenuate these metabolic changes that result in muscle loss and therefore positively affect outcomes. This paper will review the current nutrition support standards of care in the moderately to severely brain-injured population, potential routes of nutrient administration, benefit of specific nutrients, and drug-nutrient interactions of concern.

---

[14] Harborview Medical Center, University of Washington, Seattle, WA.

TABLE C-3   Chemical Messengers Effects on Inflammatory Response

Messenger	Function	Result
Cortisol	↑ gluconeogenisis ↑ proteolysis	↑ rate of muscle catabolism
Glucagon	↑ gluconeogenisis	↑ rate of muscle catabolism
Catecholamines (epinephrine, norepinephrine)	↑ insulin resistance	↑ rate of muscle catabolism
Cytokines (IL-1, IL-6, TNF)	Activates immune response ↑ RMR	↑ rate of muscle catabolism

RATIONALE FOR NUTRITION SUPPORT IN TBI

In the initial acute phase following TBI, the patient is in a hypermetabolic and catabolic state. The literature indicates energy expenditure ranges between 100–200 percent of resting metabolic rate, and this increased energy expenditure can last anywhere from one week to one year following the injury (Deutschman et al., 1986; Loan, 1999; Moore et al., 1989). During the initial acute stage of injury, glycogen stores are quickly depleted. This results in a need to use muscle proteins as a source of required glucose energy, leading to significant lean body mass catabolism (Berg et al., 2006). Non-stressed individuals lose approximately 200–300 grams of muscle per day, whereas TBI patients lose up to 1,000 grams of lean body mass per day (Loan, 1999). The major cause of this highly catabolic state is a postinjury increase in chemical messengers. These messengers include cortisol, glucagon, catecholamines, and cytokines, all of which contribute to breakdown of muscle rather than fat for energy (Table C-3) (Darbar, 2001; Loan, 1999; Moore et al., 1989; Young et al., 1988). In addition to an increase in catabolic chemical messengers postinjury, there is a decrease in anabolic hormones, such as human growth hormone (Demling, 2009). The increase in metabolic rate and resulting muscle catabolism can lead to malnutrition if not attenuated by provision of adequate nutrition support.

Inadequate nutrition support postinjury can lead to significant malnutrition. This can include significant weight loss resulting in poor outcomes including increased mortality and, increased length of hospitalization and rehabilitation. If the TBI patient is fed inadequately for one week, then this may lead to a 10 percent loss of lean body mass. If nutrition needs are not met for two weeks, then this may lead to a 30 percent loss of lean body mass, and increased mortality (Darbar, 2001). Malnourished TBI patients (BMI < 15) entering rehabilitation have a length of stay approximately 28 days longer than those who are not malnourished (Dénes, 2004).

STANDARDS OF CARE

The major principles driving the nutrition care of TBI patients include early nutrition support, provision of adequate calories (kcal) and protein, preference for enteral nutrition, use of nutrition protocols, and ongoing assessment of efficacy of nutrition support.

Evidence for early nutrition support (within the first 24–72 hours post-injury) is limited in the TBI population; however, there is growing evidence that this practice is beneficial. In one study, early nutrition support (within five days after trauma) was shown to be one of the few therapies that could positively affect two-week mortality in TBI patients (Hartl et al., 2008). Benefits of early nutrition support in other critically ill populations include lower risk of infection, decreased activation and release of inflammatory cytokines, decreased hospital and intensive care unit (ICU) length of stay, and attenuation of catabolism of skeletal muscle (McClave et al., 2009).

Determining calorie requirements is difficult in this population because many factors influence the rate of metabolism. Calorie needs may be decreased with barbiturate coma, propofol infusions, and other sedatives (Frankenfield, 2006; McCall et al., 2003; Moore et al., 1989; Rajpal and Johnston, 2009). Infection, fever, posturing, storming, and presence of other injuries may increase caloric needs (Clifton et al., 1986; Frankenfield, 2006; Moore et al., 1989; Rajpal and Johnston, 2009). Typically the energy needs are calculated by prediction formulas, which predict basal energy expenditure (BEE), such as the Harris-Benedict formula, which also includes an injury factor (Cook et al., 2008). The Brain Trauma Foundation (BTF) recommends a calorie provision of 140 percent of BEE (Bratton et al., 2007). It has been shown that prediction formulas often under- or over-predict calories, and if able, it is desirable to measure energy expenditure via indirect calorimetry. This measurement is considered the "gold standard" in determining calorie needs (Felípez and Sentongo, 2009; McClave et al., 2009; Pepe and Barba, 1999).

Protein needs are elevated in the TBI population, and the BTF guidelines suggest needs that range from 1.5–2.0 g per kg (Bratton et al., 2007). Several studies have shown variable beneficial results in delivering greater than 2 grams per kg. One study showed that when given 2.2 g of protein per kg, TBI patients corrected their negative nitrogen balance at a faster rate than those who were given less protein; however, they had increased urinary nitrogen excretion (Twyman et al., 1985).

Enterally delivered nutrition support is the preferred route of nutrient delivery if the patient's gastrointestinal (GI) tract is functioning and accessible. Benefits of enteral nutrition (EN) include the following (Artinian et al., 2006; McClave et al., 2009; Taylor et al., 1999):

- gut barrier maintenance,
- modulation of stress and immune response,
- lower risk of infection when compared to parenteral nutrition (PN) administration,
- reduction in hospital length of stay,
- lower cost of nutrition support, and
- quicker return of cognitive function and in neurosurgery patients.

Although EN support is less risky than PN support, there are still some risks associated with it. If enteral feeds are started prior to adequate resuscitation, or if GI perfusion is poor, there is an increased risk of GI tract ischemia. High infusion rates of pressors and/or sedatives, anesthetics, as well as abdominal injuries influence blood perfusion to the GI tract. Additionally, enteral feeding intolerance, such as abdominal pain, nausea, and vomiting have been described in critically ill patients, negatively affecting the rate at which patients achieve their nutritional goals.

PN is another potential route of nutrition support delivery; however, its use can result in more complications than enteral nutrition, and therefore, is not the preferred option. Risks of PN include increased risk of infection, increased cost, and increased risk of mortality (McClave et al., 2009). In the TBI population, however, it has been shown that patients on PN have fewer interruptions in feeding and their nutrition goals are reached more quickly

(Bratton et al., 2007; Young et al., 1987). One study showed that for those with head trauma, EN and PN were equally effective in meeting nutrition goals with similar infection rates and similar cost (Borzotta et al., 1994).

An assessment by a registered dietitian (RD) early in the TBI patient's admission is essential in determining nutrition goals and the nutrition plan of the TBI patient. It has been shown that implementing the RD's recommendations is correlated with decreased length of stay, higher serum albumin, and increased weight gains (Braga et al., 2006). In addition to the RD assessment, use of nutrition protocols is useful in enhancing nutrition delivery. In one study, use of the nutrition protocol increased the percentage of calories provided, and was identified as the factor having the greatest impact on successful delivery of EN in the first week of neurocritical illness (Zarbock et al., 2008).

Assessing efficacy of nutrition support is a difficult task in the ICU setting because of the confounding effects of critical illness and treatment on typical nutrition assessment parameters. Patient weights are strongly influenced by clinically induced fluid gains and losses, and are not immediately useful, although they may be more helpful in the later stages of healing. Nutrition laboratory tests are highly inaccurate in the setting of critical illness because the acute-phase response results in re-direction of the synthesis of visceral proteins toward wound healing and the immune response (McClave et al., 2009; Moore et al., 1989; Young et al., 1985, 1988). It is recommended that if albumin or transthyretin (pre-albumin) is used to assess nutrition status, C-reactive protein (CRP) must be checked as well, to determine the patient's level of inflammatory response. When CRP is elevated, this is an indication that albumin and pre-albumin will be decreased, and their use as a tool for assessment of nutrition status will not be useful. If using visceral proteins to monitor nutrition status, trends in laboratory values are more helpful compared to isolated measurements of these laboratory tests. Other indicators of adequacy of nutrition include wound healing, ability to wean from mechanical ventilation, as well as ability to participate in rehabilitative therapies.

Standards of care regarding nutrition therapy in the TBI patient are based on guidelines from various organizations including the American Dietetic Association, American Society of Parenteral and Enteral Nutrition (ASPEN), Society of Critical Care Medicine (SCCM), and Brain Trauma Foundation (BTF). The most comprehensive nutrition guidelines come from the combined efforts of ASPEN and SCCM; however, these guidelines are not specific to the TBI population. The BTF has published nutrition guidelines as well, though, because of the lack of nutrition studies in the TBI population, these guidelines are not specific. Table C-4 is a comparison of the nutrition guidelines from ASPEN/SCCM and the brain trauma foundation for moderate to severe brain injury, and may be helpful in identifying areas where more research is needed in the TBI patient population.

TABLE C-4 Comparison of ASPEN/SCCM Guidelines and BTF Guidelines

Guidelines Pertaining to	ASPEN/SCCM	BTF
Calories	No specific guidelines in TBI; Met cart gold standard	100–140 percent replacement of resting metabolism
Protein	1.2–2.0 g/kg in critical illness	15–20 percent of kcals
Timing of initiating feeds	24–48 hours following admission	No recommendation
Dosing of EN	50–65 percent of goal by day 7	100 percent of goal by day 7
EN vs. PN	EN preferred, PN only when necessary	No recommendation
Nutrition protocols	Should be implemented	No recommendation

It should be noted that currently there are no published nutrition guidelines for those with mild TBI and/or concussion.

SPECIFIC DIETS OR NUTRIENTS OF CONCERN

Specific diets or nutrients to be avoided in the TBI population are unknown, although there is some question regarding the safety of the use of the amino acid glutamine during the acute phases of TBI. During critical illness, glutamine becomes conditionally essential, and administration of exogenous glutamine in this patient population has shown some promise (McClave et al., 2009). Benefits include glutamine's anabolic/anticatabolic properties, use as an antioxidant, and use as a fuel for dividing cells. However, in the TBI population, it has been hypothesized that increased glutamine in the diet leads to increased glutamate in the interstitial fluid. Increased glutamate has been linked to high intracranial pressures and increased cerebral swelling (Cook et al., 2008; Enriquez and Bullock, 2004). Several studies have shown that feeding patients additional glutamine does increase glutamate levels in the interstitial fluid; however, more studies are needed to determine the benefit of this practice in the brain-injured population (Berg et al., 2006).

IMPORTANCE OF NUTRITIONAL FORMULATIONS

The use of immune-enhancing formulas in the critically ill population is of growing interest, and studies have shown better outcomes with the use of these formulas. Immune-modulating formulas may include higher ratio of n-3 vs. n-6 fatty acids, and/or increased provision of antioxidants including vitamins E and C, zinc, and selenium. ASPEN and SCCM recommend the use of immune-enhancing formulas in surgical and medical ICU patients, but suggest using standard formulas in populations in which there is little evidence that use of enhanced formulas improve outcomes (McClave et al., 2009). In the TBI population, evidence is lacking that these formulas provide additional benefits compared to those receiving standard formulas (Martindale et al., 2009). One study looked at early nutrition along with using an immune-enhancing formula in head injury patients, and no additional benefit was found (Minard et al., 2000). Another small study (n = 13) looked at feeding an immune-enhancing enteral formula to trauma patients, and this did not affect outcomes or levels of pro-inflammatory cytokines (Jeevanandam et al., 1999). Because of the positive results seen in other populations, larger, randomized control trials are warranted in the TBI population.

DRUG AND NUTRIENT INTERACTIONS

When devising a nutrition plan, drug-nutrient interactions should be taken into account. It is possible that calorie needs will be lower with certain medications, such as propofol, which provides 1.1 kcals of fat with each milliliter infused in addition to decreasing metabolic rate. Other medications may cause increased need for nutrients, such as vitamin D and folic acid for those on seizure prophylaxis (Felípez and Sentongo, 2009). The effect that any drug has on the GI tract should also be considered. For instance, vasopressors decrease gut perfusion; therefore, one should be cautious about aggressive nutrition regimens. Table C-5 shows a list of common drug-nutrient interactions in the TBI population. This is not a comprehensive list of all interactions; however, these are most common in the neurocritical care unit.

TABLE C-5   Common Drug/Nutrient Interactions in TBI

Drug	Nutrient Interaction
Barbiturates	Decreased metabolic rate
Propofol	• Fat kcal (n-6; pro-inflammatory) • Increased urinary excretion of zinc, iron
Seizure prophylaxis	Increased need for vitamin D, folic acid
Dilantin	Carbohydrates interfere with absorption
Vasopressors	Decreased gut perfusion

CONCLUSION

Traumatic brain injury can cause a very dramatic increase in metabolism and catabolism, resulting in extensive loss of lean body mass if adequate nutrition support is not provided. It has been shown that adequate and timely nutrition therapy can lead to positive outcomes for those with brain injury. Standards of care for nutrition support of TBI patients include early enteral nutrition if possible, measurement using indirect calorimetry rather than prediction of calories to be provided, and the use of nutrition protocols to deliver support. Because of the need for nutrition research in this population, the benefit of specific nutrients is unknown.

REFERENCES

Artinian, V., H. Krayem, and B. DiGiovine. 2006. Effects of early enteral feeding on the outcome of critically ill mechanically ventilated medical patients. *Chest* 129(4):960–967.

Berg, A., B. M. Bellander, M. Wanecek, L. Gamrin, Å. Elving, O. Rooyackers, U. Ungerstedt, and J. Wernerman. 2006. Intravenous glutamine supplementation to head trauma patients leaves cerebral glutamate concentration unaffected. *Intensive Care Medicine* 32(11):1741–1746.

Borzotta, A. P., J. Pennings, B. Papasadero, J. Paxton, S. Mardesic, R. Borzotta, A. Parrott, and F. Bledsoe. 1994. Enteral versus parenteral nutrition after severe closed head injury. *Journal of Trauma* 37(3):459–468.

Braga, J. M., A. Hunt, J. Pope, and E. Molaison. 2006. Implementation of dietitian recommendations for enteral nutrition results in improved outcomes. *Journal of the American Dietetic Association* 106(2):281–284.

Bratton, S. L., R. M. Chestnut, J. Ghajar, F. F. McConnell Hammond, O. A. Harris, R. Hartl, G. T. Manley, A. Nemecek, D. W. Newell, G. Rosenthal, J. Schouten, L. Shutter, S. D. Timmons, J. S. Ullman, W. Videtta, J. E. Wilberger, and D. W. Wright. 2007. Guidelines for the management of severe traumatic brain injury. XII. Nutrition. *Journal of Neurotrauma* 24(Suppl. 1):S77–S82.

Clifton, G. L., C. S. Robertson, and S. C. Choi. 1986. Assessment of nutritional requirements of head-injured patients. *Journal of Neurosurgery* 64(6):895–901.

Cook, A. M., A. Peppard, and B. Magnuson. 2008. Nutrition considerations in traumatic brain injury. *Nutrition in Clinical Practice* 23(6):608–620.

Darbar, A. 2001. Nutritional requirements in severe head injury. *Nutrition* 17(1):71–72.

Demling, R. 2009. Nutrition, anabolism, and the wound healing process: An overview. *Open Access Journal of Plastic Surgery* 9:65–88.

Dénes, Z. 2004. The influence of severe malnutrition on rehabilitation in patients with severe head injury. *Disability and Rehabilitation* 26(19):1163–1165.

Deutschman, C. S., F. N. Konstantinides, S. Raup, P. Thienprasit, and F. B. Cerra. 1986. Physiological and metabolic response to isolated closed-head injury. Part 1: Basal metabolic state: Correlations of metabolic and physiological parameters with fasting and stressed controls. *Journal of Neurosurgery* 64(1):89–98.

Enriquez, P., and R. Bullock. 2004. Molecular and cellular mechanism in the pathophysiology of severe head injury. *Current Pharmaceutical Design* 10(18):2131–2143.

Felípez, L., and T. A. Sentongo. 2009. Drug-induced nutrient deficiencies. *Pediatric Clinics of North America* 56(5):1211–1224.

Frankenfield, D. 2006. Energy expenditure and protein requirements after traumatic injury. *Nutrition in Clinical Practice* 21(5):430–437.

Hartl, R., L. M. Gerber, Q. Ni, and J. Ghajar. 2008. Effect of early nutrition on deaths due to severe traumatic brain injury. *Journal of Neurosurgery* 109(1):50–56.

Jeevanandam, M., L. M. Shahbazian, and S. R. Petersen. 1999. Proinflammatory cytokine production by mitogen-stimulated peripheral blood mononuclear cells (PBMCs) in trauma patients fed immune-enhancing enteral diets. *Nutrition* 15(11–12):842–847.

Loan, T. 1999. Metabolic/nutritional alterations of traumatic brain injury. *Nutrition* 15(10):809–812.

Martindale, R. G., S. A. McClave, V. W. Vanek, M. McCarthy, P. Roberts, B. Taylor, J. B. Ochoa, L. Napolitano, and G. Cresci. 2009. Guidelines for the provision and assessment of nutrition support therapy in the adult critically ill patient: Society of Critical Care Medicine and American Society for Parenteral and Enteral Nutrition: Executive summary. *Critical Care Medicine* 37(5):1757–1761.

McCall, M., K. Jeejeebhoy, P. Pencharz, and R. Moulton. 2003. Effect of neuromuscular blockade on energy expenditure in patients with severe head injury. *Journal of Parenteral and Enteral Nutrition* 27(1):27–35.

McClave, S. A., R. G. Martindale, V. W. Vanek, M. McCarthy, P. Roberts, B. Taylor, J. B. Ochoa, L. Napolitano, and G. Cresci. 2009. Guidelines for the provision and assessment of nutrition support therapy in the adult critically ill patient: Society of Critical Care Medicine (SCCM) and American Society for Parenteral and Enteral Nutrition (A.S.P.E.N.). *Journal of Parenteral and Enteral Nutrition* 33(3):277–316.

Minard, G., K. A. Kudsk, S. Melton, J. H. Patton, and E. A. Tolley. 2000. Early versus delayed feeding with an immune-enhancing diet in patients with severe head injuries. *Journal of Parenteral and Enteral Nutrition* 24(3):145–149.

Moore, R., M. P. Najarian, and C. W. Konvolinka. 1989. Measured energy expenditure in severe head trauma. *Journal of Trauma* 29(12):1633–1636.

Pepe, J. L., and C. A. Barba. 1999. The metabolic response to acute traumatic brain injury and implications for nutritional support. *Journal of Head Trauma Rehabilitation* 14(5):462–474.

Rajpal, V., and J. Johnston. 2009. Nutrition management of traumatic brain injury patients. *Support Line* 31:10–19.

Taylor, S. J., S. B. Fettes, C. Jewkes, and R. J. Nelson. 1999. Prospective, randomized, controlled trial to determine the effect of early enhanced enteral nutrition on clinical outcome in mechanically ventilated patients suffering head injury. *Critical Care Medicine* 27(11):2525–2531.

Twyman, D., A. B. Young, and L. Ott. 1985. High protein enteral feedings: A means of achieving positive nitrogen balance in head injured patients. *Journal of Parenteral and Enteral Nutrition* 9(6):679–684.

Young, A. B., L. G. Ott, D. Beard, R. J. Dempsey, P. A. Tibbs, and C. J. McClain. 1988. The acute-phase response of the brain-injured patient. *Journal of Neurosurgery* 69(3):375–380.

Young, B., L. Ott, and J. Norton. 1985. Metabolic and nutritional sequelae in the non-steroid treated head injury patient. *Neurosurgery* 17(5):784–791.

Young, B., L. Ott, D. Twyman, J. Norton, R. Rapp, P. Tibbs, D. Haack, B. Brivins, and R. Dempsey. 1987. The effect of nutritional support on outcome from severe head injury. *Journal of Neurosurgery* 67(5):668–676.

Zarbock, S. D., D. Steinke, J. Hatton, B. Magnuson, K. M. Smith, and A. M. Cook. 2008. Successful enteral nutritional support in the neurocritical care unit. *Neurocritical Care* 9(2):210–216.

Nutritional Considerations in Clinical Treatment: The Perspective of a Neurosurgeon

Jamshid Ghajar,[15] *Roger Härtl,*[16] *Linda M. Gerber,*[17] *and Jane E. McCormack*[18]

INTRODUCTION

Traumatic brain injury (TBI) remains a highly lethal injury with mortality ranging from 20–50 percent (Bulger et al., 2002; Demetriades et al., 2004; Jiang et al., 2002). Approximately 52,000 patients die from TBI each year (Sosin et al., 1995; Thurman et al., 1999) with approximately 85 percent of the deaths occurring within the first two weeks (Roberts

[15]Department of Neurological Surgery, Weill Cornell Medical College and Brain Trauma Foundation, New York, NY.

[16]Department of Neurological Surgery, Weill Cornell Medical College, New York, NY.

[17]Department of Public Health, Weill Cornell Medical College, New York, NY.

[18]Division of Trauma, Surgical Critical Care & Burn, Stony Brook University Medical Center, Stony Brook, NY.

et al., 2004). Pharmaceutical trials of TBI have failed to demonstrate any efficacy in reducing deaths (Narayan et al., 2002). Proper trauma transport systems and maintenance of cerebral perfusion and oxygenation by avoidance of hypoxemia, arterial hypotension, and intracranial hypertension reduce mortality and improves outcome (Brain Trauma Foundation, 2000; Chesnut et al., 1993; Härtl et al., 2006; Sampalis et al., 1999; Smith et al., 1990).

Currently, the metabolic status and nutritional needs of TBI patients are less of a priority than maintaining cerebral perfusion. However, TBI results in a hypermetabolic and catabolic state that increases systemic and cerebral energy requirements (Clifton et al., 1986; Deutschman et al., 1986; Hovda et al., 1995; Weekes and Elia, 1996). A recent review from the Cochrane Collaboration states that early feeding may be associated with a trend towards better outcomes after TBI (Perel et al., 2006). *The Guidelines for the Management of Severe Traumatic Brain Injury* recommend that the patient's feeding requirements should be met by the end of the first week after TBI (Brain Trauma Foundation, 2000). These recommendations were based on two small, randomized trials (Rapp et al., 1983; Taylor et al., 1999). There are no studies on the relationship of mortality to the amount and frequency of feeding in TBI patients. In the few studies done, none controlled for factors known to affect mortality from TBI, such as hypotension, age, pupillary status, and computed tomography (CT) scan findings.

The Brain Trauma Foundation (BTF) prospectively collects data on pre- and in-hospital TBI management in 20 Level I and 2 Level II trauma centers in New York state as part of a TBI quality improvement program. An analysis was conducted examining the effect of timing and quantity of nutritional support on early mortality. Early onset of nutritional support and amount of nutritional support was hypothesized to be associated with a reduced mortality at two weeks. In addition, a feeding compliance implementation program was undertaken at one of the participating hospitals to increase the net caloric intake of patients.

METHODS

The BTF designed and implemented a quality improvement initiative in New York state to improve severe TBI acute care and outcome. The program is funded by the New York State Department of Health, Division of Healthcare Financing and Acute and Primary Care Reimbursement. This program tracks pre- and in-hospital severe TBI data through an on-line Internet database called TBI-trac®. The database consists of clinical information from the prehospital environment, emergency department, the first 10 days of intensive care unit (ICU) care, and two-week mortality. When the study began in 2000, enrollment was limited to five Level I trauma centers, and this number increased to a total of 24 trauma centers in 2005, 22 of which were Level I trauma centers and 2 of which were Level II centers. This report is based on patients treated at these trauma centers between June 6, 2000 and December 31, 2005.

RESULTS

Data for 1,818 patients were entered in the database from June 6, 2000, through December 31, 2005. Patients were excluded if they had a Glasgow Coma Scale (GCS) greater than or equal to 9 on day 1 (92 patients), or a GCS motor score of 6 on day 1 (16 patients). Patients also were excluded if they had a GCS score of 3 with pupils bilaterally fixed and dilated and were not pharmacologically paralyzed (152 patients). In addition, patients were excluded for a GCS greater than or equal to 4 with pupils bilaterally fixed and dilated or missing pupillary information (93 patients), or with missing outcome assessment (51 patients). Because nutritional requirements for pediatric and adult patients are different, 153 pediatric patients less than 16 years of age were excluded. After these exclusion criteria were applied, a total of 1,261 patients were eligible for analysis.

In order to examine the effect of nutritional support within the first week after admission, only patients who had at least seven days of inpatient data (were alive for at least seven days) were analyzed. A total of 464 patients had less than seven days of data resulting in a final sample of 797 patients. Patients who had less than seven days of data were older (41.9 vs. 39.0 years, p < 0.01) and were more likely to be hypotensive on day 1 (17.6 percent vs. 13.3 percent p < 0.04) than patients with greater than seven days of data. A greater proportion of their CT scans were abnormal (84.3 percent) compared to those with greater than seven days of follow-up (74.4 percent, p < 0.001). Two-week mortality was also significantly higher when compared to those with seven or more days of records (42.0 percent vs. 9.9 percent, p < 0.0001).

Administration of feeding began in 61 percent of patients during days 1 through 3; however, 5 percent of patients were not fed during the seven-day period, and the majority (62 percent) of patients never reached 25 kcal/kg/day within seven days. No differences were found in patient characteristics or severity of illness by nutrition level achieved within the first five days of treatment. Two-week mortality by nutrition status was significantly higher among patients never fed within 5 (p = 0.0008) or seven (p < 0.0001) days. Mortality significantly decreased with increasing nutritional level such that the rate was 6.3 percent and 7.6 percent among patients fed more than 25 kcal/kg/day within five and seven days, respectively. Older age and having a high intracranial pressure (ICP) were also significantly associated with two-week mortality, while CT scan status was marginally related. The lack of correlation between hypotension and pupillary status and mortality may be explained by the specific exclusion criteria in this study; patients with bilaterally fixed and dilated pupils and GCS scores of 3 were excluded, as were patients who were not alive by day seven.

Nutrition level continued to predict two-week mortality after controlling for age, hypotension, pupillary status, initial GCS, and CT scan status. Patients not fed within five days had 2.1 times the risk of two-week mortality, while those not fed within seven days had 4.1 times the risk of two-week mortality. The amount of nutritional support given within five and seven days also contributed significantly to mortality risk. Every 10 kcal/kg decrease in nutritional support administered within five and seven days resulted in 30–40 percent increased risk of mortality (Figure C-6).

Further analysis of the relationship between ICP monitoring and early nutrition reveals that nutrition had a significant impact in patients with elevated ICP. In the first five days, patients with high ICP and without nutritional support, had a significantly increased mortality when compared to patients with intracranial hypertension who were fed (25.7 percent vs. 12.9 percent, respectively, p = 0.04). In patients who did not undergo ICP monitoring the lack of early nutritional support had an even more pronounced impact on mortality (25.8 percent vs. 6.3 percent mortality, p = 0.0004).

DISCUSSION

Current Findings

The present study adds several significant findings to the existing literature. It is the largest database that has used prospectively collected data to address the relationship between nutrition and early mortality after TBI. The main findings follow. First, any nutrition within the first five days after TBI is associated with reduced mortality. Second, there is a significant

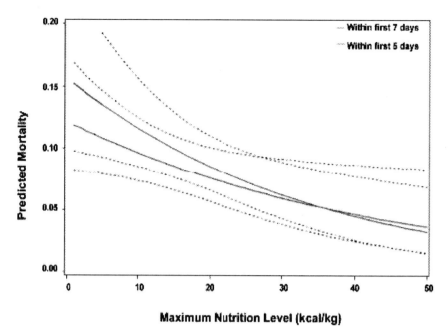

FIGURE C-6 Line graph shows the predicted mortality as a function of maximum nutrition level. Regression models were adjusted for age, hypotension status on day 1, pupil status (normal or abnormal) on day 1, initial GCS score, and CT scan findings. *Solid lines* represent the maximum amount of nutritional support, and *dashed lines* indicate the 95 percent confidence interval.
SOURCE: Härtl et al., 2008.

relationship between the maximum level of nutrition reached and mortality; every 10 kcal/kg decrease in caloric intake is associated with a 30–40 percent increase in mortality. Third, early nutrition within five days after TBI emerges as an independent factor affecting mortality even after controlling for known predictors of mortality such as arterial hypotension, age, CT diagnosis, GCS, and pupillary status. Patients who were not fed within five or seven days after TBI had a two- and four-fold increased likelihood of mortality, respectively. In addition, patients with elevated ICPs or patients who did not undergo ICP monitoring had a significantly increased mortality if they were not fed within five days after trauma when compared to patients who received nutrition. These findings demonstrate that feeding is as significant an intervention as avoidance of early arterial hypotension and hypoxia in reducing mortality from severe TBI.

How Does Feeding Affect Mortality?

Generally, nutritional support has emerged as a significant factor in improving the outcome of critically ill patients. Early initiation of enteral nutrition is associated with a lower incidence of infections, reduced length of hospital stay and possibly improved outcome in critically ill patients in surgical and medical ICUs (Marik and Zaloga, 2001). However, the mechanism by which nutrition affects outcome is unclear. One possibility is that it may provide important nutrients during a critical time period when demand exceeds available resources.

Studies have shown a rise in energy expenditure after TBI, even in paralyzed patients (Clifton et al., 1986). This hypermetabolic state after TBI may be due to systemic factors such as infection and a posttraumatic stress response, but there appears to be a cerebral component as well. There is an increase in cerebral metabolic rate for glucose in TBI possibly as a result of mitochondrial dysfunction (Merenda and Bullock, 2006). Studies in humans indicate that this increase in glucose utilization may last up to five to seven days after TBI (Bergsneider et al., 1997; Hovda et al., 1995). The significance of this cerebral hypermetabolic state is illustrated by the therapeutic effect of interventions that suppress cerebral metabolism such as barbiturate coma, hypothermia and interventions that improve blood flow and supply of nutrients such as cerebral perfusion pressure management. One of the beneficial effects of early aggressive nutritional support may be the steady supply of glucose when the brain depends on increased glucose metabolism to maintain metabolic energy balance.

Another effect of early nutrition may be its attenuation of the posttraumatic stress response and improvement of early immunological function (Bastian et al., 1998; Rovlias and Kotsou, 2000). This could result in an indirect effect on outcome mediated by a lower infection rate. A meta-analysis that compared early (within 36 hours) to delayed initiation of enteral nutrition in critically ill patients (not only TBI) demonstrated a 55 percent reduction in infection rate in patients who received early nutritional support (Marik and Zaloga, 2001). As infection rate was not collected as part of the TBI-trac® database, this relationship could not be examined. It is unlikely, however, that infection rate would have such a significant impact on two-week mortality.

Nutrition also could have an impact on the posttraumatic stress response that is associated with adverse outcome from TBI (Rovlias and Kotsou, 2000). The posttraumatic stress response is characterized by increased blood levels of glucose, lactate, catecholamines, and cortisol. In the blunt trauma population, however, early feeding within 24 hours after injury had no effect on the metabolic stress response (Eyer et al., 1993).

Arterial hypotension doubles mortality from TBI (Chesnut et al., 1993). The relationship between nutritional support and hypotension was examined based on the hypothesis that the fluid volume given with nutrition improves the patient's hemodynamic status and prevents arterial hypotension. There was, however, no relationship between arterial hypotension and nutritional support within the first five days after TBI.

Another finding in this study was that early nutritional support may have a protective effect in patients with intracranial hypertension. Results indicate that patients with high ICPs who are fed have a significantly lower mortality when compared to patients who do not receive nutritional support (12.9 percent vs. 25.7 percent, respectively). Nutritional support may protect the brain by providing large amounts of energy substrates, during a critical time period when hyperglycolysis and hyperemia are present, in an effort to maintain energy balance and cerebral ionic hemostasis (Bergsneider et al., 1997).

Why Were Patients Not Fed?

Our analysis showed that the lack of nutritional support was not related to the severity of the injury or other factors associated with outcome from TBI. Beyond this, it is difficult to determine what affected the decision not to feed patients early on. Possibilities include that patients did not tolerate enteral nutrition early after TBI and that early nutritional support may not have been given a priority by the treating physicians. Other factors that interfere with feeding and that were not registered in this database include patient transport within the hospital and enteral administration of phenytoin.

Program in Participating Trauma Center to Improve Compliance

Achieving adequate nutritional intake in this patient population is difficult, and nutritional therapy in many ICUs is suboptimal (Cahill et al., 2010). Despite best intentions many trauma centers fail to achieve adequate caloric intake. One Level 1 trauma center was consistently well below the goal of 25 kcal/kg/day, and a Quality Improvement (QI) initiative was undertaken.Its process and results are described below.

Methods

Nurse registars collect kcal/kg per patient per day into an online data base (TBI-trac®) as part of a quality initiative through the BTF. Quarterly data review demonstrated that the mean kcal/kg/day was well below goal. The QI team reviewed patient records, developed protocols, obtained attending physician consensus, monitored compliance, and revised the nutrition protocol as needed. The Nutrition Protocol was revised several times as results were analyzed. The current protocol calls for enteral feeding over 20 hours of the day, with a 4-hour time period built in for "catch up."

Results

The percentage of patients receiving nutrition by day 2 increased from 29 percent in 2007 to 50 percent in 2010. Average kcal/kg on hospital day 5 increased from a mean of 14.4 in 2007 to 28.8 in 2010 (p = 0.006, Figure C-7). The percentage of patients who received at least 25 kcal/kg on day 5 increased from 19.4 percent in 2007 to 75 percent in 2010 (p = 0.018). The percentage of patients who achieved 25 kcal/kg/day on any day within the first 5 days postinjury increased from 25.8 percent in 2007 to 91.7 percent in 2010 (p = 0.001).

Findings

A successful feeding protocol must address the unique needs of the TBI patient. Our ICU found success by building into the protocol time each day to make up or catch up if feeds were held for any reason. With this protocol we have been successful in achieving adequate nutritional intake in the severe TBI patient.

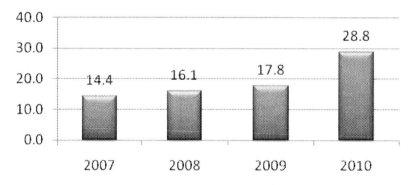

FIGURE C-7   Average kcal/kg received by patients in a Level I trauma center on hospital day 5 significantly increases from 2007 to 2010.
SOURCE: Ghajar, 2010.

CONCLUSIONS

In this severe TBI prospective database, nutritional support initiated within five days after trauma is associated with a significant reduction in two-week mortality. Furthermore, the amount of nutrition is related to mortality. These results held after controlling for other parameters known to affect mortality such as arterial hypotension, age, pupillary status, initial GCS, and CT scan findings. Thus, nutrition may be an independent predictor of mortality. A prospective, randomized trial would be necessary to confirm this finding to generate class I evidence. It is doubtful, however, that such a trial comparing nutrition vs. no nutrition will be done given the ethical implications. Together with arterial hypotension, hypoxia and intracranial hypertension, early nutritional support is one of the few therapeutic interventions that can directly affect outcome.

ACKNOWLEDGMENT

Permission obtained from *Journal of Neurosurgery* for the following article: Härtl, R., L. M. Gerber, Q. Ni, and J. Ghajar. 2008. Effect of early nutrition on deaths due to severe traumatic brain injury. *Journal of Neurosurgery* 109:50–56.

REFERENCES

Bastian, L., A. Weimann, W. Bischoff, P. N. Meier, M. Grotz, C. Stan, and G. Regel. 1998. Clinical effects of supplemental enteral nutrition solution in severe polytrauma. *Der Unfallchirurg* 101(2):105–114.

Bergsneider, M., D. A. Hovda, E. Shalmon, D. F. Kelly, P. M. Vespa, N. A. Martin, M. E. Phelps, D. L. McArthur, M. J. Caron, J. F. Kraus, and D. P. Becker. 1997. Cerebral hyperglycolysis following severe traumatic brain injury in humans: A positron emission tomography study. *Journal of Neurosurgery* 86(2):241–251.

Brain Trauma Foundation. 2000. Part 1: Guidelines for the management of severe traumatic brain injury. *Journal of Neurotrauma* 17(6–7):499–553.

Bulger, E. M., A. B. Nathens, F. P. Rivara, M. Moore, E. J. MacKenzie, and G. J. Jurkovich. 2002. Management of severe head injury: Institutional variations in care and effect on outcome. *Critical Care Medicine* 30(8):1870–1876.

Cahill, N. E., R. Dhaliwal, A. G. Day, X. Jiang, and D. K. Heyland. 2010. Nutrition therapy in the critical care setting: What is "best achievable" practice? An international multicenter observational study. *Critical Care Medicine* 38(2):395–401.

Chesnut, R. M., L. F. Marshall, M. R. Klauber, B. A. Blunt, N. Baldwin, H. M. Eisenberg, J. A. Jane, A. Marmarou, and M. A. Foulkes. 1993. The role of secondary brain injury in determining outcome from severe head injury. *Journal of Trauma* 34(2):216–222.

Clifton, G. L., C. S. Robertson, and S. C. Choi. 1986. Assessment of nutritional requirements of head-injured patients. *Journal of Neurosurgery* 64(6):895–901.

Demetriades, D., E. Kuncir, J. Murray, G. C. Velmahos, P. Rhee, and L. Chan. 2004. Mortality prediction of head abbreviated injury score and Glasgow Coma Scale: Analysis of 7,764 head injuries. *Journal of the American College of Surgeons* 199(2):216–222.

Deutschman, C. S., F. N. Konstantinides, S. Raup, P. Thienprasit, and F. B. Cerra. 1986. Physiological and metabolic response to isolated closed-head injury. Part 1: Basal metabolic state: Correlations of metabolic and physiological parameters with fasting and stressed controls. *Journal of Neurosurgery* 64(1):89–98.

Eyer, S. D., L. T. Micon, F. N. Konstantinides, D. A. Edlund, K. A. Rooney, M. G. Luxenberg, and F. B. Cerra. 1993. Early enteral feeding does not attenuate metabolic response after blunt trauma. *Journal of Trauma* 34(5):639–644.

Ghajar, J. 2010. *The perspective of a neurosurgeon.* Presented at Institute of Medicine's Workshop on Nutrition and Neuroprotection in Military Personnel, Washington, DC, June 23, 2010.

Härtl, R., L. M. Gerber, L. Iacono, Q. Ni, K. Lyons, and J. Ghajar. 2006. Direct transport within an organized state trauma system reduces mortality in patients with severe traumatic brain injury. *Journal of Trauma—Injury, Infection and Critical Care* 60(6):1250–1256.

Hovda, D. A., S. M. Lee, M. L. Smith, S. Von Stuck, M. Bergsneider, D. Kelly, E. Shalmon, N. Martin, M. Caron, J. Mazziotta, M. Phelps, and D. P. Becker. 1995. The neurochemical and metabolic cascade following brain injury: Moving from animal models to man. *Journal of Neurotrauma* 12(5):903–906.

Jiang, J. Y., G. Y. Gao, W. P. Li, M. K. Yu, and C. Zhu. 2002. Early indicators of prognosis in 846 cases of severe traumatic brain injury. *Journal of Neurotrauma* 19(7):869–874.

Marik, P. E., and G. P. Zaloga. 2001. Early enteral nutrition in acutely ill patients: A systematic review. *Critical Care Medicine* 29(12):2264–2270.

Merenda, A., and R. Bullock. 2006. Clinical treatments for mitochondrial dysfunctions after brain injury. *Current Opinion in Critical Care* 12(2):90–96.

Narayan, R. K., M. E. Michel, B. Ansell, A. Baethmann, A. Biegon, M. B. Bracken, M. R. Bullock, S. C. Choi, G. L. Clifton, C. F. Contant, W. M. Coplin, W. D. Dietrich, J. Ghajar, S. M. Grady, R. G. Grossman, E. D. Hall, W. Heetderks, D. A. Hovda, J. Jallo, R. L. Katz, N. Knoller, P. M. Kochanek, A. I. Maas, J. Majde, D. W. Marion, A. Marmarou, L. F. Marshall, T. K. McIntosh, E. Miller, N. Mohberg, J. P. Muizelaar, L. H. Pitts, P. Quinn, G. Riesenfeld, C. S. Robertson, K. I. Strauss, G. Teasdale, N. Temkin, R. Tuma, C. Wade, M. D. Walker, M. Weinrich, J. Whyte, J. Wilberger, A. B. Young, and L. Yurkewicz. 2002. Clinical trials in head injury. *Journal of Neurotrauma* 19(5):503–557.

Perel, P., T. Yanagawa, F. Bunn, I. Roberts, R. Wentz, and A. Pierro. 2006. Nutritional support for head-injured patients. *Cochrane Database of Systematic Reviews* (4):CD001530..

Rapp, R. P., D. B. Young, and D. Twyman. 1983. The favorable effect of early parenteral feeding on survival in head-injured patients. *Journal of Neurosurgery* 58(6):906–912.

Roberts, I., D. Yates, P. Sandercock, B. Farrell, J. Wasserberg, G. Lomas, R. Cottingham, P. Svoboda, N. Brayley, G. Mazairac, V. Laloe, A. Munoz-Sanchez, M. Arango, B. Hartzenberg, H. Khamis, S. Yutthakasemsunt, E. Komolafe, F. Olldashi, Y. Yadav, F. Murillo-Cabezas, H. Shakur, and P. Edwards. 2004. Effect of intravenous corticosteroids on death within 14 days in 10,008 adults with clinically significant head injury (MRC Crash Trial): Randomised placebo-controlled trial. *Lancet* 364(9442):1321–1328.

Rovlias, A., and S. Kotsou. 2000. The influence of hyperglycemia on neurological outcome in patients with severe head injury. *Neurosurgery* 46(2):335–343.

Sampalis, J. S., R. Denis, A. Lavoie, P. Fréchette, S. Boukas, A. Nikolis, D. Benoit, D. Fleiszer, R. Brown, M. Churchill-Smith, and D. Mulder. 1999. Trauma care regionalization: A process-outcome evaluation. *Journal of Trauma—Injury, Infection and Critical Care* 46(4):565–581.

Smith, J. S., L. F. Martin, W. W. Young, and D. P. Macioce. 1990. Do trauma centers improve outcome over non-trauma centers: The evaluation of regional trauma care using discharge abstract data and patient management categories. *Journal of Trauma* 30(12):1533–1538.

Sosin, D. M., J. E. Sniezek, and R. J. Waxweiler. 1995. Trends in death associated with traumatic brain injury, 1979 through 1992: Success and failure. *Journal of the American Medical Association* 273(22):1778–1780.

Taylor, S. J., S. B. Fettes, C. Jewkes, and R. J. Nelson. 1999. Prospective, randomized, controlled trial to determine the effect of early enhanced enteral nutrition on clinical outcome in mechanically ventilated patients suffering head injury. *Critical Care Medicine* 27(11):2525–2531.

Thurman, D. J., C. Alverson, K. A. Dunn, J. Guerrero, and J. E. Sniezek. 1999. Traumatic brain injury in the United States: A public health perspective. *Journal of Head Trauma Rehabilitation* 14(6):602–615.

Weekes, E., and M. Elia. 1996. Observations on the patterns of 24-hour energy expenditure changes in body composition and gastric emptying in head-injured patients receiving nasogastric tube feeding. *Journal of Parenteral and Enteral Nutrition* 20(1):31–37.

Nutrition Therapy for Patients with Traumatic Brain Injury in the Military

Kelli M. Metzger[19]

NUTRITION STATUS PRIOR TO TRAUMATIC BRAIN INJURY

Nutrition status of military service members prior to injury may vary greatly depending on the location to which they are deployed. During my deployment from December 2008

[19] Nutrition Marketing and Integration Services, Walter Reed Army Medical Center.

through November 2009, I was primarily in central Iraq. The Central Operating Bases (COBs) and Forward Operating Bases (FOBs) where I lived and those I visited in central and southern Iraq contained at least one, and sometimes several, contract-operated dining facilities. Most of these dining facilities provided four meals in a 24-hour period to serve both day- and night-shift workers. Meals at the dining facilities typically included two to four protein sources, two to four starch choices, two to three hot vegetables, salad bar, sandwich bar, specialty bar, fresh fruit, and desserts. Beverages available included water, juices, coffee, tea, sodas, ultra-high temperature (UHT) milk, and soy milk. In addition to the dining facilities, most COBs and FOBs contained at least one Army/Air Force Exchange where service members could purchase snack foods and beverages; some COBs and FOBs also housed local and American chain restaurants, which provide even more dining variety to those stationed there. Of course, many service members also received food items sent from friends and family members. Although service members at these locations have opportunities to make more healthful food choices, not all do on a regular basis. Many may be calorically nourished but lack important nutrients, particularly those associated with improved cognitive function, in their diets. In addition, some service members may be assigned to or routinely travel to more remote locations where the food choices are more limited and thus have less opportunity to obtain adequate nutrients.

MEDICAL TREATMENT OF INJURED MILITARY SERVICE MEMBERS IN THEATER AND THE UNITED STATES

Medical treatment for injured U.S. service members occurs at four echelons of care. Level 1 occurs at the unit level and includes the Battalion Aid Station and Combat Medic (Borden Institute, 2008). The combat medic provides initial treatment on the battlefield with the goal of casualty evacuation in less than an hour to at least the Level II echelon of care. Treatment in the field may consist of airway stabilization, fluid resuscitation, pain management, and brain-specific therapies. Airway management is critical in the TBI patient because of the risk of loss of consciousness impacting the ability to protect one's airway (Girard, 2007). Level II care often includes a Forward Surgical Team (FST) comprised of one orthopedic surgeon, three general surgeons, two nurse anesthetists, one critical care nurse, and technicians (Nessen, 2008). Based on location, service members evacuated from Level I care may go to either the Level II or Level III echelon of care. Level III care is provided at Army Combat Support Hospitals (CSHs), Air Force theater hospitals, and Navy ships. Level III care involves triage; resuscitation; transfusion; initial, definitive, and reconstructive surgery; postoperative care; intensive care; and patient holding capacity (Borden Institute, 2008). Depending on the length of time to stabilize a patient and flying conditions, service members may be evacuated from theater the same day they are wounded or at the latest within 72 hours. Level IV echelon of care is provided at Landstuhl Regional Medical Center (LRMC) in Landstuhl, Germany. Almost 100 percent of U.S. service members evacuated from Afghanistan and Iraq pass through LRMC for general and specialized medical and surgical care (Borden Institute, 2008). The average length of stay at LRMC is less than four days. Research conducted by the RAND Corporation (Tanielian and Jaycox, 2008) found approximately 19.5 percent of the casualties admitted to military health-care facilities in the first five years of the war in Iraq suffered from TBI. Dr. Louis French, a neuropsychiatrist at Walter Reed Army Medical Center (WRAMC), estimates that approximately 35 percent of wounded warriors entering WRAMC in the past two years suffered from some type of TBI.

INITIAL NUTRITION GOALS

A dietitian's first goal is ensuring patients receive adequate nutrition to prevent malnutrition and promote healing. A study (Härtl et al., 2008) based on information collected by the Brain Trauma Foundation in 20 Level 1 and 2 Level 2 trauma centers in New York state, found TBI patients who were not fed within five days of their injury had 2.1 times the risk of two-week mortality, while those not fed within seven days suffered 4.1 times the risk. Medical staff at LRMC typically place a nasogastric (NG) tube and initiate early enteral feeding within 24–48 hours of admission. In certain cases, such as hemodynamic instability or abdominal injury, this procedure may not be followed. The dietitians at Brooke Army Medical Center (BAMC) feed TBI patients with 2 Cal HN supplemented with glutamine, vitamin C, and selenium. According to a description by Abbott Nutrition, 2 Cal HN is a nutritionally complete, high-calorie liquid food designed to meet the increased protein and calorie needs of stressed patients and patients requiring low-volume feedings. This formula provides two calories per milliliter with 43 percent of calories from carbohydrate, 40 percent from fat, and 17 percent from protein. Dietitians at National Naval Medical Center (NNMC) also use 2 Cal HN with additional protein, glutamine, multivitamin, and Vitamin C, providing patients with 30–35 calories/kg body weight and close to 2 g/kg of protein. At WRAMC, dietitians aim for a similar calorie and protein level as NNMC, but feed with Impact Glutamine, specialized medical nutrition for surgical and trauma patients by Nestle Nutrition. Impact Glutamine contains a blend of glutamine, arginine, n-3 fatty acids, and nucleic acids providing 1.3 calories per milliliter; 46 percent of the calories are from carbohydrate, 30 percent are from fat, and 24 percent are from protein.

NUTRITION CONSIDERATIONS

In selecting the best feeding method and formulation, dietitians must consider other injuries and conditions as well as medications the patient is taking. The TBI or concurrent injuries may cause damage to the gut structure, interfering with the digestion process. If the gastrointestinal tract cannot be used to achieve nutritional goals within three days, total parenteral nutrition (TPN) should be started within 24–48 hours with a goal of reaching nutritional needs by the third or fourth day (Escott-Stump, 2008). Although parenteral nutrition may be easier than obtaining adequate enteral access, enteral nutrition has fewer incidence of complication and lower cost than parenteral with no significant differences in measured nutritional parameters (Kirby et al., 2007). Enteral feedings are preferred because they stimulate blood flow to the gastric lining mucosa and provide a comprehensive mix of macro and micronutrients. A greater number of patients tolerate jejunal feedings better than gastric feeding within 72 hours after injury (Bratton et al., 2007). A jejunal feeding also can be used to reduce gastric intolerance and residuals found in gastric feeding as well as the use of intravenous catheters required in TPN (Bratton et al., 2007). Enteral feedings should begin as soon as the patient is hemodynamically stable.

DETERMINING AND MAINTAINING ADEQUATE CALORIE LEVELS

According to research by Wilson et al. published in 2001, the nutrition goals should include attempting to reach 35–45 kcal/kg and a protein intake of 2–2.5 g/kg on day 1 or as soon as possible (Escott-Stump, 2008). Adequate calories are important to prevent malnutrition and to promote healing and recovery. The brain's function as the regulator for metabolic activity leads to a complex milieu of metabolic alterations in TBI consisting of hormonal changes, aberrant cellular metabolism, and a vigorous cerebral and systemic inflammatory response in an effort to liberate substrate for injured cell metabolism. The degree of this hypermetabolic state is proportional to the severity of injury and motor dysfunction (Fruin et al., 1986). Indirect calorimetry is the gold standard for determining the calorie needs of the patient.

NUTRIENT-DRUG INTERACTIONS

Dietitians need to keep in mind, however, that medications may affect calorie needs and/or digestion by either their effect on metabolism or the way they are packaged. For example, pentobarbital, used to induce a pharmacologic coma, reduces calorie needs to as low as 76–86 percent of predicted energy needs. Protein requirements also may be less, as reflected by a 40 percent decrease in urinary nitrogen excretion (Cook et al., 2008). Propofol, a short-acting sedative, is delivered in a lipid emulsion, and 1 mL of propofol contains approximately 0.1 g of fat (1.1 kcal). Because energy contributed from propofol may provide as much as 50 to 80 percent of resting energy expenditure (REE), nutritional requirements of patients receiving propofol over an extended period should be adjusted accordingly (Rajpal and Johnston, 2009). In addition, narcotics and neuromuscular blocking agents may slow peristalsis resulting in nausea, vomiting, gastroparesis, and ileus. Metoclopramide, erythromycin, or raglan may be used to promote gastric emptying. Until normal peristalsis resumes, however, high fiber enteral formulas should be avoided.

NUTRIENTS FOR CONSIDERATION

Once an adequate calorie level is determined and a formula is selected, the dietitian may consider adding nutrients to improve outcomes. Glutamine is an immune-enhancing nutrient that has been tested and found beneficial. Glutamine is used as a source of energy for cells of the intestinal epithelium and immune system (Falcão De Arruda and De Aguilar-Nascimento, 2004). Glutamine also supplies nitrogen for purine and pyrimidine synthesis, which are essential for cells in mitosis. The use of glutamine seems to be able to decrease the occurrence of bacterial translocation and inflammatory response, reducing the possibility of events such as systemic inflammatory response syndrome and sepsis. In a study in a hospital in Brazil (Falcão De Arruda and De Aguilar-Nascimento, 2004), enhancing enteral nutrition with glutamine and probiotics significantly reduced the incidence of infection in head trauma patients. Another potential benefit of early enteral nutrition enriched with probiotics and glutamine reduction is the period of time in the intensive care unit and the number of days requiring mechanical ventilation (Falcão De Arruda and De Aguilar-Nascimento, 2004).

Zinc is another nutrient of interest for the TBI patient. Zinc is an important co-factor for substrate metabolism, immune function, and N-methyl-D-aspartate (NMDA) receptor function (Cook et al., 2008). Because of zinc losses through the gastrointestinal tract and its role in wound healing, it may be prudent to supplement zinc in acutely injured patients (Winker and Malone, 2010). Supplementation of zinc appears to improve protein metabolism and neurologic outcome at one month after TBI (Young et al., 1996). Magnesium may also be neuroprotective because of activity at the NMDA receptor and modulation of cellular energy production and calcium influx, but supplementation of magnesium in humans has yet to yield definitive benefits (McKee et al., 2005).

Choline also may be an important nutrient for patients with TBI. Choline, a B-complex vitamin found in eggs, meat, fish, nuts, legumes, and soy, is a component of the neurotransmitter acetylcholine (Hecht, 2007). Doses of choline as high as 2,500 mg twice per day may improve memory in adults. Every cell membrane requires phosphatidylcholine; nerve and brain cells especially need large quantities for repair and maintenance (Hecht, 2007). Additional studies have found doses of choline at 100 mg and 400 mg/kg significantly reduce brain edema and breakdown of the blood-brain barrier following TBI (Hecht, 2007).

Arginine is a conditionally essential amino acid. Under usual conditions, arginine is synthesized endogenously; in stressful periods, however, endogenous synthesis is insufficient (Kirby et al., 2007). Arginine is used for protein synthesis; as part of the urea cycle; as a precursor to glutamate, proline, and polyamines; and as a substrate for creatine and nitric oxide production (Sy et al., 2006). When pharmacologic doses are given, arginine stimulates the pituitary growth hormone, insulin-like growth factor, prolactin, insulin, and other hormones, resulting in a net positive effect on wound healing and immune functions (Alexander, 1993). Arginine also is a precursor for nitrates, nitrites, and nitric oxide. Nitric oxide is important as a vasodilator, but also participates in immunologic reactions which include the ability of macrophages to kill tumor cells and bacteria. Studies have demonstrated T-cell function suppressed following major surgery or trauma. Daly and colleagues found that patients receiving 30 g/day of arginine demonstrated a quicker return to normal T-cell level compared to post-surgical patients receiving placebo (Daly et al., 1988).

NUTRITION CONCERNS IN OUTPATIENT REHABILITATION

Although initial nutrition concerns include adequate calories and supplementation of nutrients, nutrition concerns continue into rehabilitation. Patients with mild TBI may experience memory problems and difficulty concentrating, which affect their ability to perform daily activities and return to work (Miele and Bailes, 2009). Patients who sustained a moderate TBI have highly variable outcomes. Moderate brain injury survivors may suffer from cognitive or behavioral impairments that disrupt relationships, employment, or psychological well-being (Timmons and Winestone, 2009). Ninety percent of TBI patients who had good outcomes experienced memory difficulties, and 87 percent had problems performing activities of daily living (Timmons and Winestone, 2009). Despite intensive intervention, long-term disability occurs in a large portion of the survivors of severe head injury (Remig, 2010). A significant percentage of TBI patients admitted to long-term rehabilitation centers or sent home with skilled nursing support are markedly disabled and physically dependent on others for care. Many of these patients have cognitive and motor dysfunction; less than 33 percent are able to eat independently, and about 37 percent require either enteral or parenteral nutrition support (Cook et al., 2008).

Although some TBI patients require assistance with eating, most TBI patients regain their independence in oral feeding within six months after injury (Cook et al., 2008). Those with dental or facial fractures or a need for prolonged cervical immobilization with a hard cervical collar may experience a delay in initiation of an oral diet. Dysphagia can affect 25 to 60 percent of TBI patients and as many as 42 percent suffer from frank aspiration (McNamee et al., 2009). Speech pathologists can assess a patient's endoscopic instrumental swallowing evaluations. Based on these results, patients may require modified food and liquid consistencies for their safety (Cook et al., 2008). The overall goal is to find the least restrictive diet that promotes safe swallowing and maintains nutritional status (Kirby et al., 2007). In addition to swallowing evaluation, patients should be assessed for readiness to feed. Barriers to self-feeding include cognitive and motor planning behaviors, including impulsivity, distractibility, inability to stay on task, poor sequencing skills, lack of initiation, and inability to motor plan self-feeding (Kirby et al., 2007). Patients with other injuries also may experience difficulty eating. If limb weakness, paralysis, or amputation occur on the dominant side of the body, poor coordination resulting from a new reliance on the non-dominant side may make eating difficult and unpleasant. Small frequent feedings can help if fatigue or early satiety is a problem (Remig, 2010).

The role of the dietitian is important in the care of patients with TBI. Dietitians are needed to ensure the patient receives adequate nutrition immediately following the injury to prevent malnutrition and promote recovery. They also have a role to play as patients transition to rehabilitation centers and outpatient status. Dietitians can work with other team members to ensure the patient understands the foods they can best tolerate and help patients determine an appropriate calorie and nutrient level as they recover.

REFERENCES

Alexander, J. W. 1993. Immunoenhancement via enteral nutrition. *Archives of Surgery* 128(11):1242–1245.

Borden Institute. 2008. Trauma system development and medical evacuation in the combat theater. In *War surgery in Afghanistan and Iraq: A series of cases, 2003–2007*, edited by S. C. Nessen, D. E. Lounsbury and S. P. Hetz. Washington, DC: Office of the Surgeon General, U.S. Army.

Bratton, S., D. Chestnut, J. Ghajar, F. Hammond, O. Harris, R. Hartl, J. Schouten, L. Shutter, S. Timmons, J. Ullman, W. Videtta, J. Wilberger, and D. Wright. 2007. Nutrition. *Journal of Neurotrauma* 24(Suppl. 1):S77–S82.

Cook, A. M., A. Peppard, and B. Magnuson. 2008. Nutrition considerations in traumatic brain injury. *Nutrition in Clinical Practice* 23(6):608–620.

Daly, J. M., J. Reynolds, A. Thom, L. Kinsley, M. Dietrick-Gallagher, J. Shou, and B. Ruggieri. 1988. Immune and metabolic effects of arginine in the surgical patient. *Annals of Surgery* 208(4):512–523.

Escott-Stump, S. 2008. *Nutrition and diagnosis-related care*. 6th ed. Baltimore, MD: Wolters Kluwer Health/Lippincott Williams & Wilkins.

Falcão De Arruda, I. S., and J. E. De Aguilar-Nascimento. 2004. Benefits of early enteral nutrition with glutamine and probiotics in brain injury patients. *Clinical Science* 106(3):287–292.

Fruin, A. H., C. Taylon, and M. S. Pettis. 1986. Caloric requirements in patients with severe head injuries. *Surgical Neurology* 25(1):25–28.

Girard, P. 2007. Military and VA telemedicine systems for patients with traumatic brain injury. *Journal of Rehabilitation Research and Development* 44(7):1017–1026.

Härtl, R., L. M. Gerber, Q. Ni, and J. Ghajar. 2008. Effect of early nutrition on deaths due to severe traumatic brain injury. *Journal of Neurosurgery* 109(1):50–56.

Hecht, J. 2007. Nutraceuticals. In *Brain injury medicine: Principles and practice*, edited by N. Zasler, D. Katz, and R. Zafonte. New York: Demos Medical Publishing. Pp. 1037–1047.

Kirby, D., L. Creasy, and S. Abou-Assi. 2007. Gastrointestinal and nutritional issues. In *Brain injury medicine: Principles and practice*, edited by N. Zasler, D. Katz and R. Zafonte. New York, NY: Demos Medical Publishing. Pp. 657–671.

McKee, J. A., R. P. Brewer, G. E. Macy, B. Phillips-Bute, K. A. Campbell, C. O. Borel, J. D. Reynolds, and D. S. Warner. 2005. Analysis of the brain bioavailability of peripherally administered magnesium sulfate: A study in humans with acute brain injury undergoing prolonged induced hypermagnesemia. *Critical Care Medicine* 33(3):661–666.

McNamee, S., T. Pickett, S. Benedict, and D. Cifu. 2009. Rehabilitation. In *Neurotrauma and critical care of the brain*, edited by J. Jallo and C. Loftus. New York: Thieme. Pp. 385–403.

Miele, V., and J. Bailes. 2009. Mild brain injury. In *Neurotrauma and critical care of the brain*, edited by J. Jallo and C. Loftus. New York: Thieme. Pp. 175–207.

Nessen, S. C., D. R. Cronk, J. Edens, B. J. Eastridge, T. R. Little, J. Windsor, L. H. Blackbourne, and J. B. Holcomb. 2008. U.S. Army two-surgeon teams operating in remote Afghanistan—An evaluation of split-based forward surgical team operations. *The Journal of Trauma* 66(4 Suppl.):S37-47.

Rajpal, V., and J. Johnston. 2009. Nutrition management of traumatic brain injury patients. *Support Line* 31(1):10–19.

Remig, V. 2010. Medical nutrition therapy for neurologic disorders. In *Krause's food and nutrition therapy*. 12th ed., edited by L. Mahan and S. Escott-Stump. St. Louis, MO: Saunders, Elsevier. Pp. 1067–1101.

Sy, B., E. Dweik, and R. Sweik. 2006. Arginine and nitric oxide. In *Modern nutrition in health and disease*. 10th ed., edited by M. Shils, M. Shike, A. Ross, B. Coballero, and R. Cousins. Baltimore, MD: Lippincott, Williams, and Wilkins. Pp. 571–581.

Tanielian, T., and L. Jaycox. 2008. *Invisible wounds of war: Psychological and cognitive injuries, their consequences, and services to assist recovery.* Santa Monica, CA: RAND Corporation.

Timmons, S., and J. Winestone. 2009. Moderate brain injury. In *Neurotrauma and critical care of the brain,* edited by J. Jallo and C. Loftus. New York: Thieme. Pp. 208–219.

Winker, M., and A. Malone. 2010. Medical nutrition therapy for metabolic stress: Sepsis, trauma, burns, and surgery. In *Krause's food and nutrition therapy.* 12th ed., edited by L. Mahan and S. Escott-Stump. St. Louis, MO: Saunders, Elsevier. Pp. 1021–1041.

Young, B., L. Ott, E. Kasarskis, R. Rapp, K. Moles, R. J. Dempsey, P. A. Tibbs, R. Kryscio, and C. McClain. 1996. Zinc supplementation is associated with improved neurologic recovery rate and visceral protein levels of patients with severe closed head injury. *Journal of Neurotrauma* 13(1):25–34.

The Therapeutic Potential of Diet and Exercise to Counteract Brain Dysfunction Following Traumatic Brain Injury

Fernando Gomez-Pinilla[20]

INTRODUCTION

Traumatic brain injury (TBI) induces a state of vulnerability within neurons that survive the initial insult, and this may result in long-term deficits in higher order cognitive and intellectual functions. Advances in understanding how nutritional factors affect brain function and repair have put forward the interesting possibility that dietary therapy is a realistic strategy to reduce the type of weaknesses encountered in TBI pathology. In particular, recent studies show that the efficacy of nutritional factors after TBI is displayed at the level of processes involved in re-establishing energy homeostasis and providing structural substrates that can foster neuronal signaling. An increasing number of studies indicate that certain types of dietary factors, such as n-3 fatty acids, can positively influence molecular systems that serve synaptic function, while diets rich in saturated fats or high in calories do the opposite.

Dietary interventions have the advantage of being non-invasive, highly efficacious, and borne with a broad spectrum of action. These features provide the confidence that findings in animal models of TBI can be easily translated to human applications directed to reduce TBI pathology. This capacity contrasts with the large amount of unsuccessful clinical trials to assess the therapeutic action of many pharmacological compounds in TBI patients. This implies that the type of broad protection elicited by dietary factors can be particularly suitable to treat brain disorders characterized by multiple components (Figure C-8). For example, it is likely that the diffuse nature of TBI, can compromise fundamental and broad aspects of neuronal signaling events that are required for mental operation. Although cognitive and psychiatric disorders are a common feature in TBI patients, such as posttraumatic stress disorders, their cellular/molecular basis and treatment are poorly understood. The fact that select dietary factors support a large range of molecular mechanisms important for cognitive function and neural repair, strongly suggests that dietary therapy is a suitable strategy to promote mental health and brain plasticity after TBI.

THE METABOLIC DEPRESSION AFTER TBI

Brain metabolic depression is a common stage in the sequence of events occurring after TBI as observed in humans (Vagnozzi et al., 2008) and in animal models (Dietrich et al.,

---

[20]Departments of Neurosurgery and Integrative Biology and Physiology, University of California, Los Angeles.

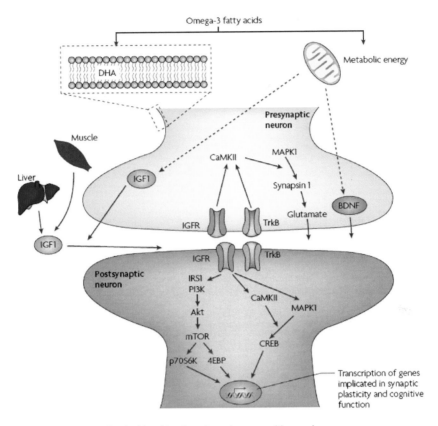

Desirable objectives to reduce cognitive and
emotional distress after TBI:
• To reduce energy crisis and promote
  membrane repair
• To elevate the potential for synaptic plasticity
• To support neuronal signaling
• To stimulate mechanisms that can provide broad
  protection
Dietary management may help accomplish
these goals.

FIGURE C-8 Synaptic transmission where most signaling events take place requires proper energy and a functional plasma membrane (disrupted by TBI).
SOURCE: Gomez-Pinilla, 2008.

1994; Hovda et al., 1991; Moore et al., 2000). The period of energy depression seems to impose a toll on the ability of the brain to maintain normal function and support repair events. It has been known that during this period, the brain is more vulnerable to a second injury. For example, it has recently been reported in the results of a pilot study performed in a cohort of athletes exposed to a single and a double concussion (Vagnozzi et al., 2008). Brain imaging based on 1H-MR spectroscopy was performed to assess the neuronal metabolic marker N-acetylaspartate (NAA) in the cerebral cortex of athletes, at different time points after concussion. Results showed that the concussion opens a temporal window of brain metabolic imbalance, the ending of which does not necessarily coincide with the improvement of clinical symptoms. Remarkably, a second concussive event occurring within the period of brain vulnerability prolonged the time required for NAA normalization by 15 days.

Experiments performed in animal models of concussion have shown similar results to those observed in humans and have revealed some of the mechanisms involved in the period of brain vulnerability. Following experimental concussion or lateral fluid percussion injury in the rat, the brain exhibits a decrease in glucose utilization lasting for up to 10 days after the injury (Ginsberg et al., 1997; Yoshino et al., 1991). During this postinjury period of metabolic depression, cells are unable to respond to physiological levels of stimulation, resulting in subsequent neurobehavioral deficits (Colle et al., 1986; Hovda et al., 1987). The energy depression seems to impose a toll on the molecular machinery that supports activity-dependent plasticity. This means that the reduced capacity for synaptic plasticity can have critical implications for the ability of the brain to start a recovery phase. Therefore, it is critical to develop strategies directed to normalize the period of metabolic depression following TBI and counteract the events that arrest proper neuronal function.

THE FUNCTION OF BRAIN-DERIVED NEUROTROPHIC FACTOR SEEMS CRUCIAL TO UNDERSTAND THE EFFECTS OF FOOD ON THE BRAIN

Brain-derived neurotrophic factor (BDNF) is an important regulator of neuronal growth and survival at different developmental stages, and it can function to enhance synaptic plasticity underlying cognitive function. As discussed in subsequent sections, experimental TBI has been shown to reduce BDNF-mediated synaptic plasticity while the action of several dietary factors on the brain has been associated with restoring the function of BDNF. Clinical studies support the importance of proper BDNF function for maintaining learning and memory capacities in humans (Egan et al., 2003; Hariri et al., 2003), i.e., individuals expressing a specific polymorphism in the BDNF gene exhibit learning impairments (Egan et al., 2003). A new line of investigations shows that the action of BDNF on synaptic plasticity is intimately related to the regulation of energy metabolism. The results of these investigations have opened new avenues to understand the mechanism of action of dietary factors on the brain. For example, it is now known that BDNF influences synaptic plasticity by acting on molecular systems important for the regulation of energy homeostasis in the hippocampus (Gomez-Pinilla et al., 2008; Vaynman et al., 2006). These actions of BDNF seem to have profound consequences for the neural control of body metabolism as animals with genetic deletion of the BDNF gene are hyperphagic and develop obesity (Lyons et al., 1999), while infusion of BDNF has been found to reduce body weight, normalize glucose levels, ameliorate lipid metabolism in diabetic rodents, and increase insulin sensitivity (Tsuchida et al., 2002). It is also notable that BDNF protein is most abundant in brain areas foremost associated with cognitive and neuroendocrine regulation, such as the hippocampus and hypothalamus.

NUTRITIONAL FACTORS WITH THE POTENTIAL TO REDUCE TBI PATHOLOGY

The potential of nutrient and/or dietary interventions to reduce TBI pathology has been demonstrated to affect at least four primary objectives to moderate cognitive and emotional distress following TBI:

- to reduce energy crisis and promote membrane repair,
- to elevate the potential for synaptic plasticity,

TABLE C-6 Main Nutrients Examined in Animal Models of TBI

Nutrient	Type of Model
Omega-3 fatty acids (DHA)	Concussion model of TBI (Mills, 2010; Wu et al., 2006, 2007)
	Models of spinal cord injury (Huang, 2007)
Curcumin (turmeric)	Concussion models of TBI (Sharma, 2010; Wu et al., 2006)
Flavonoids	Reduction of stroke in humans (Keli, 1996)
	Plaque formation in Alzehimer's Disease animal models (Joseph, 2003)
Vitamin E	Models of concussion (Wu et al., 2006, 2010)
Ketogenic diet	Models of head injury (Hu, 2009; Prins, 2005)
Dietary restriction or fasting	Models of head injury (Davis, 2008)
Caffeine	Models of head injury (Li et al., 2008)

SOURCE: Gomez-Pinilla and Ying, 2010 (workshop presentation).

- to support neuronal signaling, and
- to stimulate mechanisms that can provide broad protection.

Several dietary components that can provide some modification to these processes have been identified in the following sections (Table C-6). Some of the effective dosage for the use of select nutrients in the brain have been identified in animal models of neurological disorders. Although dosage is an important issue, it is less of a factor for the use of nutrients based on their safety profile.

n-3 Fatty Acids

The study of n-3 fatty acids have provided some of the strongest evidence for the profound effects that dietary factors can have on the brain. The n-3 is a large family of fatty acids in which the docosahexaenoic acid (DHA) is one of the most relevant forms for brain function. It is important to consider, however, that DHA may act together with other n-3 fatty acids such as eicosapentaenoic acid (EPA), which also has demonstrated neuroprotective abilities. DHA acid is a key component of neuronal membranes at sites of signal transduction at the synapse, such that its action is vital for the maintenance of neuronal structure and function (Gomez-Pinilla, 2008). Because of the inefficiency of mammals to produce DHA from precursors, supplementation of DHA in the diet is important for insuring proper function of neurons during homeostatic conditions and after injury. Evidence suggests that DHA serves to improve neuronal function by supporting synaptic membrane fluidity (Suzuki et al., 1998) and regulating gene expression and cell signaling (Salem et al., 2001). This implies that insufficient DHA can result in neuronal dysfunction affecting a broad array of functional modalities.

The literature shows positive results for the effects of DHA in the injured central nervous system. It has been found that dietary DHA when provided for a few weeks before the onset of the injury can promote resistance against the effects of brain trauma (Wu et al., 2004a, 2007). In particular, animals exposed to experimental brain trauma that had been supplemented with DHA showed nearby normal performance in the Morris water maze and nearby normal levels of BDNF-related synaptic markers in the hippocampus. DHA also has shown to overcome the effects of the injury when supplemented in the diet of animals after the injury onset, acting on the brain (Wu et al., 2004a, 2007) and spinal cord (Huang et al., 2007; Mills et al., 2010). These studies have shown that DHA can influence the injured brain by maintaining normal levels of BDNF-associated synaptic plasticity and reducing injury-related oxidative stress (Wu et al., 2007, 2008), and these DHA effects were accompanied by nearby normal cognitive abilities. As discussed in a later section, the concurrent application of exercise to animals fed on DHA dietary supplementation has been shown to have additional beneficial effects on synaptic plasticity and cognition (Wu et al., 2008).

Dietary Polyphenols

Polyphenols are found in plants and are characterized by the presence of one or more phenol groups. Curcuminoids and flavonoids are the main polyphenol subtypes with recognized actions on the brain. An inverse correlation between dietary flavonoids consumption and the incidence of stroke was found in a cohort of 552 men aged 50–69 years who were followed for 15 years (Keli et al., 1996). It has been shown that dietary supplementation of blueberry extracts for eight weeks can reverse cognitive deficits in spatial learning ability in aged rats (Andres-Lacueva et al., 2005). Blueberry extracts in the diet also have shown to reduce plaques in an Alzheimer's disease (AD) animal model (Joseph et al., 2003), apparently acting on signaling pathways important for memory formation. Although polyphenols are known for their powerful antioxidant capacity, their antioxidant effects on the brain seem to follow multiple mechanisms related to the chemistry of each flavonoid. The flavanol epicatechin found in cocoa has been shown to cross the blood-brain barrier (BBB) after ingestion in food or drink, and its consumption improved retention of spatial memory and angiogenesis in the water maze (van Praag, 2009). The property to penetrate the BBB seems to extend to other polyphenols as the flavonoid epigallocatechin gallate (Suganuma et al., 1998), and the citrus flavonoids naringenin and hesperitin (Youdim et al., 2003) have been reported to enter the brain after a gastric administration.

Curcumin

Curcumin is a major chemical component of the turmeric plant (*Curcuma longa*) and has been widely used as a spice and food preservative in India. Curcumin has shown excellent efficacy in counteracting neuronal dysfunction in several models of neurodegenerative diseases such as AD and focal cerebral ischemia (see Gomez-Pinilla, 2008 for review). Recent findings show that curcumin stimulates proliferation of embryonic progenitor cells and neurogenesis in the adult hippocampus (Kim et al., 2008). Curcumin also has been shown to protect the hippocampus and to counteract learning impairment resulting from experimental TBI, in a process involving the action of the BDNF system (Wu et al., 2006). There is substantial evidence from in vitro studies indicating that curcumin has strong antioxidant capacity exerted by increasing free radical scavengers and reducing lipid peroxidation (Wei et al., 2006). As discussed earlier, a disruption in energy metabolism is a major sequela in the acute pathology of TBI, thereby compromising synaptic function and the capacity of the brain to respond to challenges. Interestingly, recent studies have shown the potential of curcumin to restore molecular events important for energy homeostasis following TBI (Figure C-9). Study results (Sharma et al., 2010) showed that four weeks of curcumin dietary supplementation before a fluid percussion injury counteracted a decrease in the levels of AMP-activated protein kinase (AMPK), ubiquitous mitochondrial creatine kinase (uMtCK), and cytochrome c oxidase II (COX-II). These molecular systems play a crucial role in main-

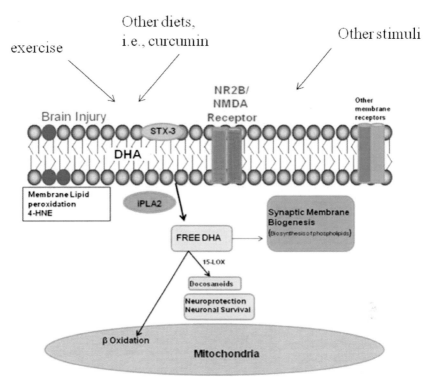

FIGURE C-9 Possible events by which TBI can affect brain function by disrupting plasma membrane homeostasis. TBI increases free radical formation in the mitochondria, thereby promoting oxidation of membrane lipids, as detected by the lipid peroxidation marker 4-HNE. These events may lead to membrane dysfunction as evidenced by reduced levels of iPLA2 with subsequent effects on membrane DHA. These events may lower membrane function as evidenced by reduced levels of STX-3 and GAP-43. The loss of membrane flexibility may compromise function of membrane embedded receptors such as the subunit NR2B of the NMDA receptor. These alterations can result in abnormal neuronal signaling, which can reduce cognitive capacity. Interventions such as exercise and curcumin with demonstrated antioxidant abilities may be able to restore membrane homeostasis and brain function after TBI. SOURCE: Modified from Sharma et al., 2010.

taining energy homeostasis; therefore, results seem to portray the capacity of curcumin to attenuate the period of metabolic dysfunction and to foster functional recovery.

Cerebral edema is a major sequela in the TBI pathology that largely contributes to reducing neuronal function and neural repair events. It has been known for a few years already that aquaporins water membrane channels play a role in edema formation after TBI (Neal et al., 2007). In agreement with its strong anti-inflammatory capacity (Menon and Sudheer, 2007), it has recently been shown that a single injection of curcumin 15 minutes prior to or 30 minutes after a cortical impact injury can reduce brain water contents and improve neurological outcome. These effects of curcumin seem associated with the blocking of aquaporin-4 expression (Laird et al., 2010). In addition, the protective effect of curcumin was associated with a significant attenuation in the acute pericontusional expression of interleukin-1b, a pro-inflammatory cytokine.

Green Tea

Green tea is rich in flavonoids (Graham, 1992) out of which the catechins epigallocatechin-gallate (EGCG), epigallocatechin (EGC), epicatechin (EC), and epicatechin-3-gallate (ECG) are the most abundant. The intake of the compound catechin has been associated with a variety of positive effects in rodents inflicted with ischemia-induced degeneration, including antioxidative, anti-inflammatory, and anti-apoptotic (Sutherland et al., 2006). In particular, a four-year follow-up study that included 5,910 individuals showed that the incidence of stroke was two-fold higher in those individuals who consumed less than 5 cups per day (Sato et al., 1989). Green tea consumption also has been related to the prevention of various structural and biochemical and behavioral characteristics of aging. For example, long-term exposure of rodents to green tea has been shown to reverse some of the degenerative effects of aging in the hippocampus (Assuncao et al., 2009; Li et al., 2009) and has shown to prevent memory regression and DNA oxidative damage in aged mice.

Resveratrol

Resveratrol is a non-flavonoid polyphenolic found in grapes, red wine, and berries. There are two isomeric forms of resveratrol, and the *trans*resveratrol (*trans*-3,4,5-trihydroxystilbene) is the biologically inactive form. A number of studies have demonstrated the antioxidant, anti-inflammatory, antimutagenic, and anticarcinogenic effects of resveratrol (de la Lastra and Villegas, 2005; Jang et al., 1997; Soleas et al., 1997). Interestingly, several epidemiological studies indicate an inverse correlation of wine consumption and the incidence of AD (Lindsay et al., 2002; Orgogozo et al., 1997; Truelsen et al., 2002). It is well-known that reducing food intake or caloric restriction extends lifespan in a wide range of species. Recently, it has been found that resveratrol can mimic certain aspects of calorie restriction such as increasing production of sirtuin proteins (Baur et al., 2006). The sirtuin is a phylogenetically conserved family of enzymes that catalyze NAD-dependent protein deacetylation, and is essential for lifespan extension elicited by caloric restriction and other stressors (Anderson et al., 2003). Interestingly, resveratrol's neuroprotective aptitude appears to be the result of its effective capability to promote caloric homeostasis acting on the mitochondria resulting in low oxidative stress and more efficient neuronal function.

Ketogenic Diet

The ketogenic diet, which is high in fat (mainly medium-chain triglycerides), moderate in protein, and low in carbohydrates, has been used for the treatment of seizure disorders for more than 50 years and has lately been regarded as protective for other types of neurological disorders. The ketogenic diet has been shown to reduce the extent of neuronal degeneration in developmental animals affected by TBI (Hu et al., 2009; Prins et al., 2005). It has recently been shown in vitro (Samoilova et al., 2010) that treatment with the ketone body D-β-hydroxybutyrate counteracts the consequences of chronic hypoglycemia, oxygen-glucose deprivation, and excitotoxicity, and that these effects are independent of seizure control. The hypothesis behind these results is that ketosis may serve as an alternative energy source during the TBI metabolic depression phase, or may help reduce metabolic stress. These ideas seem indirectly supported by the results of studies showing that reduction of calories by fasting, which is neuroprotective in animal models of TBI, elicits a stage of brain ketosis (Davis et al., 2008).

As discussed earlier, restoration of energy balance is a major goal for overcoming the pathobiology of TBI. In these terms, dietary agents that promote metabolic homeostasis or the calorie content of the diet can play crucial roles in restoring neuronal plasticity and brain function. Accordingly, strategies such as reducing the caloric content of the diet or the frequency of feeding seem to play a protective role on the brain. For example, fasting every other day has been shown to protect neurons in the hippocampus against excitotoxicity-induced death in rodent studies (Bruce-Keller et al., 1999). It can be noted that restriction of calories can increase levels of BDNF, which may contribute to support neuronal function. The effects of caloric restriction are also extended to the spinal cord. For example, it has been shown that reducing the frequency of food consumption can improve functional recovery after a partial injury to the spinal cord (Graham, 1992; Plunet et al., 2008).

Vitamin E

Vitamin E, which is naturally found in certain oils, nuts, and spinach, has shown promise in protecting the brain against the effects of TBI (Wu et al., 2010) by reducing free radical contents in the brain, which would otherwise impede optimal function of neurons. Vitamin E also has shown positive effects on reducing memory decay in aging individuals (Perkins et al., 1999). A different study in aging mice revealed the benefits of vitamin E by showing a correlation between the amount of ingested vitamin E and improved neurological performance, survival, and brain mitochondrial function (Navarro et al., 2005).

What Diets to Avoid

Although certain foods seem to contribute positively to enhance neuronal health, diets that are rich in saturated fats and sugar can do the opposite. Molteni and colleagues have shown that rats fed a diet high in saturated fats and refined sugars (similar in content to "junk food") for a period of one to two months, performed significantly worse on the spatial learning Water maze test (Molteni et al., 2002). The increased levels of oxidative stress induced by this diet result in decreased levels of hippocampal BDNF, thereby reducing cognitive abilities; however, all of these effects were counteracted by antioxidant treatment with vitamin E (Wu et al., 2004b). Even more alarming is the fact that consumption of this high-fat diet for a period of three weeks made the effects of experimental TBI worse, in terms of reducing levels of BDNF-related synaptic plasticity and protracted learning and memory ability (Wu et al., 2003). Interestingly, the application of voluntary exercise concurrent to the consumption of the diet reduced its deleterious effects on cognition and synaptic plasticity (Molteni et al., 2004).

DIET AND EXERCISE COLLABORATE TO PRESERVE MEMBRANE STRUCTURE, BRAIN METABOLISM, AND SYNAPTIC PLASTICITY

Much like a healthful diet, physical activity is thought to benefit neuronal function. According to recent studies, the combination of diet and exercise can deliver more beneficial effects than either intervention alone. Studies show that exercise applied after experimental traumatic brain injury have beneficial effects, but these effects seem to depend on the length of the postinjury resting period and the severity of the injury (Griesbach et al., 2007). Because of the potential of certain diets to restore energy homeostasis, dietary management can be regarded as an intervention that can increase the efficacy of exercise after TBI.

The complementary influence of diet and exercise on the brain can be exerted at various levels of interactions, which circumvent around mechanisms implicated with the control of energy homeostasis and synaptic plasticity (Gomez-Pinilla et al., 2008). Probably the best demonstrated interaction between exercise and diet involves the consumption of the n-3 polyunsaturated fatty acid DHA. Dietary supplementation with DHA and exercise influences hippocampal plasticity and cognitive function activating similar molecular systems, and the DHA effects are enhanced by the concurrent application of exercise (Chytrova et al., 2010; Wu et al., 2008). According to these studies, exercise seems to act on mechanisms that preserve DHA on the plasma membrane with important implications for neuronal signaling. In addition, the concurrent effects of the DHA diet and exercise involve BDNF-mediated synaptic plasticity such as the Akt signaling system (Wu et al., 2008). The results of these studies are significant and suggest the inherent capacity of the brain to benefit from the effects of DHA dietary supplementation and exercise. More in-depth studies (Gomez-Pinilla and Ying, 2010) have shown that the DHA diet and exercise exerted differential effects on molecular systems controlling important aspects of brain homeostasis, associated with food intake (obesity receptor for leptin, growth hormone receptor), energy metabolism (AMPK, SIRT1), and stress (glucocorticoid receptor, 11β-Hydroxysteroid dehydrogenase type 1), and all of them with the capacity to influence cognition. In agreement with the involvement of the hypothalamus and the hippocampus on energy homeostasis and behavior, these two regions showed distinct susceptibilities to the actions of diet and exercise. On another front, the combination of a flavonoid-enriched diet and exercise has been shown to increase the expression of genes that have a positive effect on neuronal plasticity while decreasing genes involved with deleterious processes, such as inflammation and cell death (van Praag, 2009). Exercise also has proven to be effective in reducing the deleterious effects of unhealthful diets, i.e., a diet high in saturated fat and sucrose. The concurrent exposure to exercise compensated for the effects of this diet on reducing the levels of BDNF-related synaptic plasticity and cognitive function (Molteni et al., 2004).

Control of cell energy metabolism seems to be a common denominator for the effects of foods and exercise on the brain, as several of the processes outlined above subside on the management of cellular energy. Now we know that there is a direct association between pathways associated with metabolism and synaptic plasticity, and this association can determine important aspects of behavioral plasticity such as learning and memory (Vaynman et al., 2006). Proteomic studies have revealed that voluntary exercise affects the expression pattern and post-translational modification of protein classes in the hippocampus associated with energy metabolism and synaptic plasticity (Ding et al., 2006). In particular, exercise modulates molecular systems in the brain associated with energy balance and energy transduction, which have the capacity to affect learning and memory, i.e., AMPK, ghrelin, ubiquitous mitochondrial creatine kinase (uMtCK), uncoupling protein 2 (UCP2), and insulin-like growth factor-I (IGF-I) (Gomez-Pinilla et al., 2008). The overall evidence supports the idea that select diets and exercise can influence synaptic plasticity, neuronal signaling, and cognitive function by acting on critical mediators of energy metabolism. The results of these investigations have direct implications for the therapeutic use of diet and exercise for the treatment of TBI as the pathobiology of TBI involves a period of metabolic dysfunction. Therefore, an important aspect of dietary therapy is to restore energy homeostasis, thereby increasing the capacity of the brain for plasticity.

CONCLUSIONS

The diffuse nature of TBI can compromise fundamental and broad aspects of neuronal signaling that are required for mental operation. In turn, the broad mode of action of dietary factors makes of them a unique tool that can be implemented to counteract various aspects

BOX C-1
Implications of Research on Neuroprotective Properties of Various Nutrients

- Brain trauma reduces function of neurons, many of them distant to the lesion in the brain and spinal cord; probably reducing neuronal signaling and information processing
- Select food derivatives have the capacity to restore neuronal homeostasis and to promote a suitable environment for neural repair
- Some other diets such as those rich in saturated fats and sugar can have detrimental effects on neuronal function and plasticity
- Collaborative effects of foods and exercise
- Diet and exercise can promote stable changes in the genome that can modulate the capacity of the brain to fight risks
- Therapeutic potential: strong safety profile, non-invasive, efficacy

involved in the TBI pathobiology (Box C-1). Specific diets and exercise routines have been shown in animal studies to influence select molecular systems that can make the brain more resistant to damage, facilitate synaptic transmission, and improve cognitive abilities. New evidence shows that dietary supplementations of DHA and curcumin have important actions on the mechanisms that maintain membrane physiology and neuronal signaling, and have a great potential to circumvent TBI pathobiology. Emerging studies indicate that exercise is capable of boosting the healthful effects of certain diets such as n-3 fatty acids. It also has been observed that exercise can counteract some of the deleterious effects of a saturated-fat diet on synaptic plasticity and cognitive function of rats. Therapy based on DHA, curcumin, and exercise can benefit TBI and have long-term consequences on molecular systems responsible for maintaining synaptic function, underlying higher order operations such as learning and memory, and emotions. The overall evidence indicates that the broad neuroprotection provided by diet and exercise could be implemented to counteract the diffuse nature of TBI and other neurological disorders. Although there is still much to be understood in the scientific front, there is sufficient information that can be applied to solve practical problems in the military and the community. A practical and feasible strategy in the short-term would be to use current information to implement dietary policies in the military or other institutions, and the community as a whole.

ACKNOWLEDGMENTS

This work was supported by National Institutes of Health awards NS50465, NS56413, and NS068473.

REFERENCES

Anderson, R. M., M. Latorre-Esteves, A. R. Neves, S. Lavu, O. Medvedik, C. Taylor, K. T. Howitz, H. Santos, and D. A. Sinclair. 2003. Yeast life-span extension by calorie restriction is independent of NAD fluctuation. *Science* 302(5653):2124–2126.

Andres-Lacueva, C., B. Shukitt-Hale, R. L. Galli, O. Jauregui, R. M. Lamuela-Raventos, and J. A. Joseph. 2005. Anthocyanins in aged blueberry-fed rats are found centrally and may enhance memory. *Nutritional Neuroscience* 8(2):111–120.

Assuncao, M., M. J. Santos-Marques, F. Carvalho, N. V. Lukoyanov, and J. P. Andrade. 2009. Chronic green tea consumption prevents age-related changes in rat hippocampal formation. *Neurobiology of Aging* 32(4):707–717.

Baur, J. A., K. J. Pearson, N. L. Price, H. A. Jamieson, C. Lerin, A. Kalra, V. V. Prabhu, J. S. Allard, G. Lopez-Lluch, K. Lewis, P. J. Pistell, S. Poosala, K. G. Becker, O. Boss, D. Gwinn, M. Wang, S. Ramaswamy, K. W. Fishbein, R. G. Spencer, E. G. Lakatta, D. Le Couteur, R. J. Shaw, P. Navas, P. Puigserver, D. K. Ingram, R. De Cabo, and D. A. Sinclair. 2006. Resveratrol improves health and survival of mice on a high-calorie diet. *Nature* 444(7117):337–342.

Bruce-Keller, A. J., G. Umberger, R. McFall, and M. P. Mattson. 1999. Food restriction reduces brain damage and improves behavioral outcome following excitotoxic and metabolic insults. *Annals of Neurology* 45(1):8–15.

Chytrova, G., Z. Ying, and F. Gomez-Pinilla. 2010. Exercise contributes to the effects of DHA dietary supplementation by acting on membrane-related synaptic systems. *Brain Research* 1341:32–40.

Colle, L. M., L. J. Holmes, and H. M. Pappius. 1986. Correlation between behavioral status and cerebral glucose utilization in rats following freezing lesion. *Brain Research* 397(1):27–36.

Davis, L. M., J. R. Pauly, R. D. Readnower, J. M. Rho, and P. G. Sullivan. 2008. Fasting is neuroprotective following traumatic brain injury. *Journal of Neuroscience Research* 86(8):1812–1822.

de la Lastra, C. A., and I. Villegas. 2005. Resveratrol as an anti-inflammatory and anti-aging agent: Mechanisms and clinical implications. *Molecular Nutrition and Food Research* 49(5):405–430.

Dietrich, W. D., O. Alonso, R. Busto, and M. D. Ginsberg. 1994. Widespread metabolic depression and reduced somatosensory circuit activation following traumatic brain injury in rats. *Journal of Neurotrauma* 11(6):629–640.

Ding, Q., S. Vaynman, P. Souda, J. P. Whitelegge, and F. Gomez-Pinilla. 2006. Exercise affects energy metabolism and neural plasticity-related proteins in the hippocampus as revealed by proteomic analysis. *European Journal of Neuroscience* 24(5):1265–1276.

Egan, M. F., M. Kojima, J. H. Callicott, T. E. Goldberg, B. S. Kolachana, A. Bertolino, E. Zaitsev, B. Gold, D. Goldman, M. Dean, B. Lu, and D. R. Weinberger. 2003. The BDNF Val66Met polymorphism affects activity-dependent secretion of BDNF and human memory and hippocampal function. *Cell* 112(2):257–269.

Ginsberg, M. D., W. Zhao, O. F. Alonso, J. Y. Loor-Estades, W. D. Dietrich, and R. Busto. 1997. Uncoupling of local cerebral glucose metabolism and blood flow after acute fluid-percussion injury in rats. *American Journal of Physiology* 272(6 Pt 2):H2859–2868.

Gomez-Pinilla, F. 2008. Brain foods: The effects of nutrients on brain function. *Nature Reviews. Neuroscience* 9(7):568–578.

Gomez-Pinilla, F., and Z. Ying. 2010. Differential effects of exercise and dietary docosahexaenoic acid on molecular systems associated with control of allostasis in the hypothalamus and hippocampus. *Neuroscience* 168(1):130–137.

Gomez-Pinilla, F., S. Vaynman, and Z. Ying. 2008. Brain-derived neurotrophic factor functions as a metabotrophin to mediate the effects of exercise on cognition. *European Journal of Neuroscience* 28(11):2278–2287.

Graham, H. N. 1992. Green tea composition, consumption, and polyphenol chemistry. *Preventive Medicine* 21(3):334–350.

Griesbach, G. S., F. Gomez-Pinilla, and D. A. Hovda. 2007. Time window for voluntary exercise-induced increases in hippocampal neuroplasticity molecules after traumatic brain injury is severity dependent. *Journal of Neurotrauma* 24(7):1161–1171.

Hariri, A. R., T. E. Goldberg, V. S. Mattay, B. S. Kolachana, J. H. Callicott, M. F. Egan, and D. R. Weinberger. 2003. Brain-derived neurotrophic factor Val66Met polymorphism affects human memory-related hippocampal activity and predicts memory performance. *Journal of Neuroscience* 23(17):6690–6694.

Hovda, D. A., R. L. Sutton, and D. M. Feeney. 1987. Recovery of tactile placing after visual cortex ablation in cat: A behavioral and metabolic study of diaschisis. *Experimental Neurology* 97(2):391–402.

Hovda, D. A., A. Yoshino, T. Kawamata, Y. Katayama, and D. P. Becker. 1991. Diffuse prolonged depression of cerebral oxidative metabolism following concussive brain injury in the rat: A cytochrome oxidase histochemistry study. *Brain Research* 567(1):1–10.

Hu, Z. G., H. D. Wang, L. Qiao, W. Yan, Q. F. Tan, and H. X. Yin. 2009. The protective effect of the ketogenic diet on traumatic brain injury-induced cell death in juvenile rats. *Brain Injury* 23(5):459–465.

Huang, W. L., V. R. King, O. E. Curran, S. C. Dyall, R. E. Ward, N. Lal, J. V. Priestley, and A. T. Michael-Titus. 2007. A combination of intravenous and dietary docosahexaenoic acid significantly improves outcome after spinal cord injury. *Brain* 130(Pt 11):3004–3019.

Jang, M., L. Cai, G. O. Udeani, K. V. Slowing, C. F. Thomas, C. W. Beecher, H. H. Fong, N. R. Farnsworth, A. D. Kinghorn, R. G. Mehta, R. C. Moon, and J. M. Pezzuto. 1997. Cancer chemopreventive activity of resveratrol, a natural product derived from grapes. *Science* 275(5297):218–220.

Joseph, J. A., N. A. Denisova, G. Arendash, M. Gordon, D. Diamond, B. Shukitt-Hale, and D. Morgan. 2003. Blueberry supplementation enhances signaling and prevents behavioral deficits in an Alzheimer disease model. *Nutritional Neuroscience* 6(3):153–162.

Keli, S. O., M. G. Hertog, E. J. Feskens, and D. Kromhout. 1996. Dietary flavonoids, antioxidant vitamins, and incidence of stroke: The Zutphen Study. *Archives of Internal Medicine* 156(6):637–642.

Kim, S. J., T. G. Son, H. R. Park, M. Park, M. S. Kim, H. S. Kim, H. Y. Chung, M. P. Mattson, and J. Lee. 2008. Curcumin stimulates proliferation of embryonic neural progenitor cells and neurogenesis in the adult hippocampus. *Journal of Biological Chemistry* 283(21):14497–14505.

Laird, M. D., S. Sukumari-Ramesh, A. E. Swift, S. E. Meiler, J. R. Vender, and K. M. Dhandapani. 2010. Curcumin attenuates cerebral edema following traumatic brain injury in mice: A possible role for aquaporin-4? *Journal of Neurochemistry* 113(3):637–648.

Li, Q., H. F. Zhao, Z. F. Zhang, Z. G. Liu, X. R. Pei, J. B. Wang, and Y. Li. 2009. Long-term green tea catechin administration prevents spatial learning and memory impairment in senescence-accelerated mouse prone-8 mice by decreasing A[beta]1-42 oligomers and upregulating synaptic plasticity-related proteins in the hippocampus. *Neuroscience* 163(3):741–749.

Li, W., S. Dai, J. An, P. Li, X. Chen, R. Xiong, P. Liu, H. Wang, Y. Zhao, M. Zhu, X. Liu, P. Zhu, J. F. Chen, and Y. Zhou. 2008. Chronic but not acute treatment with caffeine attenuates traumatic brain injury in the mouse cortical impact model. *Neuroscience* 151(4):1198–1207.

Lindsay, J., D. Laurin, R. Verreault, R. Hebert, B. Helliwell, G. B. Hill, and I. McDowell. 2002. Risk factors for Alzheimer's disease: A prospective analysis from the Canadian Study of Health and Aging. *American Journal of Epidemiology* 156(5):445–453.

Lyons, W. E., L. A. Mamounas, G. A. Ricaurte, V. Coppola, S. W. Reid, S. H. Bora, C. Wihler, V. E. Koliatsos, and L. Tessarollo. 1999. Brain-derived neurotrophic factor-deficient mice develop aggressiveness and hyperphagia in conjunction with brain serotonergic abnormalities. *Proceedings of the National Academy of Sciences of the United States of America* 96(26):15239–15244.

Menon, V. P., and A. R. Sudheer. 2007. Antioxidant and anti-inflammatory properties of curcumin. *Advances in Experimental Medicine and Biology* 595:105–125.

Mills, J. D., J. E. Bailes, C. L. Sedney, H. Hutchins, and B. Sears. 2010. Omega-3 fatty acid supplementation and reduction of traumatic axonal injury in a rodent head injury model. *Journal of Neurosurgery* 114(1):77–84.

Molteni, R., R. J. Barnard, Z. Ying, C. K. Roberts, and F. Gomez-Pinilla. 2002. A high-fat, refined sugar diet reduces hippocampal brain-derived neurotrophic factor, neuronal plasticity, and learning. *Neuroscience* 112(4):803–814.

Molteni, R., A. Wu, S. Vaynman, Z. Ying, R. J. Barnard, and F. Gomez-Pinilla. 2004. Exercise reverses the harmful effects of consumption of a high-fat diet on synaptic and behavioral plasticity associated to the action of brain-derived neurotrophic factor. *Neuroscience* 123(2):429–440.

Moore, T. H., T. L. Osteen, T. F. Chatziioannou, D. A. Hovda, and T. R. Cherry. 2000. Quantitative assessment of longitudinal metabolic changes in vivo after traumatic brain injury in the adult rat using FDG-microPET. *Journal of Cerebral Blood Flow and Metabolism* 20(10):1492–1501.

Navarro, A., C. Gomez, M. J. Sanchez-Pino, H. Gonzalez, M. J. Bandez, A. D. Boveris, and A. Boveris. 2005. Vitamin E at high doses improves survival, neurological performance, and brain mitochondrial function in aging male mice. *American Journal of Physiology. Regulatory, Integrative, and Comparative Physiology* 289(5):R1392–1399.

Neal, C. J., E. Y. Lee, A. Gyorgy, J. M. Ecklund, D. V. Agoston, and G. S. Ling. 2007. Effect of penetrating brain injury on aquaporin-4 expression using a rat model. *Journal of Neurotrauma* 24(10):1609–1617.

Orgogozo, J. M., J. F. Dartigues, S. Lafont, L. Letenneur, D. Commenges, R. Salamon, S. Renaud, and M. B. Breteler. 1997. Wine consumption and dementia in the elderly: A prospective community study in the Bordeaux area. *Revue Neurologique (Paris)* 153(3):185–192.

Perkins, A. J., H. C. Hendrie, C. M. Callahan, S. Gao, F. W. Unverzagt, Y. Xu, K. S. Hall, and S. L. Hui. 1999. Association of antioxidants with memory in a multiethnic elderly sample using the Third National Health and Nutrition Examination Survey. *American Journal of Epidemiology* 150(1):37–44.

Plunet, W. T., F. Streijger, C. K. Lam, J. H. Lee, J. Liu, and W. Tetzlaff. 2008. Dietary restriction started after spinal cord injury improves functional recovery. *Experimental Neurology* 213(1):28–35.

Prins, M. L., L. S. Fujima, and D. A. Hovda. 2005. Age-dependent reduction of cortical contusion volume by ketones after traumatic brain injury. *Journal of Neuroscience Research* 82(3):413–420.

Salem, N., Jr., B. Litman, H. Y. Kim, and K. Gawrisch. 2001. Mechanisms of action of docosahexaenoic acid in the nervous system. *Lipids* 36(9):945–959.

Samoilova, M., M. Weisspapir, P. Abdelmalik, A. A. Velumian, and P. L. Carlen. 2010. Chronic in vitro ketosis is neuroprotective but not anti-convulsant. *Journal of Neurochemistry* 113(4):826–835.

Sato, Y., H. Nakatsuka, T. Watanabe, S. Hisamichi, H. Shimizu, S. Fujisaku, Y. Ichinowatari, Y. Ida, S. Suda, K. Kato, et al. 1989. Possible contribution of green tea drinking habits to the prevention of stroke. *Tohoku Journal of Experimental Medicine* 157(4):337–343.

Sharma, S., Z. Ying, and F. Gomez-Pinilla. 2010. A pyrazole curcumin derivative restores membrane homeostasis disrupted after brain trauma. *Experimental Neurology* 226(1):191–199.

Soleas, G. J., E. P. Diamandis, and D. M. Goldberg. 1997. Resveratrol: A molecule whose time has come? And gone? *Clinical Biochemistry* 30(2):91–113.

Suganuma, M., S. Okabe, M. Oniyama, Y. Tada, H. Ito, and H. Fujiki. 1998. Wide distribution of [3H](–)-epigal-locatechin gallate, a cancer preventive tea polyphenol, in mouse tissue. *Carcinogenesis* 19(10):1771–1776.

Sutherland, B. A., R. M. Rahman, and I. Appleton. 2006. Mechanisms of action of green tea catechins, with a focus on ischemia-induced neurodegeneration. *Journal of Nutritional Biochemistry* 17(5):291–306.

Suzuki, H., S. J. Park, M. Tamura, and S. Ando. 1998. Effect of the long-term feeding of dietary lipids on the learning ability, fatty acid composition of brain stem phospholipids and synaptic membrane fluidity in adult mice: A comparison of sardine oil diet with palm oil diet. *Mechanisms of Ageing and Development* 101(1–2):119–128.

Truelsen, T., D. Thudium, and M. Gronbaek. 2002. Amount and type of alcohol and risk of dementia: The Copenhagen City Heart Study. *Neurology* 59(9):1313–1319.

Tsuchida, A., T. Nonomura, T. Nakagawa, Y. Itakura, M. Ono-Kishino, M. Yamanaka, E. Sugaru, M. Taiji, and H. Noguchi. 2002. Brain-derived neurotrophic factor ameliorates lipid metabolism in diabetic mice. *Diabetes, Obesity & Metabolism* 4(4):262–269.

Vagnozzi, R., S. Signoretti, B. Tavazzi, R. Floris, A. Ludovici, S. Marziali, G. Tarascio, A. M. Amorini, V. Di Pietro, R. Delfini, and G. Lazzarino. 2008. Temporal window of metabolic brain vulnerability to concussion: A pilot 1H-magnetic resonance spectroscopic study in concussed athletes—Part III. *Neurosurgery* 62(6):1286–1295; discussion 1295–1286.

van Praag, H. 2009. Exercise and the brain: Something to chew on. *Trends in Neurosciences* 32(5):283–290.

Vaynman, S., Z. Ying, A. Wu, and F. Gomez-Pinilla. 2006. Coupling energy metabolism with a mechanism to support brain-derived neurotrophic factor-mediated synaptic plasticity. *Neuroscience* 139(4):1221–1234.

Wei, Q. Y., W. F. Chen, B. Zhou, L. Yang, and Z. L. Liu. 2006. Inhibition of lipid peroxidation and protein oxidation in rat liver mitochondria by curcumin and its analogues. *Biochimica et Biophysica Acta* 1760(1):70–77.

Wu, A., Molteni R, Ying Z, and G.-P. F. 2003. A saturated-fat diet aggravates the outcome of traumatic brain injury on hippocampal plasticity and cognitive function by reducing brain-derived neurotrophic factor. *Neuroscience* 119(2):365–375.

Wu, A., Z. Ying, and F. Gomez-Pinilla. 2004a. Dietary omega-3 fatty acids normalize BDNF levels, reduce oxidative damage, and counteract learning disability after traumatic brain injury in rats. *Journal of Neurotrauma* 21(10):1457–1467.

Wu, A., Z. Ying, and F. Gomez-Pinilla. 2004b. The interplay between oxidative stress and brain-derived neurotrophic factor modulates the outcome of a saturated fat diet on synaptic plasticity and cognition. *European Journal of Neuroscience* 19(7):1699–1707.

Wu, A., Z. Ying, and F. Gomez-Pinilla. 2006. Dietary curcumin counteracts the outcome of traumatic brain injury on oxidative stress, synaptic plasticity, and cognition. *Experimental Neurology* 197(2):309–317.

Wu, A., Z. Ying, and F. Gomez-Pinilla. 2007. Omega-3 fatty acids supplementation restores mechanisms that maintain brain homeostasis in traumatic brain injury. *Journal of Neurotrauma* 24(10):1587–1595.

Wu, A., Z. Ying, and F. Gomez-Pinilla. 2008. Docosahexaenoic acid dietary supplementation enhances the effects of exercise on synaptic plasticity and cognition. *Neuroscience* 155(3):751–759.

Wu, A., Z. Ying, and F. Gomez-Pinilla. 2010. Vitamin E protects against oxidative damage and learning disability after mild traumatic brain injury in rats. *Neurorehabilitation and Neural Repair* 24(3):290–298.

Yoshino, A., D. A. Hovda, T. Kawamata, Y. Katayama, and D. P. Becker. 1991. Dynamic changes in local cerebral glucose utilization following cerebral conclusion in rats: Evidence of a hyper- and subsequent hypometabolic state. *Brain Research* 561(1):106–119.

Youdim, K. A., M. S. Dobbie, G. Kuhnle, A. R. Proteggente, N. J. Abbott, and C. Rice-Evans. 2003. Interaction between flavonoids and the blood-brain barrier: In vitro studies. *Journal of Neurochemistry* 85(1):180–192.

Resolvins and Protectins: Specialized Pro-Resolving Mediators in Inflammation and Organ Protection: Metabolomics of Catabasis

Charles N. Serhan[21]

INTRODUCTION

A highly regulated inflammatory response and its timely resolution is the ideal outcome of an acute inflammatory response essential for ongoing health. Hence the cellular and molecular mechanisms that govern natural resolution are vital. Using an unbiased metabolomic-based systems approach to profile self-limited inflammatory exudates, namely, by studying acute inflammatory responses that resolve on their own the author and colleagues identified novel potent chemical mediators. These new chemical mediators constitute a genus of specialized pro-resolving lipid mediators (SPMs) comprised of three new families coined the resolvins, protectins, and most recently the maresins biosynthesized from n-3 fatty acids. These novel local chemical signals join the lipoxin and aspirin-triggered lipoxins as potent anti-inflammatory and pro-resolving lipid mediators formed from the n-6 essential fatty acid arachidonic acid (Serhan, 2007). SPMs are each stereoselective in their actions and as a defining bioaction for this genus; each family member controls both the duration and magnitude of the inflammatory response as well as reduces leukocyte, mediated injury from within and pain signals. Mapping these endogenous resolution circuits had already provided new avenues to appreciate the molecular basis of many widely occurring diseases that are associated with uncontrolled inflammation. The focus of this review is to overview our current understanding and recent advances on the biosynthesis and actions of these novel anti-inflammatory, pro-resolving and protective lipid mediators biosynthesized from dietary essential fatty acids including eicosapentaenoic acid (EPA) and docosahexaenoic acid (DHA). Also, emphasis herein is on the neuroprotective actions of these local mediators that may be relevant in trauma and brain injury and means to enhance their local biosynthesis from the recent literature.

Currently the most widely used anti-inflammatory therapies are directed at inhibiting specific enzymes and/or antagonizing specific receptors for pro-inflammatory mediators (Brennan and McInnes, 2008). Both selective cyclooxygenase inhibitors and anti-tumor necrosis factor α (TNF-α) are examples of this clinical approach. The goal of this approach is to block the production of pro-inflammatory chemical mediators that reduce both the signs and symptoms of inflammation and local tissue damage (Brennan and McInnes, 2008; Flower, 2003). Research efforts within the author's laboratory focus on profiling self-limited inflammation and uncovering novel mechanisms that terminate the local acute inflammatory response and stimulate resolution with the return of the tissue to homeostasis in murine systems in vivo—a process known as catabasis or the return from disease or the battlefront. Identification of these biochemical and cellular processes demonstrated for the first time that the process of resolution, once considered a passive process, is actually an active, programmed process at the level of the tissue (for recent reviews see Serhan, 2007; Serhan et al., 2008). The resolution as a passive event was thought to simply burn out with the dilution of chemotactic gradients that recruit leukocytes to an infection or invading organism.

Natural resolution of self-limited challenges as well as limited second organ injury proved to be an active process in that we found evidence for temporal activation of bio-

---

[21]Center for Experimental Therapeutics and Reperfusion Injury, Harvard Institutes of Medicine, Brigham and Women's Hospital and Harvard Medical School, Boston, MA.

chemical pathways and mediators that instruct the tissue and inflammatory white cells to resolve. Research in the author's laboratory focused on the potential use of these endogenous agonists to stimulate natural resolution of inflammation rather than targeting inhibition or antagonism of inflammation. This approach also has opened a new understanding of the mechanisms underlying chronic inflammatory diseases as well as a new area in molecular pharmacology, namely resolution pharmacology. The essential n-3 fatty acids, in particular EPA and DHA, are precursors to a several families of mediators in this new genus of potent lipid mediators (LM) that are both pro-resolving and anti-inflammatory (SPM).

AN IDEAL OUTCOME

An acute inflammatory response initiated by microbial invasion or tissue damage is characterized by the cardinal signs of inflammation, i.e., heat, redness, swelling and pain (Majno, 1975). These signs and symptoms are accompanied by a well-known set of cellular microscopic events, including edema and the accumulation of leukocytes, specifically polymorphonuclear leukocytes (PMNs), followed by monocytes that differentiate locally to macrophages (Cotran et al., 1999) (Figure C-10). The local acute inflammatory response

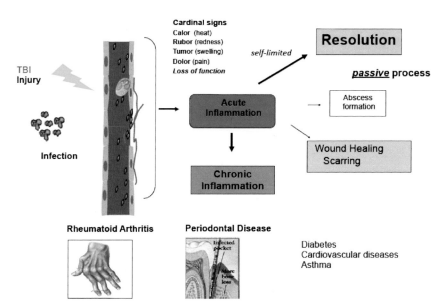

FIGURE C-10 Decision paths in acute inflammation. Several outcomes of acute inflammation caused by infection or injury are possible, including progression to chronic inflammation, tissue fibrosis and wound healing/scarring or, in the ideal scenario, complete resolution (Majno, 1975). The cardinal signs of inflammation—calor (heat), rubor (redness), tumor (swelling), dolor (pain), and loss of function—have been known as the visual signs of inflammation apparent to ancient civilizations. Chronic inflammation was viewed as the persistence of an acute inflammatory response. The chronic inflammatory diseases widely observed in the West are rheumatoid arthritis and periodontal disease. There is now considerable interest in inflammation because it is considered to be the pathophysiologic basis of many diseases that were traditionally not considered to be inflammatory in their pathobiology. These include diabetes, cardiovascular diseases, and asthma, to name a few.

is protective for the host and serves to maintain tissue homeostasis. If uncontrolled, this vital response can become deleterious for the host and the process can progress to chronic inflammation, scarring and fibrosis rather than terminate or resolve. In many cases, the fundamental cause of tissue damage is excessive leukocyte accumulation (Cassatella, 2003). In traumatic brain injury (TBI), for example excessive neutrophil infiltration amplifies local tissue damage (Cotran et al., 1999; Majno and Joris, 2004).

The Resolution Program

In self-limited resolving inflammatory reactions, leukocyte recruitment is coupled with release of local factors that prevent further or excessive trafficking of leukocytes, allowing for resolution (Serhan et al., 2000, 2002). We found that, early in the initiation phase of an inflammatory response, pro-inflammatory mediators such as prostaglandins and leukotrienes play an important role (Samuelsson et al., 1987). Monkeys fed a diet lacking essential fatty acids were found to be defective at mounting an efficient inflammatory response (Palmblad et al., 1988). This highlights the importance of arachidonate-derived eicosanoids or the n-6 essential fatty acid contribution to controlled acute inflammation. In this report from Palmblad et al. (1988), both neutrophil (PMN) chemotaxis and superoxide generation in response to the chemotactic peptide formyl-methiony-leucylphenylalanine (fMLF) were markedly abrogated when the cells were isolated from monkeys fed n-3 essential fatty acids. This is important to our appreciation of the action of dietary n-3 in non-human primates because the PMNs that normally defends the body can release reactive oxygen species ideally intended to kill invading organisms phagocytized by white cells. Instead, when they are summoned into surrounding tissues that are already damaged these cells can inadvertently spill noxious reactive oxygen species that can further destroy tissue. The finding that dietary n-3 reduces this potentially deleterious response of white cells ex vivo provides evidence from primates that leukocyte-mediated tissue damage can be reduced with dietary essential fatty acid. The molecular mechanism for this reduction in leukocyte mediated events was not known at the time of the Palmblad et al. (1988) report but appears to be related to the now known actions of the SPM (see below).

Progression from acute to chronic inflammation as in many widely occurring human diseases of concern in public health such as periodontal disease, arthritis (Koopman and Moreland, 2005), and cardiovascular disease (Libby, 2008), is widely viewed as an excess of pro-inflammatory mediators (Van Dyke and Serhan, 2006). Complete termination of an acute inflammatory insult also is pertinent for restoration of tissue homeostasis and is necessary for ongoing health. Key to this process is the complete *removal* of leukocytes from inflammatory sites without leaving remnants of the host's combat between leukocytes, invading microbes, and/or other initiators of inflammation that can seed or amplify the local inflammatory response. Evidence from the author's laboratory and many others (e.g., Morris et al., 2009) now indicates that the resolving phase of inflammation is not merely a passive process as once believed, but actively takes place as a programmed response at the tissue level (reviewed in Serhan, 2007; Serhan et al., 2008), which can be viewed as analogous to the cellular level or programmed cell death (Cohen et al., 1992). Although mononuclear cells can sometimes contribute to pro-inflammatory responses (Cotran et al., 1999), they also are critical in wound healing, tissue repair and remodeling in a non-inflammatory, non-phlogistic (not fever-causing) manner (Serhan and Savill, 2005). This important homeostatic role of monocytes and macrophages is termed efferocytosis (Tabas, 2010).

SPECIALIZED PRO-RESOLVING LIPID MEDIATORS AND NUTRITION: NOT JUST N-6 VS. N-3 IN THE CONTROL OF INFLAMMATION— A TEMPORAL PROGRESSION TO CATABASIS

The new genus of essential fatty acid-derived autacoids were coined specialized pro-resolving mediators (SPMs) because they possess families of potent anti-inflammatory, pro-resolving, and protective mediators in experimental animal models of disease (reviewed in Serhan, 2007). These include the lipoxins from n-6 arachidonic acid (Levy et al., 2001) as well as the n-3-derived resolvins, protectins, and the newly identified maresins, which are not reviewed herein (see Serhan et al., 2009). These novel families of endogenous lipid-derived mediators were originally isolated from self-limited inflammatory murine exudates captured during the natural resolution phase (Figures C-11 and C-12). Each of these local chemical mediators is actively biosynthesized via distinct cellular and in some cases transcellular, enzymatic pathways that are stereocontrolled to produce molecules that are stereoselective in their actions. Hence SPMs are potent agonists that control the duration and magnitude of inflammation by acting on specific receptors (e.g., G protein-coupled receptor [GPCR]) on separate cell populations to stimulate the overall resolution of inflammation (Serhan and Chiang, 2008).

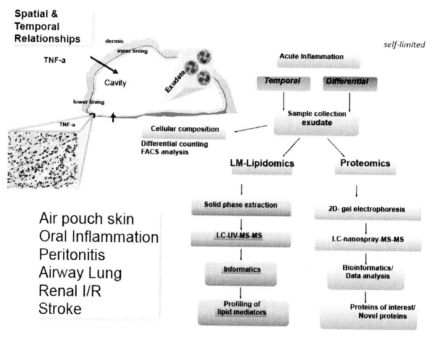

FIGURE C-11   Systems approach to metabolomics of resolution. Illustration of the systems approach taken for the differential analysis of inflammatory exudates. For these initial studies, the murine air pouch was used because it provided a convenient means to assess tissue-level responses by studying the histology as well as the temporal and spatial relationships between infiltrating leukocytes and inflammatory mediators that are initiated by pro-inflammatory stimuli such as bacteria, microbial products, or cytokines such as TNF-α. This differential temporal analysis of inflammatory exudates comparing cellular composition, lipid mediator lipidomics, and proteomics also has been carried out in oral inflammation, peritonitis, airway and lung inflammation, renal ischemia-reperfusion injury, and stroke (see text for further details).

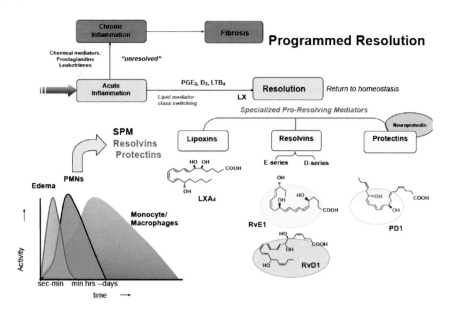

FIGURE C-12 Specialized pro-resolving mediators are generated during inflammatory resolution: ideal outcome of inflammation. Using a rigorous definition of acute inflammation and its resolution, (Cotran et al., 1999) illustrated lower left, we found that acute inflammation initiates a lipid mediator class switch from prostaglandins and leukotrienes in the initial phases to lipoxins and pro-resolving mediators to resolution and the return to homeostasis. Alternatively, an unresolved acute inflammatory response can persist and become chronic inflammation, and in this case lipid mediators such as prostaglandins and leukotrienes are elevated and lead from chronic inflammation to tissue fibrosis. Resolution is an active process switched on by specialized pro-resolving mediators (SPMs), including E-series resolvins derived from n-3 polyunsaturaed fatty acid (PUFA) eicosapentaenoic acid (Serhan et al., 2000), D-series resolvins biosynthesized from dDHA (Serhan et al., 2002; Sun et al., 2007), as well as the protectins (Serhan et al., 2002, 2006). From these results we can now consider the tissue-level events of acute inflammation as programmed resolution (see text for further details).

A systems metabolomics approach was taken using mass spectrometry to analyze the endogenous mediators and mechanisms temporally biosynthesized in vivo by exudates to actively resolve inflammation (Figure C-11). For this, the murine dorsal air pouch system proved to be very useful because self-limited inflammatory exudates could easily be obtained (Serhan et al., 2000, 2002). This system permitted direct exudate analysis in terms of lipidomics and lipid mediator metabolomic profiling (e.g., bioactive autacoids, as well as their inactive precursors and further metabolites), proteomics, and cellular composition by monitoring leukocyte trafficking. Utilizing this approach made it possible to determine when and where different families of local mediators were biosynthesized during resolution (Bannenberg et al., 2005; Serhan, 2007).

Lipoxins were the first anti-inflammatory and pro-resolving lipid mediators recognized, signaling the resolution of acute contained inflammation (Serhan, 2005). Lipoxins are lipoxygenase-derived eicosanoids derived enzymatically from arachidonic acid, an n-6 essential fatty acid that is released from phospholipid stores during inflammation (Samuelsson et al., 1987). In humans they are biosynthesized via transcellular metabolic processes engaged during leukocyte interactions with mucosal cells, i.e., epithelia of the gastrointestinal tract or bronchial tissue, and within the vasculature during platelet–leukocyte interactions

(Serhan, 2007). The murine dorsal air pouch was used to determine the formation and roles of endogenous lipoxin A_4 (LXA_4) in the resolution of acute inflammation (Levy et al., 2001). Upon initiation of inflammation with TNF-α, there was a typical acute-phase response denoted by rapid PMN infiltration preceded by generation of local prostaglandins and leukotrienes. Unexpectedly, the eicosanoids then underwent a temporal progression in local mediators we termed a "class switch". As exudates evolve, the eicosanoid profiles switch and the lipid mediators produced within the milieu of the exudate changes (Levy et al., 2001). Within the inflammatory exudate, arachidonate-derived eicosanoids changed from initial production of prostaglandins and leukotrienes to lipoxins, which halted further recruitment of neutrophils. This class switch was driven in part by COX-derived prostaglandins E_2 and D_2 that regulate the transcription of enzymes involved in lipoxin biosynthesis (Levy et al., 2001). Hence, the concept that "alpha signals omega," the beginning signals the end in inflammation was introduced (Serhan and Savill, 2005). This became evident because the appearance of lipoxins within inflammatory exudates was concomitant with the loss of PMN and resolution of inflammation (Levy et al., 2001).

In the inflammatory milieu, neutrophils undergo either apoptosis or necrotic cell death at the site of battle and must be removed. As part of the resolution circuit, lipoxins (LX) are biosynthesized (Levy et al., 2001) and signal macrophages to engulf/take up the apoptotic PMN (Godson et al., 2000). LX also proved to be potent chemoattractants for mononuclear cells, but in a non-phlogistic manner. LX activates monocyte infiltration without stimulating release of pro-inflammatory chemokines or activation of pro-inflammatory gene pathways in these cells. Thus, LX actively reduced the entry of PMN to the site of inflammation while accelerating uptake of apoptotic PMN (Serhan, 2007). LX are potent anti-inflammatory mediators that are formed and act in picogram to nanogram amounts within human tissues and in animal disease models (Serhan, 2005). They have the specific pro-resolution actions of limiting PMN recruitment, chemotaxis, and adhesion to the site of inflammation, acting essentially as a braking signal for PMN-mediated tissue injury (Morris et al., 2009; Serhan, 2005). Additionally, LX stable analogs activate endogenous anti-microbial defense mechanisms (Canny et al., 2002), and thus, unlike many other anti-inflammatory treatments, LX are not immunosuppressive.

SPMS ARE BIOSYNTHESIZED FROM THE OMEGA-3 ESSENTIAL FATTY ACIDS, EPA AND DHA

Dietary n-3 PUFA are known to carry protective effects in the cardiovascular system, many inflammatory disorders, and neural function (Leon et al., 2008; Salem et al., 2001; Simopoulos, 2008). Importantly, Hibbeln and colleagues have shown that reduced serum levels of DHA can lead to severe physiological outcomes including depression and increased suicide (1998). This reduction in circulating levels of n-3 correlated with low consumption in humans. Hence Hibbeln introduced the concept of nutritional armor to help emphasize the important role of dietary DHA and to underscore the need to balance this potential for DHA and other essential fatty acid deficits in the diet, in particular those of the military diet given the stress and potential for tissue trauma. The molecular mechanisms by which n-3 PUFAs exert their biological effects in general were incomplete and needed to be elucidated at the cellular and molecular levels. The prevailing theory on the actions of n-3 fatty acids (DHA, EPA) is that they compete for arachidonic acid in phospholipid stores, blocking the biosynthesis of eicosanoids that are pro-inflammatory such as leukotrienes and prostaglandins as well as vasoactive thromboxane (Lands, 2005). This competition between n-3 and n-6 pathways is evident with results from many studies and is demonstrable in vitro with isolated cells and enzymes with high concentrations of essential fatty acids (e.g., micro- to millimolar range) particularly DHA and EPA. New results indicate that many of the n-6 eicosanoids play important protective roles in resolution and host defense. Thus, these new findings raise critical questions regarding reducing n-6 essential fatty acid levels as relevant in human physiology. To this end, the author has addressed the question "Are the essential n-3 PUFAs such as EPA and DHA enzymatically converted locally in vivo to novel bioactive mediators? Do these local mediators serve as effectors or agonists in vivo?" Accordingly, using an unbiased metabolomic approach, mice given n-3 PUFA biosynthesized novel lipid mediators during the resolution phase of acute inflammation. These mediators are potent agonists of many responses relevant in the immune system and organ protection, particularly neuroprotection. Given the pathophysiology that accompanies TBI it is highly likely that the SPMs will have a beneficial role in TBI by limiting further tissue damage and protecting neurons from uncontrolled inflammatory cells summoned to the TBI-damaged tissue site (vide infra) (Serhan et al., 2000; 2002).

RESOLVINS: RESOLUTION-PHASE INTERACTION PRODUCTS FROM N-3 ESSENTIAL FATTY ACID

Resolvins are a family of new local mediators enzymatically produced within resolving inflammatory exudates. They were initially identified using a systems approach with LC-MS-MS-based lipidomics and informatics, and subsequently complete structural elucidation of these bioactive mediators and related compounds was achieved (Arita et al., 2005a; Hong et al., 2003; Serhan et al., 2000, 2002, 2006). The term resolvins or resolution-phase interaction products refers to endogenous compounds biosynthesized from the major n-3 fatty acids EPA and DHA, denoted E series (RvE) and D series (RvD) resolvins, respectively (Serhan et al., 2002) (Figures C-13 and C-14). Similar to lipoxins, resolvins also can be produced

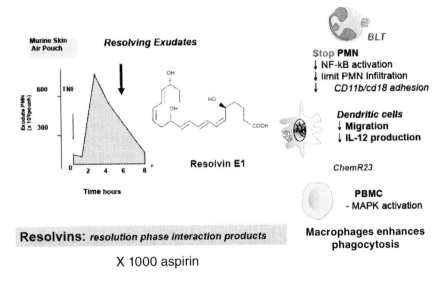

FIGURE C-13 Resolvin E1: Structure and actions. Addition of TNF to murine air pouch leads to rapid infiltration of PMN into the inflammatory exudate. As the PMN levels declined, increased production of resolvin E1 derived from EPA was first identified (Serhan et al., 2000). The complete stereochemistry and the mechanism of action for RvE1 has been established (Arita et al., 2005a, 2007). Resolvins are defined as resolution phase interaction products and proved to be, on a molar basis, log orders more potent than traditional nonsteroidal anti-inflammatory drugs including aspirin.

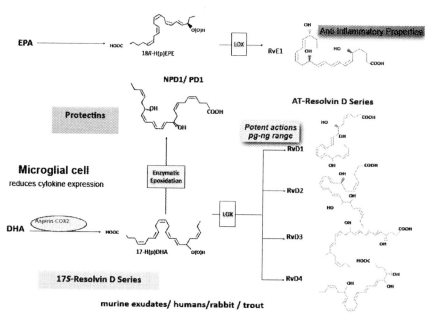

FIGURE C-14   Biosynthetic scheme of resolvins. The complete stereochemistry of RvD1 and RvD2 has been established.
SOURCE: Spite et al., 2009a; Sun et al., 2007.

by a COX-2-initiated pathway in the presence of aspirin to give "aspirin-triggered" (AT) forms. Accruing evidence indicates that resolvins possess potent anti-inflammatory and immunoregulatory actions that include blocking the production of pro-inflammatory mediators and regulating leukocyte trafficking to inflammatory sites (reviewed in Serhan et al., 2008) as well as clearance of neutrophils from mucosal surfaces (Campbell et al., 2007). Specifically, resolvins limit PMN transendothelial migration in vitro and infiltration in vivo (Serhan et al., 2002; Sun et al., 2007). The potency of these compounds is notable, with concentrations as low as 10 nM producing approximately 50 percent reduction in PMN transmigration. A more detailed description of the specific mechanistic actions of resolvins is discussed in Serhan (2007 and references cited within). Recent results established the stereochemistry and the stereoselective bioactions of RvD1, AT-RvD1, RvE1, and PD1/NPD1 (vide infra) as well as their further enzymatic inactivation because at the end of resolution these signal are "turned off" (Arita et al., 2005a; Serhan et al., 2006; Sun et al., 2007).

It is important to note that the actions of these endogenous SPM are mediated through specific receptors. RvE1 acts as an agonist on at least two GPCRs, namely ChemR23 and as a partial agonist on the LTB_4 receptor (BLT1), thus competing with LTB_4 for binding (Arita et al., 2005a, 2006). Recent research has revealed that RvE1 stimulates phosphorylation of Akt in a time- and dose-dependent manner via direct activation of ChemR23 (Ohira et al., 2009). This agonist of resolution therefore displays a distinct mechanism of action compared to LXA_4 that inhibits downstream tyrosine phosphorylation in eosinophils (Starosta et al., 2008). Additionally, a recent study identified two separate GPCRs that RvD1 specifically binds on human leukocytes, namely the LXA_4 receptor (ALX) and GPR32, an orphan receptor, which were validated using a GPCR β-arrestin coupled system (Krishnamoorthy et al., 2010). Identification of receptors for other n-3-derived SPM is in progress and is likely to be high-affinity GPCRs based on the potency of these newly discovered agonists of resolution. Thus at least two GPCRs for each SPM, RvE1, RvD1, and LXA$_4$, are shared by AT-LXA$_4$. Hence the concept that one ligand can act on a repertoire of receptors is not surprising in view of recent results on neuronal responses with the formyl peptide receptors including FPR2, peptides, and LXA$_4$, which unexpectedly evokes chemosensory actions (Riviere et al., 2009).

PROTECTINS AND NEUROPROTECTIN D1: ORGAN-PROTECTIVE MEDIATORS

In addition to D-series resolvins, DHA is also a precursor for the family of protectins. These mediators are biosynthesized via a separate pathway (Figure C-15). Protectins are distinguished by their conjugated triene-containing structure (Serhan et al., 2006). The name "protectins" was coined from the observed anti-inflammatory and protective actions in neural tissues and systems (Hong et al., 2003). The prefix *neuro*protectin gives the tissue location of its generation and local actions, such as neuroprotectin D1 (NPD1) (Mukherjee et al., 2004; Serhan et al., 2006). Like the resolvins, protectins stop PMN infiltration and enhance macrophage phagocytosis of apoptotic (dead cells) PMN (Hong et al., 2003; Serhan et al., 2006). They are biosynthesized by and act on glial cells and reduce cytokine expression (Hong et al., 2003).

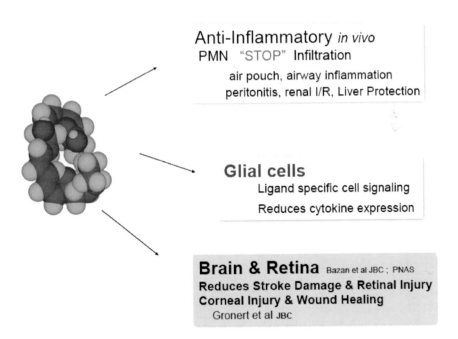

Anti-Inflammatory *in vivo*
PMN "STOP" Infiltration
air pouch, airway inflammation
peritonitis, renal I/R, Liver Protection

Glial cells
Ligand specific cell signaling
Reduces cytokine expression

Brain & Retina Bazan et al JBC ; PNAS
Reduces Stroke Damage & Retinal Injury
Corneal Injury & Wound Healing
Gronert et al JBC

FIGURE C-15 Protectins: Structure and actions. The complete stereochemistry of (NPD1) or protectin D1 (PD1) when generated in inflammatory exudates has been established (Serhan et al., 2006). NPD1 stops further neutrophilic infiltration in a number of in vivo animal systems as well as reduces microglial cell cytokine expression. These initial actions defined the biological functions and roles of PD1. In addition, in collaboration with Nicolas Bazan and colleagues, we have found that NPD1 reduces stroke damage and retinal injury (see Bazan et al., 2010).

Of special interest for this report, NPD1 reduces both retinal and corneal injury and stroke damage (Marcheselli et al., 2003), and improves corneal wound healing in mouse models (Gronert et al., 2005) (see Serhan, 2007; Serhan et al., 2008, and references cited within). DHA is well known for its role in neuronal systems and, along with arachidonic acid (AA), is a major PUFA found in the retina (Bazan et al., 2010). The available results provide the biological basis for the actions of NPD1 derived from DHA. In recent reviews we considered in detail the results obtained from several independent lines of investigation required to address the structure of the potent bioactive NPD1/PD1 (see Bazan et al., 2010). As with other bioactive mediators, such as the eicosanoids (Samuelsson et al., 1987), it is important to establish the stereochemistry of the compound and/or mediator. Notably, subtle structural changes in these and related products can be less active, inactive, or, even in some cases display opposing biologic actions as a result of subtle changes in stereochemistry that are recognized in biologic systems. To confirm the proposed basic structure and establish the complete stereochemistry, these studies on the 10,17S-docosatriene termed NPD1/PD1 included results from (a) biosynthesis studies; (b) matching of materials prepared by total organic synthesis with defined stereochemistry; and (c) the actions of these and related compounds in biological systems (Ariel et al., 2005; Hong et al., 2003; Marcheselli et al., 2010; Mukherjee et al., 2004; Serhan et al., 2002, 2006). We also consider these findings as they appeared in the literature with the goal of providing a clear and rigorous account of the evidence that supports the structure and bioactions of NPD1/PD1. Investigations along these lines were required to establish the complete structure and potent actions of NPD1/PD1 and related endogenous products biosynthesized from DHA because the small amounts of NPD1 attainable from biological systems precluded direct stereochemical analyses of the products identified in retinal pigmented epithelial (RPE) cells. For a recent review, see Bazan et al. (2010).

Briefly, the novel 10,17S-docosatriene was coined NPD1/PD1 given its potent actions *in vivo* noted above, which were identified first in Hong et al. (2003) and Serhan et al. (2002). Its basic structure was established and displayed potent anti-inflammatory actions, i.e., reducing PMN numbers in vivo and reducing the production of inflammatory cytokines by glial cells. Moreover, during the resolution phase of peritonitis, unesterified DHA levels increase in resolving exudates, where it appears to promote catabasis or the return to homeostasis following tissue insult, via conversion to D-series resolvins and 10,17S-docosatrienes (Bannenberg et al., 2005) by shortening the resolution interval of an inflammatory response in vivo (Schwab et al., 2007).

In collaboration with Dr. Bazan and colleagues at Louisiana State University, we found next that the DHA-derived 10,17S-docosatriene was generated *in vivo* in the brain during experimental stroke in the ipsilateral cerebral hemisphere following focal ischemia (Figures C-15, C-16, and C-17). We also demonstrated its potent bioactions in stroke, where NPD1/PD1 limited the entry of leukocytes, downregulated both COX-2 expression and NFκB activation, and decreased infarct volume (Figure 8 from Marcheselli et al., 2003). Of interest, 10,17S-docosatriene is also formed in the human retinal pigment epithelial cell line ARPE-19 and introduced the term *neuro*protectin D1 based on its neuroprotective bioactivity in the stroke model and RPE cells (Mukherjee et al., 2004). Also NPD1 proved to be a potent signal to *inactivate* pro-apoptotic and pro-inflammatory signaling. The capital D in NPD1 refers to its being the first identified neuroprotective mediator derived from DHA (Mukherjee et al., 2004).

In parallel to these investigations, biosynthesis and function studies were carried out with human T_H2-skewed peripheral blood mononuclear cells (PBMC) (Ariel et al., 2005). When produced by human PBMC, PD1 promotes T-cell apoptosis via the formation of lipid

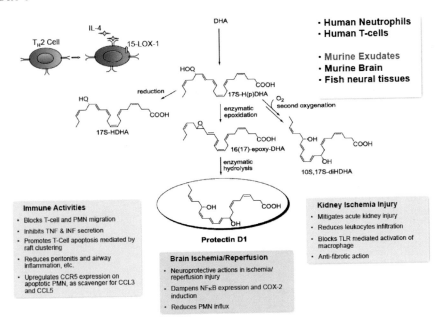

FIGURE C-16 NPD1/PD1 biosynthesis and actions. NPD1 was identified initially in murine exudates and next in murine brain cells. Fish such as trout also produce NPD1/PD1, indicating that this is a primordial structure and pathway. In the immune system, T cells skew to a Th2 cell in the presence of interleukin-4, increase their 15-LO type 1, and convert DHA to PD1. The actions of PD1 are denoted in the inset boxes. The biosynthesis of PD1 and its complete stereochemistry have been established. The conversion of DHA to PD1 enzymatically proceeds via the enzymatic epoxidation and formation of a key 16(17)-epoxy-DHA intermediate that is enzymatically converted to the complete stereochemistry required for full biological action in PD1 (see text for further details).

raft-encoded signaling complexes and reduced T-cell traffic in vivo. Matching materials prepared by total organic synthesis determined the complete stereochemistry of the PBMC DHA-derived product. NPD1/PD1 generated by human PBMC carried the complete stereo-chemistry of (10R,17S)-dihydroxydocosa-4Z,7Z,11E,13E,15Z,19Z-hexaenoic acid and was matched to the most potent bioactive product (Figure C-16) using several dihydroxytriene-containing DHA-derived products isolated from human PBMC, human PMN, and murine exudates (Ariel et al., 2005; Serhan et al., 2006).

With the stereochemistry of NPD1/PD1 established, its identification in human material was sought and found in exhaled breath condensates from human asthmatics (Levy et al., 2007) as well as in human brain tissue. NPD1 is present in both control brain tissues and at reduced levels in brain tissues from patients with Alzheimer's disease (Lukiw et al., 2005, and Table 1). In addition, PD1 is a major product in bone marrow of female rats fed EPA and DHA (Poulsen et al., 2008). PD1 is also generated in vivo during ischemia-reperfusion of renal tissues, where it has profound actions, reducing the deleterious consequences of ischemia-reperfusion in renal tissues (Duffield et al., 2006) in agreement with our earlier findings in brain tissues (Marcheselli et al., 2003).

With the complete stereochemistry and synthetic compound in hand, it was possible to demonstrate for the first time that PD1 activates resolution programs in vivo and shortens the resolution time of experimental inflammation in animal models (Schwab et al., 2007).

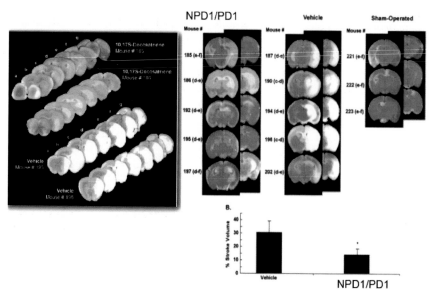

FIGURE C-17   Neuroprotective action of NPD1/PD1. NPD1 reduces stroke volume and leukocyte-mediated tissue damage in a murine model of focal ischemia in stroke. Figure is from Marcheselli et al., J. Biol. Chem. 2003; 278:43807-43817. See Bazan et al. (2010) and text for further details.

Also, with the total organic synthesis route of NPD1/PD1, it was possible to radiolabel and isolate ^{3}H-NPD1/PD1 made from the synthetic intermediate. With this radiolabel, we define for the specific binding sites present with ARPE-19 cells (K_d ~ 31 pM/mg cell protein) for ^{3}H-NPD1/PD1 as well as specific binding to human neutrophils (K_d of ~25 nM) (Marcheselli et al., 2010).

Recent results using an LC-MS-MS profiling approach demonstrated that PD1 is made during the resolution of Lyme disease infections in mice (Blaho et al., 2009). NPD1 inhibits retinal ganglion cell death (Qin et al., 2008), is renal protective (Hassan and Gronert, 2009), and regulates adiponectin (González-Périz et al., 2009). Of interest, the double dioxygenation product 10S,17S-diHDHA, isomer of NPD1/PD1, was recently shown to have actions on platelets, reducing platelet aggregation at 0.3 µM, 1 µM, and higher concentrations (Chen et al., 2009). In peritonitis, this isomer also showed biological activity but was less potent than NPD1/PD1 (Serhan et al., 2006). It is noteworthy that NPD1/PD1 and the resolvins are produced by trout tissues including trout brain from endogenous DHA, suggesting that these structures are highly conserved from fish to humans (Hong et al., 2005) and that we still have much to learn regarding the bioactions and functions of NPD1/PD1, the D-series and E-series resolvins, and related products in human physiology and pathophysiology as well as in biological systems such as fish or in bone marrow, where the actions of NPD1/PD1 remain to be fully appreciated.

OMEGA-3 ESSENTIAL FATTY ACID AND SUBSTRATE AVAILABILITY IN RESOLUTION OF INFLAMMATION

To elucidate the role of EPA, DHA, and AA during inflammation in vivo, we studied disease models in wild-type mice that overexpress the C. elegans fat-1 gene to compare the effects of n-3 and -6 PUFAs. This gene converts n-6 PUFA into n-3, resulting in elevated tissue levels of n-3 PUFA within the fat-1 overexpressing mice. In a model of oxygen-induced retinopathy, a protective effect against pathological angiogenesis was found in the retina when there was a lower ratio of n-6:n-3 PUFA. Wild-type mice lacking the fat-1 transgene had more extensive vaso-obliteration and more severe retinal neovascularization compared with fat-1 mice (Connor et al., 2007). In mice fed n-3 PUFA, biosynthetic markers of NPD1 and RvE1 were detected in the retinal tissues. In mice without n-3 PUFA supplementation, administration of RvD1, RvE1, or NPD1 gave protection from vaso-obliteration and neovascularization (Connor et al., 2007), as well as suture-induced ocular inflammation (Jin et al., 2009). These fat-1 mice also have increased levels of resolvins and protectins in the colon and are protected from colitis (Hudert et al., 2006). In evolving exudates, rapid appearance of unesterified n-3 PUFA parallels the initial increase in edema (Kasuga et al., 2008). Thus, n-3 precursors for resolving and protectin biosynthesis in exudates become available directly from the peripheral circulation. This contrasts with the pool or storage of AA and other essential fatty acid that requires phospholipase A_2 for liberation for example in inflammatory cells (Dennis, 2000; Lands, 2005) and in retina RPE cells (Bazan et al., 2010).

SPM IN INFLAMMATORY EXPERIMENTAL DISEASE SYSTEMS

Inflammatory bowel disorders, such as colitis, are characterized by a relapsing inflammatory process as a result of local mucosal damage and abnormal mucosal responses. In a well-appreciated experimental colitis in mice, mice are challenged with either an intrarectal antigenic hapten, 2,4,6-trinitrobenzene sulfonic acid (TNBS) or to induce colitis, RvE1, which was protective against bowel inflammation (Arita et al., 2005b). With treatment of as little as 1 µg of RvE1 per mouse, there was dramatic reduction in mortality, and weight loss, and less severe histologic display of colitis, namely reduction in the associated inflammatory cells, such as PMN and lymphocytes, compared with mice with TNBS-induced colitis. RvE1 is also protective in Porphyromonas gingivalis-induced periodontal disease in rabbits, where it appears to stimulate tissue regeneration of the periodontium (Hasturk et al., 2007). Another pro-resolving action of RvE1 was evident in a murine model of fatty liver disease, where RvE1 administration to obese mice significantly alleviated hepatic steatosis and restored the loss of insulin sensitivity (Gonzalez-Periz et al., 2009).

The complete stereochemical assignment for RvD2 (Figure C-11) was recently established as 7S,16R,17S-trihydroxy-4Z,8E,10Z,12E,14E,19Z-docosahexaenoic acid (Spite et al., 2009a). RvD2 proved very potent suggesting it may have a broad role in vivo and potential application in disease. Sepsis remains a clinical challenge with increasing prevalence and mortality rates. In these cases, infection progresses rapidly unless contained and cleared by phagocytes, and epithelial and endothelial barrier dysfunction results in immune suppression, multiple-organ failure, and death. Administration of n-3 PUFA in some of these cases of sepsis has shown favorable outcomes (Singer et al., 2008), although the mechanism of action is still being studied. In an established mouse model of sepsis, initiated by "mid-grade" cecal ligation and puncture (CLP) surgery, RvD2-methyl ester (RvD2-ME; 100ng) was protective (Spite et al., 2009a). After 12 hours, mice that underwent CLP surgery had severe bacterial burden both locally within the peritoneum and systemically, which was accompanied by a significant leukocyte infiltrate to the peritoneal cavity. RvD2-ME treatment immediately following CLP significantly reduced both blood and peritoneal bacterial levels and dramatically limited local PMN influx. Septic mice were hypothermic 12 hours after CLP and displayed a drastic decrease in activity levels, whereas RvD2-treated mice remained active within their cages and their body temperatures were similar to sham-operated control mice. The proportion of mice that survived seven days following "mid-grade" CLP was approximately 36 percent. RvD2-ME was able to double the survival rates (Figure C-14). Interestingly, whereas all of the mice that did not survive in the vehicle-treated group died by 36 hours, 25 percent of the mice that died in the RvD2-treated group lived until 48 hours post-CLP, suggesting that RvD2 may increase the "therapeutic window" that could afford additional time for further interventions such as antibiotics. Further analysis of peritoneal exudates showed a "cytokine-storm" of both pro-inflammatory cytokines and other mediators associated with detrimental outcomes in sepsis, as well as elevated pro-inflammatory lipid mediators LTB_4 and PGE_2. RvD2-ME significantly blunted overzealous cytokine production and pro-inflammatory lipid mediators measured 12 hours post-CLP. Dissection of mouse inguinal lymph nodes revealed that bacteria were disseminated throughout this organ in vehicle-CLP mice, whereas RvD2 enhanced phagocyte-dependent bacterial containment and clearance. Corroboratory results were obtained in vitro with human PMN exposed to RvD2 (1 and 10 nM) that showed increased phagocytosis and killing of E. coli (Spite et al., 2009a). These novel findings highlight that RvD2 is protective in mucosal barrier breakage and leakage leading to sepsis.

A recent study found that RvE1 is also anti-infective, enhancing clearance of bacteria from mouse lungs in a model of pneumonia, leading to increased survival (Seki et al., 2010). Thus, pro-resolving mediators display anti-inflammatory, anti-fibrotic, and recently demonstrated anti-infective actions in several widely used laboratory models of inflammation (see Table C-7). Together, these results indicate SPM, i.e., resolvins, are not immunosuppressive but rather enhance the innate anti-microbial systems in phagocytes and mucosal epithelial cells (Canny et al., 2002).

STEM CELLS AND RECENT RESULTS OF INTEREST FOR TRAUMATIC BRAIN INJURY

The identification and biosynthesis of resolvins and protectins from DHA in brain (Serhan et al., 2002) and microglial cells (Hong et al., 2003), and in view of their anti-inflammatory and pro-resolving actions in acute inflammation using in vivo models, suggested that these compounds also may be active in neural tissues. Indeed, neuroprotectin D1 limited neutrophilic infiltration in ischemic brain as well as reduced pro-inflammatory gene expression, suggesting that this compound had potent neuroprotective actions in local ischemia-reperfusion in the brain (Marcheselli et al., 2003), which also was observed in renal protection (Duffield et al., 2006; Hassan and Gronert, 2009) (Figure C-15). Given the importance of neural stem cells in organ regeneration, we examined the actions of LT B_4 and LX A_4 and found that murine neural stem cells produced LT B_4 and possess leukotriene receptors. LX A_4 regulated proliferation and differentiation of these cells. Of interest, the 15-epimer isomer of LXA_4 (which is more stable in vivo as it is not inactivated as rapidly as LXA_4) reduced neural stem cell growth at concentrations as low as 1 nanomolar. Gene chip analysis demonstrated that LT B_4 and LXA_4 gave opposing gene expression profiles with neural stem cells. LTB_4 induced proliferation and differentiation of neural stem cells into neurons, and the regulatory actions of LXA_4 suggested that these new pathways may be relevant in restoring stem cells (Wada et al., 2006). Using a metabolomic approach with stem cells and evaluation of redox status, Yanes et al. recently found that NPD1 is produced, which in turn showed potent actions at the 10-nanomolar range in promoting neural differentiation as well as cardiac stem cell differentiation (Yanes et al., 2010). Hence, the local molecular response to injury and local inflammation may generate these local mediators,

LX A$_4$ and NPD1, to regulate organ stem cells to initiate tissue repair and regulate the local inflammatory response.

The neuroprotection effects of LX A$_4$ also have been confirmed and extended by others. For example, LX A$_4$ is neuroprotective in experimental stroke (Sobrado et al., 2009), and LX A$_4$ methyl ester reduces neutrophilic infiltration and protects rat brain from focal cerebral ischemia-reperfusion (Ye et al., 2010). In addition to the actions on leukocytes, LX A$_4$ also regulates cytokine production from human astrocytoma cells (Decker et al., 2009). Taken together, these findings in murine systems suggest that the arachidonic acid-derived SPMs, namely lipoxins, are neuroprotective by downregulating local inflammatory response and limiting further inflammation via tissue destruction by limiting neutrophil-mediated tissue damage. Hence, arachidonic acid as substrate and an essential fatty acid plays a role in neuroprotection and particularly one that is regulated by dietary intake of essential fatty acids. Along these lines, Huang et al. reported that intravenous and dietary DHA significantly improves spinal cord injury in rats. Improvements and neuroprotection were obtained when DHA was injected intraveneously with sustained dietary supplementation (Huang et al., 2007).

GAPS IN CURRENT KNOWLEDGE: TOO MUCH OF A GOOD THING?

Recently, using a rat model of TBI, Bailes and Mills (2010) found that dietary supplementation with DHA reduced acceleration of injury. These are encouraging findings suggesting that DHA delivery can have a neuroprotective effect, likely via the local biosynthesis of pro-resolving and anti-inflammatory mediators such as NPD1 and D-series resolvins produced from the exogenous DHA. However, there is a potential negative side for excess delivery of DHA above "optimal dietary levels," the limits of which remain unknown at present. When excess DHA is available to undergo nonenzymatic autooxidation, neurotoxic products can be produced, such as trans-4-hydroxy-2-hexenal (Long et al., 2008). Likewise, in isolated neuroblastoma cells, we recently found that resolvins and protectins are not produced from DHA by these tumor cells in vitro but rather exogenous DHA is converted to hydroperoxy acid intermediates that are cytotoxic (Gleissman et al., 2010). For a cancer cell type, this may be a beneficial approach to killing tumor cells with exogenous DHA. The point taken from these experiments is that excess DHA can lead to oxidation products that can further amplify local inflammation and tissue damage at the cellular level. Along these lines, the enzymatically produced resolvin D1 reduces inflammation initiated by lipid oxidation products (Spite et al., 2009b). Taken together, these results suggest that optimal dietary levels of DHA could enhance production of neuroprotective local mediators. Thus, a clear starting point in humans is to establish the daily dose required for DHA and the levels that ought to be considered in excess for healthy individuals. In this regard, potential gender and age differences need to be taken into consideration for future studies. In considering TBI on the battlefield, the currently available animal results suggest that intravenous delivery of DHA in addition to dietary supplementation can have neuroprotective actions. These neuroprotective actions may be mediated by enhanced local production of resolvins and protectins. Indeed, if local conversion of dietary DHA to resolvins and protectins can be established in humans with TBI and stress, then dietary DHA could speed recovery time for military personnel. Because DHA is a natural product and has been shown in many studies to be safe in humans (Lands, 2005), DHA supplementation can be recommended for military personnel. This also can open the opportunity to gain direct evidence for DHA effectiveness in clinical studies with military personnel (see below).

TABLE C-7 SPM Actions in Animal Disease Models Relevant to TBI and DHA[a]

Disease Model	Species	Action(s)	References
Resolvin E1			
Periodontitis	Rabbit	Reduces neutrophil infiltration; prevents connective tissue and bone loss; promotes healing of diseased tissues; regenerates lost soft tissue and bone	(Hasturk et al., 2006, 2007)
Peritonitis	Mouse	Stops neutrophil recruitment; regulates chemokine/cytokine production Promotes lymphatic removal of phagocytes	(Arita et al., 2005a; Bannenberg et al., 2005; Schwab et al., 2007)
Dorsal air pouch	Mouse	Stops neutrophil recruitment	(Serhan et al., 2000)
Retinopathy	Mouse	Protects against neovascularization	(Connor et al., 2007; Jin et al., 2009)
Colitis	Mouse	Decreases neutrophil recruitment and pro-inflammatory gene expression; improves survival; reduces weight loss	(Arita et al., 2005b)
Pneumonia	Mouse	Improves survival; decreases neutrophil infiltration; enhances bacterial clearance; reduces pro-inflammatory cytokines and chemokines	(Seki et al., 2010)
Resolvin D1			
Peritonitis	Mouse	Stops neutrophil recruitment	(Hong et al., 2003; Spite et al., 2009b; Sun et al., 2007)
Dorsal skin air pouch	Mouse	Stops neutrophil recruitment	(Hong et al., 2003; Serhan et al., 2002)
Kidney ischemia-reperfusion	Mouse	Protects from ischemia-reperfusion-induced kidney damage and loss of function; regulates macrophages and protects from fibrosis	(Duffield et al., 2006)
Retinopathy	Mouse	Protects against neovascularization	(Connor et al., 2007; Jin et al., 2009)
Resolvin D2			
Peritonitis	Mouse	Stops neutrophil recruitment	(Spite et al., 2009a)
Sepsis	Mouse	Improves survival; reduces pro-inflammatory cytokines; regulates neutrophil recruitment; enhances bacterial containment	(Spite et al., 2009a)
Protectin D1			
Peritonitis	Mouse	Stops neutrophil recruitment; regulates chemokine/cytokine production; promotes lymphatic removal of phagocytes; regulates T-cell migration	(Ariel et al., 2005; Arita et al., 2005a; Bannenberg et al., 2005; Schwab et al., 2007)

TABLE C-7 Continued

Disease Model	Species	Action(s)	References
Asthma	Mouse	Protects from lung damage, airway inflammation, and airway hyperresponsiveness	(Levy et al., 2007)
	Human	Protectin D1 is produced in humans and is diminished in asthmatics	(Levy et al., 2007)
Kidney ischemia-reperfusion	Mouse	Protects from ischemia-reperfusion-induced kidney damage and loss of function; regulates macrophages and is anti-fibrotic	(Duffield et al., 2006)
Retinopathy	Mouse	Protects against neovascularization	(Connor et al., 2007)
Ischemic stroke	Rat	Stop leukocyte infiltration, inhibits NF-κB and cyclooxygenase-2 induction	(Marcheselli et al., 2003)
Alzheimer's disease	Human	Diminished protectin D1 production in human Alzheimer's disease	(Lukiw et al., 2005)
Embryonic stem cells	Mouse and human	NPD1 promotes cardiac and neuronal stem cell differentiation	(Yanes et al., 2010)
Neural stem cells	Mouse	LXA$_4$ regulates neuronal stem cell gene expression and proliferation	(Wada et al., 2006)
Acute stroke (focal cerebral ischemia reperfusion)	Rat	LXA$_4$ reduces local infarct volume and apoptosis of neuronal cells; decreases lipid peroxidation and cytokine production	(Ye et al., 2010)
Traumatic brain injury (TBI)	Rat	DHA reduces damage from impact acceleration injury; reduces beta amyloid precursor protein, a marker of axonal injury	(Bailes and Mills, 2010)

[a]The actions of each of the main resolvins and protectins listed were confirmed with compounds prepared by total organic synthesis (see text and cited references for details).

SUMMARY

In summation, acute inflammation initiated by neutrophils in response to injury or microbial invasion is, ideally, a self-limited response that is protective for the host. Excessive uncontrolled inflammatory responses can lead to chronic disorders as well as further tissue injury, as in the case of TBI. Neutrophil-derived pro-inflammatory mediators, including leukotrienes and prostaglandins, can amplify this process. Within contained inflammatory exudates, we found that neutrophils change phenotype to initiate resolution and begin to biosynthesize pro-resolving and protective local mediators from essential fatty acids including AA, DHA, and EPA. There is an active catabasis to return tissues to a homeostatic healthy state from the battle of host defense to microbes during inflammatory episodes

(Bannenberg et al., 2005). SPM such as LX, protectins, and resolvins biosynthesized locally from essential fatty acids accelerate this process and the return to tissue homeostasis (Schwab et al., 2007). Each of these SPMs is temporally and spatially biosynthesized to actively regulate resolution by acting on specific receptors (Serhan et al., 2008), initiating anti-inflammatory and pro-resolving signals to terminate the inflammatory response and limit further tissue injury. Hence, dietary essential fatty acids in experimental animal models reviewed herein directly regulate the magnitude and duration of local acute inflammation via the production of potent local chemical mediators that are pro-resolving. These experimental findings in animal models that demonstrate pathophysiologic events relevant to TBI (Table C-7), taken together, suggest that increasing the n-3 essential fatty acids in military personnel to boost their n-3 status may have a positive impact on traumatic tissue injury to limit the magnitude of the response. Helping to optimize the host's response to injury and local inflammation with nutritional substrates also may represent a cost-effective means to reduce recovery times in the field. Our recent findings indicate that resolvins also are potent modulators reducing pain in murine systems (Bang et al., 2010; Sommer and Birklein, 2010; Xu et al., 2010).

The answer to the question "Is there enough evidence from TBI animal models to conclude that military personnel should boost their n-3 status to protect against the effects of TBI?" is yes, but additional information from both human and animal studies is needed to directly support the cause-and-effect relationships between increasing DHA status and reducing TBI and other indications in military personnel. Because the identification of DHA metabolome in resolution of acute inflammation with the production of potent local protective and anti-inflammatory mediators in murine systems is relatively recent (see Serhan, 2007), additional results are needed to establish cause-and-effect relationships in TBI and, for example, increased resolvins and neuroprotectins or SPM and reduced tissue inflammation and local damage. The results reviewed herein suggest that the protective actions of DHA in rat TBI (Bailes and Mills, 2010) are mediated locally by resolvins and protectins, given their potent actions in in vivo models of inflammation in animals (Table C-7).

With these metabolomic tools and structures now available in synthetic form (Serhan, 2010), these suggestions can be directly tested rigorously in the field to assess their validity for military implementation. For example, human studies are needed to establish:

- Is DHA a "green pro-drug"? Is it converted locally with trauma to D-series resolvins and protectins, which in turn are bioactive mediators that limit tissue inflammation and further tissue damage?
- What is the relationship between serum/plasma DHA levels and reduced TBI and/ or ear injury in military personnel? Is there a gender selectivity for DHA conversion, actions, and overall impact?
- Do resolvins and/or protectins from DHA mediate cellular protection and reduce TBI damage and recovery time?
- Can excess serum DHA levels lead to enhanced autooxidation pathways in stressed military personnel or protection and enhanced SPM biosynthesis?
- What are the pathway biomarkers for resolvins and protectins that can be monitored in peripheral blood of military personnel? For example, do 17-HDHA, 14-HDHA, 22-hydroxy-DHA, RvD5, 7,17-diHDHA, NPD1, RvD1, or RvD2 correlate with DHA levels and/or the degree of protection in TBI and/or ear trauma? Do they reduce recovery times for military personnel?

In addition to these human studies, mechanism of action studies can be carried out with animal experiments. These also can include direct comparisons between administration of NPD1, RvD1, RvD2 versus DHA in animal models of TBI and ear injury. The role of substrate (e.g., DHA) levelscan be assessed in transgenic mice with elevated tissue DHA such as the fat-1 mouse (Hudert et al., 2006), which show protection from inflammatory disorders as well as elevated levels of resolvins and protectins. Murine models with transgenic over-expressing proresolving receptors (Devchand et al., 2003; Krishnamoorthy et al., 2010) can be used to determine the role of resolvin receptors in protection from TBI. These animal and human studies can be implemented in parallel to increase the DHA status in military personnel in order to gain mechanistic insight and fill gaps in current knowledge of the role of essential fatty acids and n-3 status in reducing trauma and shortening the time required for recovery of military personnel.

ACKNOWLEDGMENTS

The authors thank Mary H. Small for expert assistance with manuscript preparation and the members of the laboratory and collaborators for their expertise and efforts in the reports referenced herein. Research in the author's laboratory reviewed here was supported by National Institutes of Health grants DK-074448 and GM-38765 (C.N.S).

Conflict of Interest Statement

The author is inventor on patents assigned to Brigham and Women's Hospital and Partners HealthCare on the composition of matter, uses, and clinical development of anti-inflammatory and pro-resolving lipid mediators. These are licensed for clinical development. The author retains founder stock in Resolvyx Pharmaceuticals.

ABBREVIATIONS

AA	arachidonic acid
AT-RvD1	aspirin-triggered-resolvin D1, 7S,8R,17R-trihydroxy-docosa-4Z,9E,11E,13Z,15E,19Z-hexaenoic acid
DHA	docosahexaenoic acid
EPA	eicosapentaenoic acid
LX	lipoxin
LXA_4	5S, 6R,15S-trihydroxy-7,9,13-trans-11-cis-eicosatetraenoic acid
PD1/NPD1	protectin D1/neuroprotectin D1, 10R,17S-dihydroxy-docosa-4Z,7Z,11E,13E,15Z,19Z-hexaenoic acid
PMN	polymorphonuclear leukocytes
Protectins	biosynthesized from DHA, containing conjugated triene structures and are protective mediators
PUFA	polyunsaturated fatty acid
Resolvins	structurally unique and potent bioactive local mediators; E series from EPA and D series from DHA
RvD1	resolvin D1, 7S,8R,17S-trihydroxy-4Z,9E,11E,13Z,15E,19Z-docosahexaenoic acid
RvD2	resolvin D2, 7S,16R,17S-trihydroxy-4Z,8E,10Z,12E,14E,19Z-docosahexaenoic acid
RvE1	resolvin E1, 5S,12R,18R-trihydroxy-6Z,8E,10E,14Z,16E-eicosapentaenoic acid

REFERENCES

Ariel, A., P.-L. Li, W. Wang, W.-X. Tang, G. Fredman, S. Hong, K. H. Gotlinger, and C. N. Serhan. 2005. The docosatriene protectin D1 is produced by TH2 skewing and promotes human T cell apoptosis via lipid raft clustering. *The Journal of Biomedical Chemistry* 280:43079–43086.

Arita, M., F. Bianchini, J. Aliberti, A. Sher, N. Chiang, S. Hong, R. Yang, N. A. Petasis, and C. N. Serhan. 2005a. Stereochemical assignment, anti-inflammatory properties, and receptor for the omega-3 lipid mediator resolvin E1. *The Journal of Experimental Medicine* 201:713–722.

Arita, M., M. Yoshida, S. Hong, E. Tjonahen, J. N. Glickman, N. A. Petasis, R. S. Blumberg, and C. N. Serhan. 2005b. Resolvin E1, an endogenous lipid mediator derived from omega-3 eicosapentaenoic acid, protects against 2,4,6-trinitrobenzene sulfonic acid-induced colitis. *Proceedings of the National Academies of Sciences of the United States of America* 102:7671–7676.

Arita, M., S. Oh, T. Chonan, S. Hong, S. Elangovan, Y.-P. Sun, J. Uddin, N. A. Petasis, and C. N. Serhan. 2006. Metabolic inactivation of resolvin E1 and stabilization of its anti-inflammatory actions. *The Journal of Biomedical Chemistry* 281:22847–22854.

Arita, M., T. Ohira, Y. P. Sun, S. Elangovan, N. Chiang, and C. N. Serhan. 2007. Resolvin E1 selectively interacts with leukotriene B_4 receptor BLT1 and chemR23 to regulate inflammation. *Journal of Immunology* 178:3912–3917.

Bailes, J. E., and J. D. Mills. 2010. Docosahexaenoic acid (DHA) reduces traumatic axonal injury in a rodent head injury model. *Journal of Neurotrauma* 27(9):1617–1624.

Bang, S., S. Yoo, T. J. Yang, H. Cho, Y. G. Kim, and S. W. Hwang. 2010. Resolvin D1 attenuates activation of sensory transient receptor potential channels leading to multiple anti-nociception. *British Journal of Pharmacology* 161:707–720.

Bannenberg, G. L., N. Chiang, A. Ariel, M. Arita, E. Tjonahen, K. H. Gotlinger, S. Hong, and C. N. Serhan. 2005. Molecular circuits of resolution: Formation and actions of resolvins and protectins. *Journal of Immunology* 174:4345–4355.

Bazan, N. G., J. M. Calandria, and C. N. Serhan. 2010. Rescue and repair during photoreceptor cell renewal mediated by docosahexaenoic acid-derived neuroprotectin D1. *Journal of Lipid Research* 51:2018–2031.

Blaho, V. A., M. W. Buczynski, C. R. Brown, and E. A. Dennis. 2009. Lipidomic analysis of dynamic eicosanoid responses during the induction and resolution of Lyme arthritis. *The Journal of Biomedical Chemistry* 284:21599–21612.

Brennan, F. M., and I. B. McInnes. 2008. Evidence that cytokines play a role in rheumatoid arthritis. *Journal of Clinical Investigation* 118(11):3537–3545.

Campbell, E. L., N. A. Louis, S. E. Tomassetti, G. O. Canny, M. Arita, C. N. Serhan, and S. P. Colgan. 2007. Resolvin E1 promotes mucosal surface clearance of neutrophils: A new paradigm for inflammatory resolution. *The Journal of the Federation of American Societies for Experimental Biology* 21:3162–3170.

Canny, G., O. Levy, G. T. Furuta, S. Narravula-Alipati, R. B. Sisson, C. N. Serhan, and S. P. Colgan. 2002. Lipid mediator-induced expression of bactericidal/permeability-increasing protein (bpi) in human mucosal epithelia. *Proceedings of the National Academies of Sciences of the United States of America* 99:3902–3907.

Cassatella, M. A., ed. 2003. *The neutrophil*. Vol. 83, *Chemical Immunology and Allergy*. Basel: Karger.

Chen, P., B. Fenet, S. Michaud, N. Tomczyk, E. Véricel, M. Lagarde, and M. Guichardant. 2009. Full characterization of PDX, a neuroprotectin/protectin D1 isomer, which inhibits blood platelet aggregation. *FEBS Letters* 583:3478–3484.

Cohen, J. J., R. C. Duke, V. A. Fadok, and K. S. Sellins. 1992. Apoptosis and programmed cell death in immunity. *Annual Review of Immunology* 10:267–293.

Connor, K. M., J. P. SanGiovanni, C. Lofqvist, C. M. Aderman, J. Chen, A. Higuchi, S. Hong, E. A. Pravda, S. Majchrzak, D. Carper, A. Hellstrom, J. X. Kang, E. Y. Chew, N. N. Salem, Jr., C. N. Serhan, and L. E. H. Smith. 2007. Increased dietary intake of omega-3-polyunsaturated fatty acids reduces pathological retinal angiogenesis. *Nature Medicine* 13:868–873.

Cotran, R. S., V. Kumar, and T. Collins, eds. 1999. *Robbins pathologic basis of disease*. 6th ed. Philadelphia: W.B. Saunders Co.

Decker, Y., G. McBean, and C. Godson. 2009. Lipoxin A_4 inhibits IL-1beta-induced IL-8 and ICAM-1 expression in 1321N1 human astrocytoma cells. *American Journal of Physiology. Cell Physiology* 296:1420–1427.

Dennis, E. A. 2000. Phospholipase A_2 in eicosanoid generation. *American Journal of Respiratory and Critical Care Medicine* 161:S32–S35.

Devchand, P. R., M. Arita, S. Hong, G. Bannenberg, R.-L. Moussignac, K. Gronert, and C. N. Serhan. 2003. Human ALX receptor regulates neutrophil recruitment in transgenic mice: Roles in inflammation and host-defense. *The Journal of the Federation of American Societies for Experimental Biology* 17:652–659.

Duffield, J. S., S. Hong, V. Vaidya, Y. Lu, G. Fredman, C. N. Serhan, and J. V. Bonventre. 2006. Resolvin D series and protectin D1 mitigate acute kidney injury. *Journal of Immunology* 177:5902–5911.

Flower, R. J. 2003. The development of COX2 inhibitors. *Nature Reviews Drug Discovery* 2(3):179–191.

Gleissman, H., R. Yang, K. Martinod, M. Lindskog, C. N. Serhan, J. I. Johnsen, and P. Kogner. 2010. Docosahexaenoic acid metabolome in neural tumors: Identification of cytotoxic intermediates. *The Journal of the Federation of American Societies for Experimental Biology* 24:906–915.

Godson, C., S. Mitchell, K. Harvey, N. A. Petasis, N. Hogg, and H. R. Brady. 2000. Cutting edge: Lipoxins rapidly stimulate nonphlogistic phagocytosis of apoptotic neutrophils by monocyte-derived macrophages. *Journal of Immunology* 164:1663–1667.

González-Périz, A., R. Horrillo, N. Ferre, K. Gronert, B. Dong, E. Moran-Salvador, E. Titos, M. Martinez-Clemente, M. Lopez-Parra, V. Arroyo, and J. Claria. 2009. Obesity-induced insulin resistance and hepatic steatosis are alleviated by omega-3 fatty acids: A role for resolvins and protectins. *The Journal of the Federation of American Societies for Experimental Biology* 23(6):1946–1957.

Gronert, K., N. Maheshwari, N. Khan, I. R. Hassan, M. Dunn, and M. L. Schwartzman. 2005. A role for the mouse 12/15-lipoxygenase pathway in promoting epithelial wound healing and host defense. *Journal of Biological Chemistry* 280:15267–15278.

Hassan, I. R., and K. Gronert. 2009. Acute changes in dietary omega-3 and omega-6 polyunsaturated fatty acids have a pronounced impact on survival following ischemic renal injury and formation of renoprotective docosahexaenoic acid-derived protectin D1. *Journal of Immunology* 182:3223–3232.

Hasturk, H., A. Kantarci, T. Ohira, M. Arita, N. Ebrahimi, N. Chiang, N. A. Petasis, B. D. Levy, C. N. Serhan, and T. E. Van Dyke. 2006. RvE1 protects from local inflammation and osteoclast mediated bone destruction in periodontitis. *The Journal of the Federation of American Societies for Experimental Biology* 20:401–403.

Hasturk, H., A. Kantarci, E. Goguet-Surmenian, A. Blackwood, C. Andry, C. N. Serhan, and T. E. Van Dyke. 2007. Resolvin E1 regulates inflammation at the cellular and tissue level and restores tissue homeostasis in vivo. *Journal of Immunology* 179:7021–7029.

Hibbeln, J. R. 1998. Fish consumption and major depression. *Lancet* 351:1213.

Hong, S., K. Gronert, P. Devchand, R.-L. Moussignac, and C. N. Serhan. 2003. Novel docosatrienes and 17s-resolvins generated from docosahexaenoic acid in murine brain, human blood and glial cells: Autacoids in anti-inflammation. *Journal of Biological Chemistry* 278:14677–14687.

Hong, S., E. Tjonahen, E. L. Morgan, L. Yu, C. N. Serhan, and A. F. Rowley. 2005. Rainbow trout (*Oncorhynchus mykiss*) brain cells biosynthesize novel docosahexaenoic acid-derived resolvins and protectins—mediator lipidomic analysis. *Prostaglandins & Other Lipid Mediators* 78:107–116.

Huang, W. L., V. R. King, O. E. Curran, S. C. Dyall, R. E. Ward, N. Lal, J. V. Priestley, and A. T. Michael-Titus. 2007. A combination of intravenous and dietary docosahexaenoic acid significantly improves outcome after spinal cord injury. *Brain Research* 130:3004–3019.

Hudert, C. A., K. H. Weylandt, J. Wang, Y. Lu, S. Hong, A. Dignass, C. N. Serhan, and J. X. Kang. 2006. Transgenic mice rich in endogenous n-3 fatty acids are protected from colitis. *Proceedings of the National Academies of Sciences of the United States of America* 103:11276–11281.

Jin, Y., M. Arita, Q. Zhang, D. R. Saban, S. K. Chauhan, N. Chiang, C. N. Serhan, and R. Dana. 2009. Anti-angiogenesis effect of the novel anti-inflammatory and pro-resolving lipid mediators. *Investigative Ophthalmology and Visual Science* 50(10):4743–4752.

Kasuga, K., R. Yang, T. F. Porter, N. Agrawal, N. A. Petasis, D. Irimia, M. Toner, and C. N. Serhan. 2008. Rapid appearance of resolvin precursors in inflammatory exudates: Novel mechanisms in resolution. *Journal of Immunology* 181(12):8677–8687.

Koopman, W. J., and L. W. Moreland. 2005. *Arthritis and allied conditions: A textbook of rheumatology.* 15th ed. Philadelphia, Pa.; London: Lippincott Williams & Wilkins.

Krishnamoorthy, S., A. Recchiuti, N. Chiang, S. Yacoubian, C.-H. Lee, R. Yang, N. A. Petasis, and C. N. Serhan. 2010. Resolvin D1 binds human phagocytes with evidence for pro-resolving receptors. *Proceedings of the National Academies of Sciences of the United States of America* 107:1660–1665.

Lands, W. E. M. 2005. *Fish, omega-3 and human health.* 2nd ed. Champaign, IL: AOCS Press.

Leon, H., M. C. Shibata, S. Sivakumaran, M. Dorgan, T. Chatterley, and R. T. Tsuyuki. 2008. Effect of fish oil on arrhythmias and mortality: Systematic review. *British Medical Journal* 337:a2931.

Levy, B. D., C. B. Clish, B. Schmidt, K. Gronert, and C. N. Serhan. 2001. Lipid mediator class switching during acute inflammation: Signals in resolution. *Nature Immunology* 2:612–619.

Levy, B. D., P. Kohli, K. Gotlinger, O. Haworth, S. Hong, S. Kazani, E. Israel, K. J. Haley, and C. N. Serhan. 2007. Protectin D1 is generated in asthma and dampens airway inflammation and hyper-responsiveness. *Journal of Immunology* 178:496–502.

Libby, P. 2008. Role of inflammation in atherosclerosis associated with rheumatoid arthritis. *American Journal of Medicine* 121(10 Suppl. 1):S21–31.

Long, E. K., T. C. Murphy, L. J. Leiphon, J. Watt, J. D. Morrow, G. L. Milne, J. R. H. Howard, and M. J. Picklo, Sr. 2008. Trans-4-hydroxy-2-hexenal is a neurotoxic product of docosahexaenoic (22:6; n-3) acid oxidation. *Journal of Neurochemistry* 105:714–724.

Lukiw, W. J., J. G. Cui, V. L. Marcheselli, M. Bodker, A. Botkjaer, K. Gotlinger, C. N. Serhan, and N. G. Bazan. 2005. A role for docosahexaenoic acid-derived neuroprotectin D1 in neural cell survival and Alzheimer disease. *Journal of Clinical Investigations* 115:2774–2783.

Majno, G. 1975. *The healing hand: Man and wound in the ancient world.* Cambridge, MA: Harvard University Press.

Majno, G., and I. Joris. 2004. *Cells, tissues, and disease: Principles of general pathology.* 2nd ed. New York: Oxford University Press.

Marcheselli, V. L., S. Hong, W. J. Lukiw, X. Hua Tian, K. Gronert, A. Musto, M. Hardy, J. M. Gimenez, N. Chiang, C. N. Serhan, and N. G. Bazan. 2003. Novel docosanoids inhibit brain ischemia-reperfusion-mediated leukocyte infiltration and pro-inflammatory gene expression. *Journal of Biological Chemistry* 278:43807–43817.

Marcheselli, V. L., P. K. Mukherjee, M. Arita, S. Hong, R. Antony, K. Sheets, N. Petasis, C. N. Serhan, and N. G. Bazan. 2010. Neuroprotectin D1/protectin D1 stereoselective and specific binding with human retinal pigment epithelial cells and neutrophils. *Prostaglandins Leukotrienes and Essential Fatty Acids* 82:27–34.

Morris, T., M. Stables, A. Hobbs, P. de Souza, P. Colville-Nash, T. Warner, J. Newson, G. Bellingan, and D. W. Gilroy. 2009. Effects of low-dose aspirin on acute inflammatory responses in humans. *Journal of Immunology* 183:2089–2096.

Mukherjee, P. K., V. L. Marcheselli, C. N. Serhan, and N. G. Bazan. 2004. Neuroprotectin D1: A docosahexaenoic acid-derived docosatriene protects human retinal pigment epithelial cells from oxidative stress. *Proceedings of the National Academies of Sciences of the United States of America* 101:8491–8496.

Ohira, T., M. Arita, K. Omori, A. Recchiuti, T. E. Van Dyke, and C. N. Serhan. 2009. Resolvin e1 receptor activation signals phosphorylation and phagocytosis. *Journal of Biological Chemistry* 285:3451–3461.

Palmblad, J., R. W. Wannemacher, N. Salem, Jr., D. B. Kuhns, and D. G. Wright. 1988. Essential fatty acid deficiency and neutrophil function: Studies of lipid-free total parenteral nutrition in monkeys. *The Journal of Laboratory and Clinical Medicine* 111(6):634–644.

Poulsen, R. C., K. H. Gotlinger, C. N. Serhan, and M. C. Kruger. 2008. Identification of inflammatory and pro-resolving lipid mediators in bone marrow and their profile alteration with ovariectomy and omega-3 intake. *American Journal of Hematology* 83:437–445.

Qin, Q., K. A. Patil, K. Gronert, and S. C. Sharma. 2008. Neuroprotectin D1 inhibits retinal ganglion cell death following axotomy. *Prostaglandins Leukotrienes and Essential Fatty Acids* 79:201–207.

Riviere, S., L. Challet, D. Fluegge, M. Spehr, and I. Rodriguez. 2009. Formyl peptide receptor-like proteins are a novel family of vomeronasal chemosensors. *Nature* 459(7246):574–577.

Salem, N., Jr., B. Litman, H. Y. Kim, and K. Gawrisch. 2001. Mechanisms of action of docosahexaenoic acid in the nervous system. *Lipids* 36(9):945–959.

Samuelsson, B., S. E. Dahlen, J. A. Lindgren, C. A. Rouzer, and C. N. Serhan. 1987. Leukotrienes and lipoxins: Structures, biosynthesis, and biological effects. *Science* 237(4819):1171–1176.

Schwab, J. M., N. Chiang, M. Arita, and C. N. Serhan. 2007. Resolvin E1 and protectin D1 activate inflammation-resolution programmes. *Nature* 447:869–874.

Seki, H., K. Fukunaga, M. Arita, H. Arai, H. Nakanishi, R. Taguchi, T. Miyasho, R. Takamiya, K. Asano, A. Ishizaka, J. Takeda, and B. D. Levy. 2010. The anti-inflammatory and proresolving mediator resolvin E1 protects mice from bacterial pneumonia and acute lung injury. *Journal of Immunology* 184(2):836–843.

Serhan, C. N., guest ed. 2005. Special issue on lipoxins and aspirin-triggered lipoxins. *Prostaglandins Leukotrienes and Essential Fatty Acids* 73(3–4):139–321.

Serhan, C. N. 2007. Resolution phases of inflammation: Novel endogenous anti-inflammatory and pro-resolving lipid mediators and pathways. *Annual Reviews in Immunology* 25:101–137.

Serhan, C. N. 2010. Novel resolution mechanisms in acute inflammation: To resolve or not? *American Journal of Pathology* 177(4):1576–1591.

Serhan, C. N., and N. Chiang. 2008. Endogenous pro-resolving and anti-inflammatory lipid mediators: A new pharmacologic genus. *British Journal of Pharmacology* 153(Suppl. 1):S200–215.

Serhan, C. N., and J. Savill. 2005. Resolution of inflammation: The beginning programs the end. *Nature Immunology* 6:1191–1197.

Serhan, C. N., C. B. Clish, J. Brannon, S. P. Colgan, N. Chiang, and K. Gronert. 2000. Novel functional sets of lipid-derived mediators with antiinflammatory actions generated from omega-3 fatty acids via cyclooxygenase 2-nonsteroidal antiinflammatory drugs and transcellular processing. *Journal of Experimental Medicine* 192:1197–1204.

Serhan, C. N., S. Hong, K. Gronert, S. P. Colgan, P. R. Devchand, G. Mirick, and R.-L. Moussignac. 2002. Resolvins: A family of bioactive products of omega-3 fatty acid transformation circuits initiated by aspirin treatment that counter pro-inflammation signals. *Journal of Experimental Medicine* 196:1025–1037.

Serhan, C. N., K. Gotlinger, S. Hong, Y. Lu, J. Siegelman, T. Baer, R. Yang, S. P. Colgan, and N. A. Petasis. 2006. Anti-inflammatory actions of neuroprotectin D1/protectin D1 and its natural stereoisomers: Assignments of dihydroxy-containing docosatrienes. *Journal of Immunology* 176:1848–1859.

Serhan, C. N., N. Chiang, and T. E. Van Dyke. 2008. Resolving inflammation: Dual anti-inflammatory and pro-resolution lipid mediators. *Nature Reviews. Immunology* 8:249–261.

Serhan, C. N., R. Yang, K. Martinod, K. Kasuga, P. S. Pillai, T. F. Porter, S. F. Oh, and M. Spite. 2009. Maresins: Novel macrophage mediators with potent anti-inflammatory and pro-resolving actions. *Journal of Experimental Medicine* 206:15–23.

Simopoulos, A. P. 2008. The importance of the omega-6/omega-3 fatty acid ratio in cardiovascular disease and other chronic diseases. *Experimental Biology and Medicine (Maywood, NJ)* 233(6):674–688.

Singer, P., H. Shapiro, M. Theilla, R. Anbar, J. Singer, and J. Cohen. 2008. Anti-inflammatory properties of omega-3 fatty acids in critical illness: Novel mechanisms and an integrative perspective. *Intensive Care Medicine* 34(9):1580–1592.

Sobrado, M., M. P. Pereira, I. Ballesteros, O. Hurtado, D. Fernández-López, J. M. Pradillo, J. R. Caso, J. Vivancos, F. Nombela, J. Serena, I. Lizasoain, and M. A. Moro. 2009. Synthesis of lipoxin A_4 by 5-lipoxygenase mediates PPARgamma-dependent, neuroprotective effects of rosiglitazone in experimental stroke. *Journal of Neuroscience* 29(12):3875–3884.

Sommer, C., and F. Birklein. 2010. Fighting off pain with resolvins. *Nature. Medicine* 16:518–520.

Spite, M., L. V. Norling, L. Summers, R. Yang, D. Cooper, N. A. Petasis, R. J. Flower, M. Perretti, and C. N. Serhan. 2009a. Resolvin D2 is a potent regulator of leukocytes and controls microbial sepsis. *Nature* 461:1287–1291.

Spite, M., L. Summers, T. F. Porter, S. Srivastava, A. Bhatnagar, and C. N. Serhan. 2009b. Resolvin D1 controls inflammation initiated by glutathione-lipid conjugates formed during oxidative stress. *British Journal of Pharmacology* 158:1062–1073.

Starosta, V., K. Pazdrak, I. Boldogh, T. Svider, and A. Kurosky. 2008. Lipoxin A_4 counterregulates GM-CSF signaling in eosinophilic granulocytes. *Journal of Immunology* 181(12):8688–8699.

Sun, Y.-P., S. F. Oh, J. Uddin, R. Yang, K. Gotlinger, E. Campbell, S. P. Colgan, N. A. Petasis, and C. N. Serhan. 2007. Resolvin D1 and its aspirin-triggered 17R epimer: Stereochemical assignments, anti-inflammatory properties and enzymatic inactivation. *Journal of Biological Chemistry* 282:9323–9334.

Tabas, I. 2010. Macrophage death and defective inflammation resolution in atherosclerosis. *Nature Reviews in Immunology* 10:36–46.

Van Dyke, T. E., and C. N. Serhan. 2006. A novel approach to resolving inflammation. *Scientific American presents Oral and Whole Body Health*: 42–45.

Wada, K., M. Arita, A. Nakajima, K. Katayama, C. Kudo, Y. Kamisaki, and C. N. Serhan. 2006. Leukotriene B_4 and lipoxin A_4 are regulatory signals for neural stem cell proliferation and differentiation. *The Journal of the Federation of American Societies for Experimental Biology* 20:1785–1792.

Xu, Z.-Z., L. Zhang, T. Liu, J.-Y. Park, T. Berta, R. Yang, C. N. Serhan, and R.-R. Ji. 2010. Resolvins RvE1 and RvD1 attenuate inflammatory pain via central and peripheral actions. *Nature Medicine* 16:592–597.

Yanes, O., J. Clark, D. M. Wong, G. G. Patti, A. Sánchez-Ruiz, H. P. Benton, S. A. Trauger, C. Desponts, S. Ding, and G. Siuzdak. 2010. Metabolic oxidation regulates embryonic stem cell differentiation. *Nature Chemical Biology* 6(6):411–417.

Ye, X.-H., Y. Wu, P.-P. Guo, J. Wang, S.-Y. Yuan, Y. Shang, and S.-L. Yao. 2010. Lipoxin a_4 analogue protects brain and reduces inflammation in a rat model of focal cerebral ischemia reperfusion. *Brain Research* 1323:174–183.

Potential Efficacy and Mechanism of Action of the Flavanol (–)-Epicatechin in Acute Brain Trauma[22]

Sylvain Doré[23]

OVERVIEW

One objective of this research effort over the years has been to provide an integrated mechanism for research into the potential benefits, mechanism(s), and optimal doses of plant-derived flavonoids for the prevention or mitigation of neurologically based illness.

[22] This work is supported in part by grants from the National Institutes of Health R21AT005085, 1R21AT005246.

[23] Center for Translational Research in Neurodegenerative Disease, University of Florida College of Medicine.

Although many of the polyphenols and flavonoids have been suggested to provide neuro-protection via direct antioxidant properties, we propose that some of these compounds, instead, activate an endogenous cellular pathway that builds resistance to free radical and inflammatory brain damage. More specifically, we have recently reported that the flavanol, (–)-epicatechin, which is naturally enriched in some standardized dark chocolate products, may protect the brain after a stroke by increasing cellular signals already known to protect nerve cells from damage. Ninety minutes after feeding mice a single modest dose of epicatechin, we induced an ischemic stroke by almost entirely cutting off blood supply to the animals' brains. In the animals that had ingested the epicatechin, we found they had suffered significantly less brain damage than those that had not received the compound. Although most treatments against stroke in humans must be given within a 2- to 3-hour time window to be effective, epicatechin appeared to limit further neuronal damage when given to mice 3.5 hours after a stroke, but not at 6 hours after a stroke. We further showed that intra-cellular Nrf2/heme oxygenase 1 pathways appear to be of importance because eliminating one or the other abolished most protective epicatechin effects. Thus, by using preclinical models, we can begin to address the efficacy and mechanisms of action, necessary first steps in planning translational clinical tests in humans and helping health-care providers and the public understand how such bioactive nutrients may have both preventive and therapeutic beneficial effects. This work provides an understanding of the pathways by which natural bioactive compounds such as epicatechin can shield nerve cells in the brain from damage provoked by stroke, brain trauma, or age-related neurodegenerative disorders.

BACKGROUND

Polyphenols are found in most plant-derived foods and beverages, and add to the sensory and nutritional qualities of foods. More than 8,000 polyphenolic structures have been identified, but edible plants contain only several hundred of those known (Bravo, 1998; Manach et al., 2004; Ross and Kasum, 2002). They are often involved in the plant's defensive response against different types of stress, such as ultraviolet radiation, pathogens, and physical damage (Bravo, 1998; Manach et al., 2004). Because plants usually produce these polyphenols as a defensive mechanism, environmental conditions, such as soil type, sun exposure, and rainfall, along with other characteristics such as genetic factors, germination, degree of ripeness, processing and storage, and species variety, can affect the polyphenol concentration (Bravo, 1998; Manach et al., 2004; Ross and Kasum, 2002). Even pieces of fruit from the same tree can have substantial differences in their polyphenol concentrations, owing to diverse exposures to sunlight or other environmental factors. Because of the large variability, the content of polyphenols in foods is usually poorly characterized (Manach et al., 2004).

All polyphenols contain an aromatic ring with one or more hydroxyl group. Most also have at least one sugar residue (a glycoside) attached to the hydroxyl groups. They are classified into different groups depending on the number of phenol rings and chemical groups bound to the rings (Bravo, 1998; Manach et al., 2004; Ross and Kasum, 2002). Polyphenols are found in a wide range of molecular sizes. For example, phenolic acids are simple compounds, whereas the tannins are highly polymerized molecules (Bravo, 1998). Flavonoids make up most of the polyphenols and form the most biologically active group in mammals (Bravo, 1998). Table C-8 summarizes the main classes of polyphenols, some representative phenolics in the groups, and their dietary sources.

Polyphenols are usually recognized for their purported antioxidant capabilities. In test tubes, polyphenols (often at high pharmacological levels) can react with radicals to form

TABLE C-8 Major Subclasses of Polyphenols, Compounds, and Food Sources

Polyphenol Group	Representative compounds	Common sources
Flavonoid		
Flavonols	Quercetin, myricetin, kaempferol	Onions, apples, kale, red wine, green and black tea, broccoli, berries
Flavanones	Hesperetin, naringenin, eriodictyol, tangeretin	Citrus fruit, tomatoes, mint
Flavanols-Flavan-3-ol (proanthocyanidins and catechins)	Epicatechin, epigallocatechin, epicatechin-3-gallate	Apricots, green and black tea, red wine, peanut skins, chocolate
Anthocyanins	Cyanidin, pelargonidin, malvidin, dephinidin	Berries, grapes, wine, tea, eggplant, cabbage, beans, onions, radishes
Isoflavones	Genistein, diadzein, glycitein (phytoestrogens)	Lentils, chickpeas, alfalfa, clover, flaxseed, soybeans
Flavones	Apigenin, luteolin, diosmetin, tangeretin, nobiletin, sinensetin, wogonin	Parsley, thyme, celery, citrus fruit rind
Phenolic acid		
Benzoic acid derivative	Gallic acid, vanillic, syringic, hydroxybenzoic	Tea, strawberries, raspberries, blackberries, black radish, onions
Cinnamic acid derivative	p-coumaric, caffeic, ferulic, sinapic acids, vanillin, syringaldehyde, p-hydroxybenzaldehyde	Blueberries, kiwis, plums, cherries, apples, cereal grains, coffee
Lignan	Secoisolariciresinol	Linseed, lentils, cereals, garlic, asparagus, carrots, pears, prunes
Stilbene	Resveratrol	Grapes, red wine
Saponin	Ginsenoside	Ginseng root
Other	Curcumin	Turmeric

polyphenol radicals, which are more stable and less reactive because of the ability of the phenol group to absorb extra electrons. Most polyphenols are conjugated by methylation, sulfation, or glucuronidation during metabolism. The antioxidant capability can be determined by the type of conjugate and its location on the polyphenol structure (Bravo, 1998; Esposito et al., 2002; Manach et al., 2004; Nijveldt et al., 2001; Williams et al., 2004). In addition to their antioxidant ability, at high concentrations the polyphenols can inhibit the activities of several enzymes, including lipoxygenase, cyclooxygenase, xanthine oxidase, phospholipase A_2, ATPases, aldole reductase, phoshodiesterases, topoisomerase I and II, protein kinase C, phosphoinositide 3-kinase, protein kinase B (Akt/PKB), and mitogen-activated protein kinases (Esposito et al., 2002; Korkina and Afanas'ev, 1997; Nijveldt et al., 2001; Skibola and Smith, 2000; Williams et al., 2004). Some polyphenols have weak estrogenic properties, and others can inhibit the enzymes involved in estrogen metabolism, aromatase, and 17β-hydroxysteroid oxidoductase (Skibola and Smith, 2000).

The reduction of several diseases has been linked to polyphenols. Cardioprotection and a reduction in the incidence of certain types of cancer have been correlated with consumption of phenolic antioxidants (Bravo, 1998; Ross and Kasum, 2002; Skibola and Smith, 2000). Evidence also indicates that polyphenols have antiallergenic, antiviral, antibiotic, antidiarrheal, antiulcer, and anti-inflammatory properties. Polyphenols have been used to treat hypertension, vascular fragility, allergies, and hypercholesterolemia (Bravo, 1998; Korkina and Afanas'ev, 1997; Nijveldt et al., 2001), and have been implicated in the prevention of neurodegenerative diseases by their ability to protect neurons against oxidative stress. Even ascorbate, at concentrations 10-fold higher than those of the polyphenols, did not offer as much neuroprotection (Esposito et al., 2002; Williams et al., 2004). Polyphenols attenuate ischemia–reperfusion injury, suggesting that they might interfere with nitric oxide synthase activity, thereby inhibiting lipid peroxidation, decreasing the number of immobilized leukocytes during reperfusion, and reducing complement activation, resulting in a diminished inflammatory response (Nijveldt et al., 2001). In addition to their antioxidant actions, they also influence neuroprotective and neurorestorative signal transduction mechanisms (Williams et al., 2004).

Epidemiological studies show an inverse relationship between stroke and polyphenol consumption (Ross and Kasum, 2002). The dietary intake of polyphenols varies greatly among different societies. Isoflavone intake from soy consumption ranges from 20 to 240 mg/day for Asians and from 1 to 9 mg/day in the United States and Western populations (Manach et al., 2004; Skibola and Smith, 2000). Agricultural practices also can affect dietary intake of polyphenols. A region where a particular plant is grown will probably have the greatest consumption (Manach et al., 2004). The total consumption of flavonols, flavanones, flavanols, and isoflavones in Western cultures is estimated to be 100 to 150 mg/day. An accurate estimate of dietary intake of all polyphenols ingested is difficult to attain because of poor characterization of polyphenols in foods and the great variability of polyphenol concentration and "quality" within foods (Manach et al., 2004).

DISEASE STATES THAT ARE POTENTIALLY PREVENTABLE OR TREATABLE WITH FLAVONOIDS

Inflammatory Pain

Chronic pain is a leading cause of disability and high health-care costs in North America, Europe, and Australia. Although it is likely to be a significant problem in the developing countries as well, epidemiological data are not easily accessible. A recent systematic review of 13 studies reported the prevalence of chronic pain in developed nations to range from 10 percent to 55 percent (Harstall and Ospina, 2003). These data indicate a higher prevalence of chronic pain among females than males. It is estimated that the annual cost of medical care and lost productivity in the United States as a result of chronic pain is estimated at $120 billion (Harstall and Ospina, 2003). With the aging of the "baby boomers," the incidence and cost of pain management is likely to increase. Pain practitioners have recognized that chronic pain is not merely a symptom, but is a disease with far-reaching consequences on several aspects of life: mood, concentration, motor performance, sleep, and social relations.

Arthritis ranks among the most common chronic pain conditions in the elderly, with studies suggesting that about half of Americans over 65 years suffer from the disease (CDC, 2003; Feinglass et al., 2003). Although the elderly have the highest risk, approximately two-thirds of those afflicted with arthritis are below 65 years old. A third of the 66 million Americans with arthritis must restrict their daily activities because of pain (Verbrugge and Juarez, 2006). A variety of disease states, such as rheumatoid arthritis, osteoarthritis, ankylosing spondylitis, lupus, and inflammatory bowel disease (e.g., Crohn's disease and ulcerative colitis), are associated with inflammation of joints, resulting in pain, swelling, and loss of function in the affected limbs. Felson (2004) recently reviewed factors associated with pain in those with osteoarthritis. Those with pain were more likely to have effusions, bone marrow edema, synovitis and synovial hypertrophy, and tendinitis and bursitis around the joint. Policy reports from the U.S. Department of Health and Human Services in 2000 called for more research on this common disabling condition.

In terms of overall burden on the population, arthritis ranks high in America and worldwide for medical costs, lost income, and lost years of disability-free life (Murry and Lopez, 1996; Reginster, 2002). Analysis of data from the National Health Interview Survey Disability Supplement Phase Two revealed that arthritis-disabled individuals get out less often than other disabled individuals, and have more disabilities related to personal care, household management, physical tasks, transportation, and work (Verbrugge and Juarez, 2006). The disabilities result in fatigue, long task time, and pain. At the beginning of this century, it was estimated that arthritis treatment in America would exceed 2 percent of the gross domestic product, with estimated medical care costs for people with arthritis of $15 billion annually and total costs (medical care and lost productivity) of almost $65 billion annually (Felson et al., 2000).

Ischemia and Hemorrhagic Stroke

Stroke

Stroke is a major cause of morbidity and mortality across all industrialized countries. It is the third leading cause of death in America and the number one cause of adult disability. A stroke occurs when a blood clot blocks an artery or when a blood vessel breaks, interrupting blood flow to an area of the brain. When either of these things happens, brain cells begin to die and brain damage occurs. As brain cells die, speech, movement, and memory can be lost. How a stroke patient is affected depends on the location of the stroke in the brain and the extent of brain damaged. For example, someone who has a small stroke may experience only minor problems, such as weakness of an arm or leg, whereas larger strokes may cause unilateral paralysis or loss of speech. Some people recover completely from strokes, but more than two-thirds of survivors will have some type of disability.

Types of Stroke

Ischemic Stroke   Although blood clotting is normal and essential for stopping blood loss from wounds, in the case of stroke, blood clots are dangerous because they can block arteries and cut off blood flow, a process called *ischemia*. Ischemia can be caused by embolic and thrombotic strokes. In an *embolic stroke*, a blood clot forms somewhere in the body (usually the heart) and then travels through the bloodstream to the brain, where it eventually travels to a blood vessel small enough to block its passage. The clot lodges there, blocking the blood vessel and causing a stroke. The medical term for this type of blood clot is *embolus*. In *thrombotic stroke*, blood flow is impaired because of blockage to one or more of the arteries that supply blood to the brain. The process leading to this blockage is known as *thrombosis*. Ischemic strokes also can occur as the result of an unhealthy blood vessel clogged with a buildup of fatty deposits and cholesterol. The body regards these buildups as multiple tiny, repeated injuries, and reacts as it would to bleeding from a wound; it responds by forming clots. Initial treatment for ischemic stroke involves removing the blockage and restoring blood flow. Tissue plasminogen activator (t-PA) is a medication that can break up blood clots and restore blood flow when administered within three hours of the event.

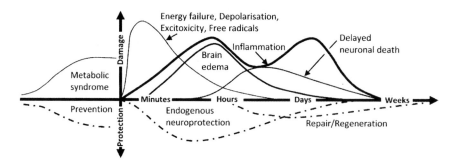

FIGURE C-18 Simplified pathobiology of stroke-induced damage, endogenous repair, and regeneration.
SOURCE: Adapted from Dirnagl et al., 1999.

Hemorrhagic Stroke Strokes caused by the breakage or rupture of a blood vessel in the brain are called *hemorrhagic strokes*. Hemorrhages can be caused by a number of disorders that affect the blood vessels, including long-standing high blood pressure and cerebral aneurysms (weak or thin spots in the vessel wall). Aneurysms, usually present at birth, develop over a number of years, and usually do not cause detectable problems until they break. There are two types of hemorrhagic stroke: *intracerebral* and *subarachnoid*. In an intracerebral hemorrhage, primarily caused by hypertension, bleeding occurs from vessels within the brain itself. In a subarachnoid hemorrhage, an aneurysm bursts in a large artery on or near the thin, delicate membrane surrounding the brain. Blood spills into the area around the brain, thereby contaminating the cerebral spinal fluid that normally surrounds the brain. Treatment for hemorrhagic stroke usually requires surgery to relieve intracranial pressure caused by bleeding. Most of the damage caused by this type of stroke results from the physical disruption of brain tissue. Surgical treatment for hemorrhagic stroke caused by an aneurysm or defective blood vessel can prevent additional strokes. Surgery may be performed to seal off the defective blood vessel and redirect blood flow to other vessels that supply blood to the same region of the brain. Endovascular treatment involves inserting a long, thin, flexible tube (catheter) into a major artery, usually in the thigh, guiding it to the aneurysm or the defective blood vessel, and inserting tiny platinum coils, called *stents*, into the blood vessel through the catheter. Stents support the blood vessel to prevent further damage and additional strokes.

It is likely that the most effective therapeutic intervention should begin as soon as possible after the onset of stroke (Figure C-18). Considering that most stroke patients seek treatment after several hours, an intervention that could limit inflammation and delayed neuronal cell death (apoptosis-like) would be highly desirable. Flavonoids could fill this need by inducing the endogenous system, such as heme oxygenase, which we and others have shown to have antioxidant, anti-inflammatory, and anti-delayed-cell-death activity.

PUTATIVE MECHANISMS OF FLAVONOIDS

It is estimated that 80 percent of strokes are preventable, but there are no simple solutions. Some measures include not smoking, exercising regularly, maintaining an appropriate body weight, and limiting dietary intake of salt, alcohol, and saturated fat. People with hypertension, diabetes, or high cholesterol can reduce their risk for stroke through proper medication and appropriate lifestyle modifications.

A vast amount of recent literature proposes that it is the polyphenols in numerous natural extracts that provide the beneficial effects, and that the benefits are mainly attributable to their potential to act as antioxidants. Among the polyphenols, the most abundant, and those with the greatest bioactivity, are the flavonoids, which are found in natural extracts, plants, and fruits. The antioxidant properties of natural extracts could be associated with the presence of flavonoids. We propose that the antioxidant properties likely result from the initiation of a cascade of intracellular events that lead to activation of endogenous antioxidant pathways. We believe that this mechanism is the most likely, as flavonoids do not reach sufficient plasma levels to neutralize free radicals directly. Consequently, the flavonoids are likely to stimulate an intracellular signaling pathway that leads to cytoprotection (Figure C-19).

Several genes and proteins have been shown to be potential targets of flavonoids. Heme oxygenase (HO) is a strong candidate. We have shown that several polyphenols are potent inducers of HO protein levels, activity, and cytoprotection (Zhuang et al., 2003). The main function of HO is to cleave heme (iron-protoporphyrin-IX). That reaction liberates iron and generates carbon monoxide and biliverdin, which are rapidly converted to bilirubin. Modulation of HO activity and levels most likely provides cytoprotection against free radical damage through degradation of heme (a prooxidant) into biliverdin/bilirubin (antioxidants). Using in vitro and in vivo models, we have shown that HO can be neuroprotective (Doré, 2002). Heme oxygenase and its metabolites also have been associated with antiapoptotic and anti-inflammatory actions, and are known to have a vasodilatory effect.

Several other enzymatic systems have been suggested to be either directly or indirectly

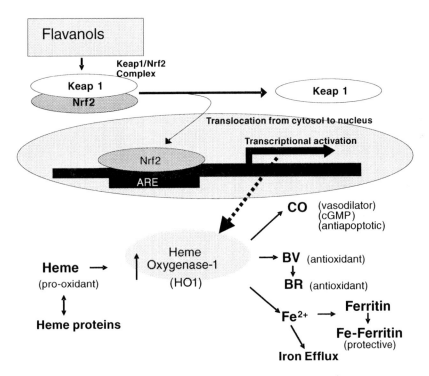

FIGURE C-19 As a working hypothesis, we have proposed that flavonoids can be protective by enhancing the levels of heme oxygenase and, consequently, its multiple beneficial functions.
NOTE: ARE = antioxidant response element, BV = biliverdin, BR = bilirubin, CO = carbon monoxide, Fe^{2+} = ferrous iron, Keap 1 = Kelch-like ECH-associated protein 1, Nrf2 = NF-E2-related factor 2.

modified by different members of the flavonoid family. For example, inflammation and carcinogenesis cause upregulation of cyclooxygenase-2 (COX-2) and tumor necrosis factor alpha (TNFα), which consequently lead to increased production and release of pro-inflammatory prostaglandins and cytokines. The inflammatory response can then activate and sensitize nearby nerve fibers, and result in persistent pain and hyperalgesia (Abbadie, 2005; Mantyh et al., 2002; Sorkin et al., 1997; Watkins et al., 1994; Woolf et al., 1997). Hence, prophylactic or therapeutic interventions aimed at inhibiting COX activity can lead to cytoprotection. A number of flavonoids have shown promising anti-inflammatory properties. For example, using animal models of cancer and inflammation, investigators demonstrated that flavonoids in tea suppress arachidonic acid metabolism, leukotriene production, and COX activity (Huang et al., 2006; Metz et al., 2000). Cyanidin-3-glucoside from blackberries was efficacious in inhibiting COX-2 and TNF expression, an effect that led to inhibition of carcinogenesis (Cooke et al., 2006; Ding et al., 2006). Our published and preliminary studies indicate that flavonoids, such as (–)-epicatechin and cyanidin-3-glucoside, have significant COX-1 and COX-2 inhibitory activities (Seeram et al., 2001). Because COX-1 inhibition can lead to deleterious effects such as gastric bleeding, and COX-2 inhibition has anti-inflammatory effects, it is important to clearly determine the effect of flavonoids on COX enzyme activity from both a therapeutic and safety standpoint.

Here, we propose that the protective properties of flavonoids primarily stem from HO-1 induction, through which they provide the brain with resistance to a variety of neurological stresses (Figure C-20). Flavonoids have been shown to affect cerebral blood flow, cell death, and inflammatory processes, all of which are important therapeutic targets, because they are known to be factors in the development of acute and/or chronic neurodegenerative diseases. These vascular properties become especially important when considering that reduction in cerebral blood flow and lack of oxygen, followed by a reperfusion phase are likely to affect specific neurons and/or the cell types that are particularly vulnerable to free radical damage. Consequently, preventing cell death is likely to have a beneficial effect on the rate of neuroinflammation and its consequences. Considering their actions and favorable effects, one can make a valid hypothesis that polyphenol flavonoids could precondition neurons against induced stress damage.

RATIONALE

One of the most popular explanations given for the benefits of bioactive nutrients is that they have antioxidant properties, but recent conflicting results reported in the literature question the validity of such general statements. Therefore, we have decided to concentrate on better understanding the purported properties of the functional foods by using various methodologies and models. Also, in numerous natural extracts, polyphenols are often cited as the main biologically active (or bioactive) components. Considering the wide variety of compounds included in the polyphenol class, we have decided to focus on the flavonoids. We already have demonstrated the neuroprotective efficacy of some flavonoids, and have developed a working hypothesis to be tested and developed in cellular and in vivo models. The research design of this endeavor will allow us to determine the efficacy of preventive and therapeutic protocols, and optimize the time course and doses with the preclinical models. That information then can be put to the challenge in a clinical trial.

Our research thus far has focused on the effect of flavonoids in ischemic stroke, though such work could be extended to other brain trauma. Again, taking into consideration the purported anti-inflammatory and antioxidant abilities of flavonoids, their actions are likely to have significant influence on the outcome of ischemia in the brain, an organ especially vul-

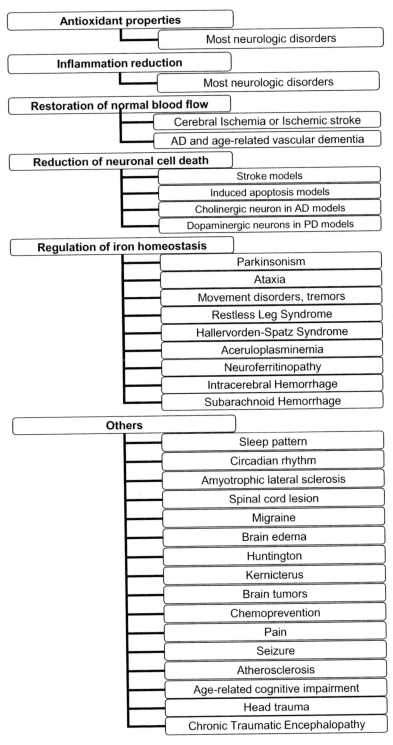

FIGURE C-20 Non-exhaustive list of potential neurological benefits of regulating HO-1 with polyphenols.
SOURCE: Updated from Doré, 2005.

nerable to inflammatory and oxidative stress injury. One of the richest flavonoid-containing foods is cocoa. It has been suggested for centuries to have medicinal properties. It appears to possess nearly twice the antioxidant level of red wine and up to three times that of green tea. The flavonoids in cocoa are principally flavanols, such as epicatechin and catechin. Based on reports that flavonoids have cardioprotective effects through blood flow regulation, their consumption has been suggested for use as potential preventive medicine and for treatment of neurological disorders. Brain cell death in acute and chronic neurodegenerative conditions is suggested to be mediated by free radical damage. Flavonoid structures normally lead one to predict their antioxidant properties, but the underlying cellular mechanisms have not been found. Knowing that the HO enzyme plays various roles in oxidative stress, blood flow, and cell death, we tested the hypothesis that HO activity could participate in flavonoid neuroprotective function. Preliminary results reveal that cultured neurons treated with flavonoids induce HO-1 expression. Pretreatment of neurons is sufficient to provide protection, demonstrating that co-treatment during induced oxidative stress is not necessary. This finding suggests that flavonoids may not be the direct cause of the protection, but that they might induce a neuroprotective pathway. The protective effect of the flavonoids is abolished by an HO inhibitor or a protein synthesis inhibitor. Therefore, specific HO-1 induction may be a novel mechanism by which flavonoids are protective. Our results show that cocoa flavanols affect stroke outcomes. In parallel, we have been investigating mechanisms of action in cultured neurons derived from wild-type control and knockout mice. This was one of the first studies to show a specific pathway by which cocoa-derived flavanol compounds can protect neurons in culture and in the brain. The study also revealed a mechanism by which those compounds might provide the brain resistance in acute and/or chronic neurological disorders.

DISCUSSION

Although the general public is targeted daily with claims that a "natural" compound will reduce inflammation, lessen cognitive decline, boost memory, prevent neurological diseases, etc., individuals and practitioners have the right to know what is effective and what is the proper dose. Moreover, although most claims of efficacy are based on potential antioxidant and anti-inflammatory properties, the most recent critical reviews suggest that such statements are probably inaccurate. There is also the misconception that because these extracts are natural, they do not have side effects, and that the more one consumes, the more benefits one would receive. When these extracts are used in clinical trials, it is important to know the appropriate dose range and maximal dose to be tested. Researchers should take advantage of well-established preclinical models to apply rigorous scientific testing to address these issues. Our goals over the years have been to examine alternative hypotheses regarding the direct antioxidant actions of phytochemicals. We have been investigating an indirect mechanism by which bioactive compounds could build intracellular or organ resistance to free radical damage. Stimulation of an endogenous defense pathway would then attenuate inflammatory and cell death cascades.

Our emphasis here has been based on several factors:

- *Elucidating the underlying mechanisms of action of nutraceutical therapies will facilitate their integration into conventional medical care.* Thus, our goal has been to focus on addressing and testing mechanisms of action based on the most recent research. Accumulation of laboratory data has allowed us to develop hypotheses to be tested, notably on the role of the transcriptional factor Nrf2 and HO as an antioxidant-protective enzyme. We believe that identifying the potential mechanisms of action can contribute to better acceptance and integration of nutraceutical therapies into conventional medicine. The information will be of benefit to both patients and practitioners.

- *Mechanistic studies of nutraceutical therapies will improve the identification of key study endpoints and, thus, will strengthen the design of nutraceutical clinical trials.* Preventive medicine is a strategy by which natural or synthetic chemicals or biological agents are used to prevent health or medical problems before they arise. Despite advances in the treatment of numerous neurological disorders, morbidity and mortality remain high. Because most neurological diseases have no cure, prevention strategies can save many lives. Epidemiological data have suggested that numerous natural, biologically based practices may prevent diseases. Studies in our research laboratories have provided evidence that natural extracts and isolated compounds can be beneficial. Because preventive clinical trials typically require thousands of patients and decades of follow-up, it is important to consider the development of suitable surrogate markers that can be used to monitor the effect of bioactive treatment on a short-term and long-term basis. Efforts from various teams have been devoted to identifying key endpoints and testing potential surrogate markers. Such tools would help the research community to design future clinical trials of nutraceuticals.
- It has been postulated that the *use of adequately defined products and optimal dosage schedules in studies decreases the risk of failures that might discourage further research into otherwise promising modalities.* Therefore, for optimal study design, it is important to: (a) determine active ingredients, pharmacology, bioavailability, and optimal dosing; (b) identify surrogate markers; and (c) assess study feasibility. The goal is that outcomes of such studies will form the basis for designing larger trials with an enhanced ability to detect a meaningful positive effect, if any, of the therapy under study.

Thus, to investigate the mechanisms of action, we have been focusing on one family of active ingredients present in numerous bioactive nutrients—the flavanols and their metabolites. By examining specific compounds, we can test specific hypotheses and potential actions. In so doing, we can better address pharmacology, bioavailability, and optimal dosing of the compounds. Appropriate support will allow various teams of investigators, including our own, to continue designing optimal protocols to use a given compound, will potentially help us to identify surrogate markers, and will certainly allow us to improve feasibility and determine the therapeutic and preventive efficacy of given members of the flavonoid family. We also understand that by testing an active ingredient to better address mechanisms of action, it is also important, in most cases, to test naturally enriched standardized extracts.

In the literature, recent results from various clinical trials of natural biologically active approaches have yielded negative data. These negative results have raised concerns, especially regarding appropriate dosages. Negative results are informative; however, carefully conducted dose-response studies that use preclinical models are needed. In response to the goals of this specific Institute of Medicine study, it is important to use and further develop preclinical models to begin resolving some of these issues that are often associated with bioactive nutraceutical research.

The general public and funding agencies are paying close attention to biologically based practices, including foods and food components, dietary supplements, and functional foods. One of the purported active ingredients often cited in food supplements is a group of compounds called polyphenols. To limit the complexity of this wide family of compounds, we will first focus our efforts on a subset of the polyphenols that is postulated to provide the main bioactivity: the flavonoids. We already have reported substantial evidence regarding the neuroprotective effects of flavonoids in both in vitro and in vivo models, though we recognize that additional research is most likely required. Once mechanisms of action have been better explored and delineated, the plan will be to test these natural compounds and/or enriched extracts. We believe that results from this research endeavor could be applied to various acute neurodegenerative disorders.

CONCLUSIONS

Bioactive nutrients often are used because of their purported beneficial properties, such as free radical scavenging and/or inhibition of enzymes involved in the inflammatory cascade. Although these beneficial effects have been shown in test tubes or in cultured cells, we and others believe that the mechanism responsible for these effects is not through direct neutralization of free radicals. It is unlikely that any of the bioactive compounds or their metabolites reach sufficient levels in the bloodstream to directly fend off free radical-induced cellular damage or inhibit enzymes. Thus, the specific mechanisms of action of most of these compounds are still unknown. Based on our ongoing research, we have been proposing that these compounds, even at very low levels in the organism, would be sufficient to initiate an intracellular defense against environmental or pathological stress. Our central working hypothesis is that flavanols, instead of acting as direct antioxidants, stimulate the Nrf2 pathway and induce an antioxidant/protective enzyme, such as HO-1, thus providing cellular and tissue resistance to damage generated by oxidative stress. We already have found that HO-1 is inducible by the flavanols. HO has been characterized as an antioxidant enzyme that catalyzes the degradation of heme, a prooxidant, into the antioxidants, biliverdin and bilirubin.

By addressing optimal doses, limitations, side effects, and mechanisms of action, such research could help both the general public and health-care providers make informed decisions on whether or not the given biologically active modalities should be accepted for prevention or as adjunct treatment for specific medical conditions. Multidisciplinary approaches, including disciplines such as neurobiology, pharmacology, imaging, biomarkers, and cellular/molecular biology, should be encouraged. We believe that the synergistic projects proposed have potentially high impact and present innovative concepts. The goal is that such efforts would result in synergistic discoveries and optimal plans for the most rigorously executed, randomized clinical trials.

REFERENCES

Abbadie, C. 2005. Chemokines, chemokine receptors and pain. *Trends in Immunology* 26(10):529–534.

Bravo, L. 1998. Polyphenols: Chemistry, dietary sources, metabolism, and nutritional significance. *Nutrition Reviews* 56(11):317–333.

CDC (Centers for Disease Control and Prevention). 2003. Public health and aging: Projected prevalence of self-reported arthritis or chronic joint symptoms among persons aged ≥ 65 years—United States, 2005–2030. *Morbidity and Mortality Weekly Report* 52(21):489–491.

Cooke, D., M. Schwarz, D. Boocock, P. Winterhalter, W. P. Steward, A. J. Gescher, and T. H. Marczylo. 2006. Effect of cyanidin-3-glucoside and an anthocyanin mixture from bilberry on adenoma development in the ApcMin mouse model of intestinal carcinogenesis—relationship with tissue anthocyanin levels. *International Journal of Cancer* 119(9):2213–2220.

Ding, M., R. Feng, S. Y. Wang, L. Bowman, Y. Lu, Y. Qian, V. Castranova, B. H. Jiang, and X. Shi. 2006. Cyanidin-3-glucoside, a natural product derived from blackberry, exhibits chemopreventive and chemotherapeutic activity. *The Journal of Biological Chemistry* 281(25):17359–17368.

Dirnagl, U., C. Iadecola, and M. A. Moskowitz. 1999. Pathobiology of ischaemic stroke: An integrated view. *Trends in Neurosciences* 22(9):391–397.

Doré, S. 2002. Decreased activity of the antioxidant heme oxygenase enzyme: Implications in ischemia and in Alzheimer's disease. *Free Radical Biology & Medicine* 32(12):1276–1282.

Doré, S. 2005. Unique properties of polyphenol stilbenes in the brain: More than direct antioxidant actions; gene/protein regulatory activity. *Neuro-Signals* 14(1–2):61–70.

Esposito, E., D. Rotilio, V. Di Matteo, C. Di Giulio, M. Cacchio, and S. Algeri. 2002. A review of specific dietary antioxidants and the effects on biochemical mechanisms related to neurodegenerative processes. *Neurobiology of Aging* 23(5):719–735.

Feinglass, J., C. Nelson, T. Lawther, and R. W. Chang. 2003. Chronic joint symptoms and prior arthritis diagnosis in community surveys: Implications for arthritis prevalence estimates. *Public Health Reports* 118(3):230–239.

Felson, D. T. 2004. Risk factors for osteoarthritis: Understanding joint vulnerability. *Clinical Orthopaedics and Related Research* 427 (Suppl.):S16–S21.

Felson, D. T., R. C. Lawrence, P. A. Dieppe, R. Hirsch, C. G. Helmick, J. M. Jordan, R. S. Kington, N. E. Lane, M. C. Nevitt, Y. Zhang, M. Sowers, T. McAlindon, T. D. Spector, A. R. Poole, S. Z. Yanovski, G. Ateshian, L. Sharma, J. A. Buckwalter, K. D. Brandt, and J. F. Fries. 2000. Osteoarthritis: New insights. Part 1: The disease and its risk factors. *Annals of Internal Medicine* 133(8):635–646.

Harstall, C., and M. Ospina. 2003. How prevalent is chronic pain? *Pain Clinic Updates* 11(2).

Huang, M. T., Y. Liu, D. Ramji, C. Y. Lo, G. Ghai, S. Dushenkov, and C. T. Ho. 2006. Inhibitory effects of black tea theaflavin derivatives on 12-o-tetradecanoylphorbol-13-acetate-induced inflammation and arachidonic acid metabolism in mouse ears. *Molecular Nutrition and Food Research* 50(2):115–122.

Korkina, L. G., and I. B. Afanas'ev. 1997. Antioxidant and chelating properties of flavonoids. *Advances in Pharmacology* 38:151–163.

Manach, C., A. Scalbert, C. Morand, C. Remesy, and L. Jimenez. 2004. Polyphenols: Food sources and bioavailability. *American Journal of Clinical Nutrition* 79(5):727–747.

Mantyh, P. W., D. R. Clohisy, M. Koltzenburg, and S. P. Hunt. 2002. Molecular mechanisms of cancer pain. *Nature Reviews. Cancer* 2(3):201–209.

Metz, N., A. Lobstein, Y. Schneider, F. Gosse, R. Schleiffer, R. Anton, and F. Raul. 2000. Suppression of azoxymethane-induced preneoplastic lesions and inhibition of cyclooxygenase-2 activity in the colonic mucosa of rats drinking a crude green tea extract. *Nutrition and Cancer* 38(1):60–64.

Murry, D. J., and A. D. E. Lopez. 1996. The global burden of disease: A comprehensive assessment of mortality and disability from disease, injuries, and risk factors in 1990 and projected to 2020. In *Global Burden of Disease and Injury Series, Vol. I*. Cambridge, MA: Harvard School of Public Health.

Nijveldt, R. J., E. van Nood, D. E. van Hoorn, P. G. Boelens, K. van Norren, and P. A. van Leeuwen. 2001. Flavonoids: A review of probable mechanisms of action and potential applications. *American Journal of Clinical Nutrition* 74(4):418–425.

Reginster, J. Y. 2002. The prevalence and burden of arthritis. *Rheumatology (Oxford)* 41(Suppl. 1):3–6.

Ross, J. A., and C. M. Kasum. 2002. Dietary flavonoids: Bioavailability, metabolic effects, and safety. *Annual Review of Nutrition* 22:19–34.

Seeram, N. P., R. A. Momin, M. G. Nair, and L. D. Bourquin. 2001. Cyclooxygenase inhibitory and antioxidant cyanidin glycosides in cherries and berries. *Phytomedicine* 8(5):362–369.

Skibola, C. F., and M. T. Smith. 2000. Potential health impacts of excessive flavonoid intake. *Free Radical Biology & Medicine* 29(3–4):375–383.

Sorkin, L. S., W. H. Xiao, R. Wagner, and R. R. Myers. 1997. Tumour necrosis factor-alpha induces ectopic activity in nociceptive primary afferent fibres. *Neuroscience* 81(1):255–262.

Verbrugge, L. M., and L. Juarez. 2006. Profile of arthritis disability: II. *Arthritis and Rheumatism* 55(1):102–113.

Watkins, L. R., E. P. Wiertelak, L. E. Goehler, K. P. Smith, D. Martin, and S. F. Maier. 1994. Characterization of cytokine-induced hyperalgesia. *Brain Research* 654(1):15–26.

Williams, R. J., J. P. Spencer, and C. Rice-Evans. 2004. Flavonoids: Antioxidants or signalling molecules? *Free Radical Biology & Medicine* 36(7):838–849.

Woolf, C. J., A. Allchorne, B. Safieh-Garabedian, and S. Poole. 1997. Cytokines, nerve growth factor and inflammatory hyperalgesia: The contribution of tumour necrosis factor alpha. *British Journal of Pharmacology* 121(3):417–424.

Zhuang, H., Y. S. Kim, R. C. Koehler, and S. Doré. 2003. Potential mechanism by which resveratrol, a red wine constituent, protects neurons. *Annals of the New York Academy of Sciences* 993:276–286; discussion 287–278.

Overview of Therapeutics for Traumatic Brain Injury

Edward D. Hall[24]

INTRODUCTION

The pathophysiology of traumatic brain injury (TBI) is divisible into two components. The first component is the "primary" mechanical injury to the brain tissue involving the shearing, stretching, or twisting of neuronal axons and dendrites and vascular elements. The only way to minimize this primary mechanical insult involves avoidance of the injury or the use of protective head gear to minimize any blunt impact or penetrating trauma to the skull and brain contained within. The only therapeutic approach to compensating for the brain damage done by the primary mechanical event involves finding a means to (1) stimulate the process of neurogenesis to form new neurons to replace those that have been lost or angiogenesis to form new blood vessels to restore adequate tissue perfusion and oxygen delivery, (2) to enhance the regeneration of the new axons from injured, but surviving, neuronal cell bodies, or (3) to somehow increase the plasticity of the axons and nerve terminals of surviving (i.e., uninjured) neurons so that they can branch and form new synaptic connections to functionally compensate for the degenerated cells and their lost postsynaptic connections. Although a number of pharmacological and gene therapeutic approaches for achieving each of these options are under investigation, the translation of these to clinical use is still many years away.

The second component of the TBI-induced brain damage involves a complex pathophysiological cascade of events that is set in motion by the primary injury, develops over the first seconds, minutes, hours, and days, and leads to progressive "secondary" microvascular, neuronal, and glial cell degeneration. This cascade has been shown to be extraordinarily complex, and the individual molecular events are linked through a number of feed-forward and feed-back pathways. However, based upon our knowledge of much of the secondary injury process, a number of therapeutic targets have been identified by which posttraumatic brain damage can be attenuated either pharmacologically, targeting individual secondary injury mechanisms, or by induction of brain cooling (i.e., moderate local or systemic hypothermia; decrease in brain temperature from ~37 to 33°C), which has been shown to simultaneously interfere with multiple secondary injury molecular targets.

Although TBI can victimize active individuals at any age, most injuries occur in young adults in the second and third decades of life. This includes a large number of blast-induced TBIs to our war fighters in the Iraq and Afghanistan theaters in the War on Terror mainly caused by improvised explosive devices (IEDs). Moreover, the majority of civilian and military TBI patients now survive their neurological insults owing to improvements in emergency, neurological intensive care and surgical treatments. Nevertheless, the need for intensive rehabilitation and the reality of prolonged disability exacts a significant toll on the individual, his or her family, and society. Effective ways of maintaining or recovering function could markedly improve the outlook for those with TBI enabling higher levels of independence and productivity. However, at present, there are no clinically proven and Food and Drug Administration-approved pharmacological therapies for acute treatment of TBI patients aimed at mitigating the damaging neurological effects of their injuries. Moreover, the efficacy and optimal application of moderate systemic hypothermia remains to be established. Nevertheless, the possibility of an effective "neuroprotective" treatment

---

[24]Spinal Cord & Brain Injury Research Center, University of Kentucky College of Medicine.

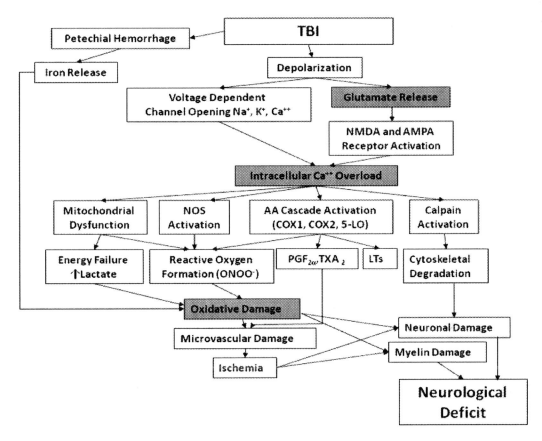

FIGURE C-21 Schematic of posttraumatic secondary injury showing the cascade of pathophysiological and pathochemical players and their inter-relationships. Reprinted with permission from Hall.
NOTE: AA = arachidonic acid; AMPA = α-amino-3-hydroxy-5-methyl-4-isoxazolepropionic acid; COX1 = cyclooxygenase 1; COX2 = cyclooxygenase 2; LTs = leukotrienes; NMDA = N-methyl-D-aspartic acid; NOS = nitric oxide synthase; ONOO⁻ = peroxynitrite; PGF$_{2\alpha}$ = prostaglandin 2α; TBI = traumatic brain injury; TXA$_2$ = thromboxane A$_2$; 5-LO = 5-lipoxygenase
SOURCE: Hall, 2007.

is derived from the fact that although some of the neurodegeneration is due to the primary mechanical trauma, the majority of posttraumatic damage is the result of secondary events that exacerbate the effects of the primary injury. Figure C-21 displays a schematic diagram that includes many of the key molecular players in secondary injury that have been experimentally targeted by pharmacological neuroprotective drug candidates and in the case of glutamate receptor-medicated excitotoxicity, intracellular calcium (Ca^{2+}) overload, and reactive oxygen-induced oxidative damage have been the subject of clinical trials during the past 2 decades.

However, as shown in Table C-9, several compounds that have targeted these mechanisms in phase II and III clinical trials in moderately and/or severely injured TBI patients have failed to produce a significant improvement in survival and neurological outcomes.

TABLE C-9 Compounds That Have Failed to Produce an Overall Improvement in Phase III (or large Phase II) TBI Trials

Compound and Pharmaceutical Sponsor	Mechanism(s) of Action
Nimodipine (Nimotop; Bayer)	L-type Ca^{2+} channel blocker
Selfotel (CGS19755; Ciba-Geigy)	competitive NMDA antagonist
D-CPP-ene (Sandoz)	competitive NMDA antagonist
Aptiganel (CNS1102; Cambridge Neuroscience)	non-competitive NMDA antagonist
CP 101,606 (Traxoprodil; Pfizer)	non-competitive NR2B subtype selective NMDA antagonist
PEG-SOD (PEG-orgatine; Sterling-Winthrop)	free radical scavenger
Tirilazad (U-74006F, Freedox; Upjohn)	lipid peroxidation inhibitor
Dexanabinol (HU211; Pharmos)	non-competitive NMDA antagonist; antioxidant; TNF-α inhibitor

MAJOR FINDINGS FROM THE 2008 NIH COMBINATION THERAPIES FOR TBI WORKSHOP

The failure of these clinical trials to demonstrate the clinical effectiveness of these various neuroprotective agents has been attributed to a number of shortcomings in discovery, development, and clinical testing including (1) an insufficient understanding of the secondary injury mechanisms, time courses, and inter-relationships, (2) inadequate preclinical testing in regards to dose-response, definition of therapeutic blood levels, optimal duration of treatment and the therapeutic post-TBI time window in which it is possible to interrupt the targeted injury mechanism, and (3) poorly conceived clinical trial design, insensitive endpoints, and lack of recognition that not all TBIs have the same pathophysiological characteristics (i.e., there are subgroups of TBI patients that might selectively respond to particular types of drugs) (Narayan et al., 2002). In regard to the possibility that particular drugs may be effective in some types of TBIs, the antioxidant/lipid peroxidation inhibitor tirilazad, listed in Table C-9, has been reported to significantly improve survival in male TBI patients who displayed traumatic subarachnoid hemorrhage (tSAH) despite the fact that this subgroup effect was statistically obscured in the overall group of moderate and severe TBI patients enrolled in the trial (Marshall et al., 1998). Similarly, there is evidence that the L-type Ca^{2+} channel blocker nimodipine may also be selectively effective in tSAH patients (Harders et al., 1996).

Recommendations from the 2008 National Institutes of Health (NIH) Combination Therapies for TBI Workshop

In addition to the reasons for the disappointing failures of past TBI therapeutic trials already mentioned, it has been suggested that the multi-factorial post-TBI secondary injury cascade (Figure C-21) may require treatment with a combination of therapeutic agents that simultaneously interrupt the cascade at multiple points in order to achieve a clinically significant effect in human TBI. This possibility was considered in detail at an NIH workshop held in 2008 from which several recommendations were elaborated (Margulies and Hicks, 2009). The objectives of the workshop were to:

1. identify promising therapies (mainly pharmacological) that would logically be expected to produce an additive neuroprotective effect when combined,
2. consider the challenges involved in preclinical and clinical testing of combination treatments, and

3. optimize strategies for developing combination therapies or single agents that may be capable of affecting multiple secondary injury mechanisms simultaneously.

Table C-10 lists some of the leading therapeutic approaches that were identified by the workshop attendees.

The combination therapy workshop also detailed several recommendations related to the future preclinical and clinical testing of combination therapies for TBI. These include

1. selecting combinations that target different and complimentary mechanisms of action,
2. validating surrogate markers to monitor treatment effects in animal models and humans,
3. developing in vitro, animal, and clinical platforms for coordinated studies across laboratories,
4. using efficient designs for preclinical and clinical trials and data analysis,
5. becoming informed of FDA regulations that need to be considered in moving toward TBI clinical trials with combinations of single agents that may only be effective when used together (similar to many cancer chemotherapeutic strategies),
6. adopting a uniform standard of care for clinical trials, and mimicking those standards in preclinical studies, and
7. establishing a shared database of positive and negative clinical and preclinical data.

Evidence that a combination of two mechanistically distinct neuroprotective drugs might achieve a significantly better degree of neuroprotective efficacy than each monotherapy has been observed in at least one instance. A phase III clinical trial in aneurysmal SAH showed that the combined use of the Ca^{2+} channel blocker nimodipine and the lipid peroxidation inhibitor tirilazad resulted in significantly greater decrease in mortality and an improvement in the distribution of Glasgow Outcome Scale scores compared to that observed in patients treated with nimodipine alone (Kassell et al., 1996).

INTRINSIC DIFFERENCES IN POSTTRAUMATIC BRAIN AND SPINAL CORD NEUROPATHOLOGY AND IMPLICATIONS FOR NUTRITIONAL INTERVENTIONS FOLLOWING INJURY

The major structural difference between the brain and spinal cord is that the former has a higher ratio of gray matter (containing neuronal cell bodies, dendrites, and synaptic connections) to white matter (composed of myelinated axonal fiber tracks) while the spinal cord has a higher white to gray matter ratio. In other words, compared to the brain, which is an exceedingly complicated structure, the spinal cord is predominantly a cable that carries sensory information from the periphery up to the brain and brain-initiated motor commands down to the muscles of the body. However, despite this difference in structural and functional complexity, an extensive body of research accumulated over the past three decades has demonstrated that there is a great deal of overlap in the molecular pathophysiology of TBI and spinal cord injury (SCI). All of the leading molecular mechanisms involved in secondary injury following acute TBI also are implicated in the secondary injury after SCI. These include glutamate-mediated excitotoxicity, intracellular Ca^{2+} overload, and free radical-induced oxidative damage. Indeed, the TBI secondary injury cascade schematic shown in Figure C-21 is essentially accurate for SCI.

Recent research in my own laboratory has compared the time course of reactive oxygen species oxidative damage in rodent models of TBI and SCI and finds that this secondary injury mechanism is initiated during the first posttraumatic hour in both instances. In the case of the injured brain, oxidative damage products tend to peak during the first 3 hours and return to the preinjury baseline by 24–48 hours (Deng et al., 2007). In contrast, oxidative damage products do not peak in the injured spinal cord until 24 hours, but they persist for at least a week (Carrico et al., 2009). Similarly, the peak of brain mitochondrial oxidative damage and bioenergetic dysfunction occurs at 12 hours after injury (Singh et al., 2006), but not until 24 hours in the case of mitochondrial isolated from the injured spinal cord (Sullivan et al., 2007). Despite these time course differences, acute treatment with the reactive oxygen scavenger tempol is able to attenuate oxidative damage and preserve mitochondrial function equally well in both TBI and SCI (Deng-Bryant et al., 2008; Xiong and Hall, 2009). On the other hand, additional studies have shown that spinal cord mitochondria produce more reactive oxygen species compared to brain mitochondria (Sullivan et al., 2004), and spinal cord mitochondria are more sensitive to bioenergetic impairment by oxidative damage products than are brain mitochondria (Vaishnav et al., 2010). What these differences mean from a translational perspective in regard to trying to achieve neuroprotective effects with either acute postinjury pharmacological antioxidant administration or the prophylactic protective effects of preinjury dietary antioxidant (e.g., alpha tocopherol, ascorbic acid, CoQ10) intake is that while these strategies should be effective in either TBI or SCI, it may take larger doses and a longer duration of treatment to achieve protection after SCI.

LEADING ANTIOXIDATION, ANTI-INFLAMMATORY THERAPEUTICS FOR TBI AND THEIR APPLICABILITY TO BLAST INJURIES

The study of blast-induced TBI is a relatively new aspect of neurotrauma research that has taken off during the past few years largely because of its prevalence in the War on Terror. However, the available pathophysiological data obtained from animal models of blast injuries strongly suggest that the pathophysiological secondary injury cascade after blast TBI includes most, if not all, of the molecular mechanisms that have been documented to occur in mechanical blunt impact or penetrating types of TBI. For instance, studies in blast TBI models thus far have confirmed that the general features of mechanical TBI including diffuse axonal injury, glutamate-mediated excitotoxicity, free radical generation and oxidative damage, disruption of Ca^{2+} homeostasis, calcium-activated proteolysis, blood-brain barrier breakdown, tissue hemorrhage, cerebral vasospasm, inflammation, and altered brain metabolism also are seen in blast-induced TBI (Margulies and Hicks, 2009). Thus, even though preclinical studies focused on blast injuries have been mainly directed at model development and description of neuropathology and pathophysiology, rather than experimental therapeutics, it is reasonable to predict that as the blast TBI field moves forward, single or combination therapies (see Table C-10) that are demonstrated to be neuroprotective or neurorestorative in models of mechanical trauma and in humans, also might be useful for the treatment of blast TBI.

Findings on Creatine and TBI and Applicability to Blast Injuries

Creatine is an amino acid that is endogenously produced in the liver, kidney, and pancreas from the precursor amino acids glycine, methionine, or arginine by the action of the enzyme creatine kinase. Creatine monohydrate has been used extensively by athletes as a performance-enhancing supplement and been shown to increase creatine levels in brain as well as muscle tissue (Andres et al., 2008). The creatine kinase/phosphocreatine system plays a major role in neuronal energy metabolism, and creatine supplementation has been shown

TABLE C-10 Currently Promising TBI Therapies—Interventions with Some Reasonable Amount of Preliminary Preclinical or Clinical Data Supporting Their Neuroprotective or Neurorestorative Efficacy

Intervention	
Citicoline	membrane repair
Erythropoietin	multiple neuroprotective and neurorestorative actions
Hypothermia	inhibits many secondary injury mechanisms
Progesterone	multiple neuroprotective actions
Cyclosporine A	mitochondrial protection
Statins	increased nitric oxide produce $\rightarrow$ improved cerebral blood flow (CBF)
Hypertonic saline	improved CBF, reduce edema, etc.

to increase the process of neurogenesis (Andres et al., 2008). Moreover, creatine supplementation has been shown to be neuroprotective in animal models of hypoxic brain damage (Balestrino et al., 1999; Holtzman et al., 1998), Parkinson's disease (Matthews et al., 1998), and amyotrophic lateral sclerosis (Klivenyi et al., 1999).

Based upon these findings, there has been interest in exploring changes in brain creatine levels and the potential neuroprotective effects of creatine supplementation in the rat controlled cortical impact TBI model, which is characterized by a contusion injury. It has been reported that creatine and phosphocreatine levels are decreased in the peri-contusional cortical tissue by 35 percent (Schuhmann et al., 2003). A single study using the same rat TBI model has examined the neuroprotective effects of creatine supplementation 3 mg/g body weight for 1, 3, or 5 days before injury, and observed that creatine supplementation for 3 days reduced cortical tissue damage by 21 percent whereas 5 days caused a 36 percent decrease. These results show that the protective effects are related to the duration of supplementation, but are apparent within a few days. However, additional experiments in the same study showed that 4 weeks of dietary creatine supplementation (1 percent in the diet) could achieve a 50 percent reduction in cerebral cortical damage (Sullivan et al., 2000). Furthermore, cortical synaptic mitochondria isolated at 4 weeks from creatine-supplemented TBI animals showed significantly less free radical formation and improved mitochondrial membrane potentials, Ca^{2+} homeostasis, and adenosine triphospate (ATP) levels compared to non-supplemented brain-injured rats. A subsequent investigation by the same laboratory found that creatine-supplemented TBI rats showed significantly lower levels of brain lactate during the first 6 post-injury hours providing further evidence of neuronal mitochondrial functional preservation as a result of chronic creatine supplementation. While these results tend to support the potential brain-protective value of dietary creatine supplementation in either athletes engaged in contact sports or war fighters, additional preclinical research is needed to accurately define the creatine dose-response characteristics, the needed duration of treatment, efficacy in different types of TBI, and its safety during chronic use.

NUTRIENTS OR DIETS THAT HAVE SHOWN PROMISE AND WARRANT FURTHER RESEARCH REGARDING ACUTE NEUROPROTECTION OF IMPROVED RECOVERY FROM TBI

Beyond the potential neuroprotective benefits of dietary creatine supplementation, perhaps the most convincing body of data regarding the beneficial effects of nutrients or diets has to do with the protective effects of various compounds that possess antioxidant (i.e., free radical scavenging) properties. The phenolic compounds curcumin (Sharma et al., 2009;

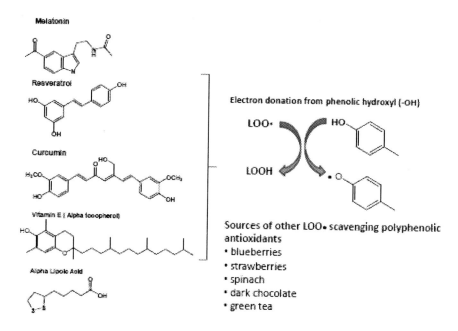

FIGURE C-22 Chemical structures of various nutraceuticals possessing antioxidant properties that are protective in preclinical neurotrauma models. Each of them has the ability to scavenge (i.e., donate an electron) to a lipid peroxyl radical (LOO•) to interrupt the process of lipid peroxidation. In the case of resveratrol, curcumin and vitamin E, the electron donation comes from the single or multiple phenolic hydroxyl groups. Moreover, certain fruits, vegetables, dark chocolate and green tea which are all high in the content of polyphenolic antioxidants have also been reported to be neuroprotective.

Wu et al., 2006), vitamin E (Badhe et al., 2007; Clifton et al., 1989; Conte et al., 2004; Flanary and Streit, 2006; Hall et al., 1992a, 1992b; Wu et al., 2010), and resveratrol (Ates et al., 2007; Sonmez et al., 2007); the indoleamine melatonin (Beni et al., 2004; Cirak et al., 1999; Mesenge et al., 1998; Ozdemir et al., 2005a, 2005b); and alpha lipoic acid (Toklu et al., 2009) have all been shown to exert a protective effect in animal models of TBI (Figure C-22). Additionally, melatonin (Gul et al., 2005; Liu et al., 2004; Samantaray et al., 2008) and vitamin E (Hall and Wolf, 1986; Hall et al., 1992b) have been reported to exert vascular and/or neuronal protective in models of SCI. In each of these cases, the protective effects were demonstrated to be due to their antioxidant properties (i.e. a reduction in oxidative damage). However, it should be noted that daily high dose supplementation with vitamin E can take as much as eight weeks of before a significant increase in central nervous system parenchymal tissue levels occurs (Machlin and Gabriel, 1982). Therefore, the full extent of the neuroprotective effects of chronic vitamin E supplementation is probably not fully developed until that time. Consistent with that, it has been shown that a chronic two-fold dietary supplementation with vitamin E required 16 weeks before cerebrovascular protection was observed in an animal model of subarachnoid hemorrhage (SAH) (Travis and Hall, 1987).

    In addition to chemically scavenging free radicals, there is increasing interest in the possibility of nutraceutically or pharmacologically inducing endogenous enzymatic antioxidant defense mechanisms. In that regard, experimental attention has recently been increasingly focused on the transcription factor Nuclear factor E2-related factor (Nrf2) which interacts with the antioxidant response element (ARE) of various cytoprotective and free radical detoxifying genes. Evidence is rapidly accumulating which shows that the induction of the Nrf2/ARE pathway is a potential therapeutic target for acute neurological injury and chronic neurodegenerative diseases (Calkins et al., 2009). An increasing number of naturally occurring or synthetic compounds have been shown to be able to induce Nrf2 activation and to exert tissue protective effects in brain and other organ systems. Nrf2 is normally repressed in the cytoplasm by binding to the Kelch-like ECH-associated protein 1 (Keap1), where it is rapidly degraded by the ubiquitin-proteasome system. However, one of the prototype Nrf2/ARE pathway activators is sulforaphane, a compound found in high concentrations in broccoli that has been demonstrated to inhibit the proteasomal degradation of Nrf2 resulting in its nuclear accumulation and hence an increased activation of Nrf2-regulated genes. In a rat TBI model, Nrf2 protein, but not mRNA levels, have been shown to increase in injured and surrounding brain areas after TBI along with an increase in mRNA levels of the antioxidant enzymes heme oxygenase-1 (HO-1) and NADPH quinone oxidoreductase-1 (NQO1). This appears to represent an endogenous neuroprotective oxidative stress response (Yan et al., 2009; Yan et al., 2008). However, this response can be pharmacologically enhanced. For instance, sulforaphane administration has been reported to protect the blood brain barrier (Zhao et al., 2007), reduce brain edema (Zhao et al., 2005) and improve cognitive recovery (Dash et al., 2009) in rodent TBI models. Curcumin, one of the phenolic radical scavengers mentioned above, has also been shown to upregulate Nrf2 levels and HO-1 expression and to protect rat brains against focal ischemia (Yang et al., 2009).

SUMMARY

Much of the damage and neurological dysfunction after TBI or SCI is not due to the effects of the primary mechanical trauma, but rather to a molecular cascade of secondary events. In animal models, these have been shown to be potentially modifiable by promptly administered pharmacological treatments that target individual secondary injury factors such as glutamate-mediated excitotoxicity, free radical production and oxidative damage, intracellular Ca^{2+} overload, mitochondrial dysfunction, etc. However, phase II and III clinical trials of compounds that target specific factors and are neuroprotective in animal models have failed to produce a significant improvement in outcome in populations of moderately or severely injured TBI patients. The only exception of note has been the observation that certain TBI patient subgroups may be selectively benefitted by certain types of compounds (e.g. reduction in mortality in patients with traumatic SAH by the antioxidant tirilazad or the L-type Ca^{2+} channel blocker nimodipine).

One of the possible reasons for the failure of various compounds to produce a convincing effect in clinical trials may be that the secondary injury cascade is too complex to be adequately inhibited by interference with a single pathomechanism. Thus, contemporary neuroprotective research includes the testing of combination pharmacotherapies that are made up of two agents that simultaneously act at complimentary target sites based upon the idea that a more robust and/or a less variable effect may be achievable. Another option along these lines is to utilize what are variously called "multi-potential," "multi-mechanistic," or "pleiotropic" compounds that possess the ability to protect the injured brain by multiple mechanisms. Two such compounds that are being examined in clinical TBI trials are the hormone progesterone and the immunosuppressive agent cyclosporine A, each of which have shown impressive neuroprotective properties in rodent TBI models.

Neuroprotective strategies that are shown to work in civilian TBIs can also reasonably be expected to be beneficial in military blast-induced TBIs and SCI in which the secondary injuries cascades are similar. In addition to monotherapies or combination therapies that might be shown to be acute postinjury treatments for civilian and military injuries in the years to come, there is also evidence that certain dietary supplements (e.g. creatine, various antioxidants, Nrf2/ARE pathway activators) may be observed to be both safe and effective for prophylactic neuroprotection in both civilians and military personnel.

REFERENCES

Andres, R. H., A. D. Ducray, U. Schlattner, T. Wallimann, and H. R. Widmer. 2008. Functions and effects of creatine in the central nervous system. *Brain Research Bulletin* 76(4):329–343.

Ates, O., S. Cayli, E. Altinoz, I. Gurses, N. Yucel, M. Sener, A. Kocak, and S. Yologlu. 2007. Neuroprotection by resveratrol against traumatic brain injury in rats. *Molecular and Cellular Biochemistry* 294(1–2):137–144.

Badhe, P., J. Thorat, B. D. Diyora, R. Mamidanna, P. Sayal, S. Badhe, and A. K. Sharma. 2007. Neuroprotective effects of vitamin E in cold induced cerebral injury in guinea pigs. *Indian Journal of Experimental Biology* 45(2):180–184.

Balestrino, M., R. Rebaudo, and G. Lunardi. 1999. Exogenous creatine delays anoxic depolarization and protects from hypoxic damage: Dose-effect relationship. *Brain Research* 816(1):124–130.

Beni, S. M., R. Kohen, R. J. Reiter, D. X. Tan, and E. Shohami. 2004. Melatonin-induced neuroprotection after closed head injury is associated with increased brain antioxidants and attenuated late-phase activation of NF-kappaB and AP-1. *The Federal American Societies for Experimental Biology Journal* 18(1):149–151.

Calkins, M. J., D. A. Johnson, J. A. Townsend, M. R. Vargas, J. A. Dowell, T. P. Williamson, A. D. Kraft, J. M. Lee, J. Li, and J. A. Johnson. 2009. The Nrf2/ARE pathway as a potential therapeutic target in neurodegenerative disease. *Antioxidants and Redox Signaling* 11(3):497–508.

Carrico, K. M., R. Vaishnav, and E. D. Hall. 2009. Temporal and spatial dynamics of peroxynitrite-induced oxidative damage after spinal cord contusion injury. *Journal of Neurotrauma* 26(8):1369–1378.

Cirak, B., N. Rousan, A. Kocak, O. Palaoglu, S. Palaoglu, and K. Kilic. 1999. Melatonin as a free radical scavenger in experimental head trauma. *Pediatric Neurosurgery* 31(6):298–301.

Clifton, G. L., B. G. Lyeth, L. W. Jenkins, W. C. Taft, R. J. DeLorenzo, and R. L. Hayes. 1989. Effect of D, alphatocopheryl succinate and polyethylene glycol on performance tests after fluid percussion brain injury. *Journal of Neurotrauma* 6(2):71–81.

Conte, V., K. Uryu, S. Fujimoto, Y. Yao, J. Rokach, L. Longhi, J. Q. Trojanowski, V. M. Lee, T. K. McIntosh, and D. Pratico. 2004. Vitamin E reduces amyloidosis and improves cognitive function in Tg2576 mice following repetitive concussive brain injury. *Journal of Neurochemistry* 90(3):758–764.

Dash, P. K., J. Zhao, S. A. Orsi, M. Zhang, and A. N. Moore. 2009. Sulforaphane improves cognitive function administered following traumatic brain injury. *Neuroscience Letters* 460(2):103–107.

Deng-Bryant, Y., I. N. Singh, K. M. Carrico, and E. D. Hall. 2008. Neuroprotective effects of tempol, a catalytic scavenger of peroxynitrite-derived free radicals, in a mouse traumatic brain injury model. *Journal of Cerebral Blood Flow and Metabolism* 28(6):1114–1126.

Deng, Y., B. M. Thompson, X. Gao, and E. D. Hall. 2007. Temporal relationship of peroxynitrite-induced oxidative damage, calpain-mediated cytoskeletal degradation and neurodegeneration after traumatic brain injury. *Experimental Neurology* 205(1):154–165.

Flanary, B. E., and W. J. Streit. 2006. Alpha-tocopherol (vitamin E) induces rapid, nonsustained proliferation in cultured rat microglia. *Glia* 53(6):669–674.

Gul, S., S. E. Celik, M. Kalayci, M. Tasyurekli, N. Cokar, and T. Bilge. 2005. Dose-dependent neuroprotective effects of melatonin on experimental spinal cord injury in rats. *Surgical Neurology* 64(4):355–361.

Hall, E. D. 2007. Stroke/traumatic brain and spinal cord injuries. In *Comprehensive medicinal chemistry II*. 2nd ed. 8 vols. Vol. 6, edited by M. Williams. Oxford, UK: Elsevier. Pp. 253–277.

Hall, E. D., J. M. Braughler, and J. M. McCall. 1992a. Antioxidant effects in brain and spinal cord injury. *Journal of Neurotrauma* 9(Suppl 1):S165–S172.

Hall, E. D., and D. L. Wolf. 1986. A pharmacological analysis of the pathophysiological mechanisms of posttraumatic spinal cord ischemia. *Journal of Neurosurgery* 64(6):951–961.

Hall, E. D., P. A. Yonkers, P. K. Andrus, J. W. Cox, and D. K. Anderson. 1992b. Biochemistry and pharmacology of lipid antioxidants in acute brain and spinal cord injury. *Journal of Neurotrauma* 9(Suppl 2):S425–S442.

Harders, A., A. Kakarieka, and R. Braakman. 1996. Traumatic subarachnoid hemorrhage and its treatment with nimodipine. German TSAH Study Group. *Journal of Neurosurgery* 85(1):82–89.

Holtzman, D., A. Togliatti, I. Khait, and F. Jensen. 1998. Creatine increases survival and suppresses seizures in the hypoxic immature rat. *Pediatric Research* 44(3):410–414.

Kassell, N. F., E. C. Haley, Jr., C. Apperson-Hansen, and W. M. Alves. 1996. Randomized, double-blind, vehicle-controlled trial of tirilazad mesylate in patients with aneurysmal subarachnoid hemorrhage: A cooperative study in Europe, Australia, and New Zealand. *Journal of Neurosurgery* 84(2):221–228.

Klivenyi, P., R. J. Ferrante, R. T. Matthews, M. B. Bogdanov, A. M. Klein, O. A. Andreassen, G. Mueller, M. Wermer, R. Kaddurah-Daouk, and M. F. Beal. 1999. Neuroprotective effects of creatine in a transgenic animal model of amyotrophic lateral sclerosis. *Nature Medicine* 5(3):347–350.

Liu, J. B., T. S. Tang, H. L. Yang, and D. S. Xiao. 2004. Antioxidation of melatonin against spinal cord injury in rats. *Chinese Medical Journal (English)* 117(4):571–575.

Machlin, L., and E. Gabriel. 1982. Kinetics of tissue alpha tocopherol uptake and depletion following administration of high levels of vitamin E. *Annals of the New York Academy of Sciences* 393:48–59.

Margulies, S., and R. Hicks. 2009. Combination therapies for traumatic brain injury: Prospective considerations. *Journal of Neurotrauma* 26(6):925–939.

Marshall, L. F., A. I. Maas, S. B. Marshall, A. Bricolo, M. Fearnside, F. Iannotti, M. R. Klauber, J. Lagarrigue, R. Lobato, L. Persson, J. D. Pickard, J. Piek, F. Servadei, G. N. Wellis, G. F. Morris, E. D. Means, and B. Musch. 1998. A multicenter trial on the efficacy of using tirilazad mesylate in cases of head injury. *Journal of Neurosurgery* 89(4):519–525.

Matthews, R. T., L. Yang, B. G. Jenkins, R. J. Ferrante, B. R. Rosen, R. Kaddurah-Daouk, and M. F. Beal. 1998. Neuroprotective effects of creatine and cyclocreatine in animal models of Huntington's disease. *The Journal of Neuroscience* 18(1):156–163.

Mesenge, C., I. Margaill, C. Verrecchia, M. Allix, R. G. Boulu, and M. Plotkine. 1998. Protective effect of melatonin in a model of traumatic brain injury in mice. *Journal of Pineal Research* 25(1):41–46.

Narayan, R. K., M. E. Michel, B. Ansell, A. Baethmann, A. Biegon, M. B. Bracken, M. R. Bullock, S. C. Choi, G. L. Clifton, C. F. Contant, W. M. Coplin, W. D. Dietrich, J. Ghajar, S. M. Grady, R. G. Grossman, E. D. Hall, W. Heetderks, D. A. Hovda, J. Jallo, R. L. Katz, N. Knoller, P. M. Kochanek, A. I. Maas, J. Majde, D. W. Marion, A. Marmarou, L. F. Marshall, T. K. McIntosh, E. Miller, N. Mohberg, J. P. Muizelaar, L. H. Pitts, P. Quinn, G. Riesenfeld, C. S. Robertson, K. I. Strauss, G. Teasdale, N. Temkin, R. Tuma, C. Wade, M. D. Walker, M. Weinrich, J. Whyte, J. Wilberger, A. B. Young, and L. Yurkewicz. 2002. Clinical trials in head injury. *Journal of Neurotrauma* 19(5):503–557.

Ozdemir, D., K. Tugyan, N. Uysal, U. Sonmez, A. Sonmez, O. Acikgoz, N. Ozdemir, M. Duman, and H. Ozkan. 2005a. Protective effect of melatonin against head trauma-induced hippocampal damage and spatial memory deficits in immature rats. *Neuroscience Letters* 385(3):234–239.

Ozdemir, D., N. Uysal, S. Gonenc, O. Acikgoz, A. Sonmez, A. Topcu, N. Ozdemir, M. Duman, I. Semin, and H. Ozkan. 2005b. Effect of melatonin on brain oxidative damage induced by traumatic brain injury in immature rats. *Physiological Research* 54(6):631–637.

Samantaray, S., E. A. Sribnick, A. Das, V. H. Knaryan, D. D. Matzelle, A. V. Yallapragada, R. J. Reiter, S. K. Ray, and N. L. Banik. 2008. Melatonin attenuates calpain upregulation, axonal damage and neuronal death in spinal cord injury in rats. *Journal of Pineal Research* 44(4):348–357.

Schuhmann, M. U., D. Stiller, M. Skardelly, J. Bernarding, P. M. Klinge, A. Samii, M. Samii, and T. Brinker. 2003. Metabolic changes in the vicinity of brain contusions: A proton magnetic resonance spectroscopy and histology study. *Journal of Neurotrauma* 20(8):725–743.

Sharma, S., Y. Zhuang, Z. Ying, A. Wu, and F. Gomez-Pinilla. 2009. Dietary curcumin supplementation counteracts reduction in levels of molecules involved in energy homeostasis after brain trauma. *Neuroscience* 161(4):1037–1044.

Singh, I. N., P. G. Sullivan, Y. Deng, L. H. Mbye, and E. D. Hall. 2006. Time course of post-traumatic mitochondrial oxidative damage and dysfunction in a mouse model of focal traumatic brain injury: Implications for neuroprotective therapy. *Journal of Cerebral Blood Flow and Metabolism* 26:1407–1418.

Sonmez, U., A. Sonmez, G. Erbil, I. Tekmen, and B. Baykara. 2007. Neuroprotective effects of resveratrol against traumatic brain injury in immature rats. *Neuroscience Letters* 420(2):133–137.

Sullivan, P. G., J. D. Geiger, M. P. Mattson, and S. W. Scheff. 2000. Dietary supplement creatine protects against traumatic brain injury. *Annals of Neurology* 48(5):723–729.

Sullivan, P. G., S. Krishnamurthy, S. P. Patel, J. D. Pandya, and A. G. Rabchevsky. 2007. Temporal characterization of mitochondrial bioenergetics after spinal cord injury. *Journal of Neurotrauma* 24(6):991–999.

Sullivan, P. G., A. G. Rabchevsky, J. N. Keller, M. Lovell, A. Sodhi, R. P. Hart, and S. W. Scheff. 2004. Intrinsic differences in brain and spinal cord mitochondria: Implication for therapeutic interventions. *Journal of Comparative Neurology* 474(4):524–534.

Toklu, H. Z., T. Hakan, N. Biber, S. Solakoglu, A. V. Ogunc, and G. Sener. 2009. The protective effect of alpha lipoic acid against traumatic brain injury in rats. *Free Radical Research* 43(7):658–667.

Travis, M. A., and E. D. Hall. 1987. The effects of chronic two-fold dietary vitamin e supplementation on subarachnoid hemorrhage-induced brain hypoperfusion. *Brain Research* 418(2):366–370.

Vaishnav, R. A., I. N. Singh, D. M. Miller, and E. D. Hall. 2010. Lipid peroxidation-derived reactive aldehydes directly and differentially impair spinal cord and brain mitochondrial function. *Journal of Neurotrauma* 27(7):1311–1320.

Wu, A., Z. Ying, and F. Gomez-Pinilla. 2006. Dietary curcumin counteracts the outcome of traumatic brain injury on oxidative stress, synaptic plasticity, and cognition. *Experimental Neurology* 197(2):309–317.

Wu, A., Z. Ying, and F. Gomez-Pinilla. 2010. Vitamin E protects against oxidative damage and learning disability after mild traumatic brain injury in rats. *Neurorehabilitation and Neural Repair* 24(3):290–298.

Xiong, Y., and E. D. Hall. 2009. Pharmacological evidence for a role of peroxynitrite in the pathophysiology of spinal cord injury. *Experimental Neurology* 216(1):105–114.

Yan, W., H. D. Wang, X. M. Feng, Y. S. Ding, W. Jin, and K. Tang. 2009. The expression of NF-E2-related factor 2 in the rat brain after traumatic brain injury. *The Journal of Trauma* 66(5):1431–1435.

Yan, W., H. D. Wang, Z. G. Hu, Q. F. Wang, and H. X. Yin. 2008. Activation of Nrf2-are pathway in brain after traumatic brain injury. *Neuroscience Letters* 431(2):150–154.

Yang, C., X. Zhang, H. Fan, and Y. Liu. 2009. Curcumin upregulates transcription factor Nrf2, HO-1 expression and protects rat brains against focal ischemia. *Brain Research* 1282:133–141.

Zhao, J., A. N. Moore, G. L. Clifton, and P. K. Dash. 2005. Sulforaphane enhances aquaporin-4 expression and decreases cerebral edema following traumatic brain injury. *Journal of Neuroscience Research* 82(4):499–506.

Zhao, J., A. N. Moore, J. B. Redell, and P. K. Dash. 2007. Enhancing expression of Nrf2-driven genes protects the blood brain barrier after brain injury. *Journal of Neuroscience* 27(38):10240–10248.

Glycemic Control in the Critically Ill and in Brain Injury Patients

Stanley A. Nasraway, Jr.[25]

GLYCEMIC CONTROL IN THE CRITICALLY ILL: OVERVIEW

The publication in 2001 of the now famous Leuven I trial (Van Den Berghe et al., 2001) showed that tight glycemic control in a population of surgical critically ill patients could improve survival and could reduce multiple organ failure and nosocomial infection. This past decade as witnessed a great deal research dedicated to confirming these initial findings.

Leuven I (Van Den Berghe et al., 2001) unleashed a torrent of skepticism, excitement and investigation into tight glycemic control. Google searches of "tight glycemic control" and "intensive insulin" produce 80,900 and 334,000 results, respectively. After entering a new decade, where are we? There is a great deal that we do not know, in part, because this field of discovery has been disadvantaged by inconsistencies in research methodology. Among differences in the studies are casetype selection, targeted ranges of blood glucose, inconsistency in the frequency of blood glucose monitoring, variability in the accuracy of glucometer devices used, in the methods used to define euglycemia, whether insulin dosing was driven by paper protocol or software algorithm and nonstandardization in caloric intake. Starting with Leuven I, all of the prospective studies conducted to date are vulnerable to significant methodologic criticisms (Nasraway Jr. and Rattan, 2010). We also really have no conclusive understanding on the biologic plausibility to explain how intensive insulin would decrease death or organ failure or nosocomial infection. Is it through anti-inflammatory pathways, because insulin is a vasodilator that may increase microperfusion, or by other unrealized mechanisms of action? In some ways, the scientific evolution of this field resembles that of Sepsis research from 1985–2005, in which the study of anti-inflammatory compounds was severely hindered by lack of standardization in the total treatment for patients with severe sepsis, with too many confounding and uncontrolled variables (Nasraway Jr., 1999).

---

[25]Department of Surgery, the Tufts Medical Center and the Tufts University School of Medicine.

After all of these studies, what do we actually *know*? What are the consistent threads? This is what we know with certainty:

1. Hyperglycemia is bad. Falciglia (2009) convincingly showed in an analysis of 259,040 intensive care unit (ICU) patients that hyperglycemia (glucose > 110 mg/dL) was associated with mortality independent of illness severity, type of ICU or length of stay. Consistent with the findings of others, the two-thirds of patients who are nondiabetic benefit more from insulin than do diabetics.

2. Hypoglycemia is bad. An incidental and constant observation from many studies is that severe hypoglycemia (glucose < 40 mg/dL) in a population of patients by logistic regression is associated with a 6-fold increase in death (Griesdale et al., 2009). It would not be surprising to find with additional study that even mild hypoglycemia has long lasting but subtle neurologic consequences that are not clinically evident or measured. Hypoglycemia is particularly detrimental to the brain, which neither produces nor stores glucose, but is entirely dependent upon cerebral glucose delivery.

3. Critically ill patients typically sustain large swings in blood glucose, even with insulin administration (Finney et al., 2003). Sustaining the blood glucose within a target range in a hypermetabolic patient with changing gluconeogenic drivers in a 24-hour day is enormously challenging, frequently outstripping the crude tools used at the bedside to measure blood glucose and respond to its variation in concentration.

4. Software-driven insulin dosing is better than paper-driven insulin protocols. Software integrates all of the glucose measurements and all of the previous insulin adjustments to determine the next best insulin dose. Software appears to reduce glucose variability and sustain glucose within the target range for prolonged periods of time (Juneja et al., 2009). There are now many software programs tested and/or available.

5. Handheld blood glucometers, originally intended for use by Type I diabetic outpatients in the 1980s, are not accurate enough in the ICU environment (Kanji et al., 2005), and are very laborious to use. In the United States, the Food and Drug Administration in March of 2010 hosted a public inquiry into glucose meters, after which it is redefining what it will accept in the way of accuracy by blood glucose measurement devices in the hospital setting going forward. It has asked the international standards body to reset its limits for accuracy for glucometers. Current generation handheld devices now in use will not make the cut.

6. The more frequent the blood glucose measurement, even with handheld glucometers, the less hypoglycemia experienced by patients and the tighter the glycemic control (Cook et al., 2008b). Frequency is crucial, however laborious it may be.

What Can We Expect Going Forward?

We can expect that the world will continue to use intensive insulin, but that the range that defines "tight" will be narrowed as it becomes more achievable. We can expect that there will be more emphasis on defining hypoglycemia, and in avoiding it with greater rigor. We can expect a movement towards insulin-dosing software, as the development of many programs appears to be simple, and competition will force down the cost of purchase and use. Software-insulin dosing has hidden advantages: it forces more blood glucose monitoring and also provides an instant database for analysis. We will someday be using glucometers that are engineered to be more accurate, especially in the hypoglycemic range, avoiding pitfalls in today's instruments due to chemical interferences and specific disease conditions. Importantly, these devices will be continuous or near continuous, and by their nature will be less arduous. At the same time, manufacturers will need to make these devices affordable, or their uptake will be slowed. The frequency of blood glucose measurements by these devices will dramatically make safer the continuous administration of insulin.

Improving the accuracy of blood glucose measurements and standardizing the determination of insulin dosing with better methods will produce better quality research, synergizing global convergence on tight glycemic control, reduced glucose variability and better patient outcomes.

GLYCEMIC CONTROL IN ACUTE BRAIN INJURY

Research into blood glucose management for patients with acute brain injury has been a representative microcosm of the larger field of glycemic control in the critically ill. Numerous studies have demonstrated that hyperglycemia in patients after stroke or other forms of acute brain injury is deleterious and worsens outcome (Bilotta et al., 2009; Cook et al., 2008a). Van den Berghe and colleagues (2005) retrospectively analyzed 63 patients from their original study; these patients had sustained isolated brain injury. Patients who had been randomized to intensive insulin therapy sustained decreases in the mean and maximal intracranial pressure. This, in turn, was associated with improved long-term recovery in comparison with those patients who had received conventional glycemic management.

However, a very important study examined the effects of tight glycemic control on cerebral glucose metabolism after severe brain injury. Tight glycemic control, even without systemic hypoglycemia, was associated with decreased brain glucose and increases in brain energy crises (Oddo et al., 2008). The latter was associated with an increase in death. The study has raised questions about the value of very tight glycemic control.

There have since been four prospective randomized controlled trials examining the benefits of intensive insulin in patients with subarachnoid hemorrhage (Bilotta et al., 2007), traumatic brain injury (Bilotta et al., 2008; Coester et al., 2010), or in a heterogeneous group of mechanically ventilated critically ill neurologic patients (Green et al., 2010). Overall, there were no differences in the rates of infection, neurologic recovery, or mortality rate. The results of these studies have frustrated advocates for very tight glycemic control.

It is clear that severe hyperglycemia in patients with acute brain injury is deleterious. However blood glucose concentrations which are normal, but tightly regulated, may also be deleterious with a reduction in brain glucose availability. As a result the best overall recommendation has been to achieve a broader range of glycemic control while avoiding hypoglycemia in this especially sensitive population. Bilotta et al. (2009) have suggested a blood glucose concentration target range of 80–155 mg/dL.

REFERENCES

Bilotta, F., R. Caramia, I. Cernak, F. P. Paoloni, A. Doronzio, V. Cuzzone, A. Santoro, and G. Rosa. 2008. Intensive insulin therapy after severe traumatic brain injury: A randomized clinical trial. *Neurocritical Care* 9(2):159–166.

Bilotta, F., F. Giovannini, R. Caramia, and G. Rosa. 2009. Glycemia management in neurocritical care patients: A review. *Journal of Neurosurgical Anesthesiology* 21(1):2–9.

Bilotta, F., A. Spinelli, F. Giovannini, A. Doronzio, R. Delfini, and G. Rosa. 2007. The effect of intensive insulin therapy on infection rate, vasospasm, neurologic outcome, and mortality in neurointensive care unit after intracranial aneurysm clipping in patients with acute subarachnoid hemorrhage: A randomized prospective pilot trial. *Journal of Neurosurgical Anesthesiology* 19(3):156–160.

Coester, A., C. R. Neumann, and M. I. Schmidt. 2010. Intensive insulin therapy in severe traumatic brain injury: A randomized trial. *Journal of Trauma—Injury, Infection and Critical Care* 68(4):904–911.

Cook, A. M., A. Peppard, and B. Magnuson. 2008a. Nutrition considerations in traumatic brain injury. *Nutrition in Clinical Practice* 23(6):608–620.

Cook, C. B., V. Abad, G. Kongable, Y. Hanseon, and D. McMahon. 2008b. The status of glucose control in U.S. intensive care units. *Critical Care Medicine* 36(12):A68.

Falciglia, M., R. W. Freyberg, P. L. Almenoff, D. A. D'Alessio, and M. L. Render. 2009. Hyperglycemia-related mortality in critically ill patients varies with admission diagnosis. *Critical Care Medicine* 37(12):3001–3009.

Food and Drug Administration (FDA). 2010. *FDA/CDRH public meeting: Blood glucose meters March 16–17, 2010.* http://www.fda.gov/MedicalDevices/NewsEvents/WorkshopsConferences/ucm187406.htm#transcripts (accessed November 7, 2010).

Finney, S. J., C. Zekveld, A. Elia, and T. W. Evans. 2003. Glucose control and mortality in critically ill patients. *Journal of the American Medical Association* 290(15):2041–2047.

Green, D. M., K. H. O'Phelan, S. L. Bassin, C. W. J. Chang, T. S. Stern, and S. M. Asai. 2010. Intensive versus conventional insulin therapy in critically ill neurologic patients. *Neurocritical Care* 13(3):299–306.

Griesdale, D. E. G., R. J. De Souza Rd, R. M. Van Dam, D. K. Heyland, D. J. Cook, A. Malhotra, R. Dhaliwal, W. R. Henderson, D. R. Chittock, S. Finfer, and D. Talmor. 2009. Intensive insulin therapy and mortality among critically ill patients: A meta-analysis including nice-sugar study data. *Canadian Medical Association Journal* 180(8):821–827.

Juneja, R., C. P. Roudebush, S. A. Nasraway, A. A. Golas, J. Jacobi, J. Carroll, D. Nelson, V. J. Abad, and S. J. Flanders. 2009. Computerized intensive insulin dosing can mitigate hypoglycemia and achieve tight glycemic control when glucose measurement is performed frequently and on time. *Critical Care (London, England)* 13(5).

Kanji, S., J. Buffie, B. Hutton, P. S. Bunting, A. Singh, K. McDonald, D. Fergusson, L. A. McIntyre, and P. C. Hebert. 2005. Reliability of point-of-care testing for glucose measurement in critically ill adults. *Critical Care Medicine* 33(12):2778–2785.

Nasraway Jr., S. A. 1999. Sepsis research: We must change course. *Critical Care Medicine* 27(2):427–430.

Nasraway Jr., S. A., and R. Rattan. 2010. Tight glycemic control: What do we really know, and what should we expect? *Critical Care (London, England)* 14(5):198.

Oddo, M., J. M. Schmidt, E. Carrera, N. Badjatia, E. S. Connolly, M. Presciutti, N. D. Ostapkovich, J. M. Levine, P. L. Roux, and S. A. Mayer. 2008. Impact of tight glycemic control on cerebral glucose metabolism after severe brain injury: A microdialysis study. *Critical Care Medicine* 36(12):3233–3238.

Van Den Berghe, G., K. Schoonheydt, P. Becx, F. Bruyninckx, and P. J. Wouters. 2005. Insulin therapy protects the central and peripheral nervous system of intensive care patients. *Neurology* 64(8):1348–1353.

Van Den Berghe, G., P. Wouters, F. Weekers, C. Verwaest, F. Bruyninckx, M. Schetz, D. Vlasselaers, P. Ferdinande, P. Lauwers, and R. Bouillon. 2001. Intensive insulin therapy in critically ill patients. *The New England Journal of Medicine* 345(19):1359–1367.

Mitochondrial Dysfunction Following Traumatic Brain Injury (TBI): Potential of Creatine as a Neuroprotective Strategy

Patrick G. Sullivan[26]

INTRODUCTION

Although TBI is a major healthcare problem in the United States, there are currently no pharmacological interventions approved for clinical treatment of this condition. TBI affects about 7 million individuals each year in North America. However, athletes—particularly in full-contact sports such as boxing, football, hockey and soccer—are exposed to single and repeated concussions at a much higher incidence than the general population, which can result in long-term neurological dysfunction and even death (Clark, 1998). Regardless

---

[26]Spinal Cord & Brain Injury Research Center and the Department of Anatomy & Neurobiology, University of Kentucky Chandler Medicine Center.

of rule changes, improved protective equipment, and conditioning, approximately 300,000 people still experience sport-related TBI annually (Cantu, 1997; Thurman et al., 1998). Furthermore, accumulating clinical evidence, as well as experience in contemporary military operations, suggests that substantial short-term and long-term neurologic deficits can be caused without a direct contact to the head (Cernak et al., 1999; DePalma et al., 2005; Elder and Cristian, 2009; Ling et al., 2009; Trudeau et al., 1998). With an estimated 15 percent of troops serving in Iraq sustaining some level of neurological impairment following blast exposure, TBI is the signature injury of this war and makes troops another high incident population for TBI (Hoge et al., 2008).

Although the neuropathology of TBI is not completely elucidated, several lines of evidence have demonstrated that mitochondrial dysfunction is a major feature of TBI. Mitochondria have also been found to play a pivotal role in neuronal cell survival and death following injury. Mitochondria serve as the powerhouse of the cell by maintaining ratios of adenosine triphosphate (ATP) to adenosine diphosphate (ADP) that thermodynamically favor the hydrolysis of ATP to ADP + Pi. Proton pumping by components of the electron transport system (ETS) generates a membrane potential ($\Delta\Psi$) that can then be used to phosphorylate ADP to ATP or used to sequester Ca^{2+} into the mitochondrial matrix. This allows mitochondria to act as Ca^{2+} sinks for the cell as well as to stay in tune with changes in cytosolic Ca^{2+} levels. However, excessive mitochondrial Ca^{2+} uptake following TBI can result in formation of the mitochondrial permeability transition pore (mPTP) (Sullivan et al., 2005). A consequence of mPTP formation is a loss of membrane potential, which causes the uncoupling of electron transport from ATP production. The release of pro-apoptotic molecules (i.e., cytochrome C, Smac/Diablo, and apoptosis-inducing factor) from the mitochondria is, in part, orchestrated by mPTP and leads to the activation of cellular death pathways. An additional consequence of mPTP formation is the production of reactive oxygen species (ROS), which contribute to cellular damage by oxidizing cellular proteins and lipids (Mazzeo et al., 2009). Thus, the fine line between cell survival and cell death relies on mitochondrial integrity and, ultimately, the state of mitochondria following TBI.

Creatine is a molecule that is produced both endogenously and acquired exogenously through diet where it plays a prominent role in buffering cellular energy stores by increasing levels of phosphocreatine. Thus, the creatine/phosphocreatine system can increase overall cellular bioenergetics following injury/insult by acting as an energy storehouse. Additionally, increases in creatine can stabilize creatine kinase which has been demonstrated to interact with components of the mPTP and inhibit permeability transition (Beutner et al., 1996, 1998; O'Gorman et al., 1997). Inhibition of the mPTP has been demonstrated to reduce damage following TBI (Sullivan et al., 2005). Together, these data may point to creatine as a viable prophylactic treatment for certain populations engaged in activities that increase their chance for sustaining a TBI. However, limited preclinical data is available concerning the use of creatine following TBI, making this an untapped resource that should be further explored.

TRAUMATIC BRAIN INJURY

Although treatment options designed to improve survival of their injuries are limited to minimizing acute brain edema, decreasing intracranial pressure, and the prevention of peripheral complications, there is no current treatment aimed at the loss of neural tissue that occurs following TBI. Perhaps the most insidious aspect of TBI is that it can occur without any obvious signs of injury to the patient's body. Medical reports dating back to World War I have recorded medical incidences of mysterious neurological disorders. Physicians in the British armed forces began to label the bulk of these phenomenon with the term "shell shock" (SS) (Jones et al., 2007). Although some cases were attributed to psychosis, SS was responsible for 14 percent of all discharges from the British armed forces, and accounted for over one-third of all discharges of nonwounded soldiers by 1917. The controversial definition of the disorder, its method of treatment, public controversy, and stigma over diagnosis delayed the development of treatment protocols and eventually caused the British army to ban the use of the term "shell shock" from reports. However, with the start of World War II, it became readily apparent that disavowing the existence of this disorder did not prevent another epidemic.

In response to the army regulations, alternative terminology arose in its place, such as postconcussional syndrome (PCS) or posttrauma concussion state. Physicians began realizing many of the soldiers that suffered from this concussed state had been in a close proximity to an explosion, and thus, leading them to speculate that some force was affecting neural tissue without affecting the rest of the body. It was also realized that patients with a severe head injury would present with immediate neurologic symptoms that would trend toward recovery; whereas PCS would have delayed onset of neurologic symptoms with a trend toward worsening symptoms (Jones et al., 2007). Since soldiers and civilians can often suffer immense psychiatric morbidity without realizing the need for medical treatment that normally stems from a physical injury, this delayed development of symptoms in mild to moderate TBI patients is perhaps the most unfortunate aspect of this condition. A recent online poll indicated that 42 percent of respondents who suffered a TBI failed to seek medical care (Setnik and Bazarian, 2007); a rate that is considerably higher than the Centers for Disease Control and Prevention estimate of 25 percent. It has been observed clinically that even mild or moderate TBI can require neurosurgical intervention, and any delay in treatment could prove to be costly in terms of cognitive and functional recovery (Setnik and Bazarian, 2007).

Of the more than 1.5 million military personnel deployed since 2001 to the Middle East, approximately 25 percent of the injured service members have reported brain injury. Given the statistic from the poll above, this is probably an extreme underestimate with regards to military peronnel. Unpublished data from the Department of Defense indicates that blast injuries are the leading cause of TBI in war zones; consequently, TBI has been labeled as a signature injury of the current Middle Eastern conflicts (Hoge et al., 2008). In addition to cognitive deficits, this injury population also has an increased predisposition to the development of post traumatic stress disorder (PTSD).

Within the civilian population of the United States, about 2 percent of the population (5.3 million) is currently living with disabilities that are the direct result of TBI (Langlois et al., 2006). TBI has a bimodal age distribution of incidence such that the peaks are found in young (< 25) and elderly (> 75) populations (Langlois et al., 2006; Rutland-Brown et al., 2006). Due to the high incidence and the development of chronic symptoms associated with TBI, the medical costs within the United States alone have been estimated at over $50 billion dollars per year. These dismal figures do not factor in the cost to social and family dynamics that occur following TBI. Despite being obvious that TBI is a devastating military and civilian health care problem in the United States, there are currently no pharmacological treatments approved for clinical treatment of this condition. Several lines of evidence have indicated that mitochondrial dysfunction is a prominent feature of TBI, and mitochondria are known to play a pivotal role in neuronal cell survival and death following injury. As such, there is a clear need for the development of mitochondrial-targeted neuroprotective therapies for the treatment of TBI.

MITOCHONDRIA AND TBI

Several studies in recent years have shown that mitochondria play a pivotal role in neuronal cell survival in addition to mitochondrial dysfunction being considered an early, prominent event in central nervous system (CNS) injury that can cause neuronal cell death (Fiskum, 2000; Sullivan et al., 2004, 2005). Experimental data also indicates that excitotoxicity may be the initial upstream mechanism that leads to TBI-induced neuronal cell death (Choi et al., 1990; Faden et al., 1989). In order to discuss mitochondrial dysfunction, however, we must first address normal mitochondrial function. Mitochondria are double-membraned organelles that orchestrate oxidative phosphorylation. Specifically, mitochondria act as the "powerhouses" of cells by taking products from the Krebs cycle (citric acid cycle), fatty acid oxidation, and amino acid oxidation and producing most of the cell's supply of ATP—the energy source used to power virtually all cellular functions. In fact, in the cells of evolutionarily "higher animals," greater than 95 percent of all ATP is produced by oxidative phosphorylation within mitochondria. Mitochondrial function is dependent upon the generation and maintenance of the mitochondrial $\Delta\Psi$, which is used to drive ATP production. $\Delta\Psi$ is generated by the translocation of protons across the inner mitochondrial membrane via the electron transport system (ETS), culminating in the reduction of O_2 to H_2O. This store of potential energy (the electrochemical gradient) can then be coupled to ATP production as protons flow back through the ATP synthase and complete the proton circuit. The potential can also be used to drive Ca^{2+} into the mitochondrial matrix via the electrogenic uniporter when cytosolic levels increase (Gunter et al., 1994). When cytosolic levels decrease, mitochondria pump Ca^{2+} out to precisely regulate cytosolic Ca^{2+} homeostasis.

During excitotoxic insults, such as the result of TBI, Ca^{2+} uptake into mitochondria has been shown to increase ROS production, inhibit ATP synthesis, and induce mitochondrial permeability transitions. It is important to note that inhibition of mitochondrial Ca^{2+} uptake by reducing $\Delta\Psi$ (chemical uncoupling) following excitotoxic insults is neuroprotective, emphasizing the pivotal role of mitochondrial Ca^{2+} uptake in TBI-induced neuronal cell death (Pandya et al., 2007; Sullivan et al., 2004). Studies from our group have demonstrated that changes in mitochondrial Ca^{2+} levels/cycling are coupled with increases in oxidative damage and significant mitochondrial dysfunction, which occurs acutely and is progressive for up to 48 hours postinjury (Maragos and Korde, 2004; Mbye et al., 2008; Pandya et al., 2009; Sullivan et al., 2004, 2005). The opening of the mitochondrial permeability transition pore (mPTP) is suggested to be a key mediator in this process.

While several studies have demonstrated mitochondrial failure in rodent TBI models over the past 15 years, only recently have careful time course studies been carried out to better understand the temporal profile of bioenergetic failure. In the mouse controlled cortical impact (CCI) model of TBI, we have shown that mitochondrial failure is significant by 3 hours within the cortical tissue surrounding the injury site and follows a progressive failure that peaks at 12 hours (Singh et al., 2006). The onset of mitochondrial dysfunction has been demonstrated to be even more rapid in the tissue considered to be the injury core and penumbra following CCI. In these studies, it is apparent that a significant loss of mitochondrial bioenergetics begins as early as 1 hour post-injury and continues for up to 48 hours postinjury (Gilmer et al., 2009; Pandya et al., 2007, 2009). Furthermore, mitochondrial Ca^{2+} overload, which directly initiates mPTP formation, was found to coincide with the loss of mitochondrial bioenergetics. However, both mitochondrial bioenergetics and Ca^{2+} loading were most amendable to treatment with a mitochondrial uncoupler administered within a 6 hour post-injury window (Pandya et al., 2009). Thus, these data sets show that a critical time for intervention occurs at $t < 6$ hours post-injury. In fact, in order for any mitochondrial–targeted compound to maximally rescue mitochondria at the epicenter of the injury, administration within a three hour post-injury window would be needed; while administration within the first six hours would prevent mitochondrial failure in the cortical tissue surrounding the epicenter. Given these findings, a prophylactic approach with a safe compound is very logical for persons at an increased risk for TBI, such as athletes and military personal in active war zones.

CREATINE

Creatine (N-(aminoiminomethy)-N-methyl glycine) is an amino acid endogenously produced from glycine, methionine, and arginine in the liver, kidney, and pancreas and is also supplied in diets containing meat products. While as much as 95 percent of the total pool of creatine is contained in muscle, high levels of creatine have also been demonstrated in the brain (Mujika and Padilla, 1997). For athletes, creatine is used to increase levels of phosphocreatine (which serves as a phosphate donor to generate ATP) and thereby decrease muscle fatigue during—and improve recovery after—repeated bouts of high intensity exercise (Mujika and Padilla, 1997). Importantly, creatine is also the main shuttle to transport energy from the mitochondria to locales in the cytosol via phosphocreatine. This is accomplished by generation of phosphocreatine from mitochondrial ATP in the intermembrane space via phosphocreatine kinase. Phosphocreatine can then be shuttled to various sites within the cell and used to regenerate ATP from ADP. This allows phosphocreatine to serve as a spatial/temporal buffer for ATP produced by oxidative phosphorylation in mitochondria. Higher levels of phosphocreatine therefore result in a higher reserve of ATP that is available for cells following injury and may account for the neuroprotection afforded by creatine supplementation. In fact, creatine supplementation has been placed into several human clinical trials for various CNS disorders including amyotrophic lateral sclerosis, Charcot-Marie-Tooth disease, Huntington's disease, and Parkinson's disease with mixed results (see Gualano et al., 2010, for review). In an effort to boost neuronal ATP and bioenergetics, all these trials used started creatine treatment after the disease state had been reached (Adhihetty and Beal, 2008).

It is also apparent that many of the neuroprotective functions that creatine has been shown to afford cannot be attributed to changes in cellular bioenergetics. One of the most striking examples is the anti-apoptotic effect, which has been attributed to the prevention or delay of the mPTP, that elevated creatine levels have been reported to produce (Adhihetty and Beal, 2008; Andres et al., 2008). Additionally, creatine kinase is now recognized as a component of the mPTP, and its activation inhibits the induction of the mPTP (Beutner et al., 1996; Beutner et al., 1998; O'Gorman et al., 1997). Given that bioenergetic failure and mPTP activation have been documented as key players in TBI-induced neuropathology, creatine supplementation would be expected to offer neuroprotection following experimental TBI (Sullivan et al., 2005).

CREATINE SUPPLEMENTATION AND TBI

Creatine supplementation has been shown to be neurprotective following TBI in both mice and rats. Our laboratory demonstrated in 2000 that chronic administration of creatine ameliorated cortical tissue damage by 36 percent in mice and 50 perecent in rats depending upon the regimen and dosage used during the pretreatment (Sullivan et al.). In mice, pretreatment with 3g/kg (intraperitoneal injections) for a minimum of three days prior to injury was required to demonstrate significant neuroprotection. In rats, animals that were fed a dietary supplementation of 1 percent creatine for four weeks demonstrated significant neuroprotection that was linked to improved mitochondrial bioenergetics, increased ATP levels, and an increased threshold for activation of the mPTP. Further experiments have reported that two weeks of dietary supplementation of creatine (0.5 and 1 percent) prior to injury was sufficient to significantly reduce lactate and free fatty acid levels following TBI (Scheff and Dhillon, 2004). Additionally, all animals feed a creatine supplemented diet had significantly less cortical tissue damage compared to non-supplemented controls. To date these are the only studies assessing the use of creatine for the treatment of TBI.

CLOSING REMARKS

Creatine may be a viable prophylactic treatment for TBI based on its proposed target mechanisms including stabilization of cellular bioenergetics and inhibition of mPTP activation. Yet, a Medline search using the terms "traumatic brain injury" and "creatine supplementation" yields only six hits, of which only one is relevant. This may seem surprising considering the robust neuroprotective effects demonstrated by creatine pretreatment. However, the need to preload the system with creatine (or with any other compound) has historically reduced enthusiasm for funding this line of research as it relates to the treatment of TBI. This, of course, has left many unanswered questions:

- What is the optimal dosage of creatine (i.e., dose-response)?
- What is the minimum amount of pretreatment needed, or the therapeutic window of opportunity?
- Is postinjury treatment beneficial in combination with pretreatment?
- What is the optimal route of administration?
- Can having creatine onboard enhance or hinder other neuroprotective treatments (i.e., does prophylactic creatine alter the TBI patient profile)?

Based on the safety profile of creatine and current experimental data, it is obvious that the potential for using creatine following TBI has not been explored sufficiently; however, creatine supplementation may offer a much needed therapeutic approach for targeting TBI in specific populations.

REFERENCES

Adhihetty, P. J., and M. F. Beal. 2008. Creatine and its potential therapeutic value for targeting cellular energy impairment in neurodegenerative diseases. *Neuromolecular Medicine* 10(4):275–290.

Andres, R. H., A. D. Ducray, U. Schlattner, T. Wallimann, and H. R. Widmer. 2008. Functions and effects of creatine in the central nervous system. *Brain Research Bulletin* 76(4):329–343.

Beutner, G., A. Ruck, B. Riede, and D. Brdiczka. 1998. Complexes between porin, hexokinase, mitochondrial creatine kinase and adenylate translocator display properties of the permeability transition pore. Implication for regulation of permeability transition by the kinases. *Biochimica et Biophysica Acta* 1368(1):7–18.

Beutner, G., A. Ruck, B. Riede, W. Welte, and D. Brdiczka. 1996. Complexes between kinases, mitochondrial porin and adenylate translocator in rat brain resemble the permeability transition pore. *FEBS Letters* 396(2–3):189–195.

Cantu, R. C. 1997. Athletic head injuries. *Clinics in Sports Medicine* 16(3):531–542.

Cernak, I., J. Savic, D. Ignjatovic, and M. Jevtic. 1999. Blast injury from explosive munitions. *Journal of Trauma* 47(1):96–103; discussion 103–104.

Choi, D. W., H. Monyer, R. G. Giffard, M. P. Goldberg, and C. W. Christine. 1990. Acute brain injury, nmda receptors, and hydrogen ions: Observations in cortical cell cultures. *Advances in Experimental Medicine and Biology* 268:501–504.

Clark, K. 1998. Epidemiology of athletic head injury. *Clinics in Sports Medicine* 17(1):1–12.

DePalma, R. G., D. G. Burris, H. R. Champion, and M. J. Hodgson. 2005. Blast injuries. *The New England Journal of Medicine* 352(13):1335–1342.

Elder, G. A., and A. Cristian. 2009. Blast-related mild traumatic brain injury: Mechanisms of injury and impact on clinical care. *Mount Sinai Journal of Medicine* 76(2):111–118.

Faden, A. I., P. Demediuk, S. S. Panter, and R. Vink. 1989. The role of excitatory amino acids and nmda receptors in traumatic brain injury. *Science* 244(4906):798–800.

Fiskum, G. 2000. Mitochondrial participation in ischemic and traumatic neural cell death. *Journal of Neurotrauma* 17(10):843–855.

Gilmer, L. K., K. N. Roberts, K. Joy, P. G. Sullivan, and S. W. Scheff. 2009. Early mitochondrial dysfunction after cortical contusion injury. *Journal of Neurotrauma* 26(8):1271–1280.

Gualano, B., G. G. Artioli, J. R. Poortmans, and A. H. Lancha Junior. 2010. Exploring the therapeutic role of creatine supplementation. *Amino Acids* 38(1):31–44.

Gunter, T. E., K. K. Gunter, S. Sheu, and C. E. Gavin. 1994. Mitochondrial calcium transport: Physiological and pathological relevance. *The American Journal of Physiology* 267:C313–C339.

Hoge, C. W., D. McGurk, J. L. Thomas, A. L. Cox, C. C. Engel, and C. A. Castro. 2008. Mild traumatic brain injury in U.S. soldiers returning from Iraq. *The New England Journal of Medicine* 358(5):453–463.

Jones, E., N. T. Fear, and S. Wessely. 2007. Shell shock and mild traumatic brain injury: A historical review. *American Journal of Psychiatry* 164(11):1641–1645.

Langlois, J. A., W. Rutland-Brown, and M. M. Wald. 2006. The epidemiology and impact of traumatic brain injury: A brief overview. *Journal of Head Trauma and Rehabilitation* 21(5):375–378.

Ling, G., F. Bandak, R. Armonda, G. Grant, and J. Ecklund. 2009. Explosive blast neurotrauma. *Journal of Neurotrauma* 26(6):815–825.

Maragos, W. F., and A. S. Korde. 2004. Mitochondrial uncoupling as a potential therapeutic target in acute central nervous system injury. *Journal of Neurochemistry* 91(2):257–262.

Mazzeo, A. T., A. Beat, A. Singh, and M. R. Bullock. 2009. The role of mitochondrial transition pore, and its modulation, in traumatic brain injury and delayed neurodegeneration after TBI. *Experimental Neurology* 218(2):363–370.

Mbye, L. H., I. N. Singh, P. G. Sullivan, J. E. Springer, and E. D. Hall. 2008. Attenuation of acute mitochondrial dysfunction after traumatic brain injury in mice by NIM811, a non-immunosuppressive cyclosporin A analog. *Experimental Neurology* 209(1):243–253.

Mujika, I., and S. Padilla. 1997. Creatine supplementation as an ergogenic acid for sports performance in highly trained athletes: A critical review. *International Journal of Sports Medicine* 18(7):491–496.

O'Gorman, E., G. Beutner, M. Dolder, A. P. Koretsky, D. Brdiczka, and T. Wallimann. 1997. The role of creatine kinase in inhibition of mitochondrial permeability transition. *FEBS Letters* 414(2):253–257.

Pandya, J. D., J. R. Pauly, V. N. Nukala, A. H. Sebastian, K. M. Day, A. S. Korde, W. F. Maragos, E. D. Hall, and P. G. Sullivan. 2007. Post-injury administration of mitochondrial uncouplers increases tissue sparing and improves behavioral outcome following traumatic brain injury in rodents. *Journal of Neurotrauma* 24(5):798–811.

Pandya, J. D., J. R. Pauly, and P. G. Sullivan. 2009. The optimal dosage and window of opportunity to maintain mitochondrial homeostasis following traumatic brain injury using the uncoupler FCCP. *Experimental Neurology* 218(2):381–389.

Rutland-Brown, W., J. A. Langlois, K. E. Thomas, and Y. L. Xi. 2006. Incidence of traumatic brain injury in the United States, 2003. *Journal of Head Trauma Rehabilitation* 21(6):544–548.

Scheff, S. W., and H. S. Dhillon. 2004. Creatine-enhanced diet alters levels of lactate and free fatty acids after experimental brain injury. *Neurochemical Research* 29(2):469–479.

Setnik, L., and J. J. Bazarian. 2007. The characteristics of patients who do not seek medical treatment for traumatic brain injury. *Brain Injury* 21(1):1–9.

Singh, I. N., P. G. Sullivan, Y. Deng, L. H. Mbye, and E. D. Hall. 2006. Time course of post-traumatic mitochondrial oxidative damage and dysfunction in a mouse model of focal traumatic brain injury: Implications for neuroprotective therapy. *Journal of Cerebral Blood Flow and Metabolism* 26(11):1407–1418.

Sullivan, P. G., J. D. Geiger, M. P. Mattson, and S. W. Scheff. 2000. Dietary supplement creatine protects against traumatic brain injury. *Annals of Neurology* 48(5):723–729.

Sullivan, P. G., A. G. Rabchevsky, P. C. Waldmeier, and J. E. Springer. 2005. Mitochondrial permeability transition in cns trauma: Cause or effect of neuronal cell death? *Journal of Neuroscience Research* 79(1–2):231–239.

Sullivan, P. G., J. E. Springer, E. D. Hall, and S. W. Scheff. 2004. Mitochondrial uncoupling as a therapeutic target following neuronal injury. *Journal of Bioenergetics and Biomembranes* 36(4):353–356.

Thurman, D. J., C. M. Branche, and J. E. Sniezek. 1998. The epidemiology of sports-related traumatic brain injuries in the United States: Recent developments. *Journal of Head Trauma Rehabilitation* 13(2):1–8.

Trudeau, D. L., J. Anderson, L. M. Hansen, D. N. Shagalov, J. Schmoller, S. Nugent, and S. Barton. 1998. Findings of mild traumatic brain injury in combat veterans with PTSD and a history of blast concussion. *Journal of Neuropsychiatry and Clinical Neurosciences* 10(3):308–313.

Nutritional Care of Active Duty Patients with TBI

Stephanie Sands[27]

INTRODUCTION

Traumatic brain injury (TBI) is a leading cause of death and disability in the United States. Among military personnel serving in Operation Enduring Freedom/Operation Iraqi Freedom (OEF/OIF), the likelihood of traumatic brain and other polytrauma injuries is significantly elevated. As defined by the U.S. Veterans Health Administration, polytrauma is "two or more injuries to physical regions or organ systems, one of which may be life threatening, resulting in physical, cognitive, psychological, or psychosocial impairments and functional disability" (United States Department of Veterans Affairs, 2009). Such injuries are often a result of rocket-propelled grenades, improvised explosive devises, gunshot wounds, and landmines. In 2005, the United States Congress established four Polytrauma Rehabilitation Centers, one of which is the James A. Haley Veterans' Hospital (JAHVH) in Tampa, Florida (Scott et al., 2006). This report is largely based on nutritional management and monitoring of complex variables of patients who have suffered TBI and polytrauma in the sub-acute and long-term setting at JAHVH.

SUB-ACUTE NUTRITIONAL MANAGEMENT

Following severe trauma and acute TBI, striking metabolic changes involving an accelerated catabolic rate and extensive nitrogen losses proportional to the severity of injury are common (Cook and Hatton, 2007). The hypermetabolic response is related to increases in energy expenditure, oxygen consumption, carbon dioxide production as well as primary mediators such as catecholamines, corticosteroids, and inflammatory cytokines (Berry, 2009; Esper, 2004). Because the brain functions as a regulator for metabolic activity, disruptions caused by TBI result in a cascade of hormonal modifications, irregular cellular metabolism, and dynamic cerebral and systemic inflammatory response as an effort to circulate substrate required at the cellular level. The end result of these alterations involves systemic catabolism causing an increase in basal metabolism, oxygen consumption, glycogenolysis, hyperglycemia, proteolysis, muscle wasting, and energy requirements (Cook et al., 2008). Optimal timing of nutrition, fluid, and electrolyte management may improve the overall clinical course in TBI patients. The fundamental goal of nutritional intervention is to provide adequate calories and protein sufficient to meet the demands of hypermetabolism and increased protein breakdown as a means of preserving lean body mass while maintaining skin integrity, immune function, gastrointestinal mucosal integrity, wound healing, and nitrogen balance during rehabilitation.

While providing nutritional care of polytrauma patients during the months following injury, one of the most challenging decisions is the accurate assessment and provision of essential calories as the complications related to under- or overfeeding can compromise rehabilitation prognosis. Nutrition support should be aimed toward current physiologic

---

[27]James A. Haley Veteran's Hospital.

reactions and should not exacerbate complications of the current phase (stress, catabolic, anabolic). Underfeeding can result in decreased respiratory muscle strength, decreased ventilator drive, failure to wean from mechanical ventilation, impaired organ function, immunosuppression, poor wound healing, increased risk of nosocomial infection, and low transport protein levels. This cachexia (i.e. wasting syndrome or loss of weight, muscle atrophy, fatigue, weakness, and significant loss of appetite in someone who is not actively trying to lose weight) can impact mobility, functional rehabilitation and overall length of stay as well as the development of complications such as decubitus ulcers, pneumonia, urinary tract infections, and venous thromboembolism. Among the complications of overfeeding include the risk of refeeding syndrome,[28] hyperglycemia, azotemia, hypertriglyceridemia, electrolyte imbalance, immunosuppression, alterations in hydration status, hepatic steatosis, and failure to wean from mechanical ventilation (Cook et al., 2008; Esper, 2004).

Calorie Provision

Energy expenditure has been investigated extensively and has been shown to be elevated following acute TBI (Cook and Hatton, 2007; Rajpal and Johnston, 2009). Two methods for determining energy requirements involve measurement of resting metabolic rate using indirect calorimetry (IC), or estimating energy needs with the use of predictive equations and clinical judgment. Although IC is considered the "gold standard" for determining energy expenditure in TBI, many clinicians do not have access to resources necessary to measure metabolic rate. Additionally, calorie requirements may vary day to day in this population secondary to symptoms such as sympathetic storming, fevers, or muscle contractions. More commonly, clinicians use one of more than 200 predictive equations that have been developed for estimating energy expenditure (McCarthy et al., 2008). For example, the Brain Trauma Foundation (BTF) recommends use of the Harris Benedict Equation multiplied by a stress factor of 1.4 with an observed variance of 1.2–2.5 (Bratton et al., 2007), and the American Society of Enteral and Parenteral Nutrition recommends 25–30 kcal/kg in critically ill patients. However, it should be noted that there is a limited amount of literature available following the critical care setting or for patients with further polytrauma injuries in addition to TBI. Because utilizing the above methods to determine energy expenditure can be imprecise considering the complexity of this patient population, the following variables have been observed or proven to alter metabolic rate (Berry, 2009; Cook et al., 2008; Dickerson and Roth-Yousey, 2005; Esper, 2004; Frankenfield, 2006; Rajpal and Johnston, 2009):

- Severity of trauma and additional injuries, burns, or wounds
- Time since injury, depending on the ongoing stress response and degree of healing
- Physiologic effects—blood pressure, heart rate, respiratory rate, sympathetic storming such as seen in Paroxysmal Autonomic Instability with Dystonia (Blackman et al., 2004), body temperature (diaphoresis, hyperthermia, and medically induced hypothermia)
- Physical activity (restlessness, agitation) or muscular dysfunction (posturing, dystonia)
- Level of consciousness (Glasgow Coma Score)
- Cognitive Functioning (Rancho Los Amigos Scale)
- Neuroendocrine disruption
- Sepsis and inflammatory response

---

[28] Abnormalities in fluid balance, glucose metabolism, vitamin deficiency, hypophosphatemia, hypomagnesemia, and hypokalemia in patients exposed to enteral or parenteral nutrition after a period of starvation.

- Medications: Central nervous system agents—sedatives, anticonvulsants, analgesics, narcotics, hypnotics, barbiturates; autonomic neuromuscular blocking agents; cardiovascular agents—beta-adrenergic blockers; steroids, inotropic agents.
- Ventilator support
- Thermic effect of food generated by caloric intake
- Preinjury nutritional status and/or malnutrition

Protein Requirements

Protein requirements following TBI are grossly elevated. Protein catabolism peaks 8 to 14 days after injury with documented nitrogen losses up to 30 grams per day. This extreme protein breakdown can cause a 10 percent loss of lean body mass during the first seven days of injury (Cook and Hatton, 2007; Gleghorn et al., 2005; Rajpal and Johnston, 2009). Urinary urea nitrogen (UUN) values can be monitored to determine a state of nitrogen balance. Although it is often unrealistic to obtain nitrogen balance during the first week after injury regardless of nutritional provision, nitrogen balance is an important way to measure the adequacy of caloric intake and metabolism in the weeks that follow (Esper, 2004; Rajpal and Johnston, 2009). The BTF recommends protein provision of 1.5–2.0 g/kg of body weight in TBI patients (Cook and Hatton, 2007; Cook et al., 2008). Although hepatic production of transport proteins (albumin, prealbumin, transferring) is reduced during states of inflammation regardless of nutrition, monitoring their trends can be helpful to determine recovery from the inflammatory process along with overall clinical improvement such as wound healing, infection resolution, and weaning from ventilator support. Some facilities also incorporate specific amino acids into their nutritional programs such as glutamine, arginine, or branched chain amino acids (Esper, 2004; Rajpal and Johnston, 2009).

Method of Feeding

Another area of consideration during nutritional care of TBI patients is the method of feeding. Initially, it has to be determined whether to use parenteral (PN) or enteral (EN) nutrition. It is generally accepted that EN is preferable over PN, with the exception of cases such as barbiturate coma, multiple vasopressors (risk of bowel necrosis), or prolonged periods of being supine. When it is determined that EN is desirable, many clinicians debate whether to obtain small bowel or gastric access given that there is limited consensus that postpyloric feedings have demonstrated improved outcomes. TBI patients often exhibit gastrointestinal dysfunction with increased incidences of aspiration pneumonia, diarrhea, vomiting, abdominal distention, and increased gastric residuals. Impaired gastric emptying is often present secondary to decreased lower esophageal sphincter tone, vagus nerve damage, elevated levels of endogenous opioids/endorphins, elevated intracranial pressure, or medication side effects (Cook et al., 2008; Esper, 2004; Ott et al., 1991; Rajpal and Johnston, 2009). Often nasogastric or nasoenteral tubes are placed until it is determined that longer term EN access is needed. The placement of longer term EN access via percutaneous endoscopic gastrostomy (PEG) tubes often proves successful in establishing well-tolerated feeding access (Cook and Hatton, 2007). Despite the potential feeding difficulties in many TBI patients, the majority of these patients are able to receive safe and adequate nutrition through EN. Approaches to improve EN tolerance include head of bed elevation (30–45 degrees), continuous tube feeding at low infusion rates advanced per tolerance, the use of pro-motility agents, using concentrated enteral formulas to decrease total volume, and consideration of small bowel versus gastric feeds (Cook et al., 2008).

TABLE C-11 Sample of Drug-Nutrition Interactions Common in TBI Medical Management

Medication	Examples of Nutrition Implications
Antipsychotics (Ziprasidone, Olanzapine, Risperidone)	Linked to weight gain
Barbiturates	May lower metabolic rate or cause constipation
Bisacodyl	Risk of hypocalcemia and decreased fat absorption
Bromocriptine	Potential of nausea/vomiting/constipation, elevated residuals
Carbamazepine	Increased risk of hyponatremia, can cause formation of orange rubbery precipitate when combined with water/dilatants
Corticosteroids	Risk of hyperglycemia; osteoporosis and gastric ulcer risk with chronic use
Mannitol	Monitor for hypokalemia, hypomagnesemia, hypovolemia
Metoclopramide	Possible for changes in mental status/cognition
Mirtazapine	Related to increased appetite and weight gain
Narcotic analgesics	Delayed emptying/constipation (especially in opioid usage)
Oxandrolone	Linked to elevated liver enzymes and/or lipid panel[a]
Phenytoin	Absorption may be impaired with provided with enteral nutrition, possible decline in folate, vitamin D
Propofol	Provides lipid calories (pro-inflammatory fat source)
Stimulants (Methylphenidate, Dextroamphetamine amphetamine)	May cause decreased appetite and weight loss
Vasopressors	Decreases gut perfusion
Zolpidem	May cause appetite changes, binge eating, nocturnal eating[a]

[a]Anecdotal observations noted at JAHVH; UpToDate Online 18.3.
SOURCE: Cook and Hatton, 2007.

Medication Interactions

Drug-nutrient interactions require consideration when providing medical nutrition therapy to TBI patients. Registered dietitians review patient medications as a part of nutritional assessment to identify nutritional implications. For example, enteral nutrition is typically held one to two hours before and after the administration of phenytoin to prevent absorptive changes and chelation. Other medications may lower electrolyte and micronutrient levels, or increase the risk of weight gain or loss. Table C-11 provides examples of some interactions encountered in the clinical setting.

Sample of 12 Polytrauma Patients

As discussed previously, there is a limited amount of research evaluating nutritional needs of TBI patients following the acute critical period or with multiple polytrauma injuries in addition to TBI. Figures C-23 through C-28 represent a snapshot of 12 patients in acute rehabilitation at JAHVH. The categories illustrated include patient age, time since injury, method of feeding, percent of usual body weight lost and caloric provision required to facilitate weight maintenance of weight gain of one to two pounds per week. The illustrations depict at typical distribution of patients which changes from day to day.

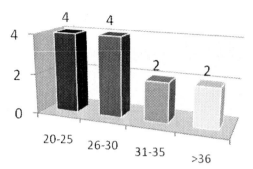

FIGURE C-23   Distribution of 12 polytrauma patients according to age (captured 9/15/2010 at JAHVH).

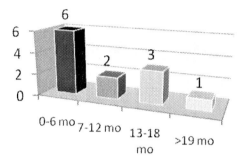

FIGURE C-24   Distribution of 12 polytrauma patients according to the number of months since injury (captured 9/15/2010 at JAHVH).

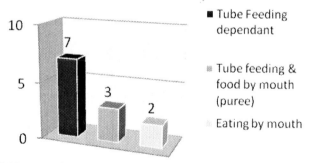

FIGURE C-25   Distribution of 12 polytrauma patients according to the method of feeding (captured 9/15/2010 at JAHVH).

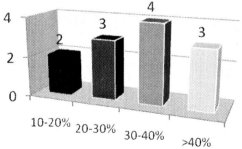

FIGURE C-26   Distribution of 12 polytrauma patients according to the percent of pre-injury weight loss since injury (captured 9/15/2010 at JAHVH).

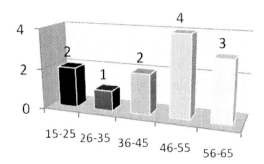

FIGURE C-27 Distribution of 12 polytrauma patients according to number of calories per kilogram to attain weight maintenance or gain (1–2 lbs per week) (captured 9/15/2010 at JAHVH).

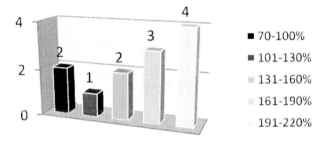

FIGURE C-28 Distribution of 12 polytrauma patients according to percent of estimated resting metabolic rate using the Harris Benedict Equation to attain weight maintenance or gain (1–2 lbs per week) (captured 9/15/2010 at JAHVH)

LONG TERM NUTRITIONAL CONSIDERATIONS

While the concerns of severe weight loss following TBI in active duty service members are significant, the opposing issue regarding unintentional weight gain has scarcely been discussed in the literature. Following TBI, changes such as alterations in the brain's regulation of hunger and satiety, neuroendocrine dysfunction, brain injury-induced hyperphagia, medication related side effects, cognitive impairments, or emotional coping may impact the ability to maintain a healthy weight. In the post-acute rehabilitation setting at JAHVH, a number of polytrauma patients experience detrimental weight gain and dyslipidemia.

Under normal conditions, the brain functions to regulate energy homeostasis by constant transmission of signals that influence energy intake and ultimately body weight (Woods and D'Alessio, 2008). Satiation signals such as cholecystokinin (CCK), glucagon-like peptide-1 (GLP-1), peptide tyrosine-tyrosine (PYY) and apolipoprotein A-IV (apo A-IV) are secreted in response to specific macronutrient stimuli. These peptides, many of which are synthesized in the brain in addition to the gastrointestinal tract, are released in response to food ingestion and act to reduce meal size. Adiposity signals, insulin and leptin, are secreted relative to the amount of body fat and are transported across the blood-brain barrier to interact with neuronal receptors predominately in the hypothalamus. Because TBI may impair the transmission of these signals, many patients experience an altered sensation of hunger and satiety.

TABLE C-12   Nutritional Implications of Post Traumatic Hypopituitarism

Hormone Insufficiency/Deficiency	Nutritional Implications
Adrenocorticotrophic hormone (ACTH) (0–19 percent of TBI patients with deficiencies)	Nausea/vomiting, abdominal pain, anorexia, weight loss, hypotension, tachycardia, hyponatremia, hypoglycemia, normocytic anemia
Growth hormone (GH) (6–33 percent of TBI patients with deficiencies)	Osteoporosis, dyslipidemia, atherosclerosis, visceral obesity, reduced lean body mass
Hypothyroidism-Thyroid stimulating hormone (TSH) (1–10 percent of TBI patients with deficiencies)	Weight gain, hypotension, myopathy, dyspnea, periorbital edema, bradycardia, normocytic anemia, mild hyponatremia
Luteinizing hormone (LH)/Follicle-stimulating hormone (FSH) (2–20 percent of TBI patients with deficiencies)	Reduced muscle mass and exercise tolerance (men), decreased breast tissue and bone mineral density (women)

SOURCE: Compiled from Schneider et al., 2007.

Disturbances of the neuroendocrine system following TBI have nutritional implications that should be considered. Schneider et al (2007) identified 19 clinical studies that report the prevalence of endocrine dysfunction ranges from 15–68 percent in TBI patients. Most researchers agree upon the association of neuroendocrine changes and the severity of brain injury, however variables such as secondary brain damage and medical complications make analysis and prediction more complicated (Rothman et al., 2007). Klose and associates (2007) reported that TBI patients with posttraumatic hypopituitarism display symptoms such as adverse lipid profiles, unfavorable body composition, and worsened perceived health-related quality of life (lowered energy, sleep, increased social isolation) compared to those with preserved pituitary function. Table C-12 reflects sample nutritional implications of post-traumatic hypopituitarism.

Although there is a paucity of information regarding brain injury-induced hyperphagia, clinicians working in TBI are likely to encounter patients with an abnormally increased appetite for and consumption of food. This can be especially problematic in a significantly impaired patient with limited self-awareness. Rao and Lyketsos (2000) describe a complex syndrome they refer to as Behavioral Dyscontrol Disorder, Major Variant. This syndrome has mood, cognitive, and behavioral manifestations in both acute and chronic stages of 5–70 percent of TBI. The behaviors reported in this report include impulsivity, aggression, hyperactivity, hyperphagia, and pica. One such scenario at JAHVH resulted in the removal of a patient-accessible family refrigerator secondary to a patient with an insatiable appetite and weight gain. This patient experienced weight gain at a rate of 15 pounds per month, with a total gain of 110 pounds over seven months. He required constant nursing supervision to prevent further instances of excessive eating and consumption of non-food substances like coffee grounds. Instances of rapid and nearly uncontrollable weight gain as described are not uncommon among this population. A multidisciplinary approach should be utilized to treat such conditions by developing environmental modification strategies, behavioral therapy, psychotherapy, and family therapy.

Another contributing factor to the weight gain experienced in the postacute setting following TBI is medication side effects. Common medications prescribed following brain injury such as antidepressants, anxiolytics, anticonvulsants, and antipsychotics may promote increased appetite and unintentional weight gain. Healthcare providers should be aware of these side effects and consider weight-neutral alternatives.

Cognitive impairments among service members who have suffered TBI greatly impact the successfulness of nutrition counseling to a degree that cannot be overstated. For example, consider how executive dysfunction may inhibit the ability to make healthful choices secondary to difficulties in planning, problem solving, organizing, sequencing, self-regulation and monitoring, judgment, set-shifting, impulse control, initiation, and motivation (Rao and Lyketsos, 2000). Tasks such as grocery shopping, reading a recipe, preparing a meal, or understanding and applying healthful eating guidelines can be nearly impossible for some patients. Furthermore, among patients with varying levels of memory impairment, the ability to remember nutritional recommendations may be compromised in addition to recalling and identifying problematic eating behaviors. The combination of impaired hunger and satiety cues as well as short-term memory loss often results in patients who cannot remember having eaten just minutes after mealtime and are likely to overeat as well.

Lastly, the emotional strain of suffering from TBI can play a significant role in the ability to make smart choices and maintain a healthy weight. Coping with symptoms such as depression, boredom, demoralization, anxiety, irritability, anger, the feeling of loss, discouragement, and posttraumatic stress disorder can lead to uncontrolled emotional eating. Additionally, families of those who have experienced a TBI are susceptible to encourage the use of food as a coping and comforting mechanism. These patients greatly benefit from a team approach to identify coping strategies and alternatives to eating as well as nutrition education to encourage healthy choices.

COMPLEMENTARY AND ALTERNATIVE MEDICINE

Incorporation of complementary and alternative medicine (CAM) into treatment regimens has become more prevalent among both acute and chronically ill patients. Many researchers are investigating the role of CAM in providing resilience to brain injury or as a treatment modality following an injury. A large portion of posttraumatic neurodegeneration is a result of secondary damage from a pathochemical and pathophysiological cascade during the first minutes, hours, and days following an injury (Hall et al., 2010). Many investigators seek to discover the optimal timing of neuroprotective substances to prevent exacerbation of damage caused by the primary injury. However, there are many challenges that come with both performing and interpreting research relating to CAM. As described by Mullin (2009):

- The majority of CAM providers are non-physician based, utilizing techniques and tools that are more experiential than evidence-based.
- CAM often focuses on treatment of symptoms, which can be subjective, rather than the underlying diagnosis of Western-based medicine.
- Blinding is often compromised and many publications labeled as randomized control trials are actually not blinded.
- Publication biases are created when investigators, reviewers, and editors submit or accept manuscripts based on the strength or direction of the findings.
    - Access to CAM literature is incomplete; one such example includes mainstream databases such as MEDLINE, which indexes only 10 percent of CAM journal worldwide.
    - Negative CAM findings are more likely to be published in mainstream medical journals, whereas most studies published in leading CAM journals have positive results.

○ Studies outside of the United States are more likely to be positive than those in the United States.

For example, while completing a PubMed literature review on supplements and TBI over the past five years, Table C-13 depicts the number of articles referenced with various supplements. It is important to note that the majority of these references utilize animal studies to answer their research question. While understanding the possibility of publication bias, one may wonder how to identify the CAM articles being published and indexed in other locations.

Clinicians attempting to provide evidence-based guidelines to patients and families are likely to encounter difficulties interpreting the literature and making recommendations. Reasons for this include the publication bias as described above, the lack of clear data, and the number of supplements being promoted. There is a copious amount of marketing which targets TBI patients anywhere along the spectrum of severity and time since injury. Patients and their families are likely to encounter or trial a number of supplements which are promoted to treat side effects of TBI or improve brain health and functioning. Table C-14 reflects a list of supplements being taken among different levels of TBI severity as disclosed by patients and families over one month at JAHVH. An especially susceptible population includes the caregivers of emerging conscious patients. Some programs seek to discover a beneficial cocktail of nutraceuticals which may assist in promoting consciousness. Incidences of patients receiving 45 different nutraceuticals, some of which are administered two or three times a day, as an effort to cause the patient to emerge have been encountered. While assisting patients in making informed decisions regarding supplements, factors should be evaluated such as the risk of causing harm if taken in excessive doses, decreasing medication side effects or modifying the action, lowering seizure threshold, instigating other deficiencies, or mislabeling or adulterating supplements.

TABLE C-13 Depiction of PubMed Literature Review of TBI and Various Supplements Over the Past 5 Years (2005–2010)

Number of Hits	Supplements Being Investigated
137	TBI and Antioxidants
53	TBI and Arginine
43	TBI and Fiber
40	TBI and Vitamins (6-B vitamins, 4-vitamin D)
36	TBI and Choline
28	TBI and Tyrosine
24	TBI and Melatonin
23	TBI and Zinc
23	TBI and CoEnzyme 10
15	TBI and Glutamine
8	TBI and Curcumin
8	TBI and Ketogenic Diet
5	TBI and Omega 3
4	TBI and Caffeine
3	TBI and Branched Chain Amino Acids
2	TBI and Lipoic acid

NOTE: The majority of TBI and CAM articles are animal studies, very few of these studies represent human research.

TABLE C-14   Illustration of Supplements Encountered Among TBI patients, Ranging from Mild to Severe Injuries (JAHVH from 8/20/2010–9/20/2010)

Antioxidant vitamins	Cinnamon	Ginseng	Omega-6 fatty acids
Apigenin	Citric Acid	Green tea	Resveratrol
B Vitamins (mega-doses)	CoEnzyme Q10	Huperzine	RNA
Baicalein Butcher's Broom	Cognitex (a-glyceryl phosphoryl choline, ginger, rosemary, phosphatidylserine, pregnolone, vinpocentine, leucoselect phytosome, wild blueberry, sensoril ashwagandha, perluxan)	Individual amino acids or blends (most commonly: branched chain, tyrosine, glutamine, arginine)	Rutin
Caffeine	Corella	Lipoic acid	Spirulina
Capsaicin	Creatine	Luteolin	St. John's wart
Carnitine (L-configuration)	Curcumin	Magnesium	Tocopherol
Carnosine (L-configuration)	D-Ribose	Milk thistle	Valarian root
Catechin	Feverfew	Mycelia extract	Vinpoceti
Choline	Ginkgo biloba	n-3 fatty acids	Zinc

CONCLUSION

Nutritional assessment, monitoring, and evaluation should be a priority throughout the course of TBI and polytrauma injuries among active-duty service members. Registered dietitians have the educational background to coordinate acute nutritional support and subacute nutritional management based on the variety of nutritional conditions prevalent following TBI. Furthermore, a multidisciplinary team approach is critical to discuss progress, treatment plans, and goals for overall best outcomes.

REFERENCES

Berry, A. 2009. Neurocritical Care 101: Learning the lingo for effective nutrition management. *Support Line* 31(6):3–11.

Blackman, J. A., P. D. Patrick, M. L. Buck, and R. S. Rust Jr. 2004. Paroxysmal autonomic instability with dystonia after brain injury. *Archives of Neurology* 61(3):321–328.

Bratton, S., D. Chestnut, J. Ghajar, F. Hammond, O. Harris, R. Hartl, J. Schouten, L. Shutter, S. Timmons, J. Ullman, W. Videtta, J. Wilberger, and D. Wright. 2007. Nutrition. *Journal of Neurotrauma* 24(1 Suppl.):S77–S82.

Cook, A., and J. Hatton. 2007. Neurological impairment. In *The A.S.P.E.N. Nutrition support core curriculum: A case-based approach-the adult patient.* 2nd ed., edited by M. Gottschlich, M. DeLegge, T. Mattox, C. Mueller and P. Worthingon. Silver Spring, MD: American Society for Parenteral and Enteral Nutrition. Pp. 424–439.

Cook, A. M., A. Peppard, and B. Magnuson. 2008. Nutrition considerations in traumatic brain injury. *Nutrition in Clinical Practice* 23(6):608–620.

Dickerson, R. N., and L. Roth-Yousey. 2005. Medication effects on metabolic rate: A systematic review (part 1). *Journal of the American Dietetic Association* 105(5):835–843.

Esper, D. 2004. Metabolic response and nutrition management in patients with severe head injury. *Support Line* 26(2):9–13.

Frankenfield, D. 2006. Energy expenditure and protein requirements after traumatic injury. *Nutrition in Clinical Practice* 21(5):430–437.

Gleghorn, E., K. Amorde-Spalding, and M. DeLegge. 2005. Neurologic diseases. In *A.S.P.E.N. Nutrition support manual.* 2nd ed., edited by R. Merritt. Silver Spring, MD: American Society for Parenteral and Enteral Nutrition. Pp. 246–250.

Hall, E. D., R. A. Vaishnav, and A. G. Mustafa. 2010. Antioxidant therapies for traumatic brain injury. *Neurotherapeutics* 7(1):51–61.

Klose, M. C., T. Watt, J. Brennum, and U. Feldt-Rasmussen. 2007. Posttraumatic hypopituitarism is associated with an unfavorable body composition and lipid profile, and decreased quality of life 12 months after injury. *Journal of Clinical Endocrinology and Metabolism* 92(10):3861–3868.

McCarthy, M. S., J. Fabling, R. Martindale, and S. A. Meyer. 2008. Nutrition support of the traumatically injured warfighter. *Critical Care Nursing Clinics of North America* 20(1):59–65.

Mullin, G. E. 2009. Issues in complementary and alternative nutrition treatments. *Nutrition in Clinical Practice* 24(5):543–548.

Ott, L., B. Young, R. Phillips, C. McClain, L. Adams, R. Dempsey, P. Tibbs, and U. Yun Ryo. 1991. Altered gastric emptying in the head-injured patient: Relationship to feeding intolerance. *Journal of Neurosurgery* 74(5):738–742.

Rajpal, V., and J. Johnston. 2009. Nutrition management of traumatic brain injury patients. *Support Line* 31(1):10–19.

Rao, V., and C. Lyketsos. 2000. Neuropsychiatric sequelae of traumatic brain injury. *Psychosomatics* 41(2):95–103.

Rothman, M. S., D. B. Arciniegas, C. M. Filley, and M. E. Wierman. 2007. The neuroendocrine effects of traumatic brain injury. *Journal of Neuropsychiatry and Clinical Neurosciences* 19(4):363–372.

Schneider, H. J., I. Kreitschmann-Andermahr, E. Ghigo, G. K. Stalla, and A. Agha. 2007. Hypothalamopituitary dysfunction following traumatic brain injury and aneurysmal subarachnoid hemorrhage: A systematic review. *Journal of the American Medical Association* 298(12):1429–1438.

Scott, S. G., H. G. Belanger, R. D. Vanderploeg, J. Massengale, and J. Scholten. 2006. Mechanism-of-injury approach to evaluating patients with blast-related polytrauma. *Journal of the American Osteopathic Association* 106(5):265–270.

United States Department of Veterans Affairs. 2009. *VA polytrauma systems of care.* http://www.polytrauma.va.gov/definitions.asp#polytrauma (accessed 10/15/10).

Woods, S. C., and D. A. D'Alessio. 2008. Central control of body weight and appetite. *Journal of Clinical Endocrinology and Metabolism* 93(11 Suppl. 1):S37–S50.

D

Glossary

Adequate Intake	The recommended average daily intake level for a nutrient, based on observed or experimentally determined approximations or estimates of intake by a group of apparently healthy people, that is assumed to be adequate. Used when there is no Recommended Dietary Allowance available.
Amygdala	Almond-shaped groups of nuclei located deep within the medial temporal lobes of the brain in complex vertebrates, including humans. The amygdala is involved in learning and memory, especially fear-related, and is central to the development of expression of conditioned fear reactions.
Angiogenesis	The process involving the growth of new blood vessels from preexisting vessels. (This term incorporates both vasculogenesis, or spontaneous blood-vessel formation; and intussusception, formation of new blood vessels by splitting off existing ones.)
Anoxia	A total decrease in level of oxygen reaching tissues of the body; an extreme form of hypoxia that can result in permanent damage.
Apoptotis	Also known as programmed cell death. Describes the biochemical events leading to characteristic morphological cell changes (blebbing, loss of cell membrane asymmetry and attachment, cell shrinkage, nuclear fragmentation, chromatin condensation, and chromosomal deoxynribonucleic acid fragmentation) and death.

Astrocytes	A subtype of glial cells that supply glucose needed for nerve activity, maintain the blood-brain barrier, maintain extracellular ion balance, and play a principal role in the repair and scarring process of the brain and spinal cord following traumatic injuries.
Astrocytosis	An abnormal increase in the number of astrocytes due to the destruction of nearby neurons, typically because of hypoglycemia or oxygen deprivation (hypoxia). Astrocytosis represents a reparative process; in some cases, it may be diffuse in a large region.
Autocoid	An organic substance, such as a hormone, produced in one part of an organism and transported by the blood or lymph to another part of the organism where it exerts a physiologic effect on that part.
Axonal sprouting	The ability of the adult brain to form new connections in areas denervated by a lesion.
Barthel Index	First published in the 1965 *Maryland State Medical Journal*, this measurement of 10 activities of daily living and mobility is used to assess physical disability.
Blood-brain barrier	A separation of circulating blood and the brain extracellular fluid in the central nervous system, with especially tight junctions around capillaries that prevent diffusion of bacteria and large, hydrophilic molecules into the cerebrospinal fluid.
Brain parenchyma	The functional part of the brain (i.e., neurons and glial cells).
Bregma	The anatomical point on the skull where the frontal and parietal bones meet, i.e., at the intersection of the coronal and the sagittal sutures.
Caudate nucleus	The caudate nuclei are located near the center of the brain, one within each hemisphere, sitting astride the thalamus. They are involved in learning and memory (feedback processing).
Cerebral edema	Excess accumulation of water in intracellular/extracellular spaces of the brain.
Cerebral ischemia	Any pathophysiological state in which there is insufficient blood flow to the brain to meet metabolic demand, which leads to depleted oxygen supply and thus the death of brain tissue. Ischemic stroke is caused by the formation of a clot that blocks blood flow through an artery to the brain.
Cerebrospinal fluid fistula	A tear between the dura and arachnoid membrane, resulting in leakage of CSF into subdural space.

Chronic traumatic encephalopathy	A progressive neurodegenerative disease believed to be caused by repeated trauma to the brain, including mild concussions and subconcussive blows. Its symptoms occur years or decades following head trauma and continue to worsen, and are distinct from the acute or postacute effects of a head injury. The early symptoms may include memory and cognitive difficulties, depression, impulse control problems, and behavior changes. Movement abnormalities are more common later; in many cases, full-blown dementia occurs.
Coma	A state in which a patient is totally unconscious, unresponsive, unaware, and unarousable.
Compressive cranial neuropathy	Cranial nerve injuries that may be caused by fractures, especially at the bottom of the skull. Damage to the facial nerve, the most commonly damaged, results in paralysis of facial muscles.
Computerized tomography (CT)	A noninvasive test combining a series of X-ray views taken from many different angles to produce cross-sectional images of bones and soft tissues. In the head, CT scans can show bone fractures, hemorrhage, hematomas, contusion, and swelling.
Contusion	Focal injuries with an area of cerebral bruising, particularly involving gray matter, in which blood leaks into extravascular space resulting in cell death and loss of tissue. Bleeding from damaged blood vessels is usually the most obvious feature on macroscopic or microscopic examination.
Diffuse axonal injury (DAI)	An injury defined by diffuse damage to axons in the cerebral subcortical parasagittal white matter, corpus callosum, brain stem, and cerebellum. The loss of connections among neurons leads to breakdown of communication.
Diffuse traumatic brain injury	A brain injury due to hypoxia, meningitis, or damage to blood vessels; can include DAI, ischemic brain injury, vascular injury, or swelling and resulting intracranial pressure. Such injuries, which may result from acceleration/deceleration injuries, are often microscopic, multifocal, and difficult to detect.
Disability Rating Scale	A functional assessment developed specifically for patients with moderate to severe traumatic brain injury (TBI).
Edema	Abnormal accumulation of fluid beneath the skin or in one or more cavities of the body.
Edema (cytotoxic)	Intracellular water accumulation in neurons, astrocytes, and microglia irrespective of the integrity of the vascular endothelial wall. It is due to the increased cell permeability for ions, ionic pump failure, and cellular reabsorption of osmotically active solutes.

Edema (vasogenic)	Caused by mechanical or autodigestive disruption or functional breakdown of the endothelial cell layer of brain vessels that are a key element of the BBB. This allows for the uncontrolled transfer of ions and proteins from the intravascular to the extravascular brain compartments, leading to water accumulation.
Estimated Average Requirement	The average daily nutrient intake level estimated to meet the requirement of half of the healthy individuals in a particular life stage and gender group.
Excitotoxicity	Excessive stimulation of glutamate receptors by neurotransmitters resulting in damage to the nerve cells. Excitotoxins like N-methyl-D-aspartate and kainic acid that bind to these receptors, as well as pathologically high levels of glutamate, can cause excitotoxicity by allowing high levels of calcium ions to enter the cell. As a result, an enzymatic cascade, including phospholipases, endonucleases, and proteases, damages cell structures and can cause cell death.
Feeney's weight-drop model	One of several methods used to induce brain trauma (primary injury is mostly focal) in rats and mice. The impact is delivered to the intact dura, causing cortical contusion and damage to the blood-brain barrier.
Focal traumatic brain injury	A focal traumatic injury results from direct mechanical forces and is usually associated with brain tissue damage visible to the naked eye. It typically has symptoms related to the damaged area of the brain; e.g., a stroke can produce focal damage associated with signs and symptoms that correspond to the part of the brain that was damaged. Focal injuries include cerebral contusions; cerebral lacerations; and epidural, subdural, intracerebral, and intraventricular hemorrhage.
Glasgow Coma Scale	A standardized test of level of consciousness and neurological function that uses three measures: eye opening, best verbal response, and best motor response. Patient assessment by the criteria of the scale yields a score between 3 (indicating deep unconsciousness) and either 14 (original scale) or 15 (the more widely used revised scale).
Glasgow Outcome Scale	A five-point score (dead, vegetative, severely disabled, moderately disabled, good recovery) given to victims of TBI postinjury. It is a very general assessment of the overall functioning of head-injury patients. It is not used in the clinical management of patients, but in research to quantify the level of recovery patients have achieved.
Hematoma	Heavy bleeding into or around the brain usually caused by damage to a major blood vessel in the head.
Hemorrhagic stroke	A stroke caused by the breakage or rupture of a blood vessel in the brain. Hemorrhages can be caused by a number of disorders that affect the blood vessels, including long-standing high blood pressure and cerebral aneurysms (weak or thin spots in the vessel wall). There are two types of hemorrhagic stroke: intracerebral and subarachnoid.
Hippocampus	One of two structures in the adult brain where neurogenesis persists.

Hydrocephalus or posttraumatic ventricular enlargement	The accumulation of cerebrospinal fluid resulting from dilation of ventricles and increase in intracranial fluid.
Hyperemia or hyperfusion	An excessive increase in blood flow to tissue(s)
Hypothalamus	The hypothalamus, an extremely complex region in the human brain, is responsible for certain metabolic processes and other activities of the autonomic nervous system, such as the control of body temperature, hunger, thirst, fatigue, sleep, and circadian cycles. The hypothalamus is located below the thalamus, just above the brain stem. It is the primary link between endocrine and nervous systems; nerves in the hypothalamus control the pituitary gland by producing neurohormones that either stimulate or suppress hormone secretions. The hypothalamic-releasing hormones, for example, stimulate or inhibit the secretion of pituitary hormones.
Hypoxia	A deficiency of oxygen reaching the tissues of the body.
Intracranial pressure	A result of swelling of the brain and accumulation of fluids due to injury.
Ischemia	The blockage of arteries and cut-off of blood flow.
Ischemia reperfusion injury	The damage to tissue caused when blood supply returns after a period of ischemia. The absence of oxygen and nutrients from blood creates a condition in which the restoration of circulation results in inflammation and oxidative damage through the induction of oxidative stress rather than restoration of normal function.
Ischemic stroke	Ischemia can be caused by embolic and thrombotic strokes. In an *embolic stroke*, a blood clot forms somewhere in the body (usually the heart), then travels through the bloodstream to the brain, where it eventually reaches a blood vessel too small to allow its passage, causing a stroke. In *thrombotic stroke*, blood flow is impaired because of blockage to one or more arteries supplying blood to the brain. Ischemic strokes can also occur as the result of an unhealthy blood vessel clogged with a buildup of fatty deposits and cholesterol.
Ketogenic diet	A diet formulated to mimic fasting, with limited glucose supply and high fat availability, that favors fatty acid oxidation, ketone body production, and utilization of ketone bodies by the brain as an alternative energy substrate.
Locked-in syndrome	A condition in which the patient is awake and aware but cannot move or communicate due to complete paralysis of the body.
Luria Memory Words test	A test used to assess the memory of elderly patients diagnosed with dementia by presenting word lists in given time periods.

Magnetic resonance imaging	A medical imaging technique that uses the property of nuclear magnetic resonance to visualize areas inside the body but that, unlike CT scans or tráditional X-rays, uses no ionizing radiation. It provides more detail and contrast than a CT scan.
Medial prefrontal cortex	The anterior part of the frontal lobes of the brain, it has been implicated in planning complex cognitive behaviors, personality expression, decision making, and moderating correct social behavior. The most typical psychological term for functions carried out by the prefrontal cortex area is executive function. Biological models suggest that a fundamental mechanism underpinning posttraumatic stress disorder involves an exaggerated response of the amygdala, which results in impaired regulation by the medial prefrontal cortex.
Modified Rankin Scale	First published in 1988, this measures activities of daily living to assess physical disability in stroke patients and is now the most commonly used clinical outcome measure for stroke clinical trials.
Morris water maze	A test widely used in behavioral neuroscience to study the psychological processes and neural mechanisms of spatial learning and memory. Animals are placed in a large circular pool of water and required to escape onto a hidden platform whose location can normally be identified only by using spatial memory.
Necrosis	The premature death of cells and living tissue. Necrosis is caused by factors external to the cell or tissue, such as infection, toxins, or trauma. Cells that die due to necrosis do not usually send the same chemical signals to the immune system that cells undergoing apoptosis do. This prevents nearby phagocytes from locating and engulfing the dead cells, leading to a buildup of dead tissue and cell debris at or near the site of the cell death.
Neuroglycopenia	A shortage of glucose (glycopenia) in the brain, usually due to hypoglycemia. Glycopenia affects the function of neurons, and alters brain function and behavior. Prolonged neuroglycopenia can result in permanent damage to the brain.
Perfusion	Process of nutritive delivery of arterial blood to a capillary bed in the biological tissue.
Polytrauma	Two or more injuries to physical regions or organ systems, one of which may be life-threatening, that result in physical, cognitive, psychological, or psychosocial impairments and functional disability.
Postconcussive syndrome	Symptoms of mild TBI that continue for longer than three months. These vary from person to person but include numerous cognitive, affective, or somatic symptoms such as headache, dizziness, balance problems, nausea, vision problems, increased sensitivity to noise and/or light, and depression, among many others.
Recommended Dietary Allowance	The average daily dietary nutrient intake level that is sufficient to meet the nutrient requirements of nearly all (97–98 percent) healthy individuals in a particular life stage and gender group.

Refractory epilepsy	Epilepsy that is resistant to treatment.
Rhinorrhea	In the context of brain injury, cerebral spinal fluid leakage from the nose.
Rotarod performance test	A performance test applied to animals that uses a rotating rod with forced motor activity being applied. It measures parameters such as riding time (seconds) or endurance, balance, and coordination.
Rotarod score	Measures performance on a Rotarod treadmill in order to assess motor coordination, and thus neurological performance, in mice and rats.
Second impact syndrome	A repeat concussion that occurs before the brain recovers from the first, usually within a short period of time (hours, days, or weeks), that results in brain swelling, permanent brain damage, and even death.
Stupor	A state of consciousness in which the patient is unresponsive but can be aroused by a strong stimulus.
Subarachnoid hemorrhage	Bleeding in the space beneath the arachnoid mater, a membrane that covers the brain. This area, called the subarachnoid space, normally contains cerebrospinal fluid. Such hemorrhage can lead to stroke, seizures, and other complications.
Synapses	The junction between the axon terminals of a neuron and the receiving cell that permits neurons to pass signals to individual target cells. Most neurons achieve their effect by releasing chemicals, the neurotransmitters, to a receiving cell.
Syndrome of inadequate secretion of antidiuretic hormone and hypothyroidism	A common fluid and hormonal imbalance occurring as a result of disruption to the pituitary, thyroid, or other glands.
Tolerable Upper Intake Level (UL)	The highest average daily nutrient intake level that is likely to pose no risk of adverse health effects to almost all individuals in the genera population. As intake increases above the UL, the potential risk of adverse effects may increase.
Vasospasm	A condition in which blood vessels spasm, leading to vasoconstriction, that can induce tissue ischemia and death (necrosis). Cerebral vasospasm may arise in the context of subarachnoid hemorrhage. Symptomatic vasospasm or delayed cerebral ischemia is a major contributor to postoperative stroke and death, especially after aneurysmal subarachnoid hemorrhage. Vasospasm typically appears four to ten days after subarachnoid hemorrhage.

Vegetative state   The condition of patients who are unconscious and unaware of their
                    surroundings but who may have a sleep-wake cycle, periods of alert-
                    ness, and periodically open eyes, unlike coma patients, and may move
                    and show reflexes. Many patients recover from this state within a few
                    weeks, but some will remain in a persistent vegetative state. It can
                    result in diffuse injury to the cerebral hemispheres without damage to
                    the lower brain and brainstem.

Ventriculostomy   Procedure to drain cerebrospinal fluid from the brain to reduce
                    intracranial pressure (mannitol and barbiturates are pharmaceutical
                    alternatives).

E

Acronyms

ACA	Acetoacetate
ACES	Army Center of Excellence, Subsistence
ACL	Acetyl-L-Carnitine
AD	Alzheimer's disease
ADA	American Dietetic Association
ADAS-Cog	Alzheimer's Disease Assessment Scale-cognitive subscale
ADP	Adenosine diphosphate
AED	Anti-epileptic drug(s)
AI	Adequate Intake
ALA	Alpha-linolenic acid
ARDS	Acute Respiratory Distress Syndrome
ALS	Amyotrophic lateral sclerosis
AMDR	Acceptable Macronutrient Distribution Range
AMP	Adenosine monophosphate
AMPK	5' AMP-activated protein kinase
AOC	Alteration of Consciousness/Mental State
ASPEN	American Society of Parenteral and Enteral Nutrition
ATP	Adenosine 5'-triphosphate
ARDS	Acute Respiratory Distress Syndrome
bAMC	Bilateral anterior medial cortex
BBB	Blood-brain barrier
BCAA	Branched-chain amino acids
BDNF	Brain-derived neurotrophic factor
BI	Barthel Index
BMI	Body Mass Index
BOH	β-hydroxyburate
BTF	Brain Trauma Foundation

Ca^{2+}	Intracellular calcium
CaEDTA	Calcium disodium ethylenediamine tetraacetate
CaMKII	Calcium/calmodulin dependent kinase I
CCI	Controlled cortical impact
CDC	Centers for Disease Control and Prevention
CDP-choline	Cytidine 5′–diphosphocholine
CI	Confidence Interval
CI	Cerebral infarction
CNS	Central nervous system
CNS	Canadian Neurological Score
COBRIT	Citicoline Brain Injury Treatment
CREB	Cyclic adenosine monophosphate response element-binding
CSF	Cerebral spinal fluid
CSWF	Continuous spikes and waves during slow sleep
CT	Computerized tomography
CTE	Chronic traumatic encephalopathy
CVA	Cerebrovascular disease
CVD	Cardiovascular disease
DAI	Diffuse axonal injury
DCI	Delayed cerebral ischemia
DFE	Dietary folate equivalents
DHA	Docosahexaenoic acid
DM	Diabetes mellitus
DMSO	Dimethyl sulfoxide
DNA	Deoxyribonucleic acid
DoD	Department of Defense
DRI	Dietary Reference Intakes
DRS	Disability Rating Scores
DVBIC	Defense and Veterans Brain Injury Center
DWI	Diffusion-weighted imaging
EAR	Estimated Average Requirements
EBG	Evidence-Based Guidelines
EDTA	Ethylene diamine teta-acetic acid (typically in the form of a salt)
EEG	Electroencephalography
EGb	*Ginkgo biloba* extract
EN	Enteral Nutrition
EPA	Eicosapentaenoic acid
ESPEN	European Society for Parenteral and Enteral Nutrition
FAST-MAG	Field Administration of Stroke Therapy—Magnesium
FFA	Free fatty acid(s)
FMD	Flow-mediated dilatation
fMRI	Functional Magnetic Resonance Imaging
FP	Fluid percussion
FSCM	Food Service Contract Management
FSMB	Food Service Management Board

GABA	Gamma-aminobutyric acid
GABA$_A$	Gamma-aminobutyric acid type A
GCS	Glasgow Coma Scale
GFAP	Glial fibrillary acidic protein
GHB	Gamma hydroxybutyrate
GOS	Glasgow Outcome Score
GRV	Gastric residual volume
GSH	Glutathione
HIF-1	Hypoxia-inducible factor 1
HR	Hazard ratio
ICP	Intracranial pressure
ICU	Intensive care unit
IED	Improvised explosive devices
IGF-I	Insulin-like growth factor
IL-1	Interleukin-1
i.m.	intramuscularly/intramuscular
IMAGES	Intravenous Magnesium Efficacy in Stroke
IOM	Institute of Medicine
IRB	Institutional Review Board
IU	International Units
i.v.	Intravenously/intravenous
JCCoE	Joint Culinary Center of Excellence
LDL	Low-density lipoprotein
LDL-c	Low-density lipoprotein cholesterol
LOC	Loss of Consciousness
LOS	Length of hospital stay
MCT	Medium-chain triglycerides
MDA	Malondialdehyde
MDRI	Military Dietary Reference Intake
Mg	Magnesium
MgSO$_4$	Magnesium sulfate
MI	Myocardial infarction
MRE	Meal, Ready to Eat
MRI	Magnetic resonance imaging
mRS	Modified Rankin Scale
MT	Metallothionein
mTBI	Mild Traumatic Brain Injury
MWM	Morris water maze
Na	Sodium
NAD$^+$	Nicotinamide adenine dinucleotide
NE	Niacin equivalents
NGF	Nerve growth factor
NHANES	National Health and Nutrition Examination Survey

NICU	Neonatal Intensive Care Unit
NIH	National Institutes of Health
NIHSS	NIH Stroke Scale
NMDA	N-methyl-D-aspartate
NO	Nitric oxide
NPD1	Neuroprotectin D1
NSE	Neuron specific enolase
NSOR	Nutritional standards for operational rations
NT-3	Neurotrophin 3
OEF	Operation Enduring Freedom
OIF	Operation Iraqi Freedom
OR	Odds ratio
Oxy-Hb	Oxy-hemoglobin
PARP	Poly (ADP-ribose) polymerase
PICO	Population, Intervention, Comparator, Outcome
PN	Parenteral Nutrition
PTA	Post Traumatic Amnesia
PTSD	Posttraumatic stress disorder
PUFA	Polyunsaturated fatty acid(s)
RCT	Randomized control trial
RDA	Recommended Dietary Allowances
RMR	Resting Metabolic Rate
RNA	Ribonucleic acid
ROS	Reactive oxygen species
RQ	Respiratory quotient
RR	Risk ratio
RXR	Retinoic acid receptor
SAH	Subarachnoid hemorrhage
SCCM	Society of Critical Care Medicine
SDNN	Standard deviation of normal RR intervals
SEM	Standard error of mean
SGZ	Subgranular zone
SIRT1	Sirtuin-1
SOD	Superoxide dismutase
SVX	Subventricular zone
TBD	To be determined
TBI	Traumatic brain injury
TEF	Thermal effect of food
TNF	Tumor necrosis factor
TPN	Total parenteral nutrition
TUNEL	Transferase-mediated biotinylated dUTP nick-end labeling
UCP	Uncoupling protein
UL	Tolerable Upper Intake Level

USARIEM   U.S. Army Research Institute of Environmental Medicine

VA   Department of Veterans Affairs
VDR   Vitamin D receptor
VDRE   Vitamin D response elements
VEGF   Vascular endothelial growth factor

WMH   White matter hypersensitivity
WRAMC   Walter Reed Army Medical Center

XO   Xanthine oxidase

Zn   Zinc

F

Committee Member Biographical Sketches

John W. Erdman, Jr., Ph.D. *(Chair)*, is Professor Emeritus of Nutrition and Food Science in the Department of Food Science and Human Nutrition and a Professor in the Department of Internal Medicine at the University of Illinois at Urbana-Champaign. His research interests include the effects of food processing on nutrient retention, the metabolic roles of vitamin A and beta-carotene, the bioavailability of minerals from foods, and the influence of food components on prostate cancer. His research regarding soy protein has extended into studies on the impact of non-nutrient components of foods such as phytoestrogens on chronic disease. Dr. Erdman has published over 160 peer-reviewed research papers. He chaired the 1988 Gordon Conference on Carotenoids, and has served as a Burroughs Wellcome Visiting Professor in Basic Medical Sciences at the University of Georgia, and the G. Malcolm Trout Visiting Scholar at Michigan State University. His awards include the Borden Award from the American Society for Nutrition and the Babcock-Hart Award from the Institute of Food Technologists. He has served on a number of Institute of Medicine (IOM) committees, including service as chair of the Standing Committee on Dietary Reference Intakes and vice chair of the Food and Nutrition Board. Dr. Erdman has served on many editorial boards, and on many program and planning committees for the American Society of Nutrition, the Institute of Food Technologists, and the National Academy of Sciences. In 1992, he was elected a fellow of the Institute of Food Technologists, and in 2003 he was elected a fellow of the American Heart Association. Dr. Erdman was elected to the IOM in 2003 and serves as chair of the standing Committee on Military Nutrition Research. Dr. Erdman received his M.S. and Ph.D. in food science from Rutgers University.

E. Wayne Askew, Ph.D., is Professor of Nutrition and the Director of the Division of Nutrition in the College of Health at the University of Utah in Salt Lake City. He teaches metabolism and sports nutrition and conducts research on nutrition and human performance. Prior to his current position at the University of Utah, he was a Medical Service Corps Officer with the U.S. Army Medical Department. His assignments included the U.S. Army Medical Research and Nutrition Laboratory, Denver, CO; Letterman Army Institute of Research, Presidio of San Francisco, CA; Tripler Army Medical Center, Honolulu, HI; and the U.S. Army Research Institute of Environmental Medicine, Natick, MA, where he was Chief of Military Nutrition Research for the U.S. Army. His research involves the study of oxidative stress, biochemical adaptations to exercise training, the role of nutrition in physical performance, assessment of nutritional status, and nutrition for human performance in environmental extremes including heat, cold and high altitude. He is a member of the American College of Sports Medicine, the American Society for Nutrition, the American Dietetic Association, the International Society for Mountain Medicine, and the Wilderness Medical Society. He has served as a member of the United States Olympic Committee Nutrition Advisory Committee and the U.S. Food and Drug Administration Advisory Committee on Food Safety. He currently serves as vice chair of the standing Committee on Military Nutrition Research. He received his Ph.D. in nutritional biochemistry from the Institute of Nutrition, Michigan State University.

Bruce R. Bistrian, M.D., Ph.D., is Professor of Medicine at Harvard Medical School and the Chief of Clinical Nutrition at Beth Israel Deaconess Medical Center. Formerly he was Co-Director of Hyperalimentation Services at New England Deaconess Hospital, and a lecturer in the Department of Nutrition and Food Science at Massachusetts Institute of Technology (MIT). Dr. Bistrian is board-certified in Internal Medicine and, from 1997–2007, in Critical Care Medicine. Dr. Bistrian's primary research interests include nutritional assessment, metabolic effects of acute infections, nutritional support of hospitalized patients, and the pathophysiology of protein-calorie malnutrition. He is a fellow of the American College of Physicians, and has received an honorary M.A. from Harvard University. Dr. Bistrian is the 2004 recipient of the Goldberger Award of the American Medical Association. Dr. Bistrian has been President of the American Society for Parenteral and Enteral Nutrition, President of the (former) American Society of Clinical Nutrition and President of the Federation of American Societies for Experimental Biology. Dr. Bistrian has served on the editorial boards of numerous nutrition and medical journals, and is the author or coauthor of over 400 articles in scientific publications. He is a member of the standing Committee on Military Nutrition Research and has served on several IOM ad hoc committees, including the Committee on Use of Dietary Supplements by Military Personnel and the Committee on Mineral Requirements for Cognitive and Physical Performance of Military Personnel. He earned his M.P.H. from Johns Hopkins University, his M.D. from Cornell University, and his Ph.D. in nutritional biochemistry and metabolism from MIT.

Joseph G. Cannon, Ph.D., is Professor in the Departments of Physiology and Biomedical Technologies and Associate Dean for Research in the College of Allied Health Sciences at the Georgia Health Science University (GHSU). Formerly, he was Professor of Applied Physiology at Pennsylvania State University. Dr. Cannon's primary research interests include the immunological mechanisms involved in bone turnover and vascular function, as well as nutritional and hormonal influences on leukocyte function. He holds the Kellett Chair in Allied Health Sciences at GHSU. Dr. Cannon has served on the editorial boards of the American Journal of Physiology and Journal of Applied Physiology and is the author or coauthor of over 100 articles in scientific publications. He is a member of the standing Committee on Military Nutrition Research and has served on the Committee on Mineral Requirements for Cognitive and Physical Performance on Military Personnel. Dr. Cannon holds a B.S. in engineering from Michigan State University, an M.S. in engineering from the University of California, Los Angeles, and a Ph.D. in physiology from the University of Michigan.

Xiang Gao, M.D., Ph.D., is Research Scientist in the Department of Nutrition at Harvard School of Public Health and Assistant Professor in the Department of Medicine at Harvard Medical School. Dr. Gao's research investigates the relationships between environmental and dietary factors and the risk of neurological diseases, such as Parkinson's disease and Restless legs syndrome. He serves as the Principal Investigator of a prospective study of restless legs syndrome funded by an R01 Research Project Grant from the National Institute of Neurological Disorders and Stroke. Dr. Gao works with data from several large, ongoing cohorts, including the Nurses' Health Study and the Health Professionals Follow-up Study. He also works on dietary pattern methodology, employing mathematical approaches to evaluate U.S. nutritional recommendations, including the Food Pyramid and the Dietary Reference Intakes. Dr. Gao has published over 60 original articles and is first or senior author on about 35. He has served on the mentoring committee of Parkinson Study Group since 2008. Dr. Gao won the Irwin H. Rosenberg Award for excellence in predoctoral research from the Jean Mayor U.S. Department of Agriculture (USDA) Human Nutrition Research Center on Aging at Tufts University in 2006, the Mentored Clinical Research Award from the Parkinson Study Group in 2007, and the Wayne A. Hening Sleep Medicine Investigator Award from the American Academy of Neurology in 2011. Dr. Gao received his M.S. from the Chinese Academy of Medical Science and Peking Union Medical College and his M.D. from Shanghai Second Medical University. He received his Ph.D. in nutritional epidemiology from Tufts University School of Nutrition Science and Policy.

Col. Michael Jaffee, M.D., began his fellowship training in sleep medicine at the San Antonio Uniformed Services Health Education Consortium (SAUSHEC) on July 1, 2010. Previously, Col. Jaffee served as National Director of the Defense and Veterans Brain Injury Center (DVBIC). Prior to his selection as DVBIC national director, Col. Jaffee served as the SAUSHEC Neurology Program Director at Wilford Hall Medical Center at Lackland Air Force Base and as the DVBIC San Antonio Site Director. He currently serves as the U.S. Air Force (USAF) Surgeon General Neurology Consultant. Col. Jaffee has served as an Aerospace Neurology Consultant at the Aerospace Consultation Service/USAF School of Aerospace Medicine and as the USAF Psychiatry Consultant on security clearance issues. His academic appointments include Assistant Clinical Professor of Neurology and Associate Clinical Professor of Psychiatry at the University of Texas Health Sciences Center and Assistant Professor of Neurology at the Uniformed Services University of the Health Sciences. He is also on the clinical faculty at the University of Virginia. Col. Jaffee serves as a Visiting Scientist to the Center for Information Technology of the National Institutes of Health (NIH). His honors and awards include being the only Department of Defense physician selected as a William Webb fellow by the Academy of Psychosomatic Medicine for excellence in advancing the understanding of the mind-body interface, citations from the U.S. Surgeon General and the Iraqi Surgeon General, and commendations from four cabinet-level departments as well as the Congressional Brain Injury Task Force. He was selected as the active-duty U.S. delegate to North Atlantic Treaty Organization for international coordination of traumatic brain injury initiatives. He has been involved in extensive research in the area of traumatic brain injury and is the author of many articles and papers. He has served on many federal panels and review boards and has been an invited speaker at many national and international conferences as well as to the Institute of Medicine. Col. Jaffee holds an M.D. from the University of Virginia School of Medicine and a B.A. from the University of Pennsylvania, as well as a B.S. in Economics from the Wharton School of Finance and Commerce. He completed residency training at Wilford Hall Medical Center where he was selected as chief resident for the departments of both Neurology and Psychiatry. He is board-certified in both neurology and psychiatry.

Robin B. Kanarek, Ph.D., is the John Wade Professor of Psychology at Tufts University. Her prior experience includes Research Fellow, Division of Endocrinology of the University of California, Los Angeles School of Medicine, and Research Fellow in Nutrition at Harvard University. Additionally, she served as Dean of the Graduate School of Arts and Sciences at Tufts University from 2002 to 2006. Dr. Kanarek's research focuses on the role of nutrition in determining brain functioning and behavior. In addition to reviewing for numerous journals, including *Science, Brain Research Bulletin, Journal of Nutrition, American Journal of Clinical Nutrition,* and *Annals of Internal Medicine,* she is a member of the editorial boards of *Physiology & Behavior* and the Tufts Diet and Nutrition Newsletter and is a past Editor in chief of *Nutrition and Behavior.* Dr. Kanarek has served on ad hoc review committees for the National Science Foundation, the NIH, and USDA nutrition research, as well as the Member Program Committee of the Eastern Psychological Association. She is a fellow of the American College of Nutrition and the International Behavioral Neuroscience Society and her other professional memberships include the American Institute of Nutrition, New York Academy of Sciences, the Society for the Study of Ingestive Behavior, and the Society for Neurosciences. She is a member of the IOM Standing Committee on Military Nutrition Research and served on the Committee on Use of Dietary Supplements by Military Personnel. Dr. Kanarek received a B.A. in biology from Antioch College, and an M.S. and a Ph.D. in psychology from Rutgers University.

Cathy W. Levenson, Ph.D., is Associate Professor of Biomedical Science and Neuroscience in the Department of Biomedical Sciences at the Florida State University College of Medicine, where she serves as the Course Director for Medical Biochemistry and Genetics. Her current research focuses on neurogenesis; her lab uses rodent models as well as cultured human neuronal precursor cells to understand the cellular and molecular mechanisms that are responsible for proliferation, survival, migration, and differentiation of adult stem cells in the brain. Dr. Levenson is a member of the Society for Neuroscience and of the American Society for Nutrition. She also served as a research associate in the laboratory of Dr. Robert Cousins at the University of Florida. She received her B.A. from the University of Virginia, her M.S. from Florida State University, and her Ph.D. from the University of Chicago.

Esther F. Myers, Ph.D., R.D., is the Chief Science Officer at the American Dietetic Association (ADA) and is an internationally known author, lecturer, educator and researcher. She is a retired member of the USAF, where she served as Chief Consultant to the Air Force Surgeon General for Nutrition and Dietetics; associate chief, Biomedical Sciences Corps for Dietetics; and flight commander, Nutritional Medicine, at the 60th Medical Group. Dr. Myers has authored several papers describing evidence analysis processes and the ADA process and coauthored a chapter on systematic reviews of evidence for *Research: Successful Approaches,* edited by Elaine Monsen. She is actively involved in research projects focusing on evaluating the impact of nutrition services in Medicare Demonstration projects, and in collaboration with Blue Cross Blue Shield of North Carolina. Dr. Myers is the ADA staff liaison with the Nutrition Care Process and Standardized Language Committee which is developing and validating terminology to reflect the nutrition care for standardized language systems and electronic health records. Prior to joining ADA, she served as a site visitor for the Commission on Accreditation for Dietetics Education, a peer reviewer for the *Journal of the American Dietetic Association,* and a member of the Health Services Research Task

Force overseeing dietetic outcomes research. She currently focuses her efforts on research activities needed for the dietetics profession and the Association as well as the ADA strategic leadership initiative in obesity and the ADA Foundation initiative, Healthy Weight for Kids. Dr. Myers has served on the Committee on the Use of Dietary Supplements by Military Personnel and the Committee on Nutrition Services for Medicare Beneficiaries. She is a member of the IOM Standing Committee on Military Nutrition Research.

Linda J. Noble, Ph.D., is Professor of Neurological Surgery and Physical Therapy and Rehabilitation Science at the University of California, San Francisco (UCSF). She holds the Alvera L. Kan Endowed Chair in the Department of Neurological Surgery, is Vice Chair of the Department of Physical Therapy and Rehabilitation Science, co-directs the Neurobehavioral Core for Rehabilitation Research, and is a Principal Investigator of the Brain and Spinal Injury Center at UCSF. Dr. Noble has an established expertise in the field of neurotrauma and hers is one of few laboratories that has developed models of both traumatic brain and spinal cord injury in the mouse that mimic the human conditions. Such modeling has provided a unique opportunity to study transgenic animals and has been used to identify specific factors that influence vascular permeability and inflammation and mediate cell injury after either traumatic spinal cord or brain injury. Dr. Noble is a member of Society for Neuroscience, the American Association for Anatomists, and the Society for Neurotrauma. She serves on the editorial boards of the *Journal of Neurotrauma* and *Developmental Neuroscience* and is a Review Editor for *Frontiers in Neurotrauma*. She currently chairs the NIH National Institute of Neurological Disorders and Stroke/National Spasomdic Dysphonia Association study section and is on the external review committee for Mission Connect, Houston, Texas. Dr. Noble served on the IOM Committee on Gulf War and Health: Brain Injury in Veterans and Long-Term Health Outcomes. She holds a B.S. from the University of Utah and the University of Nevada and a Ph.D. from the University of California, Los Angeles.

Ross D. Zafonte, D.O., is the Earle P. and Ida S. Charlton Chairman of the Department of Physical Medicine and Rehabilitation at Harvard Medical School, the Vice President of Medical Affairs at Spaulding Rehabilitation Hospital, and the Chief of Physical Medicine and Rehabilitation at Massachusetts General Hospital. Dr. Zafonte maintains a clinical practice in which he cares for patients with a wide variety of disabilities, including traumatic brain injuries, spinal cord injuries, multiple sclerosis, compressive neuropathies, spasticity, and postconcussive musculoskeletal conditions. He currently leads an NIH multisite clinical trial on the treatment of traumatic brain injury and the Traumatic Brain Injury/Post-traumatic Stress Disorder program at the Center for Integration of Medicine & Innovative Technology, which partners with the Department of Defense. Dr. Zafonte is the author of numerous publications about traumatic brain injuries and other rehabilitation topics. He has also served as an editor of several successful textbooks for the field, and has given more than 100 national and international presentations on topics in the field of rehabilitation. He is associate editor for the journals *PM&R* and the *American Journal of Physical Medicine and Rehabilitation*. Dr. Zafonte completed his residency in the Department of Rehabilitation Medicine at the Mount Sinai School of Medicine in New York City.